Dedication

To the autism community of Acadiana, especially to the Pitres, the Nettles, the Tates, the Thibodeaux, the Chacheres, and the Polotzolas, and to all those who are determined to help bring the autism epidemic to a close.

Autism

The Diagnosis, Treatment, & Etiology of the Undeniable Epidemic

John W. Oller Jr., PhD
Hawthorne Regents Professor
Department of Communicative Disorders
University of Louisiana at Lafayette
Lafayette, LA

Stephen D. Oller, PhD
Assistant Professor
Department of Biological and Health Sciences
Texas A&M University at Kingsville
Kingsville, TX

JONES AND BARTLETT PUBLISHERS
Sudbury, Massachusetts
BOSTON   TORONTO   LONDON   SINGAPORE

World Headquarters
Jones and Bartlett Publishers
40 Tall Pine Drive
Sudbury, MA 01776
978-443-5000
info@jbpub.com
www.jbpub.com

Jones and Bartlett Publishers
Canada
6339 Ormindale Way
Mississauga, Ontario L5V 1J2
Canada

Jones and Bartlett Publishers
International
Barb House, Barb Mews
London W6 7PA
United Kingdom

Jones and Bartlett's books and products are available through most bookstores and online booksellers. To contact Jones and Bartlett Publishers directly, call 800-832-0034, fax 978-443-8000, or visit our website, www.jbpub.com.

Substantial discounts on bulk quantities of Jones and Bartlett's publications are available to corporations, professional associations, and other qualified organizations. For details and specific discount information, contact the special sales department at Jones and Bartlett via the above contact information or send an email to specialsales@jbpub.com.

The authors, editor, and publisher have made every effort to provide accurate information. However, they are not responsible for errors, omissions, or for any outcomes related to the use of the contents of this book and take no responsibility for the use of the products and procedures described. Treatments and side effects described in this book may not be applicable to all people; likewise, some people may require a dose or experience a side effect that is not described herein. Drugs and medical devices are discussed that may have limited availability controlled by the Food and Drug Administration (FDA) for use only in a research study or clinical trial. Research, clinical practice, and government regulations often change the accepted standard in this field. When consideration is being given to use of any drug in the clinical setting, the health care provider or reader is responsible for determining FDA status of the drug, reading the package insert, and reviewing prescribing information for the most up-to-date recommendations on dose, precautions, and contraindications, and determining the appropriate usage for the product. This is especially important in the case of drugs that are new or seldom used.

Production Credits
Publisher: David Cella
Associate Editor: Maro Gartside
Editorial Assistant: Teresa Reilly
Senior Production Editor: Renée Sekerak
Production Assistant: Jill Morton
Marketing Manager: Grace Richards
Manufacturing and Inventory Control
  Supervisor: Amy Bacus
Composition: SNP Best-set Typesetter Ltd., Hong Kong
Cover Design: Kate Ternullo

Photo Research and Permissions Manager: Kimberly Potvin
Permissions Coordinator: Kesel Wilson
Assistant Photo Researcher: Meghan Hayes
Cover Images: Upper right, Photos.com; Middle right, ©
  Monika Gniot/ShutterStock, Inc.; Lower right, Courtesy
  of Kari Smith; Middle, Courtesy of Hestor Patout
  Bourdier; Lower left, Courtesy of Theron Pitre; Upper
  left, © Arjhargrove/Dreamstime.com
Printing and Binding: Malloy Incorporated
Cover Printing: Malloy Incorporated

Library of Congress Cataloging-in-Publication Data

Oller, John W.
  Autism : the diagnosis, treatment, & etiology of the undeniable epidemic / by John W. Oller Jr. and Stephen D. Oller.
     p. ; cm.
  Includes bibliographical references and index.
  ISBN-13: 978-0-7637-5280-4
  ISBN-10: 0-7637-5280-0
  1. Autism.   2. Autism–Treatment.   I. Oller, Stephen D.   II. Title.
  [DNLM: 1. Autistic Disorder–etiology.   2. Autistic Disorder–diagnosis.   3. Autistic Disorder–therapy. WM 203.5
O49a 2010]
  RC553.A88.O455 2010
  616.85′882–dc22
                                          2009017731

6048
Printed in the United States of America
13 12 11 10 09   10 9 8 7 6 5 4 3 2 1

Contents

Foreword

It is an honor to be asked to write a foreword, particularly one for such a valuable and scholarly contribution to the understanding of autism.

I was involved in filming with NBC, grabbing some B-roll after the serious interviews and the film crew—a producer, a cameraman, and a sound technician—were talking between takes. The cameraman noted how uncanny it was that he, the sound tech, and the producer all had nephews with Asperger syndrome. I, too, have a nephew with Asperger syndrome. Four people, none of whom had met before, were all personally impacted by this previously very rare autistic spectrum disorder, originally described, coincidentally, in only four boys in Vienna by Hans Asperger. That same week, U.K. newspaper headlines reported autistic spectrum disorders in 1 in 38 boys. A 2007 report from the California Department of Developmental Services is just in and makes for a depressing read. Examination of the epidemic growth of autism in the United States and the United Kingdom indicates, with an ominous certainty, that if you are not personally affected by autism in your family now, you will be in the future.

Few contemporary subjects have such immediate and long-term relevance to the "well-being" of the human race. A 20-year period starting in the mid-1980s—the mere blinking of an eye in the life of planet Earth—has witnessed a punctuated equilibrium in the human evolutionary continuum reflecting what I believe is a huge selection pressure on humankind. The autism epidemic is environmentally driven. There are many who believe that recent dramatic changes in early immune programming lie at the heart of this and other childhood immune system disorders. This view is not necessarily a sequela to the "hygiene" hypothesis that originally proposed a lack of exposure to environmental stressors such as infections that might be key to the recent emergence of immune-mediated diseases, but rather a proposal that an altered pattern of exposure that does not hold the substitution of infection for vaccination to be a benign influence in this process.

This new book on autism was authored by professionals in communication, and it was written for students of this subject. As the authors state, "The primary aim of this book is to apply sound logical theory to the findings of validated empirical research concerning the autism epidemic." They do so across the broadest landscape, taking the reader from autism's lackluster history in the backwaters of human idiosyncrasy to its unwelcome epidemic prominence as the fin de siècle disease—a "mind plague"—that has stolen so many lives and disrupted so many families. What appealed to me in particular is the authors' emphasis on the narrative of individual children as the bedrock of a deeper understanding of the disease.

This is not another book written about autism by someone unschooled in the subject. Rather, it is a text written by those for whom autism and the science of communication are a profession and a passion—a book grounded in analysis, reanalysis, empiricism, and logic. And it is a book that should be required reading by health agencies.

This book is unashamedly invested in the belief that the vaccine–autism story has far from run its course. Indeed, science has only just scratched the surface of this complex relationship. In parallel with the evolution of thinking in autism is the story of how enthusiasm on the one hand and fear (and its use) on the other hand—both devices of public relations—have distorted the history of vaccination and inhibited rational debate. Scientists have played their part in this journey and are by no means blameless in the distortion of the facts. I have been blamed for causing, through the media, a vaccine scare. In defense of my position and in accordance with the precautionary principle, having reviewed all the available evidence for MMR vaccine safety, I simply recommended a return to single measles, mumps, and rubella vaccines in preference to MMR and encouraged further research.

In the NBC interview, it was put to me that I was alone with a few parents in believing that the MMR vaccine was unsafe. I responded by saying that 15 years ago this was, indeed, an unusual opinion held by only a handful of physicians. I was able to say, however, that my position on the deficiencies in the relevant vaccine safety studies have now been reinforced by the systematic analysis of Dr. Thomas Jefferson and colleagues from the Cochrane Collaboration, an internationally respected body that provides independent scientific oversight. They wrote, "The design and reporting of safety outcomes in MMR vaccine studies, both pre- and postmarketing is largely inadequate" (Jefferson, Price, Demicheli, & Bianco, 2003, p. 25). In an interview with Richard Halvorsen concerning his 2007 book *The Truth about Vaccines*, one of the lead authors of the Cochrane review left no doubt as to his true feelings when he said, "The safety studies of MMR vaccine are crap. They're the best crap we have but they're still crap" (Child Health Safety, 2009 ◉). With respect to my suggested return to the protection of children with single vaccines, Jefferson and colleagues wrote, "We found limited evidence of safety of MMR compared to its single-component vaccines from low risk of bias studies" (Jefferson et al., 2003, p. 25). More recently, Dr. Lou Cooper, former head of the American Academy of Pediatrics, made the comment in *Newsweek* that "There's been grossly insufficient investment in research on the safety of immunization" (2009 ◉), and, to the Institute of Medicine, that "[Vaccine safety] research has been done on the cheap" (Wrangham, n.d. ◉).

So what has been the response of the authorities and the vaccine manufacturers to Jefferson's evidence-based approach? In the United Kingdom, the importation license for single viral vaccines was withdrawn in August 1998 at the height of demand by a justifiably concerned public, but regulators continued to deny parents the option of single-agent vaccines. Protecting policy was put before protecting children. In the United States, Merck (the sole supplier of single and combined measles, mumps, and rubella vaccines) has announced its intention to discontinue provision of single-agent vaccines.

The ability of the regulators and manufacturers to take such positions has been tenuously sustained by scientists bending the facts to the will of the Public Health Politburo. An example of this is an extraordinary quote ascribed to the authors of a recent paper by Dr. Mady Hornig and colleagues: "The work reported here eliminates the remaining support for the hypothesis that autism with GI complaints is related to MMR vaccine exposure" (Levine, 2008; Columbia University Mailman School of Public Health, 2008 ◉). Clearly at odds with this extravagant and inappropriate claim, the study actually looked at the relationship between persistent measles virus infection in poorly characterized intestinal biopsies in only five children whose clinical history (regression and onset of intestinal symptoms after MMR vaccination) identified them as being in the group of interest. The problem with this kind of compromise is that for whoever made the statement and whatever their motivation, there is no way back. They have forsaken the scientific debate for populist blog-speak and damaged the prospects of further research into an important area.

Part of what is needed in the deconstruction of the PR myth is an objective analysis of the "vast number of studies that discount an association between vaccines and autism," a line frequently employed by Dr. Paul Offit (2008) among others. This book takes a closer look at the pattern of exposure to vaccines and autism risk. A recent example of the importance of this "pattern of exposure" phenomenon comes from Kara McDonald at the University of Manitoba involving more than 11,500 children who received at least four doses of DTP (diphtheria, tetanus, and whole cell pertussis vaccine), among whom the risk of asthma was reduced by half in children whose first dose of DTP was delayed by more than 2 months (McDonald, Huq, Lix, Becker, & Kozyrskyj, 2008). The likelihood of asthma in children with delays in all three doses was reduced still further. In contrast, for those children whose first dose was given ahead of schedule, there was an estimated increased risk of asthma of 60% compared with those children who received their first dose at the recommended time. This gradient of risk associated with age of exposure is compelling and may well explain the discordance between results of other studies that sought to examine the DTP–asthma link.

As part of this deconstruction, the authors of this book have taken a look at the original flawed analysis carried out by Dr. Loring Dales, working for the California Health Services, and the CDC (Dales, Hammer, & Smith, 2001). Using Dales et al.'s data, J. W. Oller and S. D. Oller show a highly significant correlation between autism numbers and increasing uptake of vaccines over time. The data provided here support the reanalysis of Dales et al.'s data undertaken by Edwardes and Baltzan (2001), who confirmed that the rate of early MMR immunization is correlated with the incidence of autism. The correlation appears in data that were obscured in an attempted feat of graphical wizardry by Dales et al. Although the data suggest that younger age at MMR vaccination may be associated with a rise in autism at the population level, ecologic studies such as those of Dales and colleagues are of limited value when it comes to taking the question further.

In an attempt to settle this issue, CDC researchers stepped in with a case-control study comparing age at first MMR vaccination in children from the Atlanta metro area (DeStefano, Bhasin, Thompson, Yeargin-Allsopp, & Boyle, 2004). By 36 months of age, significantly more cases with autism had received MMR vaccines than controls. This association was strongest when children received the vaccine at a younger age, particularly in the 3- to 5-year age group (odds ratio = 2.34). Due to diagnostic delay, a significant proportion of this group of young children had yet to be diagnosed with autism at the time of the study, potentially underestimating this risk. In a subgroup analysis adjusted for birth weight, multiple gestation, maternal age, and maternal education, the odds ratios were increased to 3.55, however, strengthening the association between younger age of exposure to MMR and autism risk.

Why am I telling you this? Because the DeStefano et al. study has been cited as supporting the safety of MMR vaccination. The positive finding was deemed to be apparently an "artifact of vaccine requirements for special needs children." Of course, these children are actually no different from children in regular education. The argument is false, and no evidence has ever been produced to support it. Several other "negative" studies support the association between younger MMR exposure and increased autism risk (Richler et al., 2006). Even so, the "no harm from vaccines" band plays on.

It was suggested in my exchanges with NBC that the perceived response to questioning vaccine safety smacks of conspiracy theory. Although not directly relevant to the issue of vaccines, I was able to provide the production team with a recent posting on the class-action suit involving Merck and Vioxx, entitled "Drug Company Had Hit List for Doctors Who Criticized Them" (Mercola, 2009). It continued, "The international drug company Merck had a hit list of doctors who had to be 'neutralized' or discredited because they had criticized the painkiller Vioxx, a now-withdrawn drug that the pharmaceutical giant produced" (Mercola, 2009 ●).

Staff at Merck emailed each other about the list of doctors. The email, which became public during a class-action suit against the drug company, included the words "neutralize," "neutralized," and "discredit" alongside some of the doctors' names (Rout, 2009 ●). The company is alleged to have used intimidation tactics against researchers, including dropping hints that the company would stop funding their institutions and possibly even interfere with academic appointments (Rout, 2009). The article concluded with an email excerpt from a Merck employee read to the court that went as follows: "We may need to seek them out and destroy them where they live."

Who needs conspiracy? Congratulations to the authors of this text for their insights and their courage.

Finally, I should disclose that the Ollers have offered to donate any profits from sales of this book to Thoughtful House, a center for care of children with developmental disorders and research into these diseases of which I am the executive director. We are fighting to recover children with developmental disorders (autism, PDD, Asperger syndrome, ADD, ADHD, and NLD) through the unique combination of medical care, education, and research.

Andrew J. Wakefield, MB, BS, FRCS, FRCPath
Thoughtful House
Center for Children
3001 Bee Caves Road
Austin, TX 78746
http://www.thoughtfulhouse.org/index.php

Preface

A few decades ago, most ordinary citizens had no idea what autism was; they had never heard of it. Today, it seems that everyone in the world is talking about autism. Why is that? Because of media hype? Greater public awareness? Were the cases that are being diagnosed today always there but unnoticed until recently? What has changed to bring about what Edlich, Son, et al. (2007) describe as "an epidemic of neurodevelopment disorders in the United States" (p. 204)?

Logical thought shows that the upsurge in autism cannot be uncaused, but why would the Centers for Disease Control and Prevention (CDC) and other parties publicly express doubt about the existence of a growing epidemic? Why did the director of the National Immunization Program at the CDC work so hard, along with a group of 11 experts from the CDC and 40 other representatives from drug companies and the federal government, to try to make the association between autism and the neurotoxin known as thimerosal "go away" in analyses of data from the National Immunization Program's Vaccine Safety Datalink? Why have more than 5300 thimerosal-related claims for injuries that have caused autism or made it worse been filed under the Vaccine Injury Compensation Program? What is causing the upsurge in the number of persons being diagnosed with neurological and related disorders, and what can be done to help them? Is there such a thing as full recovery from severe autism?

We hope that this book not only informs college majors in communication disorders and closely related fields about the nature and causes of the autism epidemic, but also enables better understanding among private citizens and healthcare professionals about the potentially deadly and often harmful interactions of disease agents, foreign proteins, toxins, and medications to which we are commonly exposed in early childhood and later in life. We also hope that speech-language pathologists and audiologists in particular can become better informed concerning the relevant research, theory, and treatments for autism and other chronic medical conditions. We agree with Brian Jepson, who writes, "I believe that understanding autism will give us the key to unlock the mysteries of many other modern diseases" (Jepson & Johnson, 2007, p. 180). The goal is to understand what is causing such conditions so as to prevent, cure, or effectively treat them. Although this book is designed especially for majors in communication disorders headed for a career in speech-language pathology, audiology, or a related area, we believe it will be of general interest to health professionals and to all persons and families affected either directly or indirectly by autism and related diseases and disorders.

This symbol indicates that additional material can be found on the enclosed DVD.

Acknowledgments

Every book project is a team effort and this one is no exception. We must begin at home in thanking our families, especially our spouses, Mary Anne Oller and Stacy Niolon Oller, for their generous support and love throughout the arduous process of getting two books into print this summer. Both projects have involved years of work and our spouses have contributed ideas, concepts, and no small amount of research and labor. Over recent months, Mary Anne helped in gathering photos and permissions for the cover material for this book and Stacy has contributed important ideas, references, and resources for both the book and the DVD from her experience and research as a speech-language pathologist. Both of them, along with our children and, in John's case, grandchildren, were incredibly patient and understanding.

We also want to thank the families of children with autism who have shared their rich and sometimes difficult first-hand experience with the consequences of the growing epidemic. Among the many, we acknowledge the following families, each of whom contributed a photograph of one of the children with autism featured in the puzzle pieces on the cover of the book. We thank Theron and Terri Pitre and their son Ethan; Hester and Paul Bourdier II and their son Crawford; Duane and Vicki Waihi and their son Andrew, as well as the professional photographer Kari Smith, who contributed the photograph of Andrew.

In addition to the individuals who have been closest to this book project, we thank the Sertoma Club of Lafayette for cosponsoring, along with the University of Louisiana, an International Conference on Autism Spectrum at the Cajundome in Lafayette in the spring of 2007. The Sertoma Club of Lafayette also subsequently funded the bulk of a matching grant cosponsored by Sertoma International to the Autism Society of Acadiana with the senior author as Principal Investigator. That grant provided computer equipment, software, and video cameras for the study of medical protocols in the treatment of autism spectrum disorders. That grant provided some of the resources used in this work and is gratefully acknowledged. We must also mention among the key Sertoma leaders, Steve Broussard, Ron Chauffe, Paul George, Gerald Domingue, Joey LeRouge, John Nugent, Theron Pitre, Burnie Smith, and Jimmy Thomas. We also thank those families associated with our local branch of the Autism Society of America—the Autism Society of Acadiana (ASAC, an affiliate of Sertoma International). In addition to leaders of that organization whom we have already mentioned we must add Vicki, Charlie, and Katherine Nettles, and Carolyn, Ron, Jamie, Lauren, and Chris Tate.

We also thank our publishers and the team of editors with whom we have had the privilege of working with for a couple of years and especially over the last several months at Jones and Bartlett

Publishers. We must mention Dave Cella, Maro Gartside, Teresa Reilly, Jill Morton, Jill E. Hobbs, and the photo research team. We are also grateful to administrators at the University of Louisiana, Lafayette, especially Dr. Ray Authement, President Emeritus (who was in the saddle for nearly all of this ride); Dr. E. Joseph Savoie, the current President of the University of Louisiana; Dr. Steve P. Landry, Academic Vice President and Provost; Dr. C. E. Palmer, Dean of our Graduate School; and Dr. A. David Barry, Dean of the College of Liberal Arts; and at Texas A&M in Kingsville we thank Tom Fields, Interim Vice President for Academic Affairs and Graduate Studies.

Along with all the foregoing, we thank the many researchers, publishers, and colleagues who have generously shared their findings, theories, diagrams, videos, and photographs with us. Although we cannot mention all of them by name, there are some whom we cannot overlook: We are grateful to Dr. Stuart Campbell, MD, of Create Health Clinic in London, and to our colleague Dr. Linda C. Badon who introduced us to him and his work. Again, Dr. Campbell has allowed us to use his pioneering work with 4D video of unborn babies. Also, we thank Dr. Robert C. Titzer for his contributions to the understanding and teaching of literacy (also a resource discovered by Dr. Badon); David Kennedy, DDS and former President of the International Academy of Oral Medicine and Toxicology; Dr. Fritz Lorscheider, Dr. Naweed Syed, and colleagues at the University of Calgary Medical School; Dr. Vincent Carbone for his applied behavior analysis; Dr. Stephanie Cave in Baton Rouge for her pioneering work on vaccines and their components; and Dr. Andrew Wakefield of the Thoughtful House team in Austin, Texas.

Above all we thank our Creator God. In the text that follows, and on the DVD, we have explicitly thanked many other individuals who have permitted us to use their names and to quote their words. Here we must mention Clint Andrus, Amanda Blanchard, Crystal Boihem, Heidi Kidder, Melissa Fowlkes, Stephanie Grant, Rena S. Romero, Cheryl Sinner, Sharon Williams, and Sheria Williams. We also thank all our other students who participated in the pretesting and final work-up of the 600 multiple-choice items that are provided on the DVD. For invaluable help with the technical production of the DVD we thank Will Oller, as well as Taylor and Ruthie Toce. A special thank you, in the order in which material appears in the book, is owed to each of the following: For the story of Vance Walker, we thank his mother Shelly and the author/journalist Ingri Cassel; we commend and thank Lisa and J. B. Handley for their outstanding work and Web sites; Dan Hollenbeck for the excellent analyses of the growth trends in the diagnosis of autism; Aileen Mieko Smith for her Web site telling the story of Minamata disease; Jim West for his work on the etiology of polio; Dr. Robyn Cosford and colleagues for data concerning the abnormal ecosystems in the intestines of persons with autism; Dr. C. A. Wiley for allowing us to use an electron-micrograph of an HIV-infected macrophage; and T. C. Theoharides for sharing his creative work on the many complex and little understood gut–brain interactions. Finally, we should mention here that many additional specific credit lines and acknowledgments appear throughout the text and on the DVD. Thanks to everyone who has already had a part in this work and to all those users and sojourners yet to come who will share in it. We hope you benefit from and enjoy using this book and the accompanying material.

About the Authors

John W. Oller Jr., PhD, is the founder of the Applied Language and Speech Sciences PhD Program at the University of Louisiana at Lafayette. His work has focused on milestones of early childhood, with special emphasis on child language development, literacy, sociocognitive development, and disorders. His research has led to advances in the measurement of language proficiency, which is a major factor in high-stakes testing, diagnosis of disorders, and social interactions. John Oller's theory of abstraction predicted the fact that normal infants can read and demonstrate comprehension of printed words and phrases well before their first birthday and even before they are able to say them out loud. Other advances include reclassification of communication disorders across the board on a more comprehensive, simpler, and more consistent basis. This book shows that the autism epidemic is real but that it can be halted. It also shows that a paradigm shift in medicine is under way concerning the treatment of chronic diseases and disorders. Oller is a winner of the MLA Mildenberger Medal and holds one of the Doris B. Hawthorne Endowed Professorships at the University of Louisiana.

Stephen D. Oller, PhD, is a specialist in language disorders of childhood and the author of an introduction to that subject matter. He is an assistant professor at the University of Texas A&M at the Kingsville campus. He is also the author of theoretical and practical work on speech-language interventions as well as the assessment and diagnosis of communication disorders. Together with his wife, Stacy A. Oller, CCC-SLP, he has developed a training program for the Milestones Scale of Development (2006) that is discussed in Chapter 11 of this book. Stephen Oller is one of the coauthors of *Milestones: Normal Speech and Language Across the Life Span* (2006) and *Cases: Introducing Communication Disorders Across the Life Span* (2010).

chapter one

An Overview of the Book

OBJECTIVES

In this chapter, we

1. Overview the entire course.

2. Define autism in terms of its behavioral characteristics.

3. Discuss the centrality of autism to communication and developmental disorders.

4. Review several cases in some detail with the aim of getting at causes.

5. Discuss the paradigm shift from piecemeal health sciences to holistic care.

6. Review the distinctive elements of this course and its unfolding story line.

In this book, we embark on a journey that is more like a crime story than like the typical ho-hum university course. It is an excursion in investigative journalism guided by **forensic** science. The story that follows is grounded in the best and most up-to-date scientific research available. It is also based on sound theoretical advances with direct relevance to the real life and death issues of the world we live in today. It is a course about politics, big money, ethics, medicine, and law. It is about a pervasive and growing class of communication disorders that are affecting more and more children and families around the globe. It is about autism and, more specifically, the undeniable autism epidemic. The purpose of this book is to address the autism epidemic and its causation at an introductory level but without skimping on the research. We also do not shy away from complex theoretical considerations, though we aim to make them easy to understand. As you will see, the autism epidemic spills over into other disorders and disease conditions reaching out to affect the whole population of the world. It is surprising, threatening, and intriguing in many ways.

CONTENT AND PURPOSE

We begin with a discussion of what autism is and with evidence that there is a growing epidemic under way. The primary questions, then, become, What can be done to stop this epidemic and what can be done to recover those who are affected by it?

What Is Autism?

Since the first cases of autism were diagnosed by Leo Kanner in 1943, certain symptoms have been singled out as characteristic of the class of disorders called by that name. They are commonly referred to as "behavioral" and in different combinations are now also being used to define a growing class of problems also known as **pervasive developmental disorders** (**PDDs**). It is interesting that all of these PDDs are commonly equated with what are also called **autism spectrum disorders** (**ASDs**) ("Autism Spectrum Disorders," 2009 ●). As we will see in this course, autism is not only at the center of the PDDs, but, in its most common form, it also affects development severely and dramatically across the board—it is a truly pervasive disorder. Traditionally, it has been supposed that its origins are genetic. However, as we will see, this explanation is incomplete to the point of being misleading. Although the subcategories of ASDs (alias, PDDs) and all of their boundaries may be disputed, the fact that autism is central to the PDDs has never been in doubt.

In its most common form, which happens to be toward the severe end of the scale, autism is characterized by withdrawal from social relations, loss of verbal skills or failure to develop them, and exhibition of repetitive stereotypical behaviors such as hand-flapping, spinning, rocking, toe-walking, and head-banging. The previously unexplained behavioral symptoms of autism—especially the tendency toward self-stimulation up to and including self-injury, for instance—have generally been regarded as completely mysterious. Why would a child with autism engage in self-injurious head-banging to the point of rendering himself unconscious? Autism has been described as a strange and puzzling disorder with mysterious unknown causes. When asked for explanations by understandably desperate parents, the doctors have often resorted to the unsatisfying words, "We just don't know. It's a mystery."

Dr. David Feinberg, Medical Director of the Neuropsychiatric Hospital at the University of California at Los Angeles (UCLA), writes:

> Even the best minds in the field are unable to agree on answers. . . . The increasing rate is also an enigma, with many different opinions. (Feinberg, 2007, p. xii)

As reasonable as such remarks may seem, it is not difficult to see why parents find them inadequate. To researchers seeking answers, such responses are repeated calls to action. We cannot be satisfied with the implied conclusion that autism must remain a mystery.

As we look more closely into the cases of children with autism to be considered in this course, and the common symptoms they exhibit, we discover some additional common symptoms that were noted by Leo Kanner in 1943, but that were passed over as if irrelevant to the diagnosis. In the first publication on autism (Kanner, 1943), as noted by Dr. Bryan Jepson in 2007, Kanner himself found that at least 7 out of the original 11 cases that he diagnosed also had serious feeding and digestive problems—chronic vomiting, diarrhea, and more frequent infections and trips to the doctor than typically developing children (see Jepson & Johnson, 2007, pp. 14–16). If we add two other cases of children showing symptoms commonly associated with **acid reflux** and **chronic vomiting,** then as many as 9 of Kanner's original 11 cases seem to have had serious digestive tract symptoms.

In the next section, we sum up Kanner's (1943) evidence of **gastrointestinal** symptoms in his first 11 cases. We follow the work of Jepson and Johnson (2007, especially pp. 14–16) and also that of Andrew Wakefield and colleagues (see the Thoughtful House, 2009 ●). The symptoms that

Kanner recorded suggested problems of the gut that were clearly associated with well over half of the initial 11 cases that he diagnosed. Yet, in his quest to seek out the etiology of the mysterious "condition" or "syndrome" (Kanner, 1949, pp. 416–419) with "fascinating peculiarities" (Kanner, 1943, p. 216), those digestive tract symptoms were set aside and would barely be mentioned in future discussions of the definition of autism for years to come. Rutter (1978) would later describe Kanner's "careful and systematic observations on 11 children with a previously unrecognized syndrome" (p. 139), but until Wakefield and colleagues would come along, especially Jepson and Johnson (2007), neither Kanner nor any of the other authors of the manuals and books to be written would take seriously the symptoms of gut disease that Kanner observed and wrote about.

Evident Symptoms of Gut Disease

Case 1, according to Kanner, showed symptoms of abnormal gut problems. His father wrote: "Eating has always been a problem with him. He has never known a normal appetite. Seeing children eating candy and ice cream has never been a temptation to him" (Kanner, 1943, p. 216). At a later stage, the child still showed some abnormal symptoms with respect to food consumption. He was described as "chewing on paper and putting food in his hair" (p. 235). In September 1939, near his sixth birthday, his mother wrote: "He continues to eat wash and dress himself only at my insistence" (p. 221). Seven months later, in March 1940, she commented that "he feeds himself some better" (p. 221), suggesting that his eating habits were still not normal.

Case 2, when diagnosed at age 6, was "described as having large and ragged tonsils" (p. 224), which can be an indication of frequent acid reflux (see Stapleton & Brodsky, 2008).

Case 3 evidently had problems with elimination because his mother reported that "at the age of 3 weeks" she began to "train him by giving him a suppository every morning—so his bowels would move by the clock" (p. 224). It is reported that "following smallpox vaccination at 12 months . . . had an attack of fever and diarrhea . . ." (p. 224) and that he had "large tonsils and adenoids, which were removed on February 8, 1941," at the age of 3 years and 4 months (p. 225).

Case 4 is said to have "vomited a great deal during his fist year, and feeding formulas were changed frequently with little success" (pp. 226–227). His tonsils were "removed when he was 3 years old" (p. 227).

Case 5 is said to have "nursed very poorly and was put on bottle after about a week. She quit taking any kind of nourishment at 3 months. She was tube-fed five times daily up to 1 year of age. She began to eat then, though much difficulty with feeding persisted until she was about 18 months old" (p. 228). At camp, she "slid into **avitaminosis** and malnutrition" (p. 228).

For case 6, Virginia, no outstanding gut problems were reported.

Case 7 "vomited all food from birth through the third month. Vomiting then ceased almost abruptly and, except for occasional regurgitation, feeding proceeded satisfactorily" (p. 231).

Case 8 had problems during the first two months of life: "Feeding formula caused considerable concern" (p. 233), but he ate well after that. Even so, "when his infantile thumb sucking was prevented by use of mechanical devices, he gave up this behavior and instead put various other things in his mouth. On several occasions, pebbles were found in his stools. Shortly before his second birthday, he swallowed cotton from an Easter rabbit, aspirating some of the cotton so that a **tracheotomy** became necessary. A few months later, he swallowed some kerosene with no ill effects" (p. 233).

Case 9, was described by his mother as having "developed an obsession about feces and would hide it anywhere (for instance, in drawers): [He] would tease me if I walked into the room: 'You soiled your pants, now you can't have your crayons!' . . . Still not toilet trained. He never soils himself in the nursery school, always does it when he comes home. The same is true of wetting. He is proud of wetting, jumps up and down with ecstasy, says, 'Look at the big puddle *he* [Kanner's italics] made'" (p. 236).

autism? According to the Autism Developmental Disabilities Monitoring Network (2007 ◉), approximately 50% of the cases accounted for from 2000 and 2002 qualify as "intellectually disabled or mentally retarded." Thus, many of the new diagnoses are indicative of severe communication problems. So where are all these new cases coming from? What is causing the upsurge depicted in Figure 1-1? What can be done to stop it? How can individuals affected by autism, or by related disorders, best be helped?

Central to Communication and Its Disorders

Central to the study of all communication disorders are those that are developmental, and central to all of the disorders of communication that are labeled "pervasive developmental disorders" is autism. While the designations autism spectrum disorders and pervasive developmental disorders seem to suggest increasingly broader categories, as we will see in this course, both are roughly equivalent to "autism." In view of the frequency with which autism is said to be "a mystery"— see the comment by Katie Wright in her interview with David Kirby, where she says she heard that word used a thousand times (Foundation for Autism Information and Research, 2007b ◉)—it is unsurprising that there is no end in sight to the debates about what to call it and just which disorders, diseases, and conditions should be included under the scope of autism. However, it is clear that the scope of autism is much wider than many practitioners and educators have commonly supposed.

Obviously, it makes little sense to try to be extremely explicit about what "is and what is not" autism in view of the insistence by experts that we are dealing with a mystery, a puzzle, and a great deal of uncertainty. With that caveat in mind, we cannot go far wrong by applying the term "autism" to the whole of the PDD/ASD spectrum—a loose and vague classification, to say the least. Clearly, there is plenty of evidence—and widespread agreement—that the conditions loosely known as "autism" involve dramatic disruption of social connections, especially the ability to acquire and use language. It is also true that autism affects emotional balance, along with vital aspects of physical well-being and overall health such as the ability to digest and make use of common nutrients. There is also ample research evidence and concurrence among a substantial and growing number of independent research-ers, doctors, parents, and clinicians, as we will see in subsequent chapters, that autism also involves pervasive metabolic imbalances, immune system disruptions, chronic inflammation of the brain and gut, as well as electro-chemical imbalances leading to seizures in varying degrees of severity.

Autism is accompanied by full-blown, epileptic-type seizures in approximately 30% of the cases and by brain activity characteristic of seizure-like events in more than 50% of persons with autism (Kim, Donnelly, Tournay, Book, & Filipek, 2006; see also Baird, Robinson, Boyd, & Charman, 2006). As noted, 70% to 80% of individuals already diagnosed with autism have significant bowel disease (D'Souza, Fombonne, & Ward, 2006; Horvath & Perman, 2002; Jepson & Johnson, 2007, p. 87). Indeed, this finding is consistent with the initial report by Kanner in 1943. When extreme disease conditions are commonly associated with the diagnosis of autism, it becomes clear that parental concern is not only justified, but also that treatment of the disease conditions may also help to allevi-ate the diagnosed disorder. Strong evidence suggests that partial or complete recovery from autism is possible, perhaps, in a large percentage of cases (Bock & Stauth, 2007; Deth, Muratore, Benzecry, Power-Charnitsky, & Waly, 2008; Herbert et al., 2006; Jepson & Johnson, 2007; J. W. Oller et al., 2010; Pangborn & S. M. Baker, 2005, 2007).

As we will see in Chapter 2, the autism epidemic is real and cannot be explained away. It is a growing health problem of great importance and is associated with political, economic, and legal concerns of vast proportions. Autism is a major and growing quality of life issue; in fact, in cases of severe autism, it is no exaggeration to say that it is a life-threatening condition. Given that seizures or seizure-like brain abnormalities and chronic digestive problems are involved in a majority of cases,

Kanner recorded suggested problems of the gut that were clearly associated with well over half of the initial 11 cases that he diagnosed. Yet, in his quest to seek out the etiology of the mysterious "condition" or "syndrome" (Kanner, 1949, pp. 416–419) with "fascinating peculiarities" (Kanner, 1943, p. 216), those digestive tract symptoms were set aside and would barely be mentioned in future discussions of the definition of autism for years to come. Rutter (1978) would later describe Kanner's "careful and systematic observations on 11 children with a previously unrecognized syndrome" (p. 139), but until Wakefield and colleagues would come along, especially Jepson and Johnson (2007), neither Kanner nor any of the other authors of the manuals and books to be written would take seriously the symptoms of gut disease that Kanner observed and wrote about.

Evident Symptoms of Gut Disease

Case 1, according to Kanner, showed symptoms of abnormal gut problems. His father wrote: "Eating has always been a problem with him. He has never known a normal appetite. Seeing children eating candy and ice cream has never been a temptation to him" (Kanner, 1943, p. 216). At a later stage, the child still showed some abnormal symptoms with respect to food consumption. He was described as "chewing on paper and putting food in his hair" (p. 235). In September 1939, near his sixth birthday, his mother wrote: "He continues to eat wash and dress himself only at my insistence" (p. 221). Seven months later, in March 1940, she commented that "he feeds himself some better" (p. 221), suggesting that his eating habits were still not normal.

Case 2, when diagnosed at age 6, was "described as having large and ragged tonsils" (p. 224), which can be an indication of frequent acid reflux (see Stapleton & Brodsky, 2008).

Case 3 evidently had problems with elimination because his mother reported that "at the age of 3 weeks" she began to "train him by giving him a suppository every morning—so his bowels would move by the clock" (p. 224). It is reported that "following smallpox vaccination at 12 months . . . had an attack of fever and diarrhea . . ." (p. 224) and that he had "large tonsils and adenoids, which were removed on February 8, 1941," at the age of 3 years and 4 months (p. 225).

Case 4 is said to have "vomited a great deal during his fist year, and feeding formulas were changed frequently with little success" (pp. 226–227). His tonsils were "removed when he was 3 years old" (p. 227).

Case 5 is said to have "nursed very poorly and was put on bottle after about a week. She quit taking any kind of nourishment at 3 months. She was tube-fed five times daily up to 1 year of age. She began to eat then, though much difficulty with feeding persisted until she was about 18 months old" (p. 228). At camp, she "slid into **avitaminosis** and malnutrition" (p. 228).

For case 6, Virginia, no outstanding gut problems were reported.

Case 7 "vomited all food from birth through the third month. Vomiting then ceased almost abruptly and, except for occasional regurgitation, feeding proceeded satisfactorily" (p. 231).

Case 8 had problems during the first two months of life: "Feeding formula caused considerable concern" (p. 233), but he ate well after that. Even so, "when his infantile thumb sucking was prevented by use of mechanical devices, he gave up this behavior and instead put various other things in his mouth. On several occasions, pebbles were found in his stools. Shortly before his second birthday, he swallowed cotton from an Easter rabbit, aspirating some of the cotton so that a **tracheotomy** became necessary. A few months later, he swallowed some kerosene with no ill effects" (p. 233).

Case 9, was described by his mother as having "developed an obsession about feces and would hide it anywhere (for instance, in drawers): [He] would tease me if I walked into the room: 'You soiled your pants, now you can't have your crayons!' . . . Still not toilet trained. He never soils himself in the nursery school, always does it when he comes home. The same is true of wetting. He is proud of wetting, jumps up and down with ecstasy, says, 'Look at the big puddle *he* [Kanner's italics] made'" (p. 236).

Case 10 was described by his father, who said: "The main thing that worries me is the difficulty in feeding. That is the essential thing. . . . During the first days of his life he did not take the breast satisfactorily. After fifteen days he was changed from breast to bottle by did not take the bottle satisfactorily. There is a long story of trying to get food down. We have tried everything under the sun. . . . He sucks his thumb and grinds his teeth quite frequently" (p. 237). At one of his visits to Kanner, "mild obsessive trends were reported, such as pushing aside the first spoonful of every dish" (p. 238).

Case 11, Elaine, at the age of 2 years went to nursery school where she "drank the water and ate the plant when the children were being taught to handle flowers" (p. 239). There were no other bizarre symptoms of any eating or digestive disorder.

Reviewing the evidence from Kanner's first 11 cases, only Cases 6 and 11 (both girls) seem to have had no outstanding (no reported) symptoms of any kind of eating disorder, bowel disease, or digestive problems. However, the other 9 cases range from clear-cut to marginal symptoms that were reported and could be taken as indicative of gut problems. Cases 1, 4, and 7 seem to have had chronic vomiting syndrome, at least during their early years. Cases 2, 3, and 4 showed symptoms that could well point to tissue damage and inflammation from chronic acid reflux (Stapleton & Brodsky, 2008). Cases 3, 8, 9, 10, and 11 were all described as having some kind of symptom suggesting bizarre habits of eating or elimination. Thus 9 of the 11 cases seem to have had some gut-related issue that either one or both parents, or Kanner, thought worth reporting, and 7 of the 9 cases with gut-related symptoms seem to have experienced severe problems.

Such symptoms suggest the reasonable inference that autism involves a great deal more than its traditionally recognized behavioral characteristics. However, the symptoms involving the digestive tract would be set aside for about half a century following the publication of Kanner's seminal work in 1943. Parents with a child diagnosed with autism would typically be told that the digestive problems observed in their child have nothing to do with the autism diagnosis but have some other independent cause. One of our students, Heidi Kidder, who is the mother of a boy diagnosed with autism, was astonished to learn in our introductory course on communication disorders (see J. W. Oller, S. D. Oller, & Badon, 2010) that her son's chronic vomiting syndrome is a common feature of autism. Neither the pediatrician who diagnosed her son's autism nor the specialist in gastroenterology to whom he was sent because of his chronic vomiting and bloody diarrhea knew of any association between autism and gut disease. Both said the conditions were unrelated. However, the research shows that about 70% to 80% of individuals previously diagnosed with autism, when examined after the fact, are found to have disease symptoms associated with the gut (D'Souza, Fombonne, & Ward, 2006; Jepson & Johnson, 2007, p. 87; Valicenti-McDermott, McVicar, Rapin, Wershil, Cohen, & Shinnar, 2006; Wakefield, Stott, & Limb, 2006). Pediatricians should know of this association—but many evidently do not, as is pointed out in an eloquent and powerful article by Wakefield, Stott, and Krigsman (2008).

When Heidi mentioned to the doctors that according to her current reading on autism research, the seemingly interminable episodes of vomiting were almost certainly related to her son's autism, the idea was summarily dismissed by the doctors. In fact, until the number of cases of persons diagnosed with autism began to reach epidemic proportions, mainstream doctors would continue to tell parents of children with autism that there was no connection whatever with the problems they were seeing in eating habits and digestion.

In fact, with specific reference to the ongoing discussion about the association of gut disease with autism, Brian Deer, an "investigative journalist," wrote about symptoms such as persistent crying, fevers, rash, irritability, and even convulsions that "no competent doctor, acting professionally, could describe these as 'behavioral symptoms', much less hold them out as potential markers for the onset of regressive autism" (Deer, n.d., ●). Deer himself characterizes these and related symptoms as "benign" in four places in the surrounding context and he acknowledges that they are "common . . . consequences of vaccination" (Deer, n.d.). In fact, as we have already seen, Leo Kanner did describe the first 11 cases of the individuals he diagnosed with autism in behavioral terms, and he also found symptoms of gut abnormality in 9 of the 11.

Interestingly, subsequent researchers and practitioners alike would tend to ignore the gut symptoms until Wakefield called attention to them near the turn of the twenty-first century. Also, contrary to Deer's claim, symptoms of abnormal digestion and other gut disease conditions are being seriously re-examined from many different angles by competent researchers and doctors at the present time. More telling against Deer's position is the fact that no responsible parent is inclined to regard convulsions in any child, and certainly not in one of their own children, as "benign."

Controversy and Emotion

It is unsurprising that parents are upset. Katie Wright (2007), the mother of a child diagnosed with autism and the daughter of the founders of Autism Speaks (2009 🌑), descries the current situation:

> I do not want to speak to more parents who have ill, malnourished children, mentally and physically destroyed by autism. No parents should be mopping blood from their toddler's backside for two years. Parents should not be told it is normal for their autistic child to stay awake all night every night. (Jepson & Johnson, 2007, p. xx)

Over the last several decades, the number of children being diagnosed with autism, as reported under federal law from schools across the United States receiving funding under the Individuals with Disabilities Act of 1990, has grown exponentially. In the growth curve shown in Figure 1-1, the black line shows how the rate of autism diagnosis has increased steadily from 1993 to 2006; the gray line shows that the growth rate for diagnosis of all other reported categories of disorders over the same period was negligible by comparison. Why are there so many new cases diagnosed as

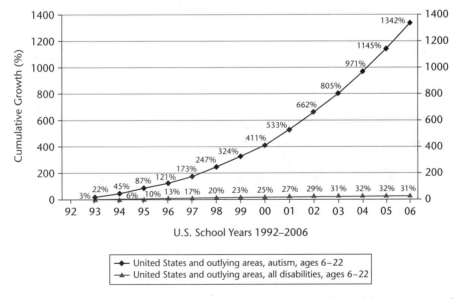

Figure 1-1 The accelerating diagnosis of autism (the black line) in the United States compared against all other reported disorders (the gray line).
Source: Retrieved April 12, 2008, from http://www.fightingautism.org/idea/autism.php. The original graph is licensed under a Creative Commons Attribution 1.0 Generic License, retrieved June 15, 2009, from http://creativecommons.org/licenses/by/1.0/. It is adapted and reprinted with the permission of Thoughtful House.

autism? According to the Autism Developmental Disabilities Monitoring Network (2007 ◐), approximately 50% of the cases accounted for from 2000 and 2002 qualify as "intellectually disabled or mentally retarded." Thus, many of the new diagnoses are indicative of severe communication problems. So where are all these new cases coming from? What is causing the upsurge depicted in Figure 1-1? What can be done to stop it? How can individuals affected by autism, or by related disorders, best be helped?

Central to Communication and Its Disorders

Central to the study of all communication disorders are those that are developmental, and central to all of the disorders of communication that are labeled "pervasive developmental disorders" is autism. While the designations autism spectrum disorders and pervasive developmental disorders seem to suggest increasingly broader categories, as we will see in this course, both are roughly equivalent to "autism." In view of the frequency with which autism is said to be "a mystery"— see the comment by Katie Wright in her interview with David Kirby, where she says she heard that word used a thousand times (Foundation for Autism Information and Research, 2007b ◐)—it is unsurprising that there is no end in sight to the debates about what to call it and just which disorders, diseases, and conditions should be included under the scope of autism. However, it is clear that the scope of autism is much wider than many practitioners and educators have commonly supposed.

Obviously, it makes little sense to try to be extremely explicit about what "is and what is not" autism in view of the insistence by experts that we are dealing with a mystery, a puzzle, and a great deal of uncertainty. With that caveat in mind, we cannot go far wrong by applying the term "autism" to the whole of the PDD/ASD spectrum—a loose and vague classification, to say the least. Clearly, there is plenty of evidence—and widespread agreement—that the conditions loosely known as "autism" involve dramatic disruption of social connections, especially the ability to acquire and use language. It is also true that autism affects emotional balance, along with vital aspects of physical well-being and overall health such as the ability to digest and make use of common nutrients. There is also ample research evidence and concurrence among a substantial and growing number of independent researchers, doctors, parents, and clinicians, as we will see in subsequent chapters, that autism also involves pervasive metabolic imbalances, immune system disruptions, chronic inflammation of the brain and gut, as well as electro-chemical imbalances leading to seizures in varying degrees of severity.

Autism is accompanied by full-blown, epileptic-type seizures in approximately 30% of the cases and by brain activity characteristic of seizure-like events in more than 50% of persons with autism (Kim, Donnelly, Tournay, Book, & Filipek, 2006; see also Baird, Robinson, Boyd, & Charman, 2006). As noted, 70% to 80% of individuals already diagnosed with autism have significant bowel disease (D'Souza, Fombonne, & Ward, 2006; Horvath & Perman, 2002; Jepson & Johnson, 2007, p. 87). Indeed, this finding is consistent with the initial report by Kanner in 1943. When extreme disease conditions are commonly associated with the diagnosis of autism, it becomes clear that parental concern is not only justified, but also that treatment of the disease conditions may also help to alleviate the diagnosed disorder. Strong evidence suggests that partial or complete recovery from autism is possible, perhaps, in a large percentage of cases (Bock & Stauth, 2007; Deth, Muratore, Benzecry, Power-Charnitsky, & Waly, 2008; Herbert et al., 2006; Jepson & Johnson, 2007; J. W. Oller et al., 2010; Pangborn & S. M. Baker, 2005, 2007).

As we will see in Chapter 2, the autism epidemic is real and cannot be explained away. It is a growing health problem of great importance and is associated with political, economic, and legal concerns of vast proportions. Autism is a major and growing quality of life issue; in fact, in cases of severe autism, it is no exaggeration to say that it is a life-threatening condition. Given that seizures or seizure-like brain abnormalities and chronic digestive problems are involved in a majority of cases, autism is clearly more than just a behavioral condition. The search for the causes of self-injurious behaviors becomes more tractable when a holistic, systems-based perspective is taken. It has been noted from the earliest diagnosed cases that autism tends to be expressed in violent mood swings that result in bizarre and often self-injurious behaviors such as head-banging and potentially harmful practices such as feces smearing by individuals well beyond the toddler stage. One mother reported that if her son's name was mentioned at the University Medical Center, everyone over there would remember him: "He was 10 years old when he smeared feces all over that place. They know who he is." While such bizarre behaviors might remain unexplained if the digestive issues and disease conditions were ignored, once they are brought into play, explanations over and above genetic factors seem to be required.

More Than a Behavioral Disorder

In the past, the bizarre behaviors associated with autism were regarded merely as genetically determined behavioral characteristics of the disorder. We now know that they are indicative of deeper and highly significant physiological imbalances. Nevertheless, at the time of this writing, autism is still diagnosed exclusively by behavioral characteristics—specifically, disruption of interpersonal relations, language loss (especially regression) or delay in acquisition, and by repetitive behaviors such as hand-flapping or even self-injurious behaviors such as head-banging. However, as we will see throughout this course, but especially in Chapters 3–5 of this book, we now have incontrovertible positive and validated research evidence from multiple sources showing that autism involves high levels of **toxicity**, **oxidative-stress**, and in a very high percentage of cases, serious problems in digestion and elimination of wastes. In about three quarters of all reported cases, gut disease of a significant and detectable level is involved (see Jepson & Johnson, 2007; Wakefield, Stott, & Krigsman, 2008).

The Primary Aim of This Book

The primary aim of this book is to apply sound logical theory to the findings of validated empirical research concerning the autism epidemic. The goal is to discover its causes in order to figure out how best to deal with it. In doing so, we must often rely on the fact-finding methods used by forensic scientists as well as by journalists and investigative reporters. As we will see, the work carries us into areas of intense controversy in politics and policy making. The story leads to secret meetings and confidential memos exchanged by high-placed officials whose stated purpose in many instances was to conceal information from the public. In some cases, individuals evidently acted on the basis of expected (and hoped-for) outcomes rather than on the basis of the unwanted evidence they came upon. They did not want to see what they found, and some, evidently, did not believe the facts even when they were staring them in the face. Others, some in positions of high responsibility, took a more active role in denying what they wished—and said in memos that have since become public— was not true. After certain expectations proved false, some officials in high places, evidently tried to shape the data to fit their preconceived notions in order to cover up problems that they wished would "go away" (Putchildrenfirst.org, 2009 ●). We will find evidence that many well-meaning pediatricians, physicians, and researchers have been trying to support their prior beliefs about vaccines and about common medical practice rather than believing the facts they actually found. It is not so much, perhaps, as Dr. Mark Hyman observes, that doctors are trying to deceive themselves and others, as that they often cannot believe what they see when the facts contrast markedly with what they expect to see. He says, "They see what they believe, rather than believe what they see" (Hyman, 2009 ●).

In the background, for individuals and families coping with the autism epidemic, as we will see especially in Chapter 2, a great deal is at stake. The story involves huge international corporations, government agencies, and public media, as well as private citizens. In this book, we rely on many research tools and resources including the Internet. Today, more than ever before, it is difficult for anyone or any group to keep secrets, even ones that were concealed behind closed doors and that were intended to be kept confidential and hidden from public view.

It is not our intention to go hunting for conspiracies or to cast blame on particular individuals. However, as independent researchers who are bound only by honor and the pursuit of truth, insofar as we are able to discern it, we are determined to follow the story and the research findings wherever they may lead. We report the facts and the research findings as we see them and we draw reasonable inferences from sound theory. Where public agencies are involved, including their officials and public employees, we do not shy away from naming names. However, when it comes to private families and individuals impacted by autism, we use names only with written permission in the shared purpose of finding the causes, putting a stop to the epidemic, and recovering persons affected by autism as much as it is possible to do so.

Disclosure: Why We Wrote the Book

We did the research and wrote this book in search of the causes of the autism epidemic. We now know what many of the offending elements are. To absolve ourselves of any profit motive, we have devoted whatever royalties may be earned by this project to a fund for the treatment of autism and related disorders as disclosed in Dr. Wakefield's Foreword to this book. We will not take a cent of profit from this book. In the course that is laid out in the pages that follow, and also in the accompanying materials contained on or hyperlinked to the DVD, users of this material will discover that the principal causes of autism are toxins, disease agents, and combinations of them. For the most part, those factors are being placed directly into the bloodstreams of younger and younger infants by physicians.

We will trace the research on such experimental uses of disease agents, toxins, and animal proteins back to a Nobel Prize awarded to Dr. Charles Richet in 1913. Richet had shown in his research with dogs, rodents, guinea pigs, and other animals that microscopic foreign particles—especially foreign biological proteins or pieces of them—introduced into the bloodstream are particularly prone to produce acute allergic reactions, especially if they happen to be injected repeatedly. The kind of hypersensitivity that he demonstrated would come to be known by the now-common term **anaphylaxis**, which Richet introduced into the forensic medical literature. For reasons to be explored in some detail in this book, toxins and foreign proteins, in addition to a great many weakened or partially destroyed disease agents, have increasingly been introduced into human populations through vaccines. The injuries caused by such injections are subtle, complex, and long-lasting, and they may or may not be expressed immediately after the injection.

There is evidence that in some cases, injuries have been sustained before birth through medications and medicinal procedures that have directly impacted one or both parents and that later have indirectly affected the baby before or after its birth. Autism is a central kind of communication disorder, and the factors involved in producing it are, as the research shows, also involved in many other diseases and disorders. In the vast majority of cases, the disease conditions to be highlighted in this course were known to parents well before (often for two or more years before) the diagnosis of autism was made by a doctor. In a minority of cases, the disease conditions were discovered after the diagnosis was made.

As a result, the traditional "it's a mystery" response to questions about causation, however valid that claim may have seemed in the past or in some of the particular present-day cases, is never an acceptable end point for parents, clinicians, or researchers. It is essential to move on to discover causes. In some cases, the causes of autism are fatal before a diagnosis is possible and in other cases they can still be fatal long after the diagnosis. When they are not fatal, we have an ethical and moral obligation nonetheless to provide the earliest possible diagnosis and to follow it with treatment that provides the best possible hope of improvement and recovery of the affected individual (see Chapters 3, 8, and 12).

CASES OF AUTISM

Although many parents did not make the connection until much later, most would wonder out loud if it was just a coincidence that the onset of autism—or something worse in the case of four-month-old Vance Walker (whom we will meet a little later in the story)—followed one or many vaccinations. That was the way it was for Dr. Jerry Kartzinel, a board-certified pediatrician. His fourth boy slipped into the world of autism after receiving his mumps, measles, and rubella (MMR) vaccine (Kartzinel, 2007, p. xv).

Kartzinel gave his son the vaccines—and for that reason he was challenged by none other than the boy's mother, who said, "You broke him; now you fix him!" The effects of autism were later described by Kartzinel in this way: "Autism, as I see it, steals the soul from a child; then, if allowed, relentlessly sucks life's marrow out of the family members, one by one. It relegates every other normal thing to utter insignificance" (p. xvi). When Jenny McCarthy asked Dr. Kartzinel what caused her own son's weakening until he had the **immune system** of a person dying from acquired immune deficiency syndrome (AIDS), Kartzinel answered in one word: "Vaccines" (McCarthy, 2007a, p. 148). Kartzinel also discussed this issue with television host Larry King, Jenny McCarthy, and others on *Larry King Live* (2007 ●). As Kartzinel pointed out at that time, the role of vaccines—specifically, their disease agents, toxins, and the foreign biological proteins that they contain—is an issue that keeps coming up in discussions of autism. Parents think vaccines are an issue, and we agree with Kartzinel and others that we must listen to them. For updates on the ongoing discussion, see *Larry King Live* (2008b, 2009 ●). The parents are the ones who are with the child before and after the relatively few minutes spent by the doctors or nurses who give the shots.

True Narratives: Real People

Getting a picture of the autism epidemic is a little like filming a war that engulfs the whole world. It is difficult to know where to point the camera. With respect to the autism epidemic, the question is how to shape this book and its accompanying DVD and the materials contained, cross-referenced, and hyperlinked there so that it will be maximally comprehensible and useful. Fictional writers dealing with such sagas commonly resort to one or more viewpoint characters that live through the events to be narrated. This story is not so different, except that the viewpoint characters here consist of a multitude of real persons—and, to one degree or another, all of us are among them.

We are in the story and it is truly unfolding as we write these words. There is nothing fictional about it. In telling the story we aim to follow some of the final advice of Dr. Randy Pausch in his famous Last Lecture at Carnegie Mellon after he was diagnosed with terminal pancreatic cancer that had spread to his liver (2009 ●). Among other things he said, "Tell the truth." We intend to do that. To that end, and for other reasons that we will spell out as we go along, we rely extensively on true narratives of real individuals. We tell about lived experience in sufficient detail to guide the forensic inferences to be drawn in discovering the causal factors emerging from the details.

Some of the stories have been previously published; others, with the permission of the persons involved, are told publicly here for the first time. If there are any errors in the telling, they are our own and are entirely unintentional. By presenting the facts of actual cases, by reporting the findings of current research, and by making reasonable inferences, our aim is to seek out the causes of the autism epidemic. Beyond that the greater goal is to halt the growth of the autism epidemic and to recover, as much as possible, the persons already affected by it. To make significant progress toward that goal, we believe it is essential to share some of the actual experiences of the people who are dealing with the autism epidemic all the time. As they say in the media, it is necessary to meet the players "up close and personal."

After introducing Hannah Poling, who was in the news a great deal beginning in March 2008, we review several other cases. We concentrate on typical rather than atypical cases, and rely on descriptions by firsthand observers. In most cases, the witnesses are the parents of the children in question. For some cases, we provide references to video links where live footage of the affected individuals can be viewed intensively by students and other users of this book.

Connecting the Qualitative and Quantitative Ends

In this course, in addition to dealing with some of the qualitative details of individual cases, we also refer throughout to the most up-to-date quantitative research studies involving substantial numbers of individuals and/or multiple measures. Of course, it is sometimes important even for measurement experts, researchers, and theoreticians to be reminded that the data points in every valid research study depend in the final analysis on real individuals who are known by or who are themselves competent observers (Borsboom, Mellenbergh, & van Heerden, 2004; Uebersax, 1988). Everything in the end depends on true narrative reports.

It is common for some epidemiologists to dismiss individual reports of particular individuals as mere anecdotes, as if that classification automatically disqualifies those reports from serious discussions. The epidemiologists holding that view need to be reminded that every valid measurement in the sciences, as has been proved in various logicomathematical ways (J. W. Oller, 1993, 1996a-b; J. W. Oller & L. Chen, 2007; Peirce, 1897; Tarski, 1949, 1956), depends on true qualitative judgments about particular individuals. There are no exceptions. The proofs cover all valid judgments and measurements in the sciences without exception. For that reason, students and instructors can confidently consider the cases presented throughout this book as reports from reliable witnesses that logically must be taken into consideration. In the final analysis, the persons affected by autism, directly and indirectly, are absolutely the most important subjects of the course. No valid research of any kind can be done without reference to actual cases. Without such cases, all so-called research and all theories are merely empty, ungrounded speculations. Self-proclaimed "experts" prone to rely on such ungrounded opinions should be regarded with profound skepticism. Every evaluator of research must keep in mind that even large-scale, data-intensive studies, at their heart, are based on unique individual reports.

To get to the bottom of the autism epidemic we require examination of actual cases and the facts pertaining to them. True narratives pertaining to such cases are absolutely indispensable. Throughout this book, as in our other book dealing with the full scope of communication disorders (see *Cases*, by J. W. Oller et al., 2010), we refer to "cases" in the sense of the actual histories of individuals with the autism diagnosis, as well as "cases" in the legal and clinical senses. Actual cases are essential to the story of the autism epidemic. Whatever **validity** it may have rests exclusively in those actual instances.

Hannah Poling

On March 7, 2008, a beautiful little red-headed nine-year-old girl with autism was introduced to the world on *Larry King Live* ("The Autism Vaccine Debate," 2008a ◐). Hannah Poling was in the news because her parents had sued the government and had ostensibly won the first major concession, or so it was incorrectly reported, in regard to a causal link between the neurotoxin thimerosal and autism. It has since been discovered that 12 cases similar to the one involving Poling had already been conceded by medical experts appointed by the Vaccine Injury Court prior to the concession in the Poling case (Kirby, 2008b ◐).

Although it is not well known, the so-called Vaccine Injury Court has an interesting history, dating back to just prior to the American Civil War. We will discuss that history and the peculiar court formerly known as the People's Court and officially called the United States Court of Federal Claims in Chapter 8. In the meantime, in connection with the case of Hannah Poling, it is useful to note that of the 2542 cases decided in favor of vaccine-injured citizens, 1254 (almost half) involved the DTP shots containing thimerosal (discussed in further detail in Chapter 3). Awards for injuries attributed to the thimerosal-containing DTP shots amounted to almost $500 million between 1988 and 2007 (Edlich, Son, et al., 2007). By July 2006, 5030 cases had been filed alleging a link between thimerosal-containing vaccines and autism. In the instance of Hannah Poling, her mother, Terry Poling, a licensed nurse and practicing lawyer, was convinced that Hannah's autism was caused in part by vaccines. Hannah became ill immediately after receiving nine vaccines in one day at a **well-baby visit** when she was 19 months of age.

A Well-Baby Visit?

The main purpose of "well-baby visits" is to perform vaccinations. In an article titled "Receipt of Well-Baby Care," the Centers for Disease Control and Prevention (CDC) explained the meaning of "well-baby" visits to the pediatrician:

> Routine well-baby care (i.e., non-illness-related visits to a health care professional during infancy) provides important opportunities to promote health in infants through timely receipt of recommended vaccinations. . . . (1994, p. 105)

Interestingly, the article goes on to say that such "non-illness-related visits" are also helpful in the "detection and treatment of diseases, and identification of potential developmental or psychosocial disorders" (p. 105). In the survey reported in this article. CDC researchers asked mothers, "How many times has your baby been to a doctor or nurse for baby shots or routine well-baby care?" Clearly, the focus is on the shots. It is vaccinations, including staying on the CDC's recommended schedule, that provide the primary motivation for "well-baby" visits. The main underlying question in the CDC study was whether infants of **low birth weight** (i.e., those weighing less than 5 pounds, 8 ounces at birth) were getting all their recommended shots. That is, did they participate in as many visits as other children? The main purpose of well-baby visits—for all babies—is to administer vaccines.

Hannah Gets Sick

In the case of Hannah Poling, within two days of her well-baby visit at the age of 19 months, she had a high fever and started a downhill slide into autism. Her mother described her from that time forward as

> . . . having a decreased level of consciousness, . . . when I would say something to her, she was very lethargic and she would not respond to me. Uh, she was very anorexic. (*Larry King Live*, March 7, 2008)

Hannah's case has been discussed in the media a great deal, and there is excellent online documentation so that we can see Hannah in her early months before autism. Thus we can observe firsthand the behavioral symptoms that characterized her autism after she received the nine vaccines.

During the interview with Larry King, Hannah is seated between her mother and father and is occupied for much of the time with a hand-held electronic device and its ear piece. She puts the ear piece in her mouth, moves it from mouth to ear, and back to her mouth. She licks it repeatedly through much of the 9.5-minute segment. At one point, she tries to remove the cord from her neck, gets assistance from her mother, and is soothed by her mother stroking her arm. When King asks, "How is she now?" her mother replies, "Autistic still."

Is Hannah Atypical?

In an article that appeared on March 7, 2008, Dr. Julie Gerberding, Director of the CDC, was quoted as saying in reference to the Poling case, "This does not represent anything other than a very special situation" ("Vaccine Settlement Complex, May Not Be First," 2008 ●). The very next day, after Hannah's case was discussed on *Larry King Live*, Gerberding appeared on *House Call with Dr. Sanjay Gupta* on CNN. While admitting she had not reviewed the details of the Poling case, she insisted, "What we can say absolutely for sure is that we don't really understand the causes of autism. . . . there really is no association between vaccines and autism." ● However, as we review the research on regressive autism following multiple vaccinations, we will see that Hannah's case of autism is actually typical in all respects relevant to the diagnosis.

Behavioral Criteria as an Impediment

It is essential to keep in mind that autism has been diagnosed behaviorally from 1943 until the present day; it has never been diagnosed by any medical tests or based on any genetic characteristics. As Stott, Blaxill, and Wakefield (2004) have noted, the "mysterious" and "unexplainable" behavioral criteria for diagnosis have, if anything, stood as "an impediment when considering mechanisms of causation" (p. 70). They refer to the classification systems used by the American Psychiatric Association in the latest edition of its *Diagnostic and Statistical Manual* (2000–2008) and by the World Health Organization in its most up-to-date *International Classification of Diseases* (1996–2009). We return to the problem of diagnosis, and more particularly to methods of determining degrees of severity in autism, in Chapter 11. For now, we should keep in mind that piecemeal diagnostic procedures are part of the problem. The behavioral criteria do not take account of the whole person, nor do they consider the multiple interacting systems of the body in the affected individual. Stott and colleagues, for that reason, suggest that the diagnostic procedures currently being applied are actually misleading. They are part of the problem, contributing to perpetuation of the "mystery," rather than to its solution.

By the age of nine years, according to Terry Poling, Hannah had already received

> . . . hundreds and hundreds of hours of applied behavioral therapy, speech therapy, **occupational therapy, physical therapy**. We had people in our home 45 hours a week for three years. She was not speaking. She had lost motor tone. She could not put food in her hand and put it up to her mouth. She did not know what her mouth was. (*Larry King Live*, 2008a)

Hannah's father, Dr. Jon Poling, a practicing neurologist, agreed that vaccines were involved in precipitating Hannah's condition.

Dov Shestack

As Jonathan Shestack and Portia Iversen found out in the case of their infant son, Dov (rhymes with "stove"), the diagnosis of autism came a long time after its onset. They knew something was wrong, but they could not find a doctor who could tell them what it was. Dov's case, just like that the Kartzinel child, involved a regression after a period of normal development. Shestack, a well-known Hollywood producer of movies such as *Father of the Bride, Dan in Real Life*, and *Ghosts of Girlfriends Past* ("Film Scouts," 1998–2009), told the story of Dov's disappearance into autism at the Autism Summit in 2003 ●; he also founded an organization devoted to finding a cure for autism.

Jon describes Dov as "adorable" and "cute." Approximately 15 months after what began as a normal childhood, however, Dov suddenly "stopped answering to his name." Jon says that Dov "had a couple of dozen words. He lost them. He stopped running to greet us when we came in the door. And it really looked like he'd disappeared in front of our eyes in the space of a couple of months." When Dov was 11 years old, "we were still trying get him back."

At first, Jon and Portia could not get a straight answer from anyone. Some experts whom they consulted denied that Dov had any kind of problem at all. So he learned and lost a few words? It was nothing to worry about. He was just a boy, and boys develop more slowly. Dov's parents got tired of hearing that "Einstein didn't speak until he was 4 years old." Finally, they talked to an individual who said the word "autism." Jon and his wife did not know what it meant. They asked, "What can you do about *that*?" The doctor replied, "There is really nothing you can do about that. You just hold on to each other and cry and get on with your own lives." Jon described the next four days of that Memorial Day weekend as the longest days of his life. He and Portia watched videotapes of their little boy over and over, asking themselves how it was that they had lost him. At the time of this writing, Dov Shestack is 12 years old and his parents are still trying to get him back. See Jon Shestack (2008) in the MSNBC video "Search for a Cure" broadcast on the *Nightly News* (●).

Evan McCarthy

More recently, people around the world have heard or read the story of Jenny McCarthy's little boy, Evan. McCarthy's book, *Louder Than Words: A Mother's Journey in Healing Autism*, was published in 2007, and she has also made her story available online (McCarthy, 2007c ●). You can hear her tell the story in person (hyperlinked on the DVD).

The journey into the black hole of autism for Jenny McCarthy began when Evan was two and a half. One day, Evan seemed to be sleeping later than usual. With a sinking feeling in the pit of her stomach, and already sensing that something was wrong, she went to check on him and found her son "struggling to breathe" (p. 2). He was having a full-blown convulsive seizure. From that day forward, Evan's descent from what had been a fairly normal development into severe nonverbal infantile autism was precipitous. He went from one life-threatening seizure to another. Over the months that followed, while spending as much as $4,000 a week on therapies, not to mention medications, hospitalizations, multiple courses of antibiotics, and countless medical procedures trying to determine what was wrong, Jenny McCarthy got the equivalent of a Google PhD in autism. Within a few months, when a neurologist tested Evan's ability to undergo treatment in the form of **intravenous immunoglobulin (IVIG)**, the preliminary tests showed that his immune system could not sustain the additional load. When she asked Dr. Kartzinel how Evan's immune system had become so damaged, he said it was because of vaccines.

We will return to the story of Evan's road to recovery later in this book. For now, it is essential to realize that the seizures he experienced, the procedures he would live through, and the persistence of his mother in pursuing answers were accompanied and motivated by the realization that the story could have had a different outcome. For many other children, the prognosis of "No hope; no way out; it's all caused by genetics; the mystery is unsolvable" would have been accepted as a sad but inevitable life sentence. From a parent's perspective, even a life sentence without parole would usually be preferred over the only other alternative—but some parents do not get the choice.

Vance Walker

At the age of four months, just prior to his well-baby visit in September 2007, Vance Walker (Figure 1-2) was a healthy little boy who had met all his normal milestones. His parents were planning an excursion to Mexico. His mother, Shelly Walker, was told that Vance had the distinction of being the youngest child in the United States to be issued a passport in that year.

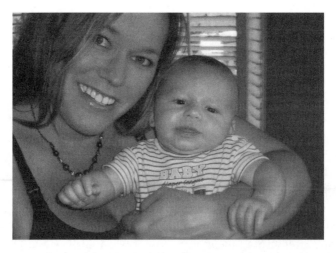

Figure 1-2   Vance Vernon Walker with his mom Shelly when he was four months old.
Source: Courtesy of *Idaho Observer* 2008.

In getting ready for his first excursion outside the United States, Vance's mother thought of the potential disease exposures south of the border. On the advice of a trusted pediatrician at Lakeside Pediatric and Adolescent Medicine in Coeur d'Alene, Idaho, on September 12, 2007, Shelly took Vance for vaccinations. She had "an uneasy feeling" about giving him so many jolts in one day, but the pediatrician said the multiple shots would do no harm. Reluctantly, she complied. It was a decision she would greatly regret.

Multiple Toxins and Disease Agents

Vance was given two injections, each of which contained multiple disease agents and various toxins. His injected vaccines consisted of **Pediarix** (developed by GlaxoSmithKline) and **Prevnar** (produced by Wyeth); he also received the oral vaccine **RotaTeq** (manufactured by Merck).

The first of the shots in the potpourri given to Vance Walker that day was Pediarix. It aims to immunize the child against diphtheria, tetanus, pertussis, hepatitis B, and three strains of the polio virus. The "prescribing information" offered by its manufacturer, GlaxoSmithKline (2008a ◉), reports the results of multiple clinical trials. It showed that the seven disease agents in the new combination shot were about twice as likely to produce a medically attended fever than when the same disease agents were administered separately but under similar conditions in all other respects. In other words, the clinical trial showed that the mixture of the vaccines brings about some interaction that is more potent than the same agents administered separately.

The Prevnar shot that Vance received contained the seven most common **pneumococcal viruses** (associated with spinal meningitis and other diseases) along with a diphtheria protein (CRM197), which closely resembles the toxin that causes diphtheria. That protein is allegedly an **antigen** that can produce immunity to diphtheria but that does not cause the disease. In the "prescribing information" for Prevnar, it is reported that in clinical trials a fever greater than 100°F (38°C) was about twice as common with both the first and second doses of Prevnar than with the usual regimen of shots without Prevnar. Thus, adding Prevnar to Pediarix increases the likelihood that the child will develop a fever higher than normal along with whatever else the interacting disease agents and other elements in the vaccines might cause.

Finally, Vance was given RotaTeq. This oral vaccine contains five distinct viruses that are supposed to inoculate a child against viral infections that are associated with vomiting and diarrhea.

The most common adverse effects reported from clinical trials of this vaccine are, in fact, diarrhea and vomiting. Block et al. (2007) also found that this combination of orally administered disease agents, like Pediarix and Prevnar, is associated with a significant increase in fevers of 100.5 °F or higher.

Too Many at a Time?

In the original article that told Vance Walker's story, Ingri Cassel (2008) counted a total of 19 disease agents. In fact, 20 disease agents were administered to Vance Walker on September 12, 2007. There were seven in the Pediarix vaccine, eight in Prevnar, and five in RotaTeq. This, of course, does not count the additional toxins and foreign animal proteins found in the vaccines along with these 20 disease agents.

The disease agents are included in the vaccines on the theory that they are potential antigens— that is, biological factors that will (theoretically, at least) produce additional immunity in the child provided that the body can handle them and defeat or eliminate them (for the history of this theory and its applications in the creation of vaccines, see Chapter 7). However, the contaminants in the vaccines that are not counted can also interact with the disease agents, and with each other, in many different and largely unexplored ways (see Hoffman, 2008 👁). Moreover, the interactions can vary depending on exceedingly complex factors of genetics, the child's current state of health, and other aspects unique to the individual. When vaccines contain multiple disease agents, they are referred to as **multivalent vaccines**. Some are also **conjugate vaccines**, in which an animal protein is used as a carrier to which one or more supposed antigens are attached.

All of the vaccines received by Vance Walker were multivalent products and, according to their prescribing information, contained additional contaminants. Vance's single dose of Pediarix also contained as much as 0.85 milligrams of aluminum, plus formaldehyde, other contaminants, and as much as 0.5% of yeast protein in addition to its seven intended disease agents. According to the CDC Web site for Pediarix (2007b), the vaccine also contains trace amounts of thimerosal ethyl mercury (see Chapter 5), which is used in manufacturing the vaccine. Assuming that it was handled correctly and shaken before administration, Vance's dose of Prevnar contained as much as 0.125 micrograms of aluminum in addition to its eight disease agents. RotaTeq contains whatever impurities were left from the cattle in which the five disease agents were cultured. It is known that the chemical reaction of aluminum and thimerosal together can produce severe tissue damage by burning (A. G. Nash, 1973). Also, if the materials are not correctly handled, settling can produce very different results across individual children because of toxins that end up in much higher concentration at the bottom of an unshaken vial.

The one critical element that is not given much attention in the prescribing information for any of the vaccines in question is their potential for participating in a multitude of possible interactions. Clinical trials confirm that combinations of disease agents are more apt to produce adverse effects such as fever, diarrhea, and vomiting (Redhead et al., 1994), but there are no trials examining all the possible interactions of the various disease agents and contaminants taken separately. The reason for this at its basis is purely mathematical. As soon as the number of potential interacting elements becomes greater than three, the cost and difficulty of doing the necessary comparisons to assess all of the possible interactions become enormous.

Thinking Through the Interactions

Of course, the cost of doing clinical trials is not the only consideration when it comes to studies of interacting chemicals inside a living body. The potential for harm, while hoping for help, can become life threatening. Setting aside the political, economical, and other considerations for a few moments, let's reflect on the biochemistry involved. All of us consume a small amount of ordinary table salt, which consists (except for contaminants!) of the chemicals sodium and chloride ("Sodium Chloride," 2009 ◐). The combinations of these chemicals, which are present at a ratio of approximately 40% sodium to approximately 60% chlorine, as we know from ordinary biochemistry, are generally useful to living organisms. However, if we combine even a small quantity of the element sodium by itself with water, it explodes. A small quantity placed in the mouth would blow your head off. Likewise, chlorine gas is potentially lethal in small concentrations. Chlorine is also the main ingredient of Clorox, which, according to the label, kills 99.9% of all bacteria with which it comes in contact. Clorox, with chlorine as its main antialgal and antifungal agent, is the product of choice used to keep many swimming pools clean. It is obvious from such simple illustrations that with chemicals, the interactions are essential.

When it comes to the complex chemical and biological agents in vaccines, drugs, foods, and the like, the reactive potentials inside a living body are vastly more complex. To say that they are astronomically complex is an oversimplification. With 20 disease agents plus an assortment of known toxins and other biological contaminants that may interact, it is a mathematical certainty that the potential interactions have never been tested adequately.

Why? With two agents—say, A and B administered simultaneously—there is just one potential interaction. If one agent is administered before the other, there are, with only two agents at least three interactions: the sort we might get with a simultaneous administration; the kind that might occur if A were administered first and then B later; and, the reverse. Setting the sequence issues aside, because they only complicate matters making the mathematical problems far greater for the drug/vaccine manufacturers, suppose we consider what is required just to test the simplest of biochemical interactions when the agents are introduced into living persons. Suppose we consider only the interaction of agents administered simultaneously (or nearly so).

Clinical trials could be arranged to assess the impact of agent A by comparing a group who received that agent with a matched group who did not receive it. To assess the impact of agent B without A, a second trial with another matched group who did not receive agent B would be required. To test the interaction of A with B, another group suitably matched against the former ones would be needed, in which group members received both A and B simultaneously. Subsequently, the results for the group receiving both A and B would have to be compared against the matched groups getting just A, just B, and neither A nor B. Assuming that all the problems of finding enough people to participate in the clinical trials could be solved, to assess the impact of just two agents (A and B) would require multiple comparisons between a minimum of four distinct matched groups. Although it is certainly possible to assess such an interaction, it should be clear that such controlled experiments are still very difficult to perform well and, therefore, are exceedingly rare.

Next, consider the case of a combination of three disease agents, toxins, or contaminants. Because no one would propose actually studying the toxins or contaminants in clinical trials with human subjects, suppose we have a vaccine containing three disease agents. The number of possible interactions to be examined would require seven distinct experimental comparisons. There are three possible interactions involving distinct pairs: A with B, A with C, and B with C. Added to these are three interactions between a pair of agents and the third agent: A with BC, B with AC, and C with AB. Finally, there is one possible interaction involving the combination of all three agents ABC. Skipping the details of the mathematical logic, as soon as the number of disease agents in a given vaccine passes the number 3, the number of interactions expands rapidly, to the point that the needed clinical trials are much too expensive and too complex to perform in practice.

As a result, when a combination of multiple disease agents, toxins, and unknown contaminants includes more than three subcomponents, the few clinical trials and experimental studies that are actually funded and carried out will be increasingly inadequate to assess the likely impact of all possible interactions. The inevitable result is that the risks associated with combining drugs, vaccines, toxins, and the like, in individual cases, remain untested and unknown. However, there is no doubt, based on the existing toxicology research and published clinical trials involving existing vaccines, that increasing the number of toxins and disease agents absolutely, with algebraic certainty, increases the possibility and likelihood of undesirable interactions.

What Happened to Vance?

On the morning of September 15, 2007, a little less than 56 hours from the time of his "well-baby" visit on September 12, Shelly Walker went to check on baby Vance. In our personal interview with her, she said she found Vance in his crib not breathing. Blood was crusted under his eyes, and dark foam was coming from his mouth onto the teddy bear blanket lying beside him. Shelly called 9-1-1, and Vance was taken to Kootenai Medical Center in Coeur D'Alene. He was pronounced dead on arrival. With her dead baby in her arms, Shelly asked, "Was this the vaccines?"

Shelly asked that an autopsy be performed. From day to day she kept asking for results so that she could find out if the vaccines were, as she suspected, the cause of her son's death. After several calls, she asked why it was taking so long; she was told that because her son's death did not involve murder or rape, it was not a priority case. Eight weeks later, Shelly finally got the results from the doctor who performed the autopsy. She was told "sometimes this happens." The cause of death was listed as the mysterious **sudden infant death syndrome** (**SIDS**).

Dr. John Iskander, speaking for the CDC, said, "The bottom line is still that we do not know what causes SIDS and the other bottom line from a number of studies is that vaccines are not the culprit" (World Now and KLXY, 2009 ☁). Although SIDS is by far the most common explanation for death following vaccinations (Braun & Ellenberg, 1997; Chock, 2008), according to the **Vaccine Adverse Events Reporting System** (**VAERS**) monitored by the CDC and the Food and Drug Administration (FDA), the standard interpretation is that the temporal association between vaccinations and infant deaths is coincidental. Nevertheless, according to careful studies, the SIDS explanation accounts for approximately half the deaths reported under VAERS (Silvers, Varricchio, Ellenberg, Krueger, Wise, & Salive, 2002).

Vaccines and SIDS

According to Braun and Ellenberg (1997), out of a total of 38,787 adverse events reported between 1991 and 1994 (estimated at less than 10% of more than 400,000 events that occurred within the time frame, according to Cave, 2001, p. xvi), here are some interesting statistics:

> Of the deaths with known age, 72.4% were reported in the first year of life, and 63.7% of these were male. The peak age for death reports was 1 to 3 months, with a gradual decline through age 9 months, after which death was relatively rare. Adverse events with onset of symptoms the day of vaccination accounted for 45.5% of total reports; 20.4% had onset of symptoms the following day. Onset within 2 weeks after vaccination was noted for 92.5% of all reports. Simultaneous administration of multiple vaccines was noted in 75.7% of reports for immunizations at ages younger than 20 years.

The vaccines received by Vance Walker—Pediarix, Prevnar, and RotaTeq—accounted for approximately half of the SIDS deaths reported in the clinical studies. In the prescribing information for Pediarix, GlaxoSmithKline (2008b ☁) claims that the SIDS rate for the United States from 1990 to 1994 was 1.2 per 1000 live births. Clinical trials reveal that administration of multiple disease agents and toxins on a single occasion is more apt to do harm (GlaxoSmithKline, 2008a; CDC, 2008f ☁). However, the published documents put out by the CDC or by pharmaceutical companies in connection with clinical trials of vaccines generally argue that multivalent vaccines actually cut the observed rate of SIDS by half (see Vennemann, Hoffgen, Bajanowski, Hense, & Mitchell, 2007). It appears that this result has been achieved in part by simply dividing the number of SIDS deaths into groups under the general heading of "sudden unexpected infant death" (pointed out to us by Melissa Fowlkes and Clint Andrus; also see CDC, 2008f).

The claim that infant deaths from SIDS are declining because of greater use of multivalent vaccines conflicts with studies of the VAERS data, which reveal that approximately 75% of the adverse events reported involve vaccines containing multiple disease agents (Wise et al., 2004). Based on this finding, if all else were kept equal, it would seem that the vaccines containing multiple disease agents—as required by logic with near algebraic certainty—are more likely to produce an adverse event than a vaccine containing only one disease agent. To claim that adding more disease agents and/or toxins to a vaccine does not increase its risk, or that it lowers the risk, is to propose an unlikely hypothesis. Yet this is what the CDC has asked the public to believe.

Lightning Struck Three Times in the Same Place?

By insisting on an autopsy for her child, Shelly Walker discovered that two other boys taken in for the "well-baby" visits within the same month at the same clinic in Coeur D'Alene, Idaho, also died within a week of their vaccinations. The other babies who died during the same time period in a sparsely populated community in Idaho were David Waddel and Paiyton Ames. All three reported for their fourth-month "well-baby" visit in the same clinic.

Is it just a coincidence that the median age of death for infants who typically die of SIDS happens to be around the four-month mark, at the time of the recommended well-baby visit to the doctor (Silvers, Ellenberg, Wise, Varricchio, Mootrey, & Salive, 2001)? Or could the stress produced by multivalent vaccines—with 20 disease agents in the case of Vance Walker—be causing the deaths? It has been proposed by Lonsdale (2001) that some form of stress combined with a genetic predisposition is the probable cause of SIDS. Could the vaccines be causing the stress?

A Link with Autism?

Interestingly, the current line of research suggests very strongly that autism, like SIDS, is caused mainly by combinations of toxins and disease agents coming especially from vaccinations and medical procedures. Autism, like SIDS, is most common in genetically vulnerable individuals who have difficulty in eliminating toxins or handling challenges to their immune systems (Dietert & Dietert, 2008). Among the known toxins that are involved is thimerosal; among the disease agents, there are viruses and combinations of other disease agents that act as triggers for the expression of autism.

Is it also just a coincidence that the rate of autism diagnosis has increased concurrently with the increasing number of toxins and disease agents being injected into the bodies and/or bloodstreams of younger and younger children? Although other sources of toxins can affect unborn babies and young children in detrimental ways, the main sources of high-density toxins affecting unborn babies, neonates, and children up to the age of six years are medications, with vaccines topping the list. It is, therefore, essential to examine vaccines critically.

ADDRESSING THE DENIAL

CDC experts have acknowledged that diagnoses of autism are increasing, but they deny that this trend represents evidence of an epidemic. In addressing this issue, the CDC (n.d.) published the following statement:

> While it is clear that more children than ever before are diagnosed as having an ASD, it is unclear how much of this increase is due to changes in how we identify and diagnose ASDs, or whether this is due to a true increase in **prevalence**.

A real increase in prevalence would mean that there are actually more individuals per capita who are being affected by autism than there were in the past. The CDC has expressed doubt that there is a real increase in autism cases, falling back to genetics as the underlying causal basis for autism. It is not uncommon for medical research teams to simply acquiesce to the theory that autism is mainly, if not exclusively, a genetic disorder, as Steyaert and De la Marche (2008) do in their recent article:

> ASD is a disorder with mainly genetic causes and recent insights show that a variety of genetic mechanisms may be involved, i.e. single gene disorders, copy number variations and polygenic mechanisms. (p. 1091)

In fact, if genetic factors were the whole explanation for the "autism epidemic," then the CDC, FDA, the American Academy of Pediatrics (AAP), and the pharmaceutical companies would presumably be off the hook. After all, those organizations have no direct control over anyone's genetic inheritance from their parents.

Although genetic factors must certainly be involved in the causation of autism, genes are also known to be impacted by certain toxins. Even if genetics is the best of all the theories for what is causing autism, we must go deeper: What has caused the abnormalities in the genetics? When that question is asked, it becomes clear that the genetic explanation is necessarily incomplete.

Autism as a Problem of Communication

The foundation of health—physiologically, socially, and logically—is successful communication at all levels, from the genes upward to bodily proteins, cells, tissues, organs, individual persons, and communities. Communication is as essential to genetics as it is to communities and nations. From beginning to end, and at all levels in between, every complex system depends on successful communication. When communication systems break down, disease, disorder, and all sorts of problems arise.

The focal problems of autism, as we have seen from its initial diagnosis by Kanner, have been about communication and interaction. In a minority of the cases currently being diagnosed, disorders are relatively mild. In most cases, however, the impact is severe. In the worst-case scenario, the person dies. Traditionally, such a death has been attributed to some unknown cause, such as SIDS, or to some other factor; even so, as we will see later in this book, there can be no reasonable doubt that the same injuries that cause the disease and disorder conditions associated with autism can cause death in severe instances. The fact that factors causing autism can also cause death will be plainly established later in this book by solid empirical evidence and by logic that cannot be refuted.

For Survivors, Autism Is an Adult Disorder

Children with autism who survive, unless they are recovered, become adults with autism. For that reason, autism is not just a childhood condition. It is also an adult disorder resulting in long-term social burdens as well as enormous economic costs over the long haul. As the number of diagnosed cases of autism grows, the cost to society also escalates. As a result, autism is a central problem for health professionals, policy makers, and all ordinary citizens.

Autism is of special interest and importance to speech-language pathologists and audiologists. The story to be told about autism is, we believe, inevitably pushing the medical community, pharmaceutical companies, government agencies, and private citizens to reconceptualize health care in general. It is becoming increasingly obvious that we must consider the health of the *whole body* in its behavioral, social, political, and economic contexts. Piecemeal approaches that look to isolated parts of the larger connected context are condemned to incompleteness. In the complex systems of communication at issue, the interactions are crucial.

To the extent that public policies of vast agencies, such as the U.S. Public Health Service with its subagencies including the CDC, the FDA, and the international WHO, are already deeply involved, a comprehensive, holistic, and global perspective is essential. We must also think in terms of the whole life span of individuals and of causes and effects that range across generations.

When the effects of a neurotoxin (such as thimerosal) or foreign animal proteins are at issue, the idea of looking for the final outcome within a few days after one or several injections is inadequate. With **genotoxic effects**, which can extend across generations, the idea of considering symptoms within days, weeks, or months defines too narrow a time range. The effects of foreign proteins and toxins can range across the life span. Thus, if **genotoxins** such as thimerosal are implicated in causation of autism, we must consider impacts that may also reach across generations.

The Ongoing Paradigm Shift

The complex nature of the autism epidemic, it seems, is causing a **paradigm shift** in the health sciences. The trend is toward a more consistent, simpler (in the sense of being more abstract), and more comprehensive (holistic) view of our bodies and our interactions with the world. The goal is to make sense of all the facts, including some that have been assembled from a great multitude of piecemeal, fragmented, disconnected, cross-disciplinary studies. The new paradigm stresses complex systems of internal and external communication systems. As the vast diversity of such systems and their interactions come into focus, they are forcing a reexamination of the fractionated view of health that has characterized the medical sciences, especially during the last couple of centuries and particularly within the last several decades. Just as the genetic system has to communicate with the body's proteins, and cells, tissues, and organ systems have to communicate with each other within the body, it is necessary for health science professionals to communicate across disciplines. Speech and language pathology make no sense without biochemistry, and nothing in the health sciences makes much sense without genetics and linguistics.

In this book we are concerned specifically with the autism epidemic. Nevertheless, for reasons that will become clear as we proceed, we focus on the internal health of the body as a whole. We must examine its defenses against invading disease agents, its systems for dumping or quarantining harmful toxins, and the way such systems interact. We will discover that "health," in every reasonable sense of the word, is utterly dependent on communication systems beginning with genetics and extending through the entire systematic hierarchy from atoms to molecules, to cells, to organ systems, and to the body as a whole. When internal communications in the immune system and the body's biochemistry break down, the health of the body deteriorates. When external communications break down, especially the skilled movements and articulate gestures of speech and language, social relations are adversely affected.

When both internal and external communications are disrupted simultaneously, extreme social and behavioral problems become evident, just as they are in autism. Of course, just because behavioral symptoms appear in a disorder does not necessarily mean that those symptoms account for or explain the disorder. A more complete explanation must tell why the symptoms occur. Without such a deeper and more abstract account, all the observations in the world about symptoms will not lead to any solution to the underlying problems of which the symptoms are merely indicative. For all of the foregoing reasons, approaches to autism that focus exclusively on symptoms are certain to leave it a mystery forever. We must look to causes.

Does Tobacco Ring Any Bells?

Just as the tobacco companies were motivated to deny the association of smoking, chewing, or otherwise exposing human beings to the well-known **carcinogens** (cancer-producing agents) in tobacco, some government agencies and corporate entities in the pharmaceutical and healthcare industries are highly motivated to protect themselves against the liabilities implicit in discovering the factors that are causing the autism epidemic.

The easiest way to dispose of all the potential liabilities associated with autism would be to show that the epidemic itself is unreal, imaginary, or something other than what it appears to be. If the epidemic did not exist, then it could not have been nor be caused by anything except imagination. Conversely, if a growing epidemic exists, then some combination of factors must be causing it. As we will see in subsequent chapters of this book, the CDC, pharmaceutical companies, and certain professional medical organizations have stood shoulder to shoulder in supporting the denial theme. In the meantime, vaccines, **dental amalgam**, and other toxins are implicated as potential causative agents, as we will see in Chapters 2–6. In Chapter 7, we examine the reasons for the faith placed in vaccines by their supporters; in Chapters 8 and 9, we will see how the repeated reassurances by vaccine promoters have only deepened public doubts. The evidence continues to implicate toxins and disease agents as the primary causal triggers of the autism epidemic. In Chapter 10, we consider the theory of the tipping point as argued by many current theoreticians, though none more cogently than Dr. Brian Jepson (see Jepson & Johnson, 2007). Jepson (2007a, 2007b ●) has also made his case in person for the possibility of radically changing the course of autism.

Throughout this book, but especially in Chapters 11 and 12, we present a more holistic, systems-oriented view of the etiology, diagnosis, and treatment of autism. In the vast majority of cases, children who manifest symptoms of autism have reached and surpassed what Jepson calls the "toxic tipping point."

We go on to consider the research and case histories that demonstrate why there is reasonable hope that the autism epidemic can be halted and that many individuals can be recovered. Unsurprisingly, the large and growing body of research already shows clearly that treatments are more effective when they address causal factors. There is also good news here for the pharmaceutical companies, the professional medical organizations, and healthcare practitioners in general. By pinpointing the key factors involved in producing autism, we will be much more capable of preventing, curing, or at least holding it at bay in many, if not all, cases. Discovering the causes, however, is crucial. Clearly, the upsurge in the number of diagnosed cases of autism is not imaginary and cannot be uncaused.

Toxins Remain at the Center

Confidence in the life-saving power of medicines in general and vaccines in particular has helped to sustain the argument that the benefits of vaccines vastly outweigh any potential for harm. However, the aura of beneficence should not color our judgment when examining the potential of vaccines, medicines, and medical procedures to do harm. Along that line we recommend the award-winning even-handed documentary book, *Evidence of Harm: Mercury in Vaccines and the Autism Epidemic: A Medical Controversy* (Kirby, 2005), and follow-up stories by the same author (Kirby, 2008a, 2008b, 2008c; and R. F. Kennedy & Kirby, 2009 ●).

As the controversy over vaccines plays out in the media and in the courts, independent toxicology research and sound reasoning continue to show that autism, a host of other neurological conditions (e.g., **scleroses**, **dystrophies**, **diabetes**, **epilepsy**, and **dementias** such as those associated with **Alzheimer's disease** and **Parkinson's disease**), and various forms of gut disease are unquestionably linked to toxins, disease agents, and foreign proteins, many of which are being deliberately injected into the bloodstreams of millions of infants, toddlers, children, and adults. Also, tons of neurotoxic mercury in dental amalgam are being placed in the mouths of dental patients worldwide. The American Dental Association has claimed that in 2006 more than 70 million fillings of dental amalgam, equivalent to approximately 12 metric tons of mercury, were placed in the mouths of Americans alone (Needleman, 2006). The total amount being carried around in this form inside human bodies has been estimated to account for approximately 55% of the world's total industrial mercury (Barr, 2004).

Thimerosal: Still Used in Vaccines

Although the public demand to get the toxins, especially mercury, out of childhood vaccines was met with tacit compliance in a published statement by the CDC and the AAP in 1999, many of the stockpiles of shots being used in the United States still contain the offending **ethyl mercury** (thimerosal) and many more of the vaccines being used in developing nations contain it (for instance, see Marques, Dorea, Fonseca, Bastos, & Malm, 2007).

Dr. Paul Offit (2007) not only acknowledges, but actually advocates the continued use of thimerosal, particularly in flu shots, in the United States and around the world. According to Offit, this chemical is completely harmless. The deaths and illnesses associated with vaccines, in his view, are purely coincidental (Gupta, 2008 ●). Offit says in the interview with Sanjay Gupta that vaccines do not cause autism. He says it is just a statistical fact that before the vaccine some of the children are okay, but afterward not. Elsewhere, he has argued that it would be safe to give neonates as many as 10,000 disease agents in one shot (Offit, 2008; Offit et al., 2002). He affirms the recent reassessment by the CDC Advisory Committee on Immunization Practices (2006) that thimerosal is safe for infants and the unborn babies of pregnant women.

We will revisit these claims in Chapters 4–6 where we review the toxicology research especially on thimerosal. It has recently been pointed out that Offit benefits from money earned and donated by the vaccine manufacturer Merck. He is the creator of the rotavirus vaccine RotaTeq, manufactured by Merck, and holds the patent on it. He also occupies a $1.5 million research chair at Children's Hospital of Philadelphia funded by Merck (Attkisson, 2008 ●).

Thimerosal: Recommended by CDC and WHO, and Used Abroad

In 2007, the Chilean government issued a statement saying that thimerosal is safe in vaccines and that its health agencies plan to keep on using it (Muñoz et al., 2007). This position is consistent with the stance taken by the WHO that thimerosal does not pose a health risk. Contrary to the public recommendation by the CDC and AAP, that thimerosal should be eliminated from all vaccines as soon as possible, it is still being used worldwide. Although thimerosal, as a preservative, has been removed from many vaccines in the mandated U.S. series of vaccinations, as mentioned earlier, it can still be found in existing stockpiles in this country and is used in the manufacture of new vaccines for non-U.S. markets.

Just as the vaccine manufacturers and their supporters have claimed that mercury is safe in vaccines, so the American Dental Association insists that it is safe to put 12 metric tons of methyl mercury per year in the mouths of patients. These "silver fillings" are actually half **methyl mercury** by weight.

Is either of these common practices safe? Are the watchdogs of public safety—the CDC and FDA in particular—sufficiently protecting the public interest? A similar question arises with respect to the medical organizations that are ethically obliged to guard the well-being of their patients. Are the American Academy of Pediatrics, the American Dental Association, and other professional medical societies honoring the long-standing requirements of the Hippocratic Oath, especially the caveat of doing no harm? We consider ethical and legal aspects of these questions in more detail in Chapter 3.

Essentially all of the healthcare professional organizations subscribe to the ethical standard requiring them, above all else, to protect the patient/client. The American Speech-Language-Hearing Association policy stresses that "speech-language pathologists and audiologists agree to the overarching principle of holding the patient's welfare paramount" (Chabon, Hale, & Wark, 2008, p. 26).

Among the outstanding questions, however, is whether and to what extent professional healthcare organizations and their members are actually providing the best possible care for individual patients rather than serving as representatives of other corporate interests.

Anticipating the Rest of the Story

In this chapter, we have introduced the "mysteries" (more accurately, controversies) surrounding the diagnosis of autism. In Chapter 2, we show that the autism epidemic is real. Throughout all of the chapters in this book, the focus is on **etiology**. What is causing the exponential growth in diagnosed cases of autism and a host of related neurological disorders, and what can be done about them? The voices of the families affected, as we can see from the cases already examined, are understandably urgent. Meantime, government agencies, medical groups, professional organizations, and pharmaceutical companies are devoting huge sums to advertising drugs, vaccines, and health care in various forms of sponsored "research."

Many of the sponsored articles and research studies have the ostensible purpose of trying ever so diligently, but altogether unsuccessfully, to find links between toxins in vaccines, dental amalgam, and drugs with autism. In reality, the underlying purpose of many of these "searches" for causes of disorders is to defend the claim that no relationship can be found between the neurological and other problems in autism, for instance, and the toxins being placed in patients' bodies by medical practitioners. Meanwhile, the fact that recommended vaccines contain potent toxins such as mercury, aluminum, formaldehyde, and other preservatives (including the major component of automobile antifreeze), not to mention multiple disease agents consisting of viruses, bacteria, protein fragments, extraneous biological contaminants from animals, and additional unstudied animal viruses, suggests that vaccines may be playing a significant role in the etiology of the ongoing epidemic of neurological and self-immune diseases. One of the most devastating manifestations of the many diseases linked to these toxins, proteins, and contaminants in vaccines and other medicines and medical procedures is autism.

WHAT IS DIFFERENT ABOUT THIS BOOK

There are several features in this book and its accompanying DVD that are not common to books or courses about the autism epidemic or about communication disorders in general:

1. For one, the whole book unfolds like a narrative and we ordinary citizens, our own children and theirs, are characters at risk in the true story as it is developing.
2. The material is user-friendly for instructors because it is user-friendly for students.
3. Students love it because of its importance to them personally and because of its readability, interest, and learnability.
4. Instructor's want to use it because the book and DVD are well designed easy to teach, and because students love it.
5. The research and theory in this book are up-to-date and the best available.
6. This book and DVD use the Internet, the Web of Science, Medline, and all the resources of our modern technologies. The selected Internet sources especially are being reviewed, in many instances, on a daily basis by many competent individuals.
7. This book plus user-friendly digital study materials, contained or linked on the DVD, is further enhanced by:
   a. A PowerPoint Summary for each chapter that makes lecture preparation and classroom work fun, colorful, and 100% relevant to the course.
   b. A searchable copy of an expanded table of contents (a greatly abridged version of the book) with hyperlinked URLs and playable media files; open-ended Study and Discussion

Questions at the end of each chapter providing for essays, class discussions, further research, and testing.

c. A complete Glossary of technical terms, the entire list of References, and an Index of subjects and authors that make it easy to find definitions, crucial threads of inference, and to track down researchers and theoreticians who are pursuing answers to remaining questions.

d. An *Instructor's Manual* containing a pretested series of 600 Multiple Choice Study Questions that are presented in sequence and cross-referenced to pages of the unfolding text (provided in Acrobat, MS Word, and WordPerfect formats enabling construction of any number of distinct "machine scorable" tests.

e. Prefabricated tests, 12 of them consisting of 50 items for each chapter; 6 tests of 100 items each covering consecutive pairs of chapters; and 5 tests of 200 items each over the entire course. These tests are provided in Acrobat format for convenient printing and use by instructors.

f. There is a section in the *Instructor's Manual* showing how the Study and Discussion Questions can be used to verify comprehension of material in the Multiple Choice Study Questions provided on the DVD.

g. An introduction to the Web of Science, Medline, and Wikipedia is also provided in the *Instructor's Manual* showing how and why these resources are invaluable.

On the whole, the materials for the course are self-explanatory, but a few points need emphasis.

It's a Narrative

Our own research on communication and learning shows that narrative organization is foundational (Badon, 1993; J. W. Oller, L. Chen, N. Pan, & S. D. Oller, 2005; S. D. Oller, 2005; N. Pan & L. Chen, 2005). It is essential to human experience, learning, recall, retention, and our ability to make sense of what we have learned. That organization, together with the relevance, depth, and up-to-date research presented here, is the most distinctive feature of this book. Teachers and students alike can get excited about this narrative *because they are in it*. The risks at stake are real and they are *our risks*. They affect our own children, their children, and us.

The most important difference, which cannot be overemphasized, is that the ongoing (actually developing) story is true. It concerns the largest and most pressing problem confronting health professionals worldwide and especially in the United States today. The autism epidemic is unfolding before our eyes in our newspapers, on the television, in YouTube broadcasts, in classrooms, clinics, hospitals, homes, and neighborhoods everywhere.

It's Easy to Teach

Students love this book because it presents facts they need and want to know. They are sometimes shocked but always motivated by what they are learning, and they are never bored or offended by the honesty and intensity of the ongoing discussion. They want to understand the autism epidemic because they are living through it. They are just like theoreticians in wanting to get to the bottom of what is causing this epidemic so that they can understand how to protect themselves and their loved ones. Many of our students have chosen communication disorders, a closely related area such as nursing, or a premed program as their field of study because they or someone they care about has been affected by autism or a related disorder.

The Facts Are Intelligible and Amazing

The evidence, research, and theory in this book are all presented at an introductory level so that all users can understand and benefit from the ongoing discussion. Most of our students, and many seasoned instructors, never dreamed that industrial mercury, a heavy metal that is highly **neurotoxic** in concentrations as sparse as parts per billion and fatal in parts per million, is found in dental amalgam, the silvery metal material used commonly in dental tooth restorations. As we have noted, although these restorations are commonly called "silver fillings," they contain approximately 50% elemental mercury by weight. The American Dental Association continues to hold that the mercury in amalgam is safe and stable, and that nearly 90% of practicing dentists continue to use it. Similarly, students are often amazed to discover that as recently as 2006, contrary to its stated plan in 1999 to eliminate thimerosal from all vaccines "as soon as possible," the CDC has advocated requiring flu shots, some still containing thimerosal, for all U.S. infants at birth, including preterm babies of low birth weight. Thimerosal is even claimed to be safe for unborn children still in their mothers' wombs (CDC Advisory Committee on Immunization Practices, 2006).

The CDC also advocates giving the HepB (hepatitis B) vaccine at birth to all babies. This particular vaccine is controversial because the disease against which it supposedly protects babies is a sexually transmitted one. The fact that babies at birth are not being exposed to sexual intercourse is just one of the major reasons for the controversy. The recommended procedure, according to the CDC, is to expose all babies at birth to multiple disease agents and toxins and then to reexpose them an additional 35 times at a minimum to many other disease agents and toxins before their sixth birthday. But does this policy really make sense?

In addition, the CDC has publicly agreed (in 1999) with statements by the WHO advocating the use of thimerosal-containing vaccines in developing nations around the world. Although the CDC has vacillated in its domestic position within the United States, agency personnel now say they prefer the vaccines with thimerosal (see CDC, 2008c ●). According to published statements, the CDC and WHO are working toward regimens with increasing numbers of vaccines, including ones containing thimerosal, for all children either at birth or as soon as possible afterward, irrespective of their birth weight. Meanwhile, as the number of vaccinations continues to escalate, so does the diagnosis of autism.

Real Cases

If you are a human who is being touched in any way by the autism epidemic or by the issues related to it, this book and this course are for you. By relating sound research and theory to real-life cases, healthcare providers who work through this course will be better able to provide much-needed information, help, guidance, and therapy in homes and neighborhoods, schools, clinics, and hospitals to the persons most affected.

The Harvard Case-Based Problem-Solving Approach

We follow the "Harvard model" of case-based problem solving (Mostaghimi et al., 2006; Tosteson, Adelstein, & Carver, 1994) for several reasons. First, such an approach is consistent with what we know of language acquisition and valid learning in general. It focuses on the primary protagonists— the persons affected by autism and related disorders and their families—who provide continuity to the story that is unfolding before our eyes.

As the research shows, the most effective teaching is grounded in true representations of actual persons, things, events, and situations in the real world. We identify with Jenny McCarthy at the neurologist's office. When he said, "I'm sorry but your son has autism," after a few moments, Jenny said, "Well, you know, I believe my son is trapped inside. I'm not settling for this. He's trapped inside and all these little characteristics that I thought were Evan's personality . . . were just autism. So he's lost and I said to myself that day, I'm gonna get 'im out. I'm gonna get 'im out—and that started the journey" (McCarthy, 2007a ●).

Real-life cases move us to action. They give us the energy to get up early and stay up late. They motivate us to spend our own resources and to do whatever it takes to make things better. Real-life cases must also be examined closely if we are to answer critical questions about diagnosis, causation, and intervention.

The One-Minute Writing Exercise

As we note in the *Instructor's Manual* we recommend the routine of asking students to write a sentence or two at the end of each class related to the material that was covered during that particular session. We usually ask them to write at least a sentence about whatever they found the most interesting, controversial, or in need of further discussion. We urge instructors to read the comments after each session. Students are insightful and well able to think critically about the material in this book. They are also eager to learn and to contribute to the course from their own experience. One of the comments most commonly voiced by many of our own students (such as Matthew Chiasson, Heidi Kidder, Melissa Fowlkes, and Stephanie Grant) at the end of each class meeting is that they "can't wait to come back for the next class meeting!" (We thank these individuals for permission to mention them by name.)

Find the Causes, Stop the Epidemic, Recover the Children

Families of individuals affected by autism cannot afford the luxury of another half-century or more of statistical epidemiological research. It is not enough to advocate increasing the number of caregivers, or enhancing the resources and facilities dedicated to the treatment of autism and related communication disorders, or improving the pay of persons who administer the treatment. It is not enough to train more and more professionals to provide more and more care and treatment. It is not enough to raise public awareness about communication disorders or to inform the public and professionals about the emotional, economic, and personal costs associated with autism and related communication disorders.

As desirable as any or all of those objectives may be, the highest and best goal, as implied by the American Speech-Language-Hearing Association (ASHA) in its Code of Ethics, is to discover the causes of autism so as to cure, prevent, or lessen its negative impacts. We must aim for finding the causes, stopping the epidemic, and recovering the children. We cannot settle for less.

In this course, we aim for the jugular vein of the autism epidemic. We must first find out what is causing the epidemic if we are to stop it. For many children who would otherwise be affected by autism, understanding its etiology can prevent them from developing this disorder. For others already affected, understanding the etiology can keep them from being further injured and may enable many of them to be recovered, or at least greatly helped.

SUMMING UP AND LOOKING AHEAD

In this chapter we have seen why the very existence of the autism epidemic and its causation are emotionally and politically charged. From what we have already considered it appears that autism is central to communication disorders in general. We reviewed the cases of Hannah Poling, Dov Shestack, Evan McCarthy, and Vance Walker, among others—putting faces on the autism epidemic. In this chapter we also overviewed critical features of the course. Among its distinctive elements are the narrative style, as well as the historical depth and currency of the research reported. Because of the narrative style, the real cases discussed, the up-to-date research findings from published literature, and application of the most powerful Internet and media tools, this book is easy to teach and learn from. It is also different from many other books because of its reliance on the case-based model of learning through problem solving. In the next chapter, we discuss all of the popular arguments that have been proposed to explain away the autism epidemic. Among them are the arguments of the CDC and some of its collaborators that the autism epidemic may be a product of better diagnosis coupled with publicity, hype, and imagination.

STUDY AND DISCUSSION QUESTIONS

1. Discuss the symptoms of gut disease observed in Kanner's first 11 patients diagnosed with autism.

2. Why is the genetic explanation for autism powerless to account for the increasing number of diagnosed cases over the last three decades?

3. Have you observed or known of situations where an undesired result was difficult to comprehend? Discuss the process of some folks "seeing what they believe rather than what they see" in relation to the autism epidemic. If such a problem exists, how can it be cured?

4. What is your reaction to the idea that interactions of toxins and disease agents coming to us from medicines and medical procedures can cause chronic diseases as well as autism?

5. What connection is there between Dr. Richet's findings that won him a Nobel Prize in 1913 and Dr. Kartzinel's appearance on *Larry King Live* in 2008 with Jenny McCarthy? How does SIDS figure in the discussion?

6. In what ways are the cases of children such as Hannah Poling, Evan McCarthy, Dov Shestack, and Vance Walker typical or atypical? What did all of them have in common? As you reflect on this question, how do you feel about Dr. Julie Gerberding's reaction to the out-of-court concession made by the government in the Poling case?

7. Why is it unlikely that all of the potential interactions of vaccines, toxins, and drug components will be tested prior to marketing these agents to the general public?

8. Is it just a coincidence—as the CDC argues—that Pediarix, Prevnar, and RotaTeq account for approximately half of all SIDS deaths reported in clinical studies? Do you find the government's arguments about SIDS and vaccines persuasive? Why or why not?

9. What is wrong with piecemeal approaches to health care and the health sciences?

10. In your judgment, how plausible is Dr. Offit's claim that neonates ought to be able to handle 10,000 disease agents at a time? If you agree, why so? If not, why not?

chapter two

Is There an Autism Epidemic?

OBJECTIVES

In this chapter, we

1. Discuss the psychology of the denial of illness and show how it has been a factor in dealing with the autism epidemic on a grand scale.

2. Establish that ordinary citizens are being affected by autism in greater numbers.

3. Analyze evidence that the increased prevalence of autism is the cause of growing public awareness, rather than the reverse.

4. Show that the defining criteria for the diagnosis of autism have changed little and cannot account for the increasing number of cases being diagnosed.

5. Review the theories of broadening criteria, public awareness, diagnostic substitution, intellectual giftedness, and genetics as bases for explaining away the autism epidemic.

6. Discuss evidence showing that factors other than genetic ones are causing the growing prevalence of autism.

Autism, according to the data reported in Figure 1-1, is the fastest-growing diagnosis of all the childhood disorders and diseases. The American Academy of Pediatrics, on its Web page titled "Facts for Parents About Vaccine Safety," says, "The apparent increase in autism may be due to a combination of factors. For example, more and more behaviors and disorders are being included in the definition of ASD than in the past. Also, the public and the medical profession recognize these disorders more often" (AAP, 2008 ◕). In this chapter we show that the autism epidemic is real. The initial reaction of parents whose children have been diagnosed with autism is often "This just can't be true. Surely this cannot happen to our child." Similarly, both government agencies and corporate entities in the private-sector health industries tend to deny the growing epidemic that is taking place on a much larger scale. Government agencies, pharmaceutical companies, and professional organizations such as the AAP have almost universally taken the position that there is no real autism epidemic.

In this chapter, we explore why theories of increased public awareness, the broadening of criteria for diagnosis, strict genetic models, and various other competitors fail to explain the facts at hand. We also show why those alternative theories—like much of the sponsored research designed to make the problem "go away"—amount at best to wishful thinking. Of course, we would prefer for one or several of the alternatives to be true. However, diagnosis of a problem, and the realization that there is a real problem, if there is one, is the first step toward finding a way to solve it. If there is an autism epidemic, we need to know. If not, there would be no need to make it go away. Interestingly, everyone admits that there has been a tremendous growth in the diagnosis of autism. The question is which of the various competing explanations, or which combination of them, best accounts for that upsurge.

THE UPSURGE IN THE NUMBER OF CASES

The number of diagnosed cases of autism—no matter how that number is arrived at—has been growing rapidly. The number of cases being diagnosed for each 100,000 persons in the United States population has been rising since 1993 on a smooth upward curve (refer back to Figure 1-1). Many have wondered out loud, or pretended at least to wonder, if the rising rate is real. Everyone who has considered the implications has hoped that the apparent increase in persons with autism might be the result of some kind of illusion, a misinterpretation of some sort. An epidemic is an undesirable situation: No one wants it.

As mature thinkers know, it doesn't do any good to say there is no epidemic unless that statement is, in fact, true. The question is whether the facts justify the denial of an autism epidemic.

Rising Prevalence or Illusion?

It is widely acknowledged that there has been an upsurge in the number of individuals being diagnosed with autism (D. B. Campbell et al., 2006; Muhle, Trentacoste, & Rapin, 2004). D. B. Campbell et al. wrote in 2006 that "there has been a dramatic increase in the diagnosis of autism" (p. 16834). Muhle, Trentacoste, and Rapin (2004) pointed out that by 1997, the increase in the number of diagnosed cases between 1991 and 1997 already amounted to "an astonishing 556% reported increase in pediatric prevalence," making autism a more common childhood disorder than "spina bifida, cancer, or **Down syndrome**" (p. E472). Although the CDC has repeatedly questioned whether there is any real increase in the number of autism cases, the agency's own studies (Autism Developmental Disabilities Monitoring Network, 2007; CDC, 2008d) show that the rate of autism diagnosis is higher than ever before—and still climbing.

As a result, we really must address two questions here:

- Why are the diagnoses still skyrocketing?
- Why are government agencies such as the CDC ambivalent about whether the increase is real?

The answers to these two questions are intimately intertwined, and both have to do with causal factors that are being—inadvertently, it seems—sponsored by the government, pharmaceutical companies, and professional medical organizations. If the denial of the autism epidemic were valid, all of the problems would essentially be resolved. Vested interests would avoid the liability associated with the most likely known and suspected causes of the autism epidemic. It is not so much the autism epidemic itself that is being denied by these vested interests, but rather the most likely causes of that epidemic are what really scare them. It is these causes that the responsible parties aim to deny.

An Accelerating Rate of Diagnosis

There is no doubt that the diagnosis of autism is on the rise. Figure 1-1 summarized the statistics gathered over a 14-year period under the Individuals with Disabilities Education Act (IDEA) and the subsequent No Child Left Behind Act (see P. W. D. Wright, P. D. Wright, & Heath, 2007). Compared with all other disorders that have been tracked under IDEA and NCLB, diagnosed cases of autism spectrum disorders are increasing more rapidly than any other category. The autism category, in fact, is growing much faster than all the other categories combined. Although the data in Figure 1-1 reach only to 2006, studies released by the CDC on February 9, 2007, showed the rate still rising.

Many sources confirm the continuing rise in the number of diagnosed cases, and many of these sources take seriously the notion that we are in the middle of a worldwide epidemic of autism (e.g., Cannell, 2008; Deth et al., 2007; Ghanizadeh, 2008; Hughes, 2008; Ichim et al., 2007; Jepson & Johnson, 2007; Kern & Jones, 2006; J. W. Oller et al., 2010; Rapin & Tuchman, 2008; Silverman & Brosco, 2007). Interestingly, some of the publications pointing to the growing increase in the rate of diagnosis of autism are being produced by the CDC. That agency has also expressed official doubt that information concerning the rising number of diagnosed cases is correct. On the one hand, the CDC has denied that there is any real increase in the number of cases of autism, so as to defend the continuing use of thimerosal in vaccines on the world market; on the other hand, it has indicated that the number of cases of autism continued to rise even after the offending neurotoxin thimerosal was supposedly removed from vaccines in the United States following the AAP and CDC recommendations published in 1999 (e.g., see AAP & Public Health Service, 1999; Fombonne, 2008 ●). Of course, as we have already noted, thimerosal was not actually removed from all vaccines even after 2002; indeed, it continued to be part of some flu vaccines and many vaccines still being used on the world market even in 2009 (see CDC, 2009 ●).

The CDC's response to such observations (Offit, 2007, 2008) has been to deny that there was ever any harm from thimerosal. This agent has been used in many multidose vaccines mandated for children in the United States since the 1930s, though it was used more extensively from approximately 1977 to 2002. Thimerosal is still being used in the manufacture of various vaccines for the world market and in flu shots in particular. The latter vaccines are still marketed in the United States, where they are recommended as safe for infants, low-birth-weight (premature) babies, and pregnant mothers (CDC Advisory Committee on Immunization Practices, 2006; also see CDC, 2008d). The CDC and related federal agencies, as well as the pharmaceutical companies manufacturing the vaccines, have maintained all along that there is no correlation between neurological disorders such as autism and the mercury (or any other ingredients and contaminants) in vaccines. Approximately 30 vaccines—about half of them containing thimerosal —were mandated for U.S. children until 2001 (Cave, 2001). Since then, six new ones have been added to the mandated series; approximately 200 additional new vaccines are being developed and several are in the pipeline for approval to be added to the mandatory vaccination schedule.

A Predicted Downturn in Thimerosal Adverse Effects After 2008

Because cohorts of children continued receiving mercury-containing vaccines until 2002, the toxin's effects would still be evident in six-year-old children starting school through 2008. In the school reporting systems under IDEA and NCLB, therefore, the full impact of the reduction in exposure to thimerosal in the United States should not be felt until 2009 and later. Even so it may be difficult to detect on account of the addition of other toxins, disease agents, and their interaction through the growing list of mandatory vaccines.

In spite of the ambivalence of the policies concerning thimerosal, a downward trend in its adverse effects may have already begun. In 2006, Geier and Geier reported substantial evidence of a downturn in reported adverse events from vaccines that formerly contained thimerosal in two large data sources: the Vaccine Adverse Event Reporting System (VAERS—a national database) and the California Department of Developmental Services (CDDS) database. The downturn might potentially show up in these sources sooner than in the schools because adverse events must be reported within a few days or weeks at most from the time of the vaccination to qualify as an "adverse event" under the current policies. The data examined by the Geiers took into account the adverse events reported on a quarterly basis from 1994 through 2005 (see D. A. Geier & M. R. Geier, 2006d). Their analysis showed that after the recommended, and partially implemented, ban on thimerosal in 1999, the number of reported adverse events from vaccinations declined in both of these large databases.

Meanwhile, the debate about what is causing the autism epidemic continues (J. P. Baker, 2008). In 2007, Paul Offit, a member of the CDC Advisory Committee on Immunization Practices and co-inventor of Merck's RotaTeq, a rotavirus vaccine, published a defense of thimerosal in the *New England Journal of Medicine*. He claimed that the form of mercury in thimerosal is harmless and unrelated to the autism epidemic. In addition, Offit argued that removing thimerosal from any vaccine was unnecessary, that such an action alarmed the public, and that it should never have been recommended by the CDC and AAP. Perhaps not surprisingly, he contended that thimerosal should continue to be used in flu shots and other vaccines. Offit agreed with the CDC and AAP that "the current levels of thimerosal will not hurt children" and pointed out the contradiction in their suggestion that "reducing those levels will make safe vaccines even safer." Finally, he marveled at the 1999 statement by the CDC and AAP that "while our current immunization strategies are safe, we have an opportunity to increase the margin of safety" (as cited by Offit, 2007, p. 1278).

According to Offit, "Critics wondered how removing something that hadn't been found to be unsafe could make vaccines safer" (p. 1278). Interestingly, this would be true of critics on all sides of the issues at stake. Some critics of the CDC/AAP decision thought it was unjustified while others based on the toxicology research, especially with various forms of mercury including thimerosal (see Chapters 4–6), believed that the decision was actually a pretense in the first place. Toxicologists and researchers in the latter group have demonstrated in many studies that thimerosal is extremely neurotoxic. Those results are not refuted by contrary expert opinions. The results of toxicology are not at all doubtful as we will see in Chapters 4–6 and are not subject to refutation by opinions.

But what Offit seemed to acknowledge was that the CDC's self-contradictions raise reasonable doubts. Thimerosal cannot be both harmful and harmless at the same time in the same individuals. The CDC and AAP have argued, nonetheless, that it can be both ways. Herein is the essential problem they have created for themselves. The preliminary findings of D. A. Geier and M. R. Geier (2006a), along with a longstanding substantial series of studies in toxicology, all suggest that the CDC and AAP self-contradiction can only be removed by admitting that they were half right in their 1999 recommendation. It is sensible to quit using thimerosal in any vaccines or internal medicines. The CDC/AAP recommendation was right in this respect. As an examination of the toxicology research shows, however, they were wrong in claiming that thimerosal did not do harm in the past and that it is not doing harm now.

Theories to Explain Away the Autism Epidemic

The foregoing confusion leads to at least one of the motivations for denying the autism epidemic: Many of the proponents of using thimerosal in vaccines and in other medicines are sincere in their hope and belief that it has done no harm. Parents of children with a diagnosis of autism, of course, may view this position with skepticism. Most assuredly, some highly placed officials and corporate beneficiaries of vaccination policies really think they are seeing what they expect to see, even when the facts contradict their beliefs. Others—including some people in positions of high responsibility—persisted in denials of the vaccine–autism link long after it became clear that they had been mistaken from the beginning. An escape route was simply to deny the existence of an epidemic. If the autism epidemic did not really exist, it certainly could not be caused by any combination of components in vaccines or any other medicines or medical procedures that they had promoted and used.

At least five theories have been proposed to justify the denial of the autism epidemic. According to many, the "autism epidemic" is mainly a matter of perception and semantics. The most popular idea along this line is that the definition of autism has been evolving and has become progressively broader, to the point that it now includes a far larger number of individuals in its sweep. We will deal with this so-called **theory of the broadened definition** first.

A second idea, related to the first, is that education and raised public awareness have led to better detection and diagnosis of autism. This **theory of public awareness** claims that there is no real increase in autism, but rather that doctors, school officials, and parents are noticing more cases because they know better than ever before what to look for.

Related to both of those theories is a third idea—that the increasing number of cases being diagnosed as autism were formerly called something else. This is the **theory of diagnostic substitution**. One possible motive for changing the diagnosis in this way is to get more money for therapy, child care, medicines, and the like. Accordingly, some have suggested that the "autism epidemic" is really an illusion that can be explained away entirely by taking into consideration the alleged shrinking of numbers in other diagnostic categories, such as "mental retardation" (e.g., Down syndrome) and the **learning disabled** category.

Yet another explanation is the **theory of intellectual diversity**, which suggests that autism is not really a disorder, illness, or disease condition, but rather a form of intellectual, linguistic, and social difference. To say there is an "autism epidemic," according to the theory of intellectual diversity, would make about as much sense as supposing that there is a "giftedness epidemic."

Finally, in the background, there is the longstanding assumption that autism, in the final analysis, will turn out to be caused entirely by genetic factors (e.g., see Steyaert & De la Marche, 2008). This idea may be called the **genetic theory of autism**. According to proponents of this theory, because there is no such thing as a "genetic epidemic," an "autism epidemic" is not possible either.

According to any one or any combination of the foregoing theories, the so-called autism epidemic must be relegated to the realm of fiction (as argued by Fombonne, 2001, and Gernsbacher, Dawson, & Goldsmith, 2005). In the final analysis, according to them, it must be a creation of the public imagination. But do any of these arguments, or any combination of them, provide a valid and reasonably complete explanation for the upsurge in diagnoses that is known to be occurring? Let's examine these theories one by one and consider both their separate and combined explanatory power.

EVOLUTION OF THE CRITERIA FOR DIAGNOSIS

Many authors—for example, Fombonne (1996, 1999, 2003a, 2003b, 2008), Gillberg (1999), Gillberg, Cederlund, Lamberg, and Zeijlon (2006), Lawton (2005), and Posserud, Lundervold, and Gillberg (2006), to mention only a few—invoke the theory of the broadened definition as the primary explanation for the "alleged" autism epidemic. This theory is usually combined with one or several of the other theories that have been proposed to minimize what is supposed to be only an apparent epidemic. To adequately assess the validity of that proposal and all of its accompanying arguments, it is necessary to review the evolution of the diagnosis of autism.

The Term and Its Roots

The term "autism," which is derived from the Latin *autismus* and the Greek root *autos*, meaning "self," was used in 1910 by Paul Eugen Bleuler in his description of certain symptoms associated with a **psychosis** for which he proposed the new term **schizophrenia**.[1] To this day, schizophrenia is characterized mainly by a loss of connection with reality. Bleuler is credited with having coined both of the terms "schizophrenia" and "autism" in that same year, 1910. Although Bleuler was evidently the first author to use the term "autism" more or less in its modern sense, the meaning with reference to the "new syndrome" would be described 33 years later by an American professor, the Johns Hopkins physician and psychiatrist Leo Kanner. He elaborated and applied the term "autism" in a more specific manner, reflecting his belief that he was reporting the discovery of an entirely new psychiatric disorder.

At about the same time, an Austrian medical doctor and psychiatrist, Hans Asperger, was working with a similar syndrome in Europe. Asperger's first publication on the subject did not appear until 1944, approximately a year after the first paper by Kanner on autism. Asperger had started his medical career at the University Children's Hospital in Vienna in 1932 but had moved to the psychiatric hospital in Leipzig, Germany, in 1934. While Kanner was working with 11 patients in the United States that he diagnosed with the "new syndrome" that he called "autism," Asperger was treating a smaller but similar group of patients in Europe for what would eventually come to be regarded as a milder form of the same disorder. Asperger's description of the syndrome was first published in 1944, but he, too, used the crucial term "autism."

In 1910, Bleuler had used the term "autism" merely to refer to certain symptoms of schizophrenia arising in adults. In 1943, however, Kanner believed that he was describing a "new syndrome" of unknown causes. As Kanner saw it, the difference between autism and the previously described schizophrenias was the onset of autism in infancy or early childhood. For that reason, he proposed the descriptive phrase "early infantile autism" to express the diagnosis. Kanner (1949) stressed that autism was distinct from the already known schizophrenias precisely because of the onset of what is now sometimes called "Kanner-type autism" before 30 months of age. However, in 1949 Kanner wrote of autism, "The basic nature of its manifestations is so intimately related to the basic nature of **childhood schizophrenia** as to be indistinguishable from it" (p. 419). He went on to say in the same article:

> I do not believe that there is any likelihood that early infantile autism will at any future time have to be separated from the schizophrenias . . . schizophrenic withdrawal can and does begin as early as in the diaper stage. . . . It also confirms the observation, made of late by many authors, that childhood schizophrenia is not so rare as was believed as recently as twenty years ago. (pp. 419–420)

The association of autism with schizophrenia, though the subject of a longstanding controversy, has been a persistent and recurrent theme right up to the present day. For many years, however, "infantile autism" would also be called, or at least would not be sharply distinguished from what Kanner (1949) called, "childhood schizophrenia." One notable feature of Kanner's 1949 paper is his anticipation of the current argument that autism has always been more common than previously thought. With that point in mind, it seems clear that Kanner himself subscribed to the view that many cases had been overlooked or misclassified prior to his time.

With this background in mind, we will see that the definition of autism has actually changed very little from the time it was first described as a "new syndrome" in 1943 by Leo Kanner. Not

---

[1] We are indebted to Cheryl Sinner, CCC-SLP, for pointing us to the Bleuler connection and for her helpful contributions to the history of the definition of the term "autism." We also want to thank Dr. Hung-Chu Lin, Nasmiye Evra Gunhan-Senol, Stephanie Grant, and Patricia Olivier for their contributions to the seminar on this subject that took place in spring 2008 at the University of Louisiana in Lafayette.

only has the definition of autism changed very little in the intervening years, but, as we will see in the following pages, almost every significant theory and controversy about autism—including those pertaining to its definition, its character, and its causes—were either anticipated in the description of the first few cases that were diagnosed or were explicitly proposed in the early writings of Kanner and Asperger. In fact, Kanner was the first to suggest the theory rejected by Rimland (1964)—namely, that parents, especially mothers, cause their children to become autistic by being cold toward them.

Autism in Early Childhood According to Leo Kanner

From 1943 until 1956, autism was generally known by the clinical descriptions of the 11 cases, none older than 11 years, first diagnosed and described in some detail by psychiatrist Leo Kanner (also see Kanner, 1944, 1946, 1949). In his earliest descriptions, and in the title of the 1943 article, Kanner stressed that "autism" was an **affective disorder**—that is, it had to do with disruption of the social aspect of communication. Symptoms pertained especially to the expression and comprehension of emotions, feelings, and their meanings. In fact, the title of Kanner's 1943 paper published in the *Nervous Child* journal was "Autistic Disturbances of Affective Contact."

In 1952, the first edition of the American Psychiatric Association's *Diagnostic and Statistical Manual of Mental Disorders* (*DSM*) was published, but did not recognize autism as a separate category. In 1956, together with Eisenberg, Kanner argued that the main symptoms of what he termed "infantile autism" were manifested in (1) difficulties in making emotional connections with other people, along with (2) stereotypical and abnormal repetitive behaviors. Kanner and Eisenberg (1956) downplayed the symptoms associated with delayed language acquisition or lost language skills, but by emphasizing the importance of broken or undeveloped social relations implicated the critical role that language played in communication. In fact, the proposed restriction on their definition would never be widely accepted or used in the diagnosis of autism as such, but would become the basis for defining "Asperger's disorder" almost half a century later. We will come to that development a little later in this chapter when we discuss the addition of Asperger's disorder to what would come to be known later on as "the autism spectrum."

The importance of language development as central to social and cognitive development is difficult to overemphasize. Language, whether obviously strange or seemingly lost in severe nonverbal individuals with autism, invariably comes into play in determining both the absence or distortion of normal social connections and the presence of abnormal interests, activities, and many of the characteristic repetitive behaviors of autism. As a result, the emphasis on this aspect of autism by Kanner and Eisenberg (1956) did not change the status quo. One of the defining features noted by Kanner back in 1943 was the tendency for the person with autism to repeat something said by someone else, even when the repeated verbal sequence was not apparently understood fully (or at all in some cases) by the individual with autism. This tendency, termed **echolalia**, is a distinctly linguistic manifestation typical of the abnormal repetitive behaviors associated with autism. So, even after Kanner and Eisenberg, the delay, loss, or absence of normal language skills invariably remained implicitly involved in the diagnosis of autism.

Foreshadowing Subsequent Discussions

We are not the first authors to note that Kanner's initial descriptions of "infantile autism" (1943, 1944, 1946, 1949) would provide the basis for essentially all future discussions and definitions of the autism spectrum. Rutter (1978) wrote that "any account of the definition of autism must start with Kanner's (1943) careful and systematic observations on 11 children with a previously unrecognized syndrome" (p. 139). In what follows, we will show that the major themes of theory and research concerning autism continue to rely fundamentally on Kanner's original descriptions.

The features of the "new syndrome" as described by Kanner (1943) stressed multiple abnormal behaviors, but especially those having to do with social relationships. The same was true for the milder form of autism that would come to be known as "Asperger syndrome." Nevertheless, for many years there would be an ongoing controversy over whether and to what extent Asperger syndrome could be distinguished from the mild form of autism that would later be called "high-functioning autism." The main feature that distinguished Asperger syndrome was that the individuals he described a year later than Kanner (see Asperger, 1944, 1968, 1979), though slower in overall development than typical children, seemed closer to the norm in their rate and maximal level of language acquisition. In some respects, they would even appear as gifted, bordering in some respects on **savantism**, having unusually well-developed specialized knowledge, vocabulary, or esoteric skills. A savant in mathematics might be able to produce a series of very large prime numbers. Other savants can perform feats of visual or musical recall in astonishing detail (e.g., drawing a scene in exquisite detail that has briefly been experienced just one time, or playing a complex musical composition after hearing it only once). Such abilities have greatly puzzled researchers from the beginning of the discovery of autism.

In 1978, summing up the characteristics of autism as detailed by Kanner, Michael Rutter barely hints at savantism in mentioning "a good rote memory" along with the more common traits of autism first described in Kanner's original writings—"failure to develop relationships with people, a delay in speech acquisition, the noncommunicative use of speech after it is developed, delayed echolalia, pronominal reversal, repetitive and stereotyped play activities, an obsessive insistence on the maintenance of sameness, a lack of imagination, [and] a good rote memory" (p. 140).

Kanner (1944, p. 212) gave an example of **delayed echolalia** where the clause "Don't throw the dog off the balcony!" was repeated in contexts very different from the one where the individual first encountered it. The later contexts had only a slight resemblance to the one in which the clause was first uttered by the person with autism. Many other examples were given of similar echolalic (repetitive linguistic) behaviors.

Pronominal reversal was also singled out by Kanner as a diagnostic feature. As he described it, pronominal reversal involves the apparent confusion of or failure to distinguish the underlying **referents** particularly of the personal pronouns "I" and "you." Kanner went on to say that this symptom was "almost **pathognomonic**" (1946, p. 242), meaning that it could almost be used all by itself as the defining feature of the syndrome. In saying this, he anticipated key aspects of a great deal of theory and research that would be developed in later years, especially with respect to what would be termed the **theory of mind** (see Baron-Cohen, 1991; Baron-Cohen, Leslie, & Frith, 1985; Charman, Baron-Cohen et al., 2000; O. Golan, Baron-Cohen, & Y. Golan, 2008), also the theory of **perspective taking** (McHugh, Y. Barnes-Holmes, & D. Barnes-Holmes, 2004), and the more developed and detailed **theory of abstraction** (J. W. Oller & Rascón, 1999; J. W. Oller et al., 2006, 2010).

The theory of mind idea came from questions about whether chimpanzees are able to take account of the perspectives of other chimps the way that human beings do (Premack & Woodruff, 1978). Later that question was applied by Simon Baron-Cohen and others to the complex of symptoms observed in autism. The question became not whether chimpanzees have a theory of mind, or whether a chimp can take account of the perspective of another chimp, but rather whether human beings with autism are able to take the viewpoint of others into consideration.

The "Almost Pathognomonic" Symptom

Kanner thought what he called "pronominal reversal" was almost the defining basis for the "new syndrome" that he proposed to call "early infantile autism." It is noteworthy that the underlying problem displayed in the symptom that he called "pronominal reversal" would prove to be of central interest to subsequent researchers. They would not all make the connection with "pronominal reversal" as Kanner described it, but they would zero in on the underlying problem of abstraction that it illustrated. It is critical, for this reason, to explain what is actually happening—or, more accurately, not happening—in what Kanner described as the "almost pathognomonic" symptom of early infantile autism. The problem, as he saw it, was manifested in a peculiar use of the personal pronouns "I" and "you."

Ordinarily, "I" is used by the producer of speech or writing to refer to himself or herself. The referent of this pronoun is spoken of as the **first person** of grammar. By contrast, "you" is the personal pronoun used to refer to the person addressed in speech or writing. Accordingly, it is referred to as the **second person** of grammar. In the "new syndrome" that Kanner was describing, the affected individual had a strong tendency to refer to himself or herself as "you" and to the person spoken to as "I." Sometimes the affected individual would refer to himself or herself as "he" or "she," thus using a **third person** pronoun. For instance, one of Kanner's patients, a boy named Paul, at age three was apparently referring to himself as "he" when he sang again and again, "He wants the telephone," while handling a toy telephone from a box of toys. Such apparent confusions of pronominal reference can arise from what Kanner termed "echolalia." Language acquisition specialists understand the latter as a tendency to repeat the **surface forms** of speech without complete comprehension.

By definition, the "surface forms" of speech, writing, or manually signed languages, as the phrase suggests, are the manifest forms that can be heard, seen, or perceived through some combination of the senses of sight, hearing, and touch. A parrot or mynah bird, for example, can often produce some of the surface forms of speech, but talking birds are evidently not fully able to relate the surface forms they produce to their contexts of use as a normal human speaker of the language would do. For instance, when a parrot says something like, "Polly want a cracker?" with a question intonation, for example, the surface form of the utterance as a question may be perfectly intelligible to an English speaker, yet the same parrot does not show comprehension of the utterance or the questioning intonation. In other words, if asked, "Who is Polly?" the parrot will not be able to answer, "I am." Or, if asked to identify a cracker, the parrot will be unable to say, "Now, there is a cracker." The parrot handles some of the surface forms of speech and is able to produce them, yet does not fully understand the referential relations involved or the intentions that conventionally accompany them when used by normal speakers of a language.

In the echolalia of autism, the failure to comprehend some of the surface forms—these would be the different personal pronouns in the cases of interest to Kanner—is evident if we examine the contexts of experience present at the time those surface forms were produced by the person diagnosed with autism. If the surface forms of the symbols "I" and "you" are not differentially connected with the speaker and listener, and changed when the roles are shifted, the child diagnosed with autism is evidently not connecting "I" with the person speaking in the manner that normal mature language users do. The person with autism appears to be failing to perform the **pragmatic mapping** (see Figure 2-1) necessary to connect the surface form of the personal pronoun "I" to the person doing the speaking. The trouble, of course, does not restrict itself in such cases merely to pronouns. It extends to highly abstract referring relations in a general way, although Kanner focused his attention on certain pronouns. (We explain the general problem at issue more completely later in this chapter in the section titled "The Crucial Role of Abstraction.")

Similarly, in echolalia, a child may be able to repeat all or part of the surface form of a segment of speech, or even a long series of segments, without performing the deeper pragmatic operations of fully associating referring terms with their meanings. An example was provided by a mother who told Kanner that when her son Paul was two years old, she was reciting the nursery rhyme about "Peter, Peter, pumpkin eater." When she dropped a sauce pan while reciting the rhyme, Paul at about age three evidently associated the surface form of the nursery rhyme, or a portion of it which he transformed into "Peten-eater," with the dropping of the sauce pan (Kanner, 1943, p. 227). Later

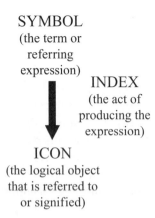

Figure 2-1 The simplest sort of pragmatic mapping relation, a symbol linked through an index to an icon.

he would repeat the portion of the rhyme on many occasions to refer to a sauce pan. This sort of phenomenon Kanner referred to as "delayed echolalia," where the surface form produced by little Paul was derived from a form he had heard long before.

Actually, however, little Paul's imperfect understanding was not strictly a repetition of the surface forms without meaning. Although he did not fully understand the nursery rhyme, and although it was peculiar to use only a few of the syllables from it to refer to a sauce pan, three-year-old Paul was already doing more than a parrot would be expected to be able to do. Paul was using language referentially, even if the pragmatic mapping of the surface symbols onto elements of experience was incomplete. It did not completely conform to the conventions of English: We do not refer to sauce pans as "Peten-eaters." However, the important thing to note in connecting "pronominal reversals" with what Kanner—we believe misleadingly—termed "delayed echolalia" is that the latter can produce the former. That is, if the child attends to and reproduces surface forms of certain utterances without understanding their referential relations fully, what Kanner called "pronominal reversal" is a guaranteed outcome. It is not, however, necessarily pathological to do this. On the contrary, it is a very normal stage in language acquisition that is commonly observed, though less persistently, in normally developing children.

For instance, if a child merely repeats when someone else says, "I will help you" (or "I helped him") or "You will hurt yourself" (or "She hurt herself") when offering help or warning the child of potential harm, the result will appear to be what Kanner called "pronominal reversal." The child, while meaning to say, "I hurt myself," is apt to come up with "You hurt yourself"; when intending "I want the telephone," he or she is apt to say, "He wants the telephone." It is not the occurrence of such phenomena in language acquisition that is pathognomonic of autism, but, if they persist, or define a plateau of development beyond which the child does not advance, then, they may indeed be symptomatic of an underlying disorder. It is the chronic, persistent aspect of a particular stage of development for longer than would normally be expected that defines such a phenomenon as characteristic of autism.

A Deeper Analysis of Pronominal Reversal

What Kanner evidently did not know is that precisely such pronominal reversals are common in normally developing toddlers at a particular stage of language acquisition (see J. W. Oller et al., 2006). In fact, the applications of "I" and "you" in such "reversals" do not actually involve any reversal except from the adult's point of view. The child is not reversing anything, but rather failing to fully understand their meaning when using the distinct pronouns as referring terms. The child is associating the pronoun with the person referred to as if it were a simpler, less abstract referring term, such as a name or a symbol requesting an action—for example, "Down!" meaning "Put me down," or "Up!" meaning "Pick me up!" Simple referring expressions, such as the name "Ginny," can refer to the child named Virginia no matter who is using it and no matter where Ginny is. Similarly, many expressions such as "Up!" or "Down!", unlike the personal pronouns, share the same sort of relative pragmatic simplicity. They also function as relatively simple referring or signifying terms with respect to the situations in which they are commonly used and understood. They involve relatively simple one-to-one mappings that are well described by Figure 2-1.

To use the personal pronouns such as "I," "you," "he," and "she" according to the usual conventions of the language, the child has to take account of who is speaking and who is being spoken to or about. In referring to the speaker as contrasted with the person spoken to or about, the child must abstract from the individual actors to the higher level of their actions. It is necessary to take the relationship between the actors into consideration. Not only does the conventional use of the personal pronouns require abstraction to a higher level, but it also requires taking account of at least two persons who are engaged in a conversation. Put simply, the perspective of more than one person must be considered. This two-part (**dyadic**) relationship involves the speaker and the person spoken to in a dynamic conversational relation. The dynamic aspect that produces the complexity for the use of the personal pronouns consists of the fact that the partners in the conversation may frequently exchange roles as speaker and listener.

To understand the dynamics and the changing pragmatic mapping relations of the pronouns "I" and "you" in an ongoing conversation, the participants need to differentiate the distinct roles and personal perspectives of the speaker and hearer, over and above the different persons who may take on these roles. The perspectives also may differ along with the roles of speaker/hearer and the persons taking on any particular perspective and/or a particular participant role. For this reason, some researchers have discussed the difficulty in perspective taking as a defining symptom of autism. What Kanner called "pronominal reversal" is just one of the symptoms covered under the scope of "perspective taking."

At a slightly higher remove, it can be argued that to keep track of turn changes between the speaker and the listener in a conversation, the child acquiring a language must consider the fact that the other person in a conversation also has a point of view different from his or her own point of view. To refer to the normal capacity to take account of another person's views, intentions, and feelings, Simon Baron-Cohen and others have proposed the phrase "theory of mind" (Baron-Cohen, 1991; Baron-Cohen et al., 1985; Charman, Baron-Cohen, et al., 2000; McHugh et al., 2004; O. Golan et al., 2008). They argue that individuals with autism have difficulty in forming a theory of mind.

All such theories about autism, looking right back to Kanner's "almost pathognomonic" symptom of pronominal reversal, as we have argued extensively elsewhere (J. W. Oller & Rascón, 1999; J. W. Oller et al., 2006, 2010), involve abstraction in a critical way. Also, all of them have a common weakness: They do not express the fact that there are always more than two levels of abstraction involved in ordinary social interactions. This point is crucial to the system of differentiating levels of severity in autism that we present in Chapter 11. For that reason, and to understand the symptoms at issue, it is important to consider the crucial role of abstraction. It turns out that the process of abstraction is indispensable to the progress a normal child makes when acquiring the so-called nonverbal systems underlying and forming the basis for the acquisition of the so-called verbal systems of language. Abstraction is the key to enriching the conception of what others have called theory of mind or perspective taking.

The Crucial Role of Abstraction

Abstraction is the mental process of separating some **logical object** of attention, thought, or imagination, where a "logical object" can be defined as a bodily thing, an event, or a relation between things and events, or a sequence of any of these, from its context(s) of existence. A logical object is whatever might be attended to, thought of, or imagined. It might be the body of a person or a physical object. The first level of abstractive separation involves no more than finding the boundaries, edges, or limits of the logical object within its context—for example, distinguishing it within the field of perception, experience, or imagination. The second level of separation involves the movement of the object within the field; an example is imagining where the object will be after it moves from its present location. The third and highest level of abstraction, the greatest degree of separation of an object from its context of existence, involves imagining or thinking of that object as removed entirely from any particular context—for example, imagining a Boeing 747 without reference to wherever it may or may not be at the moment.

It is possible to show that the first degree of abstraction must logically precede the second and that the second degree of abstraction must precede the third. The degree of abstraction preceding the first can be considered to be the zero degree of the real world. The middle degree is essential to connect the first to the third. As the process of abstraction is applied, each degree of abstraction generates a distinct level of sign systems. As each of those signs is reentered into the real world of objects, events, and relations, it enriches the possible further abstractions that can be achieved, leading to higher levels. The first products at each level provide the necessary building blocks for the formation of the signs at the next level up, and so on. Because the process of abstraction has to begin by operating on the bounded objects (e.g., persons, things, events) of the real world, it shows how and why icons (representations of bounded objects) form the essential basis for building up indexes (representations of dynamic changing relations between objects), which in turn (icons together with indexes) form the basis for building up the more abstract relations of meaningful symbols and complex constructions of languages.

The interesting thing about the theory of abstraction is that it shows how and in which order the highly complex, multilayered representational systems that constitute language are achieved. As a result, it becomes possible to predict a certain sequential progression through the multilayered system of the signs that constitute normal language acquisition. The logic of the theory of abstraction is such that it accounts for growth horizontally at any given level by adding more and more concepts at that same level. It also explains vertical growth, whereby increasing levels of abstraction above the one at hand can be attained. We will have more to say about the theory of abstraction in Chapter 11, but by keeping in mind the constructive, layered, and cyclic processes involved in abstraction, we can already be more explicit about what goes wrong in the symptom of autism that Kanner referred to as "pronominal reversal."

Revisiting "Pronominal Reversal"

The main problem in what is called "pronominal reversal" consists of a delay or a complete failure to advance from the degree of abstractness associated with the ordinary mapping of any referring term onto its object, to the more abstract level associating the personal pronouns "I" and "you" appropriately with two or more persons who may exchange roles repeatedly in a conversation.

The mapping of a name to the person named, or any conventional verbal sign to its meaning, is complicated enough. It can be thought of as diagrammed in Figure 2-1. There, a referring term (an abstract symbol), such as a name, is mapped through an intentional act (an indexical sign) onto its logical object (an iconic representation)—that is, the bodily person, scene, event sequence, or activity referred to. Figure 2-1 depicts the simplest pragmatic mapping, involving an arbitrary, conventional linguistic symbol, a word or phrase that is used to refer to or signify a logical object. As we have already noted, the logical object (the referent or whatever is signified) may be a thing, person, event, activity, or a sequence or complex arrangement of such events or objects.

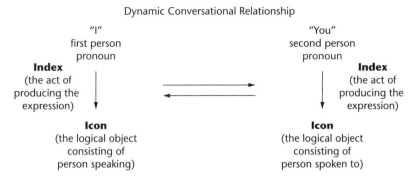

Figure 2-2 The more abstract pragmatic mapping of the first and second person pronouns to their logical objects within a dynamic conversational interaction.

It takes the normal child about five to nine months after birth just to comprehend the simplest sort of pragmatic relation between an arbitrary linguistic sign and its conventional object as depicted in Figure 2-1. A partial example of such a mapping would be the first meaningful word the child can understand. Usually, this is the child's own name or a verbal signal for a very common and salient action—for example, "bye-bye," signifying "someone leaving and someone else staying behind," or commands such as "Up!" or "Down!", meaning "Pick me up" or "Put me down," each one often accompanied by the corresponding gesture. When the child is able to produce the verbal symbol showing full command of such a pragmatic mapping relation, we usually speak of this milestone as the production of the first meaningful word. To reach this milestone usually takes several months longer than the mere comprehension of the first word. The actual production of the first meaningful, recognizable, and generalized first word—a milestone that usually follows the first meaningful comprehension of a word by about six months—is rarely attained much before the end of the first year of life or several months afterward.

The correct conventional use of the personal pronouns "I" and "you" is considerably more complex and, more importantly, is more abstract. It requires a differential mapping of "I" to the person doing the speaking, regardless who it may be that is speaking, and of "you" to the person spoken to in the dynamic dyadic conversational relation (see Figure 2-2). Such pragmatic mappings are readily constructed by adults who have mastered them, but they are much more complex than the sort of mapping shown in Figure 2-1. The conventions underlying the use of the first and second personal pronouns require taking at least two persons into consideration simultaneously, while naming them on the basis of the abstracted concept of one person as the speaker/producer and the other person as the listener/addressee. The shifting meaning of the pronouns is essential if the speaker is to correctly conform to the conventional system of mapping the personal pronouns "I" and "you" onto their referents.

The child who engages in what Kanner called "pronominal reversal" fails to associate the pronoun for the person speaking (the pronoun "I" or the first person pronoun) with the new speaker when that person changes. Similarly, when the person spoken to—who by convention is referred to with the second person pronoun "you"—shifts, the child who does not change the pronoun from "I" to "you," rather than performing a reversal or shift, is failing to do so. In fact, shifting the pronoun "I" to the new speaker and "you" to the person being spoken to, at turn changes in a conversation, requires a higher level of abstraction in language than merely referring to each person by name. By 6 to 9 months of age, the normally developing infant can comprehend different referring terms for persons, actions, and situations. About 6 months later (by about 10 to 18 months of age), the child normally becomes able to produce at least one word with sufficient clarity so that other persons can understand it and know what the child means by it. It usually takes an additional 6 months to a year (or longer) after the first word before the typically developing child (at about 24 to 30 months) will be able to correctly use conventional "shifters" (Edward Sapir, 1921) such as the first and second personal pronouns.

What Kanner called "pronominal reversal" commonly occurs in normal children anywhere from months 18 to 30 after birth (J. W. Oller et al., 2006). For that reason it can hardly be thought of as "pathognomonic" of autism, but Kanner (1943, 1944) was correct in noting that in the "new syndrome" that he was describing, verbal individuals with autism typically fail to acquire the distinctions between the personal pronouns and are apt to apply them imperfectly for a much longer period of time than is common in normal language acquisition.

Savant Traits

In fact, the full range of the remarkable behavioral symptoms of autism were quite well detailed in the early writings of Kanner. These would include **savant traits** such as "astounding vocabulary . . . excellent memory for events of several years before . . . phenomenal rote memory for poems and names, and . . . precise recollections of complex patterns and sequences" (Kanner, 1944, p. 217).

Kanner described one individual's ability to recall the details of a three-dimensional scene in the following way:

> After the lapse of several days a multitude of blocks could be rearranged in precisely the same unorganized pattern with the same color of each block turned up, with each picture or letter on the upper surface of each block facing in the same direction as before. The absence of a block or the presence of a supernumerary block was noticed immediately and there was an imperative demand for the restoration of the missing piece. If someone would remove a block, the child would struggle to get it back, going into a panic tantrum until he regained it, and then promptly and with sudden calm after the storm would return to the design and replace the block. (p. 216)

Kanner's emphasis on rote memory—that is, the ability to recall or in some way reconstruct the details of a complex scene or a script of some sort—foreshadowed an interest that would occupy many psychologists and others for years to come. In his earliest writings about autism, Kanner emphasized the special intellectual abilities that were sometimes associated with it. The term "savantism" would be applied to describe such cases and would turn out to be far more common in persons with autism than in the general population (Rimland, 1978). Of the documented cases of savantism, more than half have been persons also diagnosed with autism (Treffert & Wallace, 2002). The most peculiar aspect of savantism in autism was clearly, if insensitively, described by Kanner (1949). He wrote that some of his patients had "withdrawn to the point of functional idiocy or imbecility" although they nevertheless demonstrated "especially in their behavior with puzzles and form boards, residual oases of planned mental activity" (p. 417). Among the savants with autism who have been most studied, as correctly anticipated by Kanner's description of savant traits of autism, are individuals with amazing memories for relatively unimportant facts, the ability to say on which day a particular date on a calendar will fall many years in the future, and the like.

The character in the 1988 movie *Rain Man*, played by Dustin Hoffman, displayed some of the savant characteristics actually associated with reported cases of autism. In the movie, Raymond Babbit was portrayed as a savant with respect to certain aspects of numerical computation. He could count the number of toothpicks in a pile almost instantaneously after they were spilled in a mess on the floor. This incident was actually based on a pair of remarkable twin savants observed by Oliver

Sacks. When a box of matches was spilled, the two were correctly able to report almost instantly, just by looking at the pile of matches, that there were exactly 111 of them, and to note instantly that the number 111 was the sum of 37 + 37 + 37 (Sacks, 1990, p. 199).

These same twins, like the composite character played by Hoffman in the movie *Rain Man*, were observed on another occasion exchanging a sequence of six-digit numbers. Sacks was intrigued and wrote down some of the numbers. All of the numbers turned out to be primes. Later, with the help of a book of prime numbers, Sacks returned to present the twins with a prime number of eight digits. He reported that they paused for only about a "half-minute . . . and suddenly, simultaneously, they broke into smiles" (p. 203). Then, one of them produced a prime number of 10 digits and the other responded with one of 12.

Observers are amazed at the visual recall demonstrated by another living savant, Stephen Wiltshire. After a short ride over Rome in a helicopter—one that lasts only about 45 minutes (and part of which is filmed)—he was able to draw, over the next three days, an incredibly detailed and accurate panoramic view of Rome's skyscape ("Beautiful Minds," 2009 and "About Stephen," 2009 ●).

The puzzlement of researchers trying to figure out how such feats can be accomplished has persisted to the present day. Together with Dr. L. C. Badon, in our 2010 *Cases* book, introducing and reclassifying communication disorders from a semiotic perspective, we have suggested how overdevelopment of sensory-motor representations, accompanied by underdevelopment of higher linguistic and social representations, can, at least partially, account for the amazing specialized abilities found in "autistic savants." The discovery of such remarkable abilities can be dated clear back to Kanner (1943) and are part of the near voyeuristic intrigue that has been associated with the study of autism ever since.

Distinguishing Autism from Other Disorders

In his 1949 article, Kanner distinguished autism from various other diseases and disorders including Heller's disease, which would later be called "childhood disintegrative disorder." Kanner insisted that a significant difference was that "Heller's disease has a definite onset; the child impresses people as feeling and being sick" (p. 417); he claimed that his patients with autism, however, did not go through any such phase.

The same distinction is still part of the standard definition of autism today. However, we do not have to look far to see that the actual facts of autism, as known from the current literature, show that even Kanner had evidence to contradict his claim that illness was not involved. As described in Chapter 1, 9 of Kanner's 11 initial patients evidently had digestive problems significant enough for him to describe them in the published record. Also, we now know that regressive cases of autism are substantially—by a four to one margin—the most common kind. Typically they are preceded, as were some of Kanner's cases, by vomiting, digestive problems, bloody diarrhea, and indications of toxicity, disease, and malaise at or near the first noticed symptoms of autism. It is remarkable that practicing physicians (albeit in psychiatry) such as Kanner and Asperger did not give more attention to the signs of gut disease that were presented by their patients. Kanner noted some of the evidences in at least 9 of the 11 cases he saw, but still reached the conclusion that his patients were not feeling sick. In view of the number of cases that were deemed "nonverbal," perhaps this finding is not unexpected.

At the same time, Kanner rejected the theory, proposed by some, that early infantile autism was "basically an aphasic phenomenon related to so-called congenital word deafness" (p. 417). That theory was similar to the present-day theory of mind and word blindness alternatives proposed by Baron-Cohen and colleagues. Kanner's objection to the idea of such sensory-intellectual deficits was that he had seen word-deaf children who were shy, apprehensive, lacking in spontaneity, pathetically bewildered, and insecure. But they all responded promptly to gestures, were keenly sensitive to physiognomies [facial appearances and different facial expressions and bodily postures], and had a definite relation to their mothers, mostly one of clinging dependence. None showed the isolation, obsessiveness, and fragmentation of interests typical of early infantile autism. Certainly there are enough autistic children who have amazingly large vocabularies; one patient who was brought to me from South Africa could speak English, French, and Afrikaans. (p. 417)

Kanner (1949) also pointed out that children diagnosed with autism who are apparently nonverbal are occasionally observed producing an intelligible utterance of some complexity. For instance, one five-year-old who had reportedly never uttered a single word became agitated when a prune became stuck to the roof of his mouth said plainly, "Get it out of there!" From this and similar observations, Kanner concluded that even seemingly nonverbal children with autism "do not suffer from either **sensory [aphasia]** or **motor aphasia**" because the ones

who eventually begin to talk give evidence that during the silent period they have accumulated a considerable store of readily available linguistic material. (p. 418)

This statement by Kanner would certainly apply to the case of Ethan Kurtz more than five decades later. When Ethan's gut problems were cleared up, he began to speak plainly after a period of being "nonverbal" and socially unresponsive for about two years.

ETIOLOGY: SPECULATING ABOUT CAUSES

From the discovery and the earliest definition of autism, it was understood that the mysteriousness of this "new syndrome" was that the person affected could seem almost completely disconnected from other persons and shared experience, a trait that would justify the association of autism with schizophrenia. At the same time, the affected individual would, in most instances, retain certain abilities. Some individuals at the high-functioning end of the spectrum, such as Stephen Wiltshire, would be able to advance to a savant level, for instance, in music, memorization, computation, or just in the ability to recall a familiar space in excruciating detail.

Genuinely Mysterious and Distinct

As early investigators noted, autism was unlike mental retardation, which seemed to slow development, possibly to a halt at some point, but without distortion. Autism was also unlike disabilities affecting one or more of the senses of sight, hearing, touch, taste, smell, or balance. It was unlike the disorders commonly caused by a brain injury, such as **aphasia**. Autism did not seem to affect a focused aspect of behavior or communication (e.g., speech but not writing, or vice versa; motor skills but not cognition, or vice versa).

The "new syndrome" was characterized from the beginning by strange and unexplained distortions in the patterns of normal development in infancy and early childhood. Those distortions, it was recognized from the beginning, were definitive characteristics of the disorder. Because Kanner believed from 1943 forward that the "new syndrome" was quite different from previously described syndromes and disorders, it is unsurprising that he would be spurred to speculate about its causation.

The Full Range of Possible Causes Considered

In keeping with the psychiatry of the times, and in response to the profound influence of Sigmund Freud (1901/1975, 1915–1917/1924), the prevailing tendency among psychiatrists and clinical psychologists was to look for "non-organic" causes for what were regarded as "mental" disorders. There already was a considerable awareness of the fact that an individual's mental and emotional development was also influenced by blood lines; thus genetic factors and the "heritability" of disease conditions and disorders comprised background questions. It evidently occurred to Kanner to pursue both of these lines in exploring the etiology of the "new syndrome."

A possible causal explanation that Kanner dismissed was the notion that autism might result from some complex of organic injuries or an accumulation of them. He set that idea aside in 1949:

> ... residual oases of planned mental activity ... should deter one from thinking in terms of a degenerative organic process [p. 417]. ... Not one of the 55 patients studied has had in his infancy any disease or physical injury to which his behavior could be attributed by any stretch of the imagination. (p. 420)

Thus physical injury, disease, or cumulative organ damage were collectively dismissed as having any possible causal role in the "new syndrome."

Kanner also dismissed the idea of any hereditary (genetic) basis for autism. He wrote:

> It is customary to evaluate the hereditary element in the schizophrenias. Such an inquiry into the ancestral background of the autistic children [the 55 he had studied by this point] is entirely fruitless if one limits the investigation to overtly psychotic and hospitalized relatives [which was common practice with adult schizophrenia]. It is indeed remarkable that, with the exception of the paternal aunt of one of the children, there is no history of psychosis, at least, of committable mental disorder [one that did or could result in institutionalization in an insane asylum], in any of the antecedents. There is no instance of schizophrenia, manic-depressive psychosis, or even senile psychosis among the parents, grandparents, uncles, and aunts of the autistic children. (p. 420)

In dismissing the possibility of an organic basis along with a genetic one, Kanner shows awareness of essentially all of the possible causes for the "new syndrome" including ones originating in the following areas:

- Genetics
- Physical (organic) causes
- Linguistic, social, and/or emotional experience

Interestingly, and perhaps unsurprisingly in view of Kanner's background in psychiatry, he would settle exclusively on the third of these alternatives and would dismiss the other two. His commitment to the idea of a social and emotional basis for the causation of autism was already suggested by the title of his first paper on the subject in 1943, "Autistic Disturbances of *Affective* Contact" [emphasis added].

In dismissing genetics and physical injuries, as from poisons or diseases, and in exclusively embracing the theory that autism was a social, behavioral, and linguistic/cognitive disorder, Kanner set the stage for the perpetuation of a cascading series of omissions and errors that would characterize the treatment of autism for many years to come. He also established a context in which the absence of meaningful research into causes was virtually guaranteed to persist for another 50 years.

Dismissing Genetic Tendencies for the Refrigerator Theory

In his 1943 descriptions of his first 11 patients, it seemed that Kanner was looking for the possibility that the "new syndrome" might have a genetic basis. Later, in 1949, after seeing 44 additional cases of infantile autism, he would reject the possibility of any genetic basis, despite the fact that his own notes concerning the siblings, parents, aunts, uncles, and grandparents of his first 11 cases contained many suggestions of genetic components in the etiology of autism.

As noted by Jepson and Johnson (2007), the bizarre (and ultimately rejected) theory that autism was caused by emotional neglect of the child by his or her parents was not merely foreshadowed in Kanner's original writings (1943, 1944) but was explicitly advocated by him in 1949, though the much-despised theory would later be credited mainly to Bruno Bettelheim (1950, 1967). In 1949, Kanner dismissed all of his own considerable findings of familial tendencies toward symptoms of autism and settled on what is now regarded as one of the most hurtful ideas ever proposed concerning the etiology of autism—namely, that autism could be caused by a "mechanization of human relationships" (1949, p. 421). That idea, as even Kanner (1949, p. 426) admitted, came into immediate conflict with the fact that most of the siblings of children diagnosed with autism—approximately 93% according to D. B. Campbell et al. (2006, p. 16834)—were apparently typical in their development and unaffected by autism.

The descriptive phrase applied to Kanner's remarkable leap of inference was "the refrigerator mother theory" (and variations on this theme). The emphasis on the mother's role in the development of autism was interesting in view of the fact that Kanner was almost as critical of the fathers of his patients as of their mothers. Instead of representing evidence of a genetic factor, the affective aloofness of many of the parents described by Kanner was taken as evidence supporting the "refrigerator parent" theory. That idea can be perceived in the background of his descriptions of the history of his first 11 patients published in 1943. Although, as we have noted, the "refrigerator mother" theory would later be championed by Bruno Bettelheim, in reality Kanner was ahead of him in proposing it in a paper in 1949.

Kanner described behaviors of parents in ways that would suggest to later researchers that the parents themselves were symptomatic:

> One is struck by what I should like to call a mechanization of human relationships. Most of the parents declare outright that they are not comfortable in the presence of people. (p. 421)

Oddly, however, Kanner did not see such behaviors as evidence that the parents had some of the same genetic tendencies as their children, but rather supposed that the parents were willfully neglecting their children's need for affection. He continued:

> [M]aternal lack of genuine warmth is often conspicuous in the first visit to the clinic. . . . Many of the fathers hardly know their autistic children. . . . Many of the fathers and most of the mothers are perfectionists. Obsessive adherence to set rules serves as a substitute for the enjoyment of life. (p. 421)

Neither did Kanner seem to think of the possibility that what he saw as mechanical routines were, in part, no doubt, coping strategies forced on the parents by the nature of autism. It was Kanner himself who first noted that autism involved an "obsessive desire for the preservation of sameness" (1949, p. 416). Deviating from routines, as he documented very well, could result in major emotional meltdowns. Instead, Kanner read the routines followed by the parents as products of their own upbringing, pushing the blame clear back to the grandparents of the child with autism. Rather than seeing such routines as coping strategies, he regarded them as attempts to sustain an attitude of "perfectionism":

These people, who themselves had been reared sternly in emotional refrigerators, have found at an early age that they could gain approval only through unconditional surrender to standards of perfection. . . . (pp. 421–423)

A little farther on in the same 1949 paper, if there remained any doubt about his claim that autism is caused by cold and unfeeling parents, Kanner wrote:

Most of the patients were exposed from the beginning to parental coldness, obsessiveness, and a mechanical type of attention to material needs only. They were the objects of observation and experiment conducted with an eye on fractional performance rather than with genuine warmth and enjoyment. They were kept neatly in refrigerators which did not defrost. (p. 425)

Kanner went on to suggest that the withdrawal of the children with autism from what he described as a "frosty atmosphere" could be understood as seeking "comfort in solitude" (p. 425). Before he jumped to the conclusion that the parents were actually causing their children to withdraw from the cold reality of their homes into a form of childhood schizophrenia, Kanner produced a considerable amount of evidence supporting a significant and substantial genetic component in the etiology of autism.

It will be useful to go through the evidence of genetic factors that he amassed with respect to the first 11 cases that he diagnosed in 1943. However, in doing so, we need to bear in mind that Kanner was developing the false notion that the behaviors of the parents, rather than showing that they themselves genetically tended toward mild traits of autism, were actually causing autism in their children.

Clues Suggesting Genetics

In this section, we consider some of the details of the individual histories that Kanner published in 1943, which plainly suggest a substantial genetic component in the etiology of autism.

Kanner described the parents and close relatives of the children with the "new syndrome" as highly intelligent, socially aloof, sometimes peculiar, obsessive, withdrawn, possibly regarding themselves as superior, and so on. To see how these observations were developed, we need to review, again one by one, the first 11 cases described by Kanner. At first look, it might seem that he was looking for evidence of the **heritability** of autism—that is, evidence that the autism syndrome, like schizophrenia, tends to run in family lines, but on closer examination it comes out that he was more likely building a basis for his conclusion that the parents were causing the autism in their own children. Nevertheless, his descriptions of the family history of most of his cases strongly suggest heritable genetic tendencies running in families.

Kanner referred to one or both of the parents of Cases 1–4 as "obsessive," "peculiar," or "absent" (pp. 217–228). He said nothing about the attitudes or habits of the parents or any relatives of Case 5, but he stressed that the brother of Case 6 (a girl named Virginia), who was himself a "severe stutterer," had burst into tears as he described his own father (and Virginia's) as a man that never spoke except to scold. According to Kanner's description, Philip "felt that all his life he had lived in a frosty atmosphere—with two inapproachable strangers" (p. 230). The father, himself a psychiatrist, is said to have volunteered that he "never liked children" and that Virginia's mother was "not by any means the mother type. Her attitude [toward a child; Kanner's interpolation] is more like that toward a doll or a pet than anything else" (Kanner, 1943, p. 230).

Of Case 7, Kanner wrote that the boy's father, a psychiatrist, was "a man of unusual intelligence, sensitive, restless, introspective, taking himself very seriously, not interested in people." Kanner said

one developed on an international level and the other mainly in the United States. They developed somewhat independently at first, but converged increasingly from 1968 forward.

Historical Context of the Discovery and Definition of Autism

In 1942, the third edition of the *International Statistical Classification of Diseases, Injuries, and Causes of Death* (*ICD-3*) had appeared without mentioning the term "autism" because the "syndrome" had not been discovered, defined, nor diagnosed as yet. From the very beginning, the purpose of the *ICD* series was to classify diseases—that is, "morbid" conditions, and especially those linked to causes of death. The First International Conference on the subject had taken place in 1900 in Paris where the first *ICD* was adopted. At that conference, it was decided to revise the list of recognized diseases at international meetings to occur every ten years thereafter.

In 1946, an Interim Commission of the World Health Organization was entrusted with the job of preparing the next "decennial" revision of the *ICD*. This would be the sixth revision of a list first established in a preliminary form in 1900. Prior to that time there was a long and complex history of various lists, leading through both the League of Nations (established in 1919) and the United Nations (established in 1946). For the international list, from the beginning practically everything depended on the cooperation of member nations as well as the quality and extent of their medical records. The sixth revision of the *ICD* (*ICD-6*) was approved at the close of the International Conference for the Sixth Revision of the International Lists of Diseases and Causes of Death, which took place in Paris in 1948.

By the time of the publication of *ICD-7* in 1957, it was already well appreciated that achieving "a standard of classification of disease and injury for statistical purposes" was both essential and fraught with difficulty. The authors noted in the Introduction to *ICD-7* that diseases could be classified and named from many different points of view, including how the body was affected, how the condition developed and progressed over time, and, of course, what caused the disease (i.e., etiology).

The *ICD-7* authors stressed, quoting extensively from William Farr in 1856 in the *Sixteenth Annual Report* of the Registrar General of England and Wales, that any classification of diseases seeks meaningful generalizations and may, for a given purpose, group diseases called by different names together or distinguish ones that are "likely to be confounded with each other" (WHO, 1957, p. viii). Nevertheless, the main point of a classification was made clear: to "facilitate the statistical study of disease phenomena" (p. viii). For this purpose, "miscellaneous categories should be kept to a minimum" (p. ix). Farr's system of classification had been recommended as early as 1860 by none other than the famed Florence Nightingale (p. xv). However, the authors of *ICD-7* noted that because "the medical entries on sickness records, hospital records, and death certificates are certain to be of mixed terminology," they "cannot be modernized or standardized by the wave of any magician's wand" (p. ix). Compromises, rather than "a strictly logical arrangement" would be required "between classifications based on etiology, anatomical site, age, and circumstance of onset, as well as the quality of information available on medical reports" (p. ix). The goal was "a common basis of classification for general statistical use" (p. ix). Cutting through to the heart of the matter: The primary underlying reason to do a classification was and remains to discover the causes of diseases and disorders so as to make our lives longer and better.

Of autism, *ICD-7* (WHO, 1957) took no special notice. Unless the **schizophrenia praecox**, the childhood type of schizophrenia, were to be counted as the precursor of what Kanner would later call "autism," it was not mentioned at all. The *ICD* series sought to provide a classification with "mutually exclusive" subcategories that would be "sufficiently detailed for the purpose of a diagnostic index" and to "indicate the classification of synonyms if new subcategories are made" (p. xxxix). So, where was autism to fit in? And with which existing categories or subcategories was it to be regarded as synonymous, if any?

All the while, somewhat parallel efforts were being made in the United States and elsewhere to define diagnostic criteria for diseases and disorders—for instance, by the APA. That effort, it is agreed, was essential because without diagnostic criteria defining the nature of diseases and disorders in some meaningful and intelligible way, it would be utterly impossible to make sensible use of "a diagnostic index" of the sort that the authors of the *ICD* series were developing.

From 1968 to 1980

By 1968, the second edition of the APA's manual for mental disorders, *DSM-II*, had appeared. A distinctive trait of that edition of the U.S. classification system was that it supposedly brought the U.S. categories more closely into line with *ICD-8*, which appeared in the same year (Spitzer & Williams, 1987, p. xviii). Apparently, autism was still too rare and/or too little known to merit a separate place in any of the *ICD* manuals up to *ICD-8* or in either *DSM-I* or *DSM-II*. When *DSM-III* was published in 1980, the term "infantile autism" was finally included, under the scope of the newly created category of "pervasive developmental disorders" (APA, 1980, p. 86 ff).

Before 1980, as originally proposed by Kanner (1949), autism was regarded as a form of "childhood schizophrenia." The key distinguishing trait of all schizophrenias consisted of distorted, bizarre, and abnormal false beliefs about the real world. By being associated with schizophrenia, autism was classed among the psychoses—that is, mental disorders involving "gross impairment in reality testing" (APA, 1980, p. 367). Schizophrenias commonly involve reported perceptions of things or events not present (e.g., fierce dogs barking when no dogs are present), known as **hallucinations**. It can also involve greatly exaggerated states of affairs or relationships (e.g., a frail child claiming to be able to overpower older and larger siblings) or a claim to be someone of great importance (e.g., the owner of the whole neighborhood, the boss of all present, or the like); these symptoms are known as **delusions**.

Kanner's original description and definition of autism prevailed from 1943 until 1980. During this period, Asperger syndrome was not recognized as a separate category by either the *ICD* or *DSM* series.

Official Definition in 1980: *DSM-III*

In 1980 the *DSM-III* differentiated, in principle, two distinct types of PDDs based on the time of onset: (1) prior to 30 months of age or (2) after 30 months and before 12 years of age. The later onset was defined as less severe. Within each type, two distinct levels of severity were distinguished, followed by a still less severe "miscellaneous" class. The last group would account for any other cases that could not better be placed in some other *DSM-III* category or a subcategory under the PDDs.

Along with infantile autism, the *DSM-III* task force included four other diagnoses: (1) infantile autism, residual state; (2) childhood onset pervasive developmental disorder; (3) childhood onset pervasive developmental disorder, residual state; and (4) atypical pervasive developmental disorder. It is necessary to consider the criteria for each of these classifications to see how the definition of autism was evolving toward the current view of autism as a "spectrum disorder" (National Institute of Mental Health, 2008 ●).

The central and most severe of the PDDs, according to *DSM-III*, was infantile autism, whose diagnosis required five positive features and could not include any of the hallmark symptoms of schizophrenia. Specifically, this diagnosis required the "absence of delusions, hallucinations, loosening of associations, and incoherence" (APA, 1980, p. 90). Its presented features had to include the following:

- Onset before 30 months
- Pervasive lack of responsiveness to other people (autism)
- Gross deficits in language development
- If speech is present, peculiar speech patterns such as delayed echolalia, metaphorical language, or pronominal reversal
- Bizarre response to various aspects of the environment (e.g., resistance to change, peculiar interest in or attachments to animate or inanimate objects) (APA, 1980, pp. 89–90)

If the person being diagnosed once had an illness that met the criteria for infantile autism but at the time of diagnosis "no longer meets the full criteria" but still has persistent "signs of the illness" such as "oddities of communication and social awkwardness," then "infantile autism, residual state" should be diagnosed. Clearly, this category represents a less severe form of infantile autism, implying a partial recovery. However, the *DSM-III* manual warned that the course of this central variety of the PDDs is chronic and that "two-thirds remain severely handicapped and unable to lead independent lives" (p. 88). The manual said of infantile autism that it is "extremely incapacitating, and special educational facilities are almost always necessary" (p. 88).

If the onset is after the age of 30 months and before 12 years, the individual should be diagnosed with childhood-onset pervasive developmental disorder if the symptoms include "gross and sustained impairment in social relationships" plus at least three symptoms from the following: "(1) sudden excessive anxiety . . . ; (2) constricted or inappropriate affect . . . ; (3) resistance to change . . . ; (4) oddities of motor movement, such as peculiar posturing, peculiar hand or finger movements, walking on tiptoe; (5) abnormalities of speech, such as question-like melody, monotonous voice; (6) hyper- or hypo-sensitivity to sensory stimuli . . . ; (7) self mutilation, e.g., biting or hitting self, head banging"; and absence of schizophrenic symptoms. This level of PDD is seemingly less severe than infantile autism but may not be less severe than "infantile autism, residual state."

Next, if the child "once had an illness that met the criteria for childhood onset pervasive developmental disorder" but "no longer meets the full criteria" though some symptoms such as "oddities of communication and social awkwardness" persist, the diagnosis should be "childhood onset pervasive developmental disorder, residual state." The latter category would seem to correspond well to what is diagnosed currently as Asperger syndrome.

Finally, if "distortions in the development of multiple basic psychological functions that are involved in the development of social skills and language and that cannot be classified as either Infantile Autism or Childhood Onset Pervasive Developmental Disorder" are observed, the diagnosis should be "atypical pervasive developmental disorder."

Thus *DSM-III* provided five subcategories of decreasing severity under the heading of PDDs, with infantile autism of the Kanner type at the core. It also differentiated infantile autism from "schizophrenia occurring in childhood," which it asserted was characterized by "hallucinations, delusions, and loosening of associations or incoherence" (APA, 1980, p. 89), none of which was present in infantile autism. The research shows that such **psychotic symptoms** are rarely, if ever, associated with autism. Nevertheless, until 1979, the *Journal of Autism and Developmental Disorders* was known as the *Journal of Autism and Childhood Schizophrenia*. In 1979, the name of that journal, which had been established in 1971, would be changed to its current title: *Journal of Autism and Developmental Disorders*. Almost three decades after its name change, the journal still identifies both autism and childhood schizophrenia as being among the "severe psychopathologies in childhood" to which the journal is devoted (Springer, 2009 ●).

From *ICD-8* (published in 1968) forward, as noted by Spitzer (1980), there was a greater effort within the World Health Organization and the American Psychiatric Association to coordinate their diagnostic classifications. Reflecting their continuing cooperation, the whole chapter on mental disorders from *ICD-9* is reprinted in *DSM-III* as Appendix D (APA, 1980, pp. 422–423). There we see that "childhood autism," "infantile psychosis," and "Kanner's syndrome" are all listed as synonyms of "infantile autism," which in turn is distinguished from "disintegrative psychosis" (also known as **Heller's syndrome** and disintegrative childhood disorder) and from "schizophrenic syndrome of childhood" (childhood schizophrenia).

Thus the criteria for infantile autism, as laid down by Kanner (1943, 1944, 1946, 1949), stood essentially unchanged from 1943 to 1980. Autism was not included as a disorder in either *DSM-I* or *DSM-II*, and neither did it appear in any of the *ICD* manuals from the first through the eighth editions. With the publication of *DSM-III* in 1980, the essential change in the definition was the addition of levels to recognize that the disorder might have later childhood onset and that it could appear in milder forms. Asperger syndrome was still not mentioned at this point. Nonetheless, the implication that autism ranges across a spectrum from relatively severe to milder cases was certainly suggested in *DSM-III*. Of course, marked differences in degrees of severity were also noted in the earliest writings by Kanner.

DSM-III-R (1987)

In 1987, a revision of the third edition of the American manual, *DSM-III*, appeared after several years of fine-tuning. The revision was known as *DSM-III-R*, where the "R" signaled the fact that the manual had been revised. The last sentence of Spitzer's "Introduction" to *DSM-III* became the opener for *DSM-III-R*. He had stressed that each edition of the manual was merely "one still frame in the ongoing process of attempting to better understand mental disorders" (Spitzer, 1980, p. 12; Spitzer & Williams, 1987, p. xvii). The purpose of the revision was to improve the "consistency, clarity, and conceptual accuracy" of the criteria as spelled out in *DSM-III-R* (Spitzer & Williams, 1987, p. xvii). The APA had always been intended to do a revision of the *DSM* to come out at about the same time as *ICD-10*, which was to appear in 1992. However, because *DSM-IV* was delayed (it did not appear in print until 1994), it was decided to do an earlier, interim revision of *DSM-III*. The question for our present purposes is, to what extent did the revision in 1987 affect the definition and diagnosis of the "autism spectrum"? In *DSM-III-R*, the PDD category was simplified to just two subclasses: autistic disorder, described as "a severe form . . . with onset in infancy or childhood" (APA, 1987, p. 38), and the catch-all term "pervasive developmental disorder not otherwise specified" (PDDNOS; p. 39).

DSM-III-R provided a menu of 16 items (criteria for diagnosis) arranged under four subheads: (A) impairment in reciprocal social interaction, (B) impairment in verbal and nonverbal communication, (C) markedly restricted repertoire of activities and interests, and (D) onset during infancy or childhood (pp. 38–39). These four subheads merely outlined the original criteria for autism as laid out by Kanner. Except for the possibility of including cases with onset after the age of 36 months, all of the criteria came from Kanner's descriptions. The authors of *DSM-III-R*, however, required the diagnostician to note whether the case involved "childhood onset (after 36 months of age)" (p. 39). Diagnosis was made if the child met any 8 of the 16 criteria, provided that at least 2 criteria under subhead (A), plus at least 1 criterion each from (B) and (C) were also present. The list of criteria under subhead (A) included the following:

1. Marked lack of awareness of the existence or feelings of others
2. No or abnormal seeking of comfort at times of distress
3. No or impaired imitation
4. No or abnormal social play
5. Gross impairment in ability to make peer friendships (p. 38)

Under subhead (B), at least one of the following criteria had to be met:

1. No mode of communication
2. Markedly abnormal nonverbal communication
3. Absence of imaginative play
4. Marked abnormalities in the production of speech
5. Marked impairment in the ability to initiate or sustain a conversation with others, despite adequate speech (pp. 38–39)

Under subhead (C), at least one of the following criteria also had to be met:

1. Stereotyped body movements
2. Persistent preoccupation with parts of objects
3. Marked distress over changes in trivial aspects of environment
4. Unreasonable insistence on following routines in precise detail
5. Markedly restricted range of interests and a preoccupation with one narrow interest (p. 39)

PDDNOS was broadly described: "qualitative impairment in the development of reciprocal social interaction and of verbal and nonverbal communication skills, but the criteria are not met for Autistic Disorder" (p. 39). Also, delusions, hallucinations, etc., which would define a psychosis are missing. The PDDNOS diagnosis may or may not involve "restricted repertoire of activities and interests" (p. 39).

Some critics have argued that *DSM-III-R* may have made the definition of autism too flexible (see Jepson & Johnson, 2007, p. 35), although it is difficult to suppose that it involved a significant broadening of the criteria that were already in place in 1980. The essential changes were to collapse the categories "infantile autism" and "childhood onset pervasive developmental disorders" into one category to be known as "autistic disorder" in *DSM-III-R* and to simply rename the miscellaneous category called "atypical pervasive developmental order" as "pervasive developmental disorder not otherwise specified."

In the general discussion of the PDDs, the new version of the *DSM* claimed that "the criteria have been revised extensively to constitute a richer clinical description of the manifestations of the disorder at different ages" (APA, 1987, p. 414). But, as before, PDDs (with autism at the center) still involve "impairment in the development of reciprocal social interaction, in the development of verbal and nonverbal communication skills, and in the development of imaginative activity. These abnormalities are not normal for any stage of development" (p. 31). The authors of *DSM-III-R* go on to distinguish the PDDs from "mental retardation (unassociated with another disorder)," which is said to involve "generalized delays in development" (p. 31). Presumably, in pointing out the delays in mental retardation, they anticipate the APA's later statement that PDDs involve "distortions or delays in . . . intellectual skills," though they note in *DSM-III-R* that PDDs carry "in most cases . . . an associated diagnosis of Mental Retardation"(p. 33), which is "most commonly in the moderate range (IQ 35–49)" (p. 35).

Other generalized features of the PDDs mentioned in *DSM-III-R* include "a markedly restricted repertoire of activities and interests, which frequently are stereotyped and repetitive" (p. 33). There are also developmental problems in the "comprehension of meaning in language and the production of speech (in addition to problems in the social use of speech for reciprocal communication); posture and movements; patterns of eating, drinking, or sleeping; and responses to sensory input" (p. 33). All these symptoms were noted by Kanner in the 1940s. Except for detailed examples (some of them also from Kanner), there is really nothing new here. We have previously noted that the references to eating and digestive problems associated with autism were mentioned by Kanner in his description of the majority of his first 11 cases in 1943. Although "abnormalities of eating, drinking, or sleeping (e.g., limiting diet to a few foods, excessive drinking of fluids, and recurrent awakening at night with rocking)" are mentioned in the *DSM-III-R*, problems in and associated with the gut are clearly just background information. Just as Kanner did, authors of the *DSM-III-R* set aside gut problems to stress those behavioral features on which the official diagnosis was based from 1943 forward. One point that is stressed in *DSM-III-R*, though it serves only to obscure the fact that mental retardation is also "pervasive" in its impact, is that the revised manual

> recognizes only one subgroup of the general category Pervasive Developmental Disorders: Autistic Disorder, also known as Infantile Autism and Kanner's syndrome. (p. 34)

This statement, and its continuation, provide the basis for the later assertion that PDDs are equivalent to what would soon come to be referred to as "autism spectrum disorders." The manual continues immediately by saying that autistic disorder

> is merely the most severe and prototypical form of the general category Pervasive Developmental Disorders. Cases that meet the general description of a Pervasive Developmental Disorder but not the specific criteria for Autistic Disorder are diagnosed as Pervasive Developmental Disorder Not Otherwise Specified (PDDNOS). (p. 34)

Interestingly, the authors of *DSM-III-R* try to predict in advance how the newly proposed categories will be distributed when applied to persons worldwide:

> Whereas in clinical settings Autistic Disorder is more commonly seen than PDDNOS, studies in England and the United States, using criteria similar to those in this manual, suggest that PDDNOS is more common than Autistic Disorder in the general population. (p. 34)

Perhaps more severe cases are more likely to be seen in clinics, but this does not account for the fact that a high proportion of cases currently being diagnosed in the United States in school-age children (see Figure 1-1) fall toward the severe end of the spectrum.

An interesting detail that appears in *DSM-III-R* is the observation that a toddler with autistic disorder may "seem to recognize his mother primarily on the basis of smell" (p. 34). In discussing abnormalities in language development, it is noted that the child may not understand "jokes, puns, and sarcasm" (p. 34). It is also said that major depression may be diagnosed later on but is "most easily recognized in people who have sufficient speech to describe symptoms accurately" (p. 35). Of course, thoughtful readers will see that this understates the case: If severe depression occurs in nonverbal children with autism, it cannot be diagnosed by the implied requirement that the nonverbal child would have to be able to describe his or her symptoms to qualify for the diagnosis. Such an understatement reminds us of other infelicities in the manual—for example, the circular statement that "abnormalities are not normal" (p. 31) and vague statements about distinctions that are made explicitly somewhere only to be explicitly contradicted somewhere else, such as the notation that mental retardation is "general" and that it pervasively affects intellectual and social abilities (p. 28 ff), even though autistic disorder is the only subgroup in the category of pervasive developmental disorders (p. 34).

DSM-IV (1994)

In 1994, with the publication of *DSM-IV*, the class of PDDs was expanded to include Asperger syndrome and Rett's disorder as subclasses along with autistic disorder and childhood disintegrative disorder (referred to as Heller's syndrome or disintegrative disorder of childhood in *DSM-III-R*). Thus the definition of what would become known as "the autism spectrum" was theoretically expanded, but the central definition of autistic disorder was actually brought back more closely in line with the way Kanner had described it originally in 1943. The new definition of autistic disorder, however, differed in important ways from Kanner's 1949 argument that it was the same as childhood schizophrenia. The authors of *DSM-IV* wrote:

> Although terms like "psychosis" and "childhood schizophrenia" were once used to refer to individuals with these conditions, there is considerable evidence to suggest that the Pervasive Developmental Disorders are distinct from Schizophrenia. (APA, 1994, p. 66)

They do allow that individuals with PDD may sometimes later be diagnosed with schizophrenia.

For autistic disorder, which remained at the center of the PDDs, the 16 criteria offered in *DSM-III-R* were tightened to a leaner 12 and the number to be met to qualify for the diagnosis was likewise pruned from 8 to 6. As a result, the ratio of required criteria to the total number in the menu was kept the same: $8/16 = 6/12 = 1/2$. However, there was a significant narrowing of the definition of autistic disorder (pp. 70–71) in the reinstatement of the criterion of early onset as originally set out by Kanner (1943) for "early infantile autism." The *DSM-IV* requires "abnormal functioning" in "social interaction," "language as used in social communication," or "symbolic or imaginative play" with "onset prior to age 3 years" (APA, 1994, p. 71).

As in *DSM-III-R*, "impairment in social interaction" remained the most important defining trait, with the manual requiring that two of the following criteria be met to warrant a diagnosis of autistic disorder:

1. Marked impairment in the use of multiple nonverbal behaviors
2. Failure to develop peer relationships appropriate to developmental level
3. A lack of spontaneous seeking to share enjoyment, interests, or achievements with other people
4. Lack of social or emotional reciprocity (p. 70)

Under "impairments in communication," at least one of the following criteria had to be met:

1. Delay in, or total lack of the development of, spoken language
2. In individuals with adequate speech, marked impairment in ability to initiate or sustain a conversation with others
3. Stereotyped and repetitive use of language or idiosyncratic language
4. Lack of varied, spontaneous make-believe play or social imitative play appropriate to developmental level (p. 70)

Finally, under "restricted repetitive and stereotyped patterns of behavior, interests, and activities," at least one of the following criteria must be met:

1. Encompassing preoccupation with one or more stereotyped and restricted patterns of interest that is abnormal either in intensity or focus
2. Apparently inflexible adherence to specific, nonfunctional routines or rituals
3. Stereotyped and repetitive motor mannerisms
4. Persistent preoccupation with parts of objects (p. 71)

According to the authors of *DSM-IV*, "Autistic Disorder must be differentiated from *other pervasive developmental disorders*" (p. 69), Rett's disorder, childhood disintegrative disorder (formerly known as Heller's syndrome, **dementia infantilis**, and **disintegrative psychosis**), and Asperger's disorder (also known as Asperger syndrome).

In particular, Rett's disorder is to be distinguished partly by the fact that it is seen almost exclusively in females; males with the condition rarely survive to term. Rett's disorder also involves "head growth deceleration, loss of acquired purposeful hand skills and the appearance of poorly coordinated gait or trunk movements," and "difficulties in social interaction" (p. 69). The communication difficulties associated with Rett's disorder, as described by the *DSM-IV*, are supposedly distinct from autistic disorder in that the difficulties in Rett's disorder are "transient" (p. 69). Childhood disintegrative disorder is distinguished (as noted in both *DSM-III* and *DSM-III-R*) in that it is preceded by normal development up to two years, after which "a distinctive pattern of developmental regression" occurs. The only defining trait for Asperger's disorder is "the lack of delay in language development." The *DSM-IV* manual explicitly admonishes that "Asperger's Disorder is not diagnosed if criteria are met for Autistic Disorder" (p. 69).

For any diagnosis that does not fit the latter categories and that does not meet all the criteria for autistic disorder or some other defined disorder, the *DSM-IV* recommended the catch-all diagnosis of PDDNOS (pp. 77–78). This label is a miscellaneous category that accounts for cases meeting some (but not all) of the criteria for autistic disorder and yet not qualifying for any of the other four PDD categories. PDDNOS is commonly referred to as "atypical autism," where some of the symptoms are less severe and/or there is late onset (after the age of three years).

The description of Asperger's disorder in *DSM-IV* is interesting, especially in view of the controversy that persisted at least from the 1970s to the present concerning whether it is possible to distinguish Asperger's disorder from what came to be called "high-functioning autism" (HFA). Certainly, the original cases described by Asperger himself in 1944, in the final analysis, would be judged to be at the less severe end of the autism spectrum. That spectrum would be regarded as incompletely described in 1994 when the *DSM-IV* was published, but would include five subcategories. At its center, of course, was autistic disorder; on the periphery was the catch-all category PDDNOS (which had first appeared in *DSM-III-R* and in *DSM-III* was called atypical pervasive developmental disorder, and which now was said to include atypical autism). In addition to these first two categories there were three more: childhood disintegrative disorder (CDD) and the newly added categories of Rett's disorder and Asperger's disorder.

Diagnosed cases within two of these categories—CDD and Rett's disorder—remain extremely rare, so the debate about the broadening definition of autism as causing an illusory epidemic would depend greatly on whether the addition of Asperger syndrome could account for the upsurge in the number of cases depicted in Figure 1-1. Did the addition of Asperger's disorder in *DSM-IV* increase the scope of the prior definition from *DSM-III* and *DSM-III-R*? Is Asperger's disorder qualitatively distinct from the Kanner type of autism? Also, is it actually possible to distinguish cases diagnosed as Asperger syndrome from cases diagnosed with mild autism or HFA?

The fact that Kanner-type autism and Asperger syndrome are qualitatively similar was made clear by Kanner himself in 1956. When he teamed up with Eisenberg to describe the history of autism from 1943 to 1955, the pair actually wanted to limit the definition of autism to the very ones that the APA would use in 1994 when defining Asperger's disorder in *DSM-IV*. The same definition for Asperger's disorder would be kept in *DSM-IV-TR* (where the "TR" stands for "text revision"), which was published in 2000.

In the meantime, the *ICD* manual of the World Health Organization from 1968 forward was increasingly based on the APA's *DSM* series. As a result, the determination of whether the autism epidemic could be caused by a broadening definition depends largely on the role of Asperger's disorder. To see the extent to which this addition changed the definition, we need to consider the *DSM-IV-TR* manual, which appeared in 2000.

Transition to *DSM-IV-TR* (2000)

The diagnostic criteria for Asperger's disorder, as set down in *DSM-IV*, were kept in place in *DSM-IV-TR*. The only changes from *DSM-IV* to *DSM-IV-TR* involved fine points and a few nuanced distinctions that are mentioned in Appendix D of the 2000 edition (APA, 2000–2008, pp. 829–830). For instance, the requirement for PDDNOS was narrowed by specifying that difficulties must be evident in at least two (not merely one) of the major categories of criteria for autistic disorder—namely, social interaction, communication, and/or stereotyped behaviors. This change was made "to correct an error" (p. 830). It was newly noted that "some cases of Rett's Disorder are associated with a specific genetic mutation" (p. 830). In the discussion of autistic disorder, it was noted that "recent studies suggest a higher prevalence" and that "pragmatic aspects of language" have been highlighted to improve "assessment of higher-functioning individuals" (p. 830).

This last comment is interesting in view of the fact that it is at that higher level of functioning where the greatest difficulty has been encountered in differentiating autism from Asperger syndrome (Pomeroy, Friedman, & Stephens, 1991; Van Krevelen, 1971; Wing, 1981a; Wolff & Barlow, 1979). Concerning the distinction between autistic disorder and Asperger's disorder, the authors of the *DSM-IV-TR* write:

> [T]ext has been added to clarify the requirement for no clinical delays in language does not imply that individuals with Asperger's Disorder have no problems with communication. (p. 830)

The question that arises is whether the distinction has been successful. Is Asperger's disorder sufficiently different from HFA so that adding Asperger's disorder to the mix actually has the effect of greatly broadening the whole spectrum?

In fact, the criteria for Asperger's disorder in *DSM-IV* and *DSM-IV-TR* were exactly in line with the 1956 recommendation of Kanner and Eisenberg for defining the whole scope of autism. Nearly 38 years before the publication of *DSM-IV* and 44 years before the publication of *DSM-IV-TR*, they had insisted that the definition of autism needed to emphasize the importance of social relations and repetitive behaviors while minimizing the mention of language. Kanner and Eisenberg seem to have supposed that the manifestation of symptoms pertaining to social interaction and stereotyped behaviors was so completely intertwined with linguistic evidence (or lack thereof) that it was unnecessary to stress the linguistic symptoms to define the autism spectrum.

In fact, the authors of *DSM-IV* and *DSM-IV-TR*—unintentionally, it seems—took the advice of Kanner and Eisenberg (1956) not in defining autism, but rather in differentiating it from Asperger's disorder, which they were adding to the mix. To accomplish this, when adding Asperger's disorder officially to the autism spectrum, the authors of *DSM-IV* and *DSM-IV-TR* copied exactly, word for word, their own diagnostic criteria for autistic disorder under the headings of "social interaction" and "restricted repetitive and stereotyped patterns of behavior, interests, and activities," and simply applied these criteria as the main defining elements of Asperger's disorder. (Compare pages 70–71 and 77 of *DSM-IV* and page 75 of *DSM-IV-TR* with page 84.) In doing so, they merely omitted from the requirements for a diagnosis of Asperger's disorder the criteria pertaining to language development under the rubric of autistic disorder. In view of the fact that any person meeting the criteria for the newly defined Asperger's disorder would also qualify for a diagnosis under PDDNOS, it is difficult to see how the addition could possibly broaden the spectrum. On the contrary, the guidelines in *DSM-IV-TR* narrow the spectrum slightly, by requiring that qualification for a diagnosis of PDDNOS calls for symptoms in at least two of the three main sets of criteria for autistic disorder.

With respect to Asperger's disorder, the system of diagnostic criteria remained identical from *DSM-IV* to *DSM-IV-TR*, with the exception that the slightly more than two page description for Asperger's disorder in the *DSM-IV* (pp. 75–77) would be amplified to almost five pages in *DSM-IV-TR* (pp. 80–84). However, the criteria for the diagnosis of Asperger's disorder would remain the same from *DSM-IV* in 1994 to *DSM-IV-TR* in 2000. The latter manual also noted:

> Although the social deficit in Asperger's Disorder is severe and is defined in the same way as in Autistic Disorder, the lack of social reciprocity is more typically manifest by an eccentric and one-sided social approach to others (e.g., pursuing a conversational topic regardless of other's reactions) rather than social and emotional indifference. (APA, 2000–2008, p. 80)

According to *DSM-IV-TR*, a diagnosis of Asperger's disorder was appropriate when the patient had at least two of the symptoms listed under "social interaction" (making it the primary defining element) plus at least one of the symptoms described under "restricted repetitive and stereotyped patterns of behavior, interests, and activities" (APA, 1994, p. 77).

Furthermore, the diagnosis of Asperger's disorder, according to *DSM-IV-TR*, has some additional requirements to differentiate it from autistic disorder. These include the requirement that "the disturbance causes clinically significant impairment in social, occupational, or other important areas of functioning." Three exclusions are specified:

- [T]here is no clinically significant delay in language (e.g., single words used by age 2 years, communicative phrases used by age 3 years);
- [N]o clinically significant delay in cognitive development or in the development of age-appropriate self-help skills, adaptive behavior (other than in social interaction), and curiosity about the environment in childhood; . . .
- [C]riteria are not met for another Pervasive Developmental Disorder or Schizophrenia. (APA, 1994, p. 77)

COULD THE AUTISM EPIDEMIC BE IMAGINED?

With the foregoing discussion of the discovery, diagnosis, and definition of the autism spectrum in mind, we come next to the various theories that have been put forward to explain what appears to be an autism epidemic. Is the apparent epidemic just a mistaken perception of the increased number of diagnoses that are being made? Are the diagnoses attributable to increasing incidence of the disorder, or does some other explanation apply? In this section, we explore the various theories that have been proposed to explain away the epidemic.

The Theory of the Broadening Definition

The idea that the upsurge in diagnosed cases of autism could be explained by the broadened definition of autism has been advocated by some impressive researchers and authorities. For instance, Eric Fombonne, a world-renowned epidemiologist specializing in autism, has subscribed to that theory (Fombonne, 1996, 1999, 2003a, 2003b, 2008), along with Christopher Gillberg and colleagues (Gillberg, 1999; Gillberg et al., 2006; Posserud et al., 2006), and many other advocates of this position could be mentioned as well. The question is whether the theory of broadening criteria is valid.

Looking back over the history of the discovery, definition, and diagnosis of autism from 1943 forward, it is clear that the disorder has always involved three major kinds of symptoms: (1) impaired social interaction; (2) distortions in communication and language development; and (3) repetitive "stereotyped" behaviors, routines, narrowed interests, and what Kanner termed "an obsessive desire for the preservation of sameness" (1949, p. 416). The exemplary cases Kanner described in 1943 would define the range of symptoms right up to the present time. A summary of the *DSM-IV* description, which is echoed in *DSM-IV-TR*, describes the autism spectrum (alias the PDDs) in the following terms:

> severe and pervasive impairment in several areas of development: reciprocal social interaction skills, communication skills, or the presence of stereotyped behavior, interests, and activities. The qualitative impairments that define these conditions are distinctly deviant relative to the individual's developmental level or mental age. . . . (p. 65)

So how much of the increase in the rate of diagnosis of autism can be attributed to the theory of broadening criteria? The major change points can be narrowed to the years of 1987 and 1994. There was also a minor adjustment in 2000 that can be examined as well. Fortunately, we have sufficient data to examine each of these supposed change points—especially the dramatic changes of 1987 and 1994, in order to assess the validity of the broadening criteria theory as an explanation of the continuing upsurge in diagnosed cases of autism.

From 1943 until 1980, when the first official definition appeared for pervasive developmental disorders, there was essentially no change in the definition of autism. In any event, hardly any reliable statistical data (certainly not of an epidemiological kind) are available prior to 1980. After that point, infantile autism was defined as the essential core of the PDD category in *DSM-III*. In that publication, infantile autism was regarded as synonymous with childhood autism, infantile psychosis, and Kanner's syndrome and was grouped alongside but supposedly distinguished from other PDDs known as disintegrative psychosis (also known as Heller's syndrome and disintegrative childhood disorder) and from schizophrenic syndrome of childhood (childhood schizophrenia). Recall that Kanner insisted in 1949 that early infantile autism was indistinguishable from schizophrenia with a very early onset, even at the diaper stage. However, authors of the *DSM* series would consistently demand differentiation of the PDDs on the theory that each of the subcategories was distinct from the others (synonymous ones, of course, having supposedly been excluded).

In spite of the statements that the various categories under PDD must be sharply differentiated (e.g., in *DSM-IV*, p. 69, and in *DSM-IV-TR*, pp. 82–83), the entire class of pervasive developmental disorders (PDDs) would come to be commonly referred to as the autism spectrum disorders (ASDs). For instance, the National Institute of Mental Health's (NIMH) Web site on autism asserts that "the five pervasive developmental disorders"—autistic disorder, Rett's syndrome, childhood disintegrative disorder, Asperger syndrome, and pervasive developmental disorder not otherwise specified—are collectively "more often referred to today as autism spectrum disorders" (NIMH, 2008 ●). It is unsurprising that PDDs would be equated with ASDs in view of the centrality of the criteria for autism in the definition of the whole spectrum from 1980 forward. Prior to that time, as we have already documented, Kanner's original criteria prevailed.

In 1987, the categories of infantile autism and childhood-onset pervasive developmental disorders were collapsed into a single diagnosis, autistic disorder. In addition, atypical pervasive developmental disorder was renamed pervasive developmental disorder not otherwise specified. Although it is true that the criteria for the diagnosis of autistic disorder were elaborated by 16 descriptors, it is difficult to see the autism spectrum as having been broadened. Although there was essentially nothing new in the descriptors (they closely matched the descriptions of exemplary cases given by Kanner and Asperger), the nature of the disorder should have been clarified and, therefore, defined more sharply and distinctly. If that were the case, we should expect a reduction in the number of false diagnoses of PDDs in the year following the publication of the clarified system. The authors

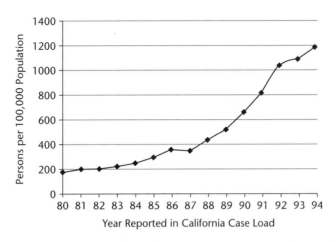

Figure 2-3 Cases of autism reported in California from 1980 to 1994. Data from an internal email between Diane Simpson and Larry Pickering at the CDC on June 11, 2001.
Source: Lisa Handley and J. B. Handley under the Freedom of Information Act, retrieved January 24, 2009, from http://www.putchildrenfirst.org/chapter4.html.

of *DSM-III-R* did say that it was their purpose in doing the revision to enhance "consistency, clarity, and conceptual accuracy" (APA, 1987, p. xvii). Conversely, if one were to suppose (falsely, we believe) that the definition of autism was broadened in 1987, then a sudden upsurge in diagnosed cases, which then leveled off in the following years, should be predicted.

Fortunately, we have some data from the most populous state in the union—California—that are directly relevant to the question at hand. Figure 2-3 shows the number of persons per 100,000 diagnosed with autism and listed in the California case load from 1980 through 1994. If the changed definition in 1987 explained the observed growth, we would expect to see an approximately flat line from 1980 until 1987 (a period during which the definition did not change), rising sharply after the definition was supposedly broadened and then leveling off within a year or two until the next major revision of the *DSM* was published in 1994. Conversely, if the criteria were sharpened and made more accurate, thereby eliminating diagnoses of autism that should have been called something else, the line should dip after 1987 and then level off. In fact, it does neither.

Figure 2-4 shows the first of the predicted patterns consistent with a broadening of the autism definition. The expected growth line is superimposed as a dotted line in the graph. The actual data, however, do not fit that prediction. Likewise, they do not fit with the notion that a sharpening of the definition would result in a downturn due to a reduction in the number of false diagnoses of autism. Thus it does not appear that changes in the definition are driving the growth curve at all. The continuing upsurge in the number of diagnosed cases of autism must have some other basis.

The data come very near fitting an exponential growth curve as shown in the solid line superimposed in Figure 2-4. Our readers can obviously judge for themselves, but it appears to us that the smooth growth curve is a better fit for the actually reported California data (per internal memos and at least one published study in *JAMA*; see Dales, Hammer, & Smith, 2001) than the sort of picture suggested by the theory of broadening criteria. A smooth growth curve, as shown earlier in Figure 1-1 (Chapter 1), which is based on national data, is quite incompatible with the theory that the increasing number of diagnosed cases is being produced by intermittent broadening of the definition of autism. In fact, as we have shown from the only authoritative documents, the definition was hardly changed from 1943 until 1980 and was adjusted very little, perhaps by restricting it, in 1987. However, any impact of the changes in the definition of autism that took place in 1987 seems to have been swallowed up in a growth trend that has some other driving force.

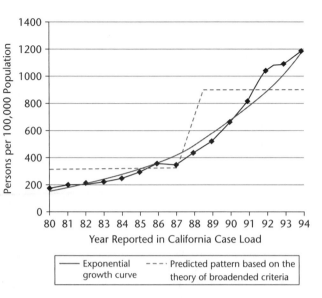

Figure 2-4 The growth pattern predicted on the basis of the theory of broadened criteria in the dotted line, the pattern actually observed in the thin line connecting the diamonds representing data points, and an exponential growth curve supplied by Microsoft's graphing program.
Source: Lisa Handley and J. B. Handley under the Freedom of Information Act, retrieved January 24, 2009, from http://www.putchildrenfirst.org/chapter4.html.

With that point in mind, we look next to see how the theory of broadening criteria fares with respect to the overhaul of the *DSM* definition that took place in 1994 with the publication of *DSM-IV*. The main change in 1994 was the addition of Asperger's disorder to the umbrella category of PDDs. In that year, the subcategory of Rett's syndrome was added. It cannot have affected the big picture very much, however, because Rett's syndrome is so rare. The other categories (autistic disorder, childhood disintegrative disorder, and PDDNOS) were not changed much.

In the 2000 text revision (*DSM-IV-TR*), it was noted that a certain "error" was corrected. The error of *DSM-IV* was to allow a person with symptoms in only one of the three major classes of criteria defining autism (i.e., social impairments, communication deficits, or repetitive behaviors) to be diagnosed with PDDNOS. Thus, in 2000, the criteria for the spectrum were slightly narrowed by requiring symptoms in more than one of the major classes to qualify an individual as having PDDNOS. Following that change to its logical conclusion, according to the view espoused by advocates of the theory that definitions are driving the upsurge and creating an illusion of an epidemic, the inclusion of Asperger's and Rett's disorders, along with the "error" of only one kind of symptom for inclusion in PDDNOS (also known as atypical autism; APA, 2000–2008, p. 84), ought to lead to a growth spike in the number of diagnosed cases in the years following 1994. Similarly, because the narrowing of the PDDNOS category was the only significant change made in *DSM-IV-TR*, if that singular change in the diagnostic criteria for PDDs in 2000 were to have any impact, it should show up as a downturn in the number of diagnosed cases in 2001. In reality, neither of these predictions was borne out.

Interestingly, the claim that broadening of criteria in 1994, especially the inclusion of Asperger's syndrome, would produce notable growth in the number of diagnosed cases of autism, can be tested by looking at the national statistics reported in Figure 1-1. If the theory that broadening the criteria (to include Asperger's and Rett's disorders) caused an illusory epidemic were valid, then the growth pattern should look like the dotted line of Figure 2-4. When we superimpose such a line on the data from Figure 1-1 (as is done in Figure 2-5), however, the dotted line does not agree at all with the actual data. Not only is there no spike in 1994, but, in fact, there is not even a detectable blip. On

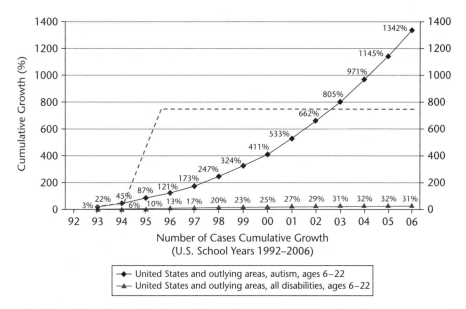

Figure 2-5 The dotted line shows the expected growth curve if the broadened criteria theory of the autism epidemic were correct.
Source: Retrieved February 11, 2008, from http://www.fightingautism.org/idea/autism.php? The original graph is licensed under a Creative Commons Attribution 1.0 Generic License, retrieved June 15, 2009, from http://creativecommons.org/licenses/by/1.0/. It is adapted, modified, and reprinted with the permission of Thoughtful House.

the contrary, the growth trend from 1993 to 2006 appears as a smooth exponential curve of the sort we added to Figure 2-4. Also, there is no dip in the line in 2001, as might be expected from the narrowing of the catch-all category of PDDNOS that took place in the 2000 text revision, in *DSM-IV-TR*. On the contrary, the growth curve seems completely unaffected by any adjustment in the definition either in 1994 or in 2000.

The Theory of Awareness: Better Detection and Diagnosis

The idea of what we will call the "awareness theory" is that more public awareness about the nature of autism could lead to better detection and diagnosis. In turn, awareness leading to keener observations could produce the illusion of an autism epidemic. This form of the awareness theory is fully accepted and advocated by Gernsbacher, Dawson, and Goldsmith (2005). It is referred to, but not accepted by, Newschaffer (2006).

This theory must be considered, keeping the background work on the theory of broadening criteria in mind. After considering the awareness theory as a possible driving force—perhaps the primary one—in the upsurge in diagnoses of autism, we will go on to consider three other theories that both Gernsbacher et al. and Newschaffer alluded to: (1) the substitution theory, which claims that the epidemic consists of diagnostic substitution of autism for some prior diagnosis; (2) the intellectual diversity theory, which states that autism is a form of diversity, even giftedness; and (3) the notion that the whole story of autism may turn out to be a genetic one. All of these theories have a common aim—namely, reaching the conclusion that there is no autism epidemic. The question is whether any one or some combination of them may be valid.

We have seen that the broadening definition theory does not fit the historical facts or the empirical evidence. Next we examine the awareness theory.

It is certainly true that public awareness of autism and other PDDs has increased. The release of movies such as *Rain Man* in 1988 and other films with autism in their story line may have been partly responsible for the upsurge in the diagnosis of autism. Of course, the popularity of such films may also demonstrate that consumers are interested in autism because increasing numbers of children are being affected by it. Films featuring autism have included the following releases:

- *Backstreet Dreams* (1990), with Brooke Shields
- *House of Cards* (1993), with Kathleen Turner and Tommy Lee Jones
- *Forrest Gump* (1994), with Tom Hanks, Robin Wright Penn, Gary Sinise, Mykelti Williamson, and Sally Field
- *Mercury Rising* (1998), with Bruce Willis, Alec Baldwin, Miko Hughes, and Kelley Hazen
- *Snow Cake* (2006), with Sigourney Weaver and Alan Rickman

Earlier films with autism as a thematic element did not garner nearly as much public interest. For instance, the 1969 movie *Change of Habit* starred Elvis Presley, Mary Tyler Moore, Barbara McNair, and Ed Asner. The French film, *L'enfant sauvage* (1969), focused on Victor, also known as the "The Wild Boy of Aveyron." The real child on whom the story was based was found living in the woods near Aveyron, France, in 1799 and may have been the earliest described case of autism (Lane, 1978). It is supposed that the parents of the child may have abandoned him in desperation.

In the last several years, novels also have incorporated the theme of autism, including the following works: John Dunning, *The Sign of the Book* (2005); Mark Haddon (diagnosed with Asperger syndrome himself), *The Curious Case of the Dog in the Night-time* (2003); Anne Bauer, *Wild Ride Up the Cupboards* (2005 ●); Marty Leimbach, *Daniel Isn't Talking* (2006; see Talese, 2009, for a review and comments ●); and Cammie McGovern, *Eye Contact* (2006). Someone has suggested that fictional stories written by parents of children with autism involve "autistic license," which we take to mean that only some of that fictional material is true to life, and some of it is just made up.

When people get to know individuals dealing with autism, all of them are motivated. Consider the story of Jason McElwain, a high school senior with HFA who had never been in a varsity game in his life, yet played four minutes in his team's last basketball game of the season (McElwain, 2006 ●). Jason had been a team helper but not a player until March 4, 2006. His friends showed up at the game, knowing the coach intended to let him suit up and play. They made signs with his picture to support him. Finally, Jason's coach decided it was time to let him play. The coach later explained what he was thinking when Jason first got the ball: "Oh please, Lord, just get him a basket." Jason missed a long shot and then a lay-up—but then hit one two-pointer plus six three-point shots in a row. He matched the team record for three-pointers in a single game while playing only four minutes. Jason made national news and even got to meet then President George W. Bush. Was the enthusiasm for his story reflective of the rising public awareness about autism? Would it have made the news if people were not already especially interested in autism?

According to the public awareness theory, there is no autism epidemic, just an increase in the number of cases that are being discovered and diagnosed. This theory claims that a sharpened understanding of the autism spectrum has produced the illusion of an epidemic. Proponents of this view suppose that the new cases of autism that are now being diagnosed in ever-increasing numbers have been there all along, but were just not being noticed until recently. In other words, greater public and professional awareness of what to look for are seen as causing a real increase in the number of persons being diagnosed, even though there has actually been no change in the actual prevalence of the disorder. According to this theory, it is not autism that is increasing, but rather its diagnosis. The awareness theory is often combined with the theory of the broadening definition.

For example, Gernsbacher, Dawson, and Goldsmith (2005) subscribe to the theory of "broadened diagnostic criteria, coupled with deliberately greater public awareness and intentionally improved case finding" (p. 55), to argue that the autism epidemic is not real. They suppose that the prevalence of autism (i.e., the proportion of cases in any sizable sample of the world's population) has always been much higher than the number of cases that have actually been diagnosed at any given time. Their idea about a relatively unchanging prevalence was foreshadowed by Kanner (1949), who identified early infantile autism in conjunction with childhood schizophrenia and then went on to say that this childhood form "is not so rare as was believed as recently as twenty years ago" (p. 421).

Could increased public awareness have created the illusion of an autism epidemic? Has the prevalence remained the same over the decades since 1943, and even before then? DeNoon (2005 ◉) argues that it was the passing of the Individuals with Disabilities Education Act (IDEA) that "assured appropriate public education for children with autism. Soon after, schools began reporting high numbers of students with autism." Although DeNoon indicates that this legislation was passed in 1991, IDEA was actually enacted in 1990. In addition, data pertaining to it generally date back to the much earlier Public Law 94–142, which was passed in 1975 (U.S. Office of Special Education Programs, 2000 ◉). The use of the acronym "IDEA" was extended retrospectively to include the Education of All Handicapped Children Act of 1975 (EHA). The IDEA legislation of 1990 (PL 101–476), which was also known as the Education of the Handicapped Act Amendments of 1990, was the precursor to the more expansive IDEA law enacted in 1997. It collected prior laws pertaining to persons with disabilities beginning with Public Law 94–142, the original EHA, and its amendments (especially PL 99–457) under the new name of IDEA. Setting the historical inaccuracy of DeNoon's summary to one side, let's consider the argument he attributes to Gernsbacher regarding public awareness and the reporting of increasing numbers of cases of autism under the IDEA law.

Gernsbacher is quoted as saying that reporting "high numbers of students with autism . . . doesn't mean there's an autism epidemic . . . any more than increased sales of petite clothing means women are getting smaller." She continues with her analogy:

> My hunch is that if we looked at the production and purchase of petite-sized clothing we'd see a greatly increasing trend in the number of petite-sized garments produced and purchased over the past two decades. Should we therefore conclude that U.S. women are getting increasingly more petite? Probably not. There was probably always a contingent of petite-sized women, and their needs are being increasingly better met. (DeNoon, 2005 ◉)

Translating this analogy back to the autism epidemic, Gernsbacher's argument is that just because more individuals are being diagnosed with autism does not mean that autism is becoming more common. Her theory is that the number of individuals who actually have autism has not changed since Kanner's time; there have just been huge numbers of individuals who were not previously diagnosed.

We can test Gernsbacher's argument against the data summed up in Figure 2-4. If her proposal were correct, there should have been a sudden upsurge in the number of diagnosed cases of autism soon after 1990, when IDEA was enacted. However, this supposition is not consistent with the IDEA data in Figure 2-4 covering the years from 1980 until 1994: There is no sudden increase in the growth pattern in the years following 1990; specifically, there is no dramatic additional acceleration of the rate of growth in 1991–1994. On the contrary, there seems to have been a slight deceleration in the general upward trend during this period. Also, the notion that IDEA could be driving the exponential growth curve associated with the autism epidemic does not explain the prior growth in diagnosed cases from 1980 to 1994. Thus the theory of Gernsbacher and colleagues appears to be inconsistent with the documented growth curve.

Next, we return to the historical inaccuracy of Gernsbacher's argument. Her reference to the law is not correct. In fact, the supposed guarantee of a "free and appropriate public education" (FAPE) for persons with disabilities was first enacted in 1975 under the Education for All Handicapped Children Act, also known as Public Law 94–142 (these laws are linked on the DVD 💿). It was this act that first mandated an "individualized education program" from which the California case loads for autism could be determined for the years covered in Figures 1-1, 2-3, 2-4, and 2-5. The original EHA of 1975 was subsequently carried forward in the Americans with Disabilities Act of 1990 (ADA) and, more comprehensively, when the same law was reenacted, expanded, and renamed as the Individuals with Disabilities Education Act of 1990 (PL 101–476), also known as the Education of the Handicapped Act Amendments of 1990.

The whole system of legislation pertaining to this field would be expanded in 1997 and yet again in 2007. However, it was IDEA 1990 that first collected the prior laws pertaining to persons with disabilities from PL 94–142, the original EHA, and its amendments, especially PL 99–457, under the new name of IDEA (for further discussion of the laws and pertinent cases, see J. W. Oller et al., 2010). The data presented in the figures in this chapter are based on the IDEA legislation from 1975 (U.S. Office of Special Education Programs, 2000 💿).

The theory that public awareness has brought about better detection and diagnosis, thereby leading to an illusory autism epidemic, also runs afoul of two other problems. One of the critical empirical problems is that the public awareness theory cannot possibly account for the increasing number of cases diagnosed at the severe end of the spectrum. Among the cases that are being newly diagnosed within a few years of birth, many are severe—and that number is both substantial and growing. Those severe cases present a peculiar problem for the theory that increased public awareness has created the illusion of an autism epidemic.

According to *DSM-III*, which presented the first official description of autism, pervasive developmental disorder—the autism spectrum with "infantile autism" at its center—is "extremely incapacitating, and special educational facilities are almost always necessary" (p. 88). *DSM-III* (APA, 1980) noted that, of all patients with this disorder, "two-thirds remain severely handicapped and unable to lead independent lives" (p. 88). If 66% of all the cases being diagnosed are *that severe*, how could such an incapacitating condition be overlooked in thousands of undiagnosed cases? The fact that the majority of cases being diagnosed under *DSM-III* from 1980 forward were described as incapable of independent survival was consistent with *DSM-III-R*, which noted that PDDs carry "in most cases . . . an associated diagnosis of mental retardation" (APA, 1987, p. 33) that is "most commonly in the moderate range (IQ 35–49)" (p. 35). Likewise, *DSM-III-R* stated that "manifestations are, in almost all cases, lifelong . . . a small minority [surely less than one-third] are able to lead independent lives" (p. 36). Similarly, *DSM-IV* describes the whole autism spectrum (alias the PDDs) as involving "severe and pervasive impairment . . . distinctly deviant relative to the individual's developmental level or mental age" (APA, 1994, p. 65). That description was repeated verbatim in *DSM-IV-TR* (APA, 2000–2008, p. 69). Both *DSM-IV* and *DSM-IV-TR* acknowledge that the condition is often accompanied by mental retardation, and both manuals use the same words in describing autistic disorder as preventing all but "a small percentage of adults" from going on "to live and work independently" (APA, 1994, p. 69; APA 2000–2008, p. 73). Both agree with the 1980 description that only in "about one-third of cases, some degree of partial independence is possible" (APA, 1994, p. 69; APA, 2000–2008, p. 73). Fast forwarding to 2007, the most recently published statistics on the distribution of persons diagnosed with autism show that approximately 50% of the cases diagnosed in 2000 and 2002 were also cognitively impaired with significant intellectual disability or mental retardation (Autism Developmental Disabilities Monitoring Network, 2007, p. 20 💿). The prognosis that autism is a lifelong condition has not changed.

How could so many severe cases of autism—individuals who are "extremely incapacitated," "distinctly deviant," and unable to live and work independently—have gone unnoticed until recently? Similarly, why are we not seeing many adolescents and adults being newly diagnosed with autism? What happened to all those lifelong cases of severe autism that were not diagnosed among children in the 1940s, 1950s, and so on? Put simply, the evidence shows that the proportion of severe cases of autism remains high in the newly diagnosed children and that the huge number of overlooked adults who ought to be roaming around unable to support themselves or carry on a conversation do not exist.

If two-thirds of the individuals diagnosed with autism (PDD) from 1980 forward were supposed to remain unable to carry on an independent life, how would tens of thousands of adults grow up in such a condition without being noticed? Where are they now? The fact that tens of thousands of adults with a debilitating form of autism have not been discovered since 1980 shows that such cases probably never existed in the first place. The upshot of this analysis: The growing number of diagnosed cases of autism in successive birth cohorts that has been extensively documented (albeit imperfectly) since 1980 is probably indicative of a true autism epidemic.

The public awareness theory also faces another problem in addition to its inability to explain the exponential growth in the diagnosis of autism, and the fact that most cases since 1980 have been too severe to be overlooked in the past. Namely, it is more plausible to suppose that the growing number of children who are receiving valid diagnoses of autism is driving increasing public awareness. It is much more reasonable to suppose that movies, TV talk shows, parental concern, and the demand to know what is causing the epidemic of autism have produced the increase in public awareness, rather than the reverse. Instead of supposing that an increase in public awareness about autism is increasing prevalence by leading to more diagnoses, it is more plausible that increasing prevalence is causing greater public awareness to grow.

Finally, if education about autism, through valid descriptions about what it is and how to detect and diagnose it, is actually advancing, how could this increase in knowledge result in "better diagnosis and detection" on the one hand, while on the other hand lead to a national illusion that the disorder most grandparents had never heard of when they were children is suddenly more common than cleft lip/palate, spina bifida, childhood diabetes, or childhood cancer, which all of them had heard of two generations ago? Is it just a consensual imagination that many more children are being diagnosed with severe, nonverbal, hand-flapping, head-banging, 24/7 autism before they reach their fourth or fifth birthday? Are doctors, clinicians, and parents who know more now than ever before about autism becoming more likely to share the joint illusion of a nonexistent epidemic? Obviously, no amount of training will make the absence of language and the presence of hand-flapping and head-banging behaviors more noticeable than they already are; they are extreme indicators of pathology.

It is simpler and more reasonable to suppose that the autism epidemic is real and has driven the greater public awareness of this disorder noted in recent years. We save the best argument for last, however, because it is so widely believed.

The Theory of Diagnostic Substitution

The diagnostic substitution theory tries to explain away the autism epidemic by suggesting that administrative officials reporting data under IDEA since 1990 have been changing the diagnosis of children in special education from mental retardation and learning disability, or from some other category such as "developmental language disorder," to autism (Bishop, Whitehouse, Watt, & Line, 2008). One possible motivation for such changes, according to Shattuck (2006) and others (as implied by Fombonne, 2008), is to get more money for therapy and/or for the persons, schools, and agencies providing it. The idea that more money has been available for the autism diagnosis than for the other categories, especially mental retardation and learning disabilities, however, is not consistent with the known facts.

The problem of funding for the treatment of autism is one faced on an almost daily basis by speech-language pathologists (as confirmed by Stacy Oller, CCC-SLP). The difficulty in getting third-party entities (e.g., insurance companies) to pay for treatment of autism spectrum disorders is that payers do not authorize (without court influence) any treatment of autism because they argue that the disorder is "hopeless" (i.e., untreatable). From that point of view, parents would be better off with a diagnosis of mental retardation (which is eligible for reimbursement) than with a diagnosis of autism. Also, true to the objection of the insurance companies, behavioral therapies commonly result in only minimal, if any, improvement in individuals diagnosed with autism. As a consequence, whereas IDEA may be paying out substantial sums to provide services in schools for autism, third-party insurers are not. Thus there does not appear to be any primary monetary motivation for a mass exodus from the mental retardation category to autism.

Nevertheless, Shattuck (2006) claims that although prevalence remains unchanged for valid cases of autism, children formerly diagnosed with mental retardation or learning disability are being shifted—presumably on an arbitrary basis—to autism. Some of these changes might occur because of errors. However, the point of Shattuck and followers is not to suggest that errors are being corrected in order to move cases into a more appropriate diagnosis. Their point is rather to dismiss the national consensus of parents and many other researchers (e.g., Newschaffer, 2006; Newschaffer, Falb, & Gurney, 2005) who suppose that the number of cases of autism has actually been rising dramatically over the last three decades.

Shattuck says in the middle of his argument that "special education trends cannot substantiate or refute the presence of an actual epidemic of autism" (2006, p. 1034). Throughout his article, and in the abstract and conclusion, however, he claims plainly that there is no autism epidemic. His argument, which is supported by others following his lead (e.g., Bishop et al., 2008; Coo, Ouellette-Kuntz, Lloyd, Kasmara, Holden, & Lewis, 2007), is that individuals formerly diagnosed with mental retardation or learning disability are being reclassified as having autism. However, Newschaffer, Falb, and Gurney (2005), in looking at birth cohorts within the same data sources relied on by Shattuck (2006), found that the trend data do show "that prevalence increases within birth cohorts through age 16" (p. e278). Also, when Newschaffer (2006) reexamined the age range of 6 to 10 years used by Shattuck (2006), he concluded, "any offset by MR [mental retardation] alone would not be complete. In addition, at ages 10 and 11, autism prevalence still increases with successive birth cohorts but MR prevalence no longer decreases consistently" (p. 1436). Figure 2-6 summarizes data from IDEA reports suggesting strongly that the increasing number of diagnosed cases, as Newschaffer and colleagues have argued, is greater for younger cohorts. (A more complete, although more complex, analysis is reported by Fightingautism.org, 2009 ◐ in the last figure on the opening page of that Web site.)

Although Shattuck looked at group trends in classification in special education on a state-by-state basis, he had no actual data on individual cases. Nonetheless, his substitution theory suggests by implication that doctors are arbitrarily changing the diagnosis of many children who were formerly assigned a different diagnostic label. This follows from the fact that the diagnosis of autism has to be made by a doctor, pediatrician, neurologist, psychiatrist, or other healthcare provider in most contexts and cannot be arbitrarily made by school personnel. Additionally, studies cited by Shattuck (2006) show "that the vast majority of children reported in the special education autism category also meet case criteria for ASD" (p. 1030). Thus it would seem that any diagnostic changes that did take place should probably be attributed to the *correction of less accurate diagnoses*. However, Shattuck does not mention that possibility. Yet, the evidence that the "vast majority of children in the special education autism category" are judged to meet the criteria for that category suggests that

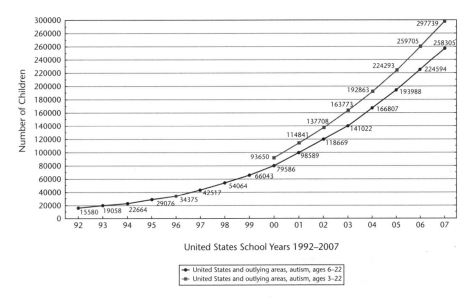

Figure 2-6 Evidence from IDEA data showing that the increase in number of diagnosed cases is greater for the younger cohorts than for older ones (for breakout by ages, see http://www.fightingautism.org/idea/autism .php? accessed May 9, 2009).
Source: Retrieved April 12, 2008, from http://www.fightingautism.org/idea/autism.php. Licensed under a Creative Commons Attribution 1.0 Generic License, retrieved June 15, 2009, from http://creativecommons .org/licenses/by/1.0/. Reprinted with the permission of Thoughtful House.

changes in diagnosis from mental retardation and learning disability to autism are probably not arbitrary, but rather are valid changes. Setting that issue to one side, the deeper question is whether Shattuck's conclusion that there is no autism epidemic is justified by his data and arguments.

In fact, Shattuck denies the possibility of his own conclusions: As we noted earlier, he says that "special education trends cannot substantiate or refute the presence of an actual epidemic of autism" (p. 1034). Nevertheless, he seems to reform this statement into a strong negative claim against any autism epidemic in his conclusion that "special education trends cannot be legitimately used to support claims of an autism epidemic" (p. 1036). In addition, Shattuck does not recognize the limitations on his analytical method or the fact that 28 states, including California, failed to show the very trend he claims as the basis for refuting the existence of an autism epidemic. Those who are counting will realize that 56% of the states Shattuck surveyed showed trends contrary to his conclusions. On the basis of relatively meager evidence of changes in diagnoses from 20 states (a minority of the whole and not including the most populous state of California), Shattuck nevertheless concludes that the autism epidemic does not exist.

Interestingly, the theories of broadening criteria and of public awareness suggest that individuals making the autism diagnosis are greatly influenced by knowing the distinctive traits and characteristics of autism. Also, Shattuck has cited research showing that the cases reported in the autism category assigned by administrative officials while reporting data under the IDEA legislation are generally correct in "the vast majority of cases" (2006, p. 1030). Thus it makes sense to suppose that the vast majority of diagnostic changes taking place are moving in the direction of more valid—not less valid— reporting. If that is the case, then it is irrelevant that cases assigned to the mental retardation and learning disability classes are diminishing, as they are in some states (certainly not in California). The only relevant question is whether the cases of autism as being reported are validly diagnosed.

Strangely, although the theory of awareness and the theory of the broadening definition try to explain away the autism epidemic by admitting that there are more valid cases of autism to be diagnosed, the diagnostic substitution theory suggests that the effects of growing awareness of autism have been overwhelmed by an arbitrary tendency to change diagnoses of mental retardation and learning disabilities to a diagnosis of autism. Of course, the definition of autism is fundamental to all questions about diagnosis. Any detection and diagnosis, and any valid knowledge or education concerning the nature of autism (or concerning any other disorder or phenomenon, for that matter), depend on how the phenomenon is defined. It follows that the definition of the autism spectrum is crucial to all theories about its prevalence. However, if the definition of autism is being applied correctly in the vast majority of instances that are called "diagnostic substitution" by Shattuck and followers, how does this practice refute the notion that the proportion of children being diagnosed is actually increasing? To the extent that diagnoses are valid, and increasing in new birth cohorts, as suggested by Newschaffer, Falb, and Gurney (2005), and as shown in Figures 1-1 and 2-3, the substitution theory is either a moot argument against an autism epidemic, or, to the extent that changes in diagnoses are valid, the substitution theory actually is itself evidence of the autism epidemic.

The Theory of Intellectual Diversity

Next there is the popular theory saying autism may be a mere form of intellectual diversity, a kind of giftedness. It is not popular, of course, with the parents dealing with autism on a 24/7 basis nor is it plausible to parents of children with severe traits of autism. No parent who has a seven-year-old child with autism who is still in diapers, no clinicians who are seeing adults with autism who are not potty-trained will be apt to accept the giftedness theory. However, if it were accepted, it would certainly rule out the possibility of an autism epidemic. Whoever heard of an epidemic of creativity or brilliance? Only when the sort of savantism noted early on by Kanner and Asperger is combined with problems of social reciprocity that are severe enough to have been called "idiocy" in the past is a "gifted individual" apt to be placed on the autism spectrum. Nevertheless, the idea has sometimes been proposed that autism is a "blessing in disguise" that should be embraced and accepted. If it were true it would rule out the possibility of an autism epidemic, so it must be examined. Is it true? Do individuals with Asperger's disorder, for instance, typically have significant intellectual advantages?

From the beginning of the diagnosis of the first cases of autism by Kanner in 1943, there was the question of where and how to account for the cases described just a little later by Asperger (1944). Were his cases to be classified along with Kanner-type autism as milder instances of the disorder? Or had Asperger described a completely different disorder? Were Asperger's cases merely milder versions of the same disorder, indistinguishable from what would come to be called high-functioning autism, or did they represent a distinct category? All of these questions would continue to be debated right up to the present day and they are central to the consideration of another theory that might, if true, be a basis for dismissing the existence of the autism epidemic.

The idea that "autism is a gift" (referred to here as the giftedness theory) did not begin with Sigourney Weaver (2007 ●). Nevertheless, Weaver evidently did make this claim in an interview concerning the person with HFA that she played in the 2006 film *Snow Cake* (see M. Evans & Pell, 2006 ●). This movie, which opened the Berlin Film Festival on February 9, 2006 (BBC News Channel, 2006 ●), shows that public awareness about autism did not begin or end with *Rain Man*.

The giftedness theory of autism is discussed and dissected by Chiang and Lin (2007). It seems almost exclusively to pertain to persons at the very high-functioning end of the spectrum. In particular, it has to do with the special abilities that have often been associated with HFA and Asperger's disorder. Chiang and Lin (2007) focused their attention on "mathematical ability" in their review. They found that most individuals diagnosed with HFA or Asperger syndrome are actually a little below average in mathematical ability, although some of them are gifted in peculiar aspects of mathematical computation.

The giftedness theory of autism brings us back full circle to the theory of the broadening definition, and especially to the role played by Asperger's disorder when it was added to the autism spectrum in 1994. We postponed the discussion of Asperger's disorder and the extent to which it is distinguishable from HFA until this point for two reasons.

First, Asperger's disorder is often credited with being the key to the broadening of the autism spectrum with the publication of *DSM-IV* in 1994, as carried over and amplified in *DSM-IV-TR* in 2000. This claim, however, hinges on the question of whether Asperger's disorder, as defined in 1994 or earlier, is actually different from, and clinically distinguishable in practice, from HFA. If the two cannot be distinguished, then the addition of Asperger's disorder as a category to the autism spectrum cannot broaden it because HFA is already part of the spectrum.

The second reason for saving the discussion of Asperger's disorder until now was that HFA and Asperger's disorder, taken together, are almost exclusively the categories that are pointed to by advocates of the theory that autism is merely a form of intellectual diversity—that is, the giftedness theory.

The critical problem that the giftedness theory cannot overcome is the severity of the social impairments that typically accompany HFA and Asperger's disorder and that cannot be compensated for by a peculiar advantage, say, in computing prime numbers, recalling complex scenes, musical compositions, or anything like these feats. Having an extreme esoteric skill hardly compensates for lost social connections. At the severe end of the autism spectrum, where the persons affected typically not only do *not* have any intellectual advantage but rather are greatly impaired, the theory of "autism as a gift" is worse than wishful thinking. It discourages any kind of effective treatment. Contemporary parent and researcher Stan Kurtz (2007) puts forth an interesting question in this regard: Would treating a gifted person for, say, pneumonia, make that individual any less gifted? By the same token, the valid gifted aspects of autism, he argues, will not be removed by lessening the impairments.

Does Adding Asperger's Disorder Broaden the Definition of Autism?

As to whether adding Asperger's disorder to the autism spectrum in 1994 actually increased its breadth, the question comes down to whether Asperger syndrome is distinct from HFA. In their 2008 studies of HFA and Asperger syndrome, R. A. Ritvo and colleagues (see R. A. Ritvo, E. R. Ritvo, Guthrie, & M. J. Ritvo, 2008; R. A. Ritvo, E. R. Ritvo, Guthrie, Yuwiler, M. J. Ritvo, & Weisbender, 2008) applied a scale that was 100% effective in distinguishing persons previously diagnosed with either HFA or Asperger syndrome from typical (normal) adults; however, their scale could not distinguish HFA from Asperger syndrome. As noted, *DSM-IV* included Asperger syndrome as one of the pervasive developmental disorders along with autistic disorder, but insisted that Asperger's disorder, autistic disorder, and PDDNOS were distinct diagnoses.

To date, however, no one has figured out a way to sharply differentiate HFA from Asperger syndrome. The 2008 studies by Ritvo and colleagues did not do so. Similarly, neither *DSM-IV-TR* nor its international counterpart, *ICD-10*, provide any basis for doing so.

The research has shown for decades that Asperger syndrome cannot be sharply distinguished either from what has been termed "autism" or from what was formerly called "childhood schizoid disorder." The so-called schizoid disorder, was another category, along with schizophrenia, that was first proposed and described by Eugen Bleuler (1908). According to Bleuler, it consisted, supposedly, of a tendency to focus attention inward rather than on the external world. In *DSM-IV-TR*, schizoid disorder is represented as distinct from "schizophrenia, a mood disorder with psychotic features" or any other "psychotic disorder, or a pervasive developmental disorder"; according to this manual, it cannot be diagnosed as caused by "a general medical condition" (APA, 2000–2008, p. 695).

The idea that adding Asperger syndrome could broaden the definition of the autism spectrum was already suspect in 1979, when Wolff and Barlow published a comparison of eight children diagnosed with schizoid disorder who were matched with eight children with autism. They showed that the clinical features of "schizoid personality disorder" were "identical in all respects with those described by Asperger" (Wolff & Barlow, 1979, p. 38).

It follows from Wolff and Barlow (1979) and the work by Ritvo and colleagues (2008) that Asperger's disorder has always been included, logically speaking, in the definition of autism. Savantism, manifested in extreme forms of peculiar gifts in computation, rote memory, musical recall, and the like, has also been noted from the very beginning. As we have already documented, Kanner had a great deal to say about the savant characteristics of some of the cases he observed. Nevertheless, it is a long stretch from the claim that some individuals have some peculiar abilities contrasting with their pervasive disabilities, to the notion that autism is merely a normal, cultural or intellectual form of diversity or giftedness.

As we have argued extensively elsewhere, when it comes to measurement in the sciences (see J. W. Oller & L. Chen, 2007) or in any kind of valid assessment, testing, or evaluation of language proficiency, intelligence, or any other ability (J. W. Oller et al., 2006), successes count a great deal more than failures. In fact, the probability of accidental success in complex communication (or computation) tasks is so slight that in most cases it completely vanishes. Therefore, the idea that HFA and Asperger syndrome may involve special oases of giftedness is certainly worth noting. In fact, it is the vast difference between those facets of development that are grossly impaired and other facets that may seem normal or even overdeveloped that is the hallmark of autism. What distinguishes the autism spectrum from what has been called "mental retardation" is that the latter has generally involved delays without the sorts of distortions in different areas of development that characterize and typify the autism spectrum.

Although there is no such thing as a giftedness epidemic, it also appears to be the case that autism cannot reasonably be construed as representing a normal form of intellectual giftedness. The research of Chiang and Lin (2007) shows that the peculiar abilities sometimes associated with Asperger syndrome do not result in mathematical ability that is outside the average range, as some had claimed. Nor is autism a respecter of cultural boundaries. The idea that autism is just another form of cultural diversity makes about as much sense as the notion that the high incidence of toxic poisoning in industrial areas is strictly a matter of culture.

Also, the idea that adding Asperger's disorder to the autism spectrum, as was done in the *DSM* manual in 1994, could account for the smooth exponential growth in the number of cases of autism being diagnosed fails as an explanation. If Asperger's disorder is not being distinguished empirically from HFA, then adding the diagnosis of Asperger's disorder to the spectrum and claiming that it increases the number of cases is like calling a subgroup of "fast horses" in a herd by two different names and supposing that in doing so we can increase the size of the herd. This logic is reminiscent of an argument reported between Abraham Lincoln and a politician who thought he could change the nature of things by calling them by different names. Knowing that his opponent was a rancher, Lincoln asked the man what appeared to be a silly question: "How many legs do you suppose a cow has?" The man allowed that the correct answer would be four. Next Lincoln said, "Suppose we were to call the cow's tail a leg. Then how many legs would the cow have?" The politician now said five. Lincoln responded, "That's where you are wrong. Calling a cow's tail a leg does not increase the number of legs on a cow." Likewise, designating persons in the PDD category by the additional descriptor "Asperger's disorder" does not increase their number. Thus the giftedness argument fails and provides no assistance to the broadening definition theory.

Looking back, the substance of the argument against the broader definition is that there have been no actual spikes in the number of diagnosed cases at the *DSM* definition change points in 1987,

1994, and 2000. Also, the evidence against the diagnostic substitution explanation is that cases in competing categories are not diminishing. The strength of the argument against the giftedness argument is that 50% to 66% of the affected individuals require institutionalization or related services. The alleged "giftedness" does not result in substantial real-world gains.

Genetics and the Autism Epidemic

Next we come to the underlying theory that forms the background and basis for the foregoing theories denying that there has been genuine growth in the number of children being diagnosed with autism. The underlying claim in all of these theories is that autism is essentially a genetic condition. That idea is recommended by Muhle, Trentacoste, and Rapin (2004), who suppose that "multiple interacting genetic factors" are, indeed, the "main causative determinants of autism" (p. e472). While Muhle and colleagues suggest that interactions between multiple genes cause idiopathic autism, they also allow that "**epigenetic** factors and exposure to environmental modifiers may contribute to variable expression of autism-related traits" (p. e472). If genetics could be the sole explanation for the etiology of autism, there could not be any autism epidemic because genetic factors do not change fast enough in the human population to produce one.

Nevertheless, the argument for a genetic basis for autism is appealing. For one thing, as noted earlier in this chapter, autism is one of the most heritable of all neurological disorders. Research continues to accumulate showing that multiple genetic abnormalities are associated with it (Alarcon, 2002; Bacchelli & Maestrini, 2006; Deth, Muratore, Benzecry, Power-Charnitsky, & Waly, 2008; Hagerman, 2006; Herbert et al., 2006; Hertz-Picciotto, Croen, Hansen, Jones, van de Water, & Pessah, 2006; Kumar & Christian, 2009; Le Couteur et al., 2006; Moy & Nadler, 2008; Pardo & Eberhart, 2007; Rapin & Tuchman, 2008; Schanen, 2006; Schellenberg et al., 2006; Yrigollen et al., 2008). However, genetics cannot be the whole story and according to Kumar and Christian (2009, p. 188) "remains enigmatic."

The fact that a genetic epidemic is an impossibility was first stated clearly by parents of children with autism, some of whom were medical professionals (Bernard et al., 2001; Shestack, 2003). It has been widely acknowledged by professional researchers that there can be no such thing as a genetic epidemic (e.g., see Barclay, 2005 ●; D. B. Campbell et al., 2006; Muhle et al., 2004). Newschaffer (2006) is quoted as saying, "If the true risk of a condition increases over a short time period, that implies that there have been changes in nonheritable risk factors, because shifts in genetic risk factors take generations to have perceptible impacts on risk trends" (see DeNoon, 2006; also see DeNoon, 2005 ●).

Because no one can reasonably deny that the number of diagnosed cases of autism is growing, and because we cannot be witnessing a logically impossible "genetic epidemic," to hold onto the it's-all-about-genetics theory it is necessary to insist, as does Shattuck (2006), that the prevalence rate of autism has always been at the currently high level. To make this claim plausible, the evident acceleration in the growth curve of autism cases being diagnosed must be either denied or explained away. In fact, Shattuck (2006) and Gernsbacher, Dawson, and Goldsmith (2005) insist that the prevalence of autism has always been about where it is now—a rate that is astronomically higher than that supposed in the 1940s, 1950s, 1960s, 1970s, 1980s, and 1990s. Shattuck uses prevalence estimates of the CDC from 2000 and 2002, which show a rate of about 1 case per 150 births as the baseline. He does not explain why he does not assume a still higher prevalence estimate, though to be consistent he should, given his argument that many undiscovered cases remain to be diagnosed. Shattuck's underlying message is that the trend toward more new cases observed from 1980 forward is just the administrative system catching up with the facts. The cases, according to Shattuck (as well as Gernsbacher and colleagues), have always been out there, but until the professionals and the general public became better educated about autism (the awareness theory), the vast majority of those cases simply went unnoticed.

Genetics Plus: Mixing and Matching

When it is pointed out that it would be difficult *not* to notice a child who cannot recognize his or her own mother, tie his or her shoes, or talk to his or her teachers (per Kirby, 2005, 2007; R. F. Kennedy & Kirby, 2009 ●), the proponents of better detection and diagnosis cite the theory of the broadening definition. When it is noted that the official *DSM-IV* definition has really not changed a scintilla since 1994, the fallback is to public awareness and better detection and diagnosis. The giftedness theory, meantime, floats on the coattails of the other theories, denying that autism should make a parent weep—it's rather a good thing. If pressed, the proponents of all those theories will suggest that the addition of Asperger syndrome to the list of autism spectrum disorders is the essential key in explaining the ongoing upsurge. Why is the rate of diagnosis still apparently accelerating? Easy—because not all the cases have been discovered yet. It is interesting that the genetic theory has been used to support all of the foregoing theories that would wash out the autism epidemic. For that reason, we left it to be considered last.

There are three fatal flaws in all of the arguments that would try to cast the autism epidemic as some sort of exclusive genetic problem, or a genetics-plus-some-fiction problem. Any one of the flaws to be mentioned next is sufficient to reject any theory of exclusive genetics causation. Any one of them also presents a solid case against any of the mix-and-match added theories that would supposedly render the it's-all-about-genetics argument more plausible. But whether we consider these three flaws singly or together, the arguments against a singular genetic explanation for autism are conclusive. They show the logical bankruptcy of any attempt to make genetics the whole explanation for the enormous increase in the number of diagnosed cases of autism and the ongoing exponential increase in autism prevalence.

Flaw 1: The Majority of Cases Are Severe

The idea that the cases have always been there but simply went unnoticed runs aground when we consider that a majority of the cases currently being diagnosed fall toward the severe end of the spectrum. In fact, all of the cases being diagnosed under the criteria from Kanner forward, but especially as noted in *DSM-IV*, are described as "severe and pervasive impairment . . . distinctly deviant relative to the individual's developmental level or mental age" (APA, 1994, p. 65). In a substantial number of the cases being newly diagnosed in birth cohorts from 1980 forward, the autism has been of an extreme severity, with many cases involving individuals who are nonverbal, are unresponsive to social interaction, and demonstrate additional symptoms of hand-flapping and self-injurious behavior. The idea that such cases are just gradually being entered into case loads, as more previously undetected cases are slowly noticed, is inconsistent with the fact that most of the cases are being diagnosed in young children and less commonly in adolescents and adults. The relative rarity of adult diagnosis can be directly inferred from the many observations concerning the average age of diagnosis, which remains in early childhood.

The notion that severe symptoms might go unnoticed by parents and teachers—not to mention pediatricians and family practitioners—beyond the first or second year in school is a remarkably implausible idea. According to this view, many patients with severe autism should have passed through adolescence and entered into adulthood during the 1980s and 1990s. There should now be tens of thousands of undiagnosed adults with severe autism who cannot support themselves or lead independent lives. The question is, as Kirby (2005, 2007; also see Jepson & Johnson, 2007) has asked, where are all these undiagnosed individuals? Surely it is true, as argued by Shattuck (2006), that some of the increase in numbers being reported under IDEA can be accounted for by changed diagnoses—specifically, from mental retardation and learning disabilities to the autism spectrum. Some of the increase can also certainly be attributed to greater public awareness of Asperger syndrome and milder forms of atypical autism classified in the PDDNOS catch-all subcategory. Nevertheless, none of the proposed theories to make the autism epidemic "go away" can explain the fact that significant increases in diagnosed cases were observed through the last three decades in successive birth cohorts, as illustrated in Figures 1-1, 2-3, and 2-6 (Newschaffer et al., 2005; Newschaffer, 2006).

Flaw 2: Positive Evidence Unexplained

A second fatal flaw in the genetic explanation for the worldwide upsurge in autism is that the genetic theory cannot explain the positive evidence that exponential growth in the number of diagnosed cases is occurring. Thus the exclusive genetic theory not only cannot produce the tens of thousands of undiagnosed adults with severe autism that are supposedly out there somewhere, as contrasted with the tens of thousands of cases of children who have already been diagnosed. Because human beings do not reproduce as fast as bacteria, fruit flies, plants, or even rabbits, a genetic theory of autism without any other interactive factors must fail.

There must be some other interactive factors besides the known and yet-to-be-discovered genetic factors. For this reason, proponents of the genetic theory of the autism epidemic require additional factors to supplement their theory. Genetic factors alone cannot even tell the whole story with respect to what are called "genetic" conditions. The theoretical work going on in genetics, toxicology, and neurobiology shows unequivocally that genetic processes are universally dependent on interactions with nutrition and other environmental factors. Herbert et al. (2006) have argued that "genetic complexity" alone appears increasingly inadequate "as evidence of systemic abnormalities (e.g., gastrointestinal and immune), increasing rates [of diagnosis,] and less than 100% monozygotic concordance" accumulate. They propose reinterpreting "autism as a multisystem disorder with genetic influence and environmental contributors" (p. 671).

Genetic explanations cannot fully differentiate the various subcategories of PDDs from other so-called communication disorders such as **attention-deficit/hyperactivity disorder** (**ADHD**), or even from adult neurological conditions such as Alzheimer's disease, Parkinson's disease, and **neuroAIDS** (Segura-Aguilar & Kostrzewa, 2006). In addition, the research shows that the environmental factors involved in triggering and exacerbating the autism spectrum affect not only essentially all of the diseases and disorders associated behaviorally with communication, but also the nervous system and the internal systems of communication involving genetics, metabolism, the immune systems, and the whole body (Jepson & Johnson, 2007). In explaining a growing theoretical consensus, Moy and Nadler (2008) point out that the "etiology [of autism] is thought to involve complex, multigenic interactions and possible environmental contributions" (p. 4). Newschaffer (2006) had already noted that

> when genetic susceptibility and environmental triggers work together, disease heritability is easily overestimated; the stage now should be set for well-reasoned, carefully designed research exploring the potential role of environmental exposures as well as genetic liability in autism etiology. (p. 1437)

It appears that epigenetic factors must be taken into consideration, and that genetics alone can no more explain the autism epidemic than a human baby could survive without a suitable nurturing environment.

Flaw 3: Not a Complete Explanation

A third and even more fundamental flaw exists in attempts to use genetics to dismiss, deny, or explain away the rising number of individuals being diagnosed with autism spectrum disorders. Genetic abnormalities associated with diseases and disorders also require explanation—that is, also have some etiology. They themselves are not uncaused. To present a genetic basis for a disorder as if it were the final word is about as final as sweeping dust under the carpet as a method of house cleaning. It only postpones the work that is needed to find a real solution. It is just a mistake in logic and a misunderstanding of **genomics** (Sanford, 2005) to suppose that locating genetic correlates of a disorder is anything like a final explanation. The genetic system that controls heritability is itself subject to multiple interactions long before the birth of any given individual. In studying the genetic etiology of diseases and disorders, the history of the family tree must be examined for cumulative environmental impacts.

Some of the factors causing cumulative genetic problems are well known. Also, ample research, mainly with rodents (Moy & Nadler, 2008), has revealed that genetic factors are greatly dependent on complex environmental interactions in general. For additional evidence on such interactions, see the work of Pabello and Lawrence (2006); Palomo, Beninger, Kostrzewa, and Archer (2003); Palomo, Archer, Beninger, and Kostrzewa (2004); and Hertz-Picciotto et al. (2006). Finally, among the known causes of genetic mutations across generations are toxins such as mercury (Crespo-Lopez, de Sa, Herculano, Burbano, & do Nascimento, 2007; L. C. Lee et al., 2006; Westphal et al., 2003) and aluminum (Lima et al., 2007). Is it just a coincidence that these toxins, along with foreign proteins, and a growing number of disease agents have been increasingly used in vaccines during the same period that witnessed exponential growth in the prevalence of multisystem disorders such as autism? The idea that the genetic material passed from one generation to the next could be a complete explanation for the increasing prevalence of autism is short-sighted. Logically, empirically, and practically, there must be a great deal more to the story.

SUMMING UP AND LOOKING AHEAD

The number of diagnosed cases of autism has been following a relatively smooth exponential growth curve at least since 1980, when it was first described as a distinct clinical entity, and continuing through 2006. Since 1943, the autism spectrum disorders have been defined in terms of severe and pervasive behavioral symptoms of distorted (abnormal) development. Typical cases have been severe from Kanner's first 11 patients, with a minority (fewer than one third) being able to lead independent lives. In this chapter, we examined five theories aimed at explaining away the autism epidemic.

The theory of the broadened definition failed because in fact the definition of autism has changed very little since 1943 until now. The idea that adding Asperger syndrome to the spectrum, which was officially done in 1994, could account for the growing number of cases of autism being diagnosed was shown to be false. The theory that greater public awareness could explain the upward growth curve of autism and has produced an illusory upsurge in cases was shown to be implausible because it is more likely that the greater awareness is the result of the increasing prevalence of autism rather than the reverse. Also, the diagnostic substitution theory failed for two reasons: for one, keener awareness ought to make the diagnosis more—rather than less—valid and in such a climate of better understanding diagnostic substitutions ought to result in truer reporting, rather than the illusion of a worldwide epidemic. Although the giftedness theory makes a valid point about savantism, it also stresses one of the striking manifestations of the abnormal distortions that characterize autism and it only applies to the relatively mild end of the spectrum, leaving two thirds of the problem, or more, unaccounted for. Finally, we saw in this chapter that the genetic theory of autism is incomplete.

To explain the increasing prevalence of autism in successive birth cohorts at least from 1980 forward, it is necessary to look to factors that interact with each other and that arise over and above genetic factors. The toxins and disease agents in medical procedures, as sanctioned by government, industry, and the medical profession, are implicated. Despite their efforts to make the autism epidemic go away, it appears to be real. In the next chapter, we consider documentary evidence obtained under the Freedom of Information Act (1966–2007) that suggests that highly placed officials working for and with the CDC have tried to keep evidence of the autism epidemic and its suspected causes from the public view.

STUDY AND DISCUSSION QUESTIONS

1. Consider Offit's claim that the neurotoxin thimerosal, as used in vaccines, has never done any harm. What evidence or motives could be behind his claim? Why do you think the claim is valid or invalid?

2. Why would an agency of the government—for instance, the CDC—offer contradictory views about thimerosal (e.g., that it ought to be removed from vaccines; that it has been removed from vaccines; and that thimerosal never did any harm and it ought to be used worldwide in vaccines)?

3. What real changes in the criteria for diagnosing autism have been made?

4. Why is "pronominal reversal," as described by Kanner, a likely phenomenon in normal early child language development?

5. Discuss the theory of mind and perspective-taking explanations of autism. Compare them with the theory of abstraction (see also the discussion of the theory of abstraction in Chapter 11).

6. What does the research show about the theory that Asperger syndrome is a form of giftedness?

7. Does adding Asperger's disorder to the autism spectrum broaden it? Why or why not?

8. What evidence can be used to test the various theories that aim to explain away the autism epidemic?

9. How can we account for the increase in awareness concerning autism? Can that increase explain the observed growth in diagnosed cases? If so, how? Or, why not?

10. In the final analysis, what is wrong with the idea that genetic predisposition allows us to dismiss the evident autism epidemic?

chapter three

Seeking Causes

OBJECTIVES

In this chapter, we

1. Review data suggesting a link between autism and the mercury and other toxins in vaccines.

2. Discuss discoveries about autism made by the CDC and by private citizens.

3. Review public proclamations related to the impact of known neurotoxins on autism.

4. Consider the behavioral definition of autism and purported uncertainty about its causes.

5. Discuss the requirements of common sense, medical ethics, and logic in discovering the causes of autism so as to enable recovery from this disorder.

6. Consider documentary evidence of what parents of children diagnosed with autism have discovered and why there is hope for recovery.

Having shown in Chapter 2 that there has been a real increase in the prevalence of autism spectrum disorders, it makes sense to turn our attention to the causes of this class of disorders. As we will see, the facts of the autism epidemic have led to a situation where the public is increasingly demanding accountability not only of medical practitioners, but also of the CDC and FDA. Interestingly, high-placed officials in the U.S. Public Health Service have admitted that the greatest progress so far in seeking out causes and developing effective interventions for autism have come from parent groups and the independent research they have funded. This point was made in the introduction of Jon Shestack by Tom Insel, then the director of the National Institute of Mental Health, at the 2003 Autism Summit in Washington, D.C. ◯ We will see in this chapter that many children have been recovered from severe autism to the point that they have become indistinguishable from neurotypical children. It was parents of children with autism who founded the Autism

Research Institute, Cure Autism Now, Defeat Autism Now, the Autism Genetics Resource Exchange, Autism Speaks, and Talk About Curing Autism. To make their way toward a more hopeful future, the parents had to make their own advances, often in the face of opposition and criticism from members of government agencies (especially the CDC and FDA), professional organizations, and pharmaceutical companies.

THE LONG ARM OF THE LAW

Well before people began to talk about an autism epidemic, it became increasingly apparent that vaccines were implicated in neurological disorders and that they were suspiciously associated with sudden infant death syndrome (SIDS). The concern about vaccines, which dates back at least to 1969, was more than just hyped-up anxiety (Shattuck, 2006; Gernsbacher et al., 2005). By the early 1980s, vaccines were so widely implicated in neurological problems and in SIDS that the public outcry led to an act of Congress in 1986. In years to come, research on vaccine injuries would confirm that parents are better sources of information about adverse events in many respects than are the healthcare providers who deliver the vaccinations (Silvers, Varricchio, et al., 2002).

The National Childhood Vaccine Injury Act of 1986

In the 1980s, it became increasingly clear that vaccines were not always associated with wellness. Too many deaths occurred on the heels of a round of vaccinations. About half of those deaths were recorded as SIDS, as is still the case today (Braun & Ellenberg, 1997; Silvers, Ellenberg et al., 2001; Silvers, Varricchio, et al., 2002). That mysterious undefined illness was only loosely described at a conference in 1969 as follows:

> the sudden death of any infant or young child, which is unexpected by history, and in which a thorough postmortem examination fails to demonstrate an adequate cause of death. (Bergman et al., 1970, p. 18)

Was it merely a coincidence that an increasing number of such "unexplained" deaths happened after the administration of the new multivalent diphtheria/tetanus/pertussis (DTP) vaccine? When the 1986 legislation was passed, the concern about the preservative thimerosal, which was present in the standard DTP shots, had yet to reach a critical level. However, the number of lawsuits dealing with claims of vaccine injuries did reach a crisis level in the 1980s, and the furor was sufficient to lead to passage of the National Childhood Vaccine Injury Act in 1986 (Public Law 99-660).

This legislation is important to the story of autism because the increasing number of injuries that precipitated its enactment typically involved neurological communication disorders such as autism or sometimes SIDS. The facts of the unfolding story would lead from real and pretended ignorance, to wishful thinking, and even to evidence of even less admirable roles played by the CDC, FDA, professional medical organizations, and the pharmaceutical industry. The explanations of injuries offered by the official watchdog agencies supposedly protecting the public from injuries would reveal inconsistencies that would strain the limits of common sense—yet the narrative is true and the key facts are a matter of public record.

At least from 1980 forward, the rates of autism diagnosis began to assume the form of an exponential growth curve (refer back to Figures 1-1 and 2-3). Autism was rapidly becoming the fastest-growing diagnosis of all childhood disorders and diseases. In Chapter 2, we summed up the evidence that autism involves significant genetic factors, even as we showed why it must also involve other epigenetic interactions. In the 1990s, parent groups and independent researchers inferred that environmental toxins were playing a role in the increased rate of autism diagnoses. Because of the vast literature on the toxicity of metals such as lead, mercury, aluminum, cadmium, and manganese, all

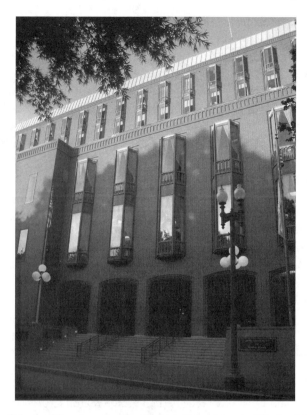

Figure 3-1 Photograph of the building housing the United States Court of Federal Claims, also known as the Vaccine Injury Court since 1986.
Source: Courtesy of Anne Marie Kelly.

possible sources of such contaminants were implicated, including pesticides, food preservatives, and the like. In the background, when the U.S. Congress amplified the National Childhood Vaccine Injury Act of 1986 by redesignating the existing "People's Court"—the U.S. Court of Federal Claims, originally established in 1856—as the "Vaccine Injury Court" in 1988, the notion that vaccines were a source of toxins began to be examined by a few research-oriented parents.

In 1988, Congress established the National Vaccine Injury Compensation Program (VICP) to be adjudicated by the newly designated "Vaccine Injury Court." The new program allowed persons seeking redress and compensation under the 1986 Vaccine Injury Act—provided they met a fairly stringent list of requirements (see the section titled "A Special Statute of Limitations for Vaccine Injuries")—to be heard in the Vaccine Injury Court. This court, formerly known as the "People's Court," remains the only legal forum in the United States where individuals can seek reparations from the federal government for wrongs done to them by the federal government. This special court has its own distinct procedures and rules. Its original purpose was enunciated by President Abraham Lincoln in the Annual Message to Congress in 1861:

> It is as much the duty of Government to render prompt justice against itself, in favor of citizens, as it is to administer the same between private individuals. (Lincoln, 1861 ●)

This sentence is engraved on the building where the court is housed (see Figure 3-1).

According to its original, idealistic purpose, the Vaccine Injury Court was not supposed to protect the interests of government, pharmaceutical companies, federal agencies, or the large and powerful professional trade associations of medicine, dentistry, and so on, but rather to protect the rights of individual private citizens against wrongs done by the government itself. In 1986, under the Vaccine Injury Act, however, the mission of the People's Court was interpreted in a way that would protect the manufacturers of vaccines, and the government agencies that promote their use, from suits filed in civil courts by individual citizens. At the time of the enactment of the 1986 law, the civil suits that were being filed in other courts had reached a critical mass, and Congress sought to redirect these complaints to the People's Court.

The idea of the Vaccine Injury Act was to provide **no-fault** compensation to the parents or advocates for any child injured by a licensed and/or federally mandated vaccine. In a no-fault system, no person or agency is accused of doing anything wrong that could be punished by law. This approach differs dramatically from what happens in traditional courts, where contests involve accusations of harm done by one party to another. In the People's Court, instead of a plaintiff, there is a **petitioner**; likewise, instead of a **defendant**, there is a **respondent**. There is no jury, and the person who decides the case is not a judge or jury of the usual kind, but rather a **Special Master**—a lawyer appointed by the court. Individual cases of alleged vaccine injuries can be heard by a single individual acting as the sole arbiter of the decision; in other words, the Special Master is the whole jury and the judge rolled into one person.

To get on the legal schedule for the Vaccine Injury Court, the following requirements must be met:

> (1) . . . the injured person must have received a vaccine manufactured by a vaccine company located in the U.S. and returned to the U.S. within 6 months after the date of vaccination . . . [and] to be eligible to file a claim, the effects of the person's injury must have lasted for more than 6 months after the vaccine was given; or (2) resulted in a hospital stay and surgery; or (3) resulted in death. (National Vaccine Injury Compensation Program, 2008 ●)

A Suspected Link of Vaccines to Autism

We have already noted that the vaccine injuries leading up to the VICP commonly involved the sorts of neurological problems and impairments associated with disorders on the autism spectrum. Also, as would be noted repeatedly in the various editions of the *DSM* from 1987 forward, the most common cases of autism were severe—approximately one in five then and perhaps as many as four in five now (see Pangborn, 2005, p. 149)—tended to involve a normal course of development up to about 15 to 18 months of age, followed by a regression into severe autism. In Kanner's Case 3, the boy's mother said, "Following smallpox vaccination at 12 months, he had an attack of fever and diarrhea from which he recovered in about a week"; on a visit two months before his third birthday, she said, "I can't be sure just when he stopped the imitation of word sounds . . . he has gone backward mentally gradually for the last two years" (Kanner, 1943, p. 225). It is not clear whether she made the connection with the vaccine, but her account suggests that the descent into autism began soon after the smallpox vaccination.

The idea that **encephalopathic conditions**, of which autism is certainly one, could be caused by injections containing foreign proteins and/or other toxins goes back to a much earlier line of research pursued by Charles Richet, who received the Nobel Prize in Physiology or Medicine in 1913 (see Hoffman, 2008). Richet was honored for his work in a branch of research that is still being pursued today with a variety of methods (Deth et al., 2008; Hertz-Picciotto et al., 2006; Ming, Stein, Brimacombe, Johnson, Lambert, & Wagner, 2005). In his Nobel lecture of 1913, Richet summed up research from 1902 forward, showing that injections of extremely minute quantities of foreign proteins from the blood or tissue of another species, or other known toxins, can generate hypersensitivity leading to **anaphylactic encephalopathy**. In less severe cases, the results of the poisoning by injection would include fever, vomiting, and diarrhea. All of these effects are common symptoms of autism (from Kanner's cases to the present) and also of well-known adverse reactions to vaccinations (Block et al., 2007; Braun & Ellenberg, 1997; Wise et al., 2004).

Richet and his contemporary researchers had discovered that the effects of soluble proteins and toxins injected into the bloodstream increase from one injection to the next, and that this increase is an extremely general phenomenon:

> Instead of applying only to toxins and toxalbumins [proteins or fluids from an animal], it held good for all proteins, whether toxic at the first injection or not. . . . A dog when injected previously even with the smallest dose, say of 0.005 liquid per kilo, immediately showed serious symptoms: vomiting, blood diarrhea, syncope [fainting], unconsciousness, asphyxia and death. This basic experiment was repeated at various times and by 1902 we were able to state three main factors which are the corner-stone of the history of anaphylaxis: (1) a subject that had a previous injection is far more sensitive than a new subject; (2) that the symptoms characteristic of the second injection, namely swift and total depression of the nervous system, do not in any way resemble the symptoms characterizing the first injection; (3) a three or four week period must elapse before the anaphylactic state results. This is the period of incubation. (Richet, 1913)

We will examine the research on the role of toxins and vaccines in autism especially in Chapters 5 and 6. Here, however, we emphasize that parental concerns about the possibility that vaccines were somehow involved in the increasing prevalence of autism were grounded in experience. In fact, the study of anaphylaxis—that is, hypersensitivity producing neurological consequences—had a long history prior to the Vaccine Injury Act of 1986.

In addition, we must note that the VICP includes some provisions that have tended to exclude many cases where the regression into autism seems to have been legitimately linked to vaccinations. In some of those instances, parents misunderstood the law by supposing that the reporting of a problem under the Vaccine Adverse Event Reporting System (also established by Congress in connection with the Vaccine Injury Act) would trigger the initiation of a VICP claim. It does not: The two systems are independent and disconnected. Two entirely separate reports are required, and a VICP claim must meet certain requirements, including being subject to a stringent **statute of limitations**.

A Special Statute of Limitations for Vaccine Injuries

If any given vaccine injury claim is not filed within three years of the onset of symptoms, the case cannot ever be filed, nor can it ever be heard in the Vaccine Injury Court. This statute is "special" in that it prevents a claim from being filed by or on behalf of an injured person who discovers at, say, age six, that an injury sustained in infancy from a mandated vaccine resulted in the diagnosis of autism more than three years after the injury occurred. That person will not receive any kind of compensation under the Vaccine Injury Act. Such a limitation is unusual because most civil suits dealing with injuries that can be shown to have been caused by another individual or by a corporation, for instance, are not limited in this way (see analysis by attorney Jeff Z. Sell, 2006 ⬤).

In neurological disorders such as autism, which have accounted for the majority of the VICP cases since the late 1980s, it has often been difficult for parents to get a timely diagnosis for their child. In many cases, it took years to get a diagnosis—and even more time for a substantial number of parents to begin to notice that the onset of symptoms was commonly occurring after one or several routine vaccinations. Among the children excluded by the statute of limitations were the twin boys of attorney Jeff Z. Sell. Both boys developed autism after receiving the DPT vaccination with thimerosal, but it took more than three years to get a diagnosis and to discover the connection. When seeking to get on the docket for the U.S. Federal Court of Claims, Sell (2006) ran into a wall:

> A claim must be filed under the VICP within three (3) years of when the first symptoms occurred. This rule is inflexible. . . . It does not matter that a child's parents did not know about this program, or that they did not know that their child's injuries were related to the vaccine. . . . Most states also have laws which toll (i.e., stop) the running of the statute of limitations while someone is under a disability. . . . In many states a child who is injured does not even have to file a case until sometime after they reach majority [at age 18 or 21 depending on the state].

But in the case of the federal law governing vaccine injuries, if a diagnosis is delayed, or if a case is not filed within three years of the onset of symptoms, no case can ever be filed—even if it should become known that vaccines caused lifelong problems.

According to attorney Tom Powell, speaking in the U.S. Court of Federal Claims on June 11, 2007, the original purpose of the Vaccine Injury Act was threefold:

> The first was to protect manufacturers [of vaccines] from civil liability. The second was to encourage vaccines to be used and administered and developed, and the third was to provide a fair, just, speedy and generous compensation program for those children, hopefully a small number, ideally rare, [with] . . . expected adverse reactions to vaccines. (U.S. Court of Federal Claims, 2007 ◉)

The new law was especially important to persons with neurological conditions such as autism, whose symptoms are known to be caused or exacerbated by toxins, disease agents, and accidental components. The government has described these components as "adventitious agents" (FDA/CBER, 2008 ◉) that end up in vaccines and then are placed in children's bodies. The vaccinations are usually mandated by state laws in accordance with federal requirements imposed from above. As discussed in detail in Chapter 7, for the vaccines to be effective in producing immunity, they must generally contain at least some portion of the agents that are believed to cause the diseases that the vaccines are supposed to prevent. The theory is that any given disease agent (or part of one) that is included in the vaccine will serve as an effective antigen thus stimulating the body's immune system to produce antibodies against that particular agent or ones like it that are associated with the disease in question.

In the 1980s and afterward, DTP vaccines, along with the hepatitis vaccine and the vaccine for *Haemophilus influenzae* B (Hib), all contained thimerosal as a preservative agent. In the manufacturing process, vaccines are also known to acquire biological proteins, viruses, and other contaminants from the animals—chickens, ducks, rabbits, dogs, monkeys—used in producing them (Cave, 2001, p. 38). One virus of considerable interest among the 40-plus viruses that have been catalogued as originating in monkeys used in the manufacture of vaccines is **simian virus 40 (SV40)**, to which we return in Chapter 10. We will see there that the concerns of parents of children with autism and of independent researchers are not unfounded.

Watchdogs or Collaborators?

Watchdog agencies (especially the CDC and FDA) as well as members of the pharmaceutical industry and professional medical associations involved in promoting the use of vaccines and dental amalgam have all too often taken refuge in the claim that autism is an unsolvable mystery. All the while, everyone has hoped that the medical procedures in question could be exonerated. No one has wanted vaccines to be implicated in causing harm. And who would have dreamed that tons of neurotoxic material would be placed in the mouths of unsuspecting dental patients by dentists? Would we expect pediatricians to knowingly inject poisons into infants? Could all the concern be generated by over-protective, misguided parents? If we take seriously any or all of the explanations that would suggest the autism epidemic is an imaginary phenomenon, we might suppose that the parents of children with autism, as well as the groups they formed to study and treat autism, must be mistaken.

To dismiss parents' concerns about vaccines and toxins, however, would require ignoring the long and extensive history of toxicology demonstrating the association of toxins with neurological disorders. Independent researchers and theoreticians (as we saw in Chapter 2) have consistently come to the conclusion that toxins are involved in autism and are a contributing factor in the increasing prevalence of neurological diseases and disorders. All too often that line of research—especially in toxicology—seems to have been ignored by pharmaceutical companies and professional medical organizations, which have continued promoting the use of mercury in vaccines and in dental amalgam. All of this information would be eventually discovered by parents and the independent researchers who would join them in researching the causes of autism. Increasingly, they would come to focus on the role of toxins, disease agents, foreign proteins, and the known and potential interactions of such agents.

Legal battles would follow on the heels of many independent claims of injury. Suits filed under the Freedom of Information Act would bring to light formerly secret memoranda from public officials. Some of the relevant data and facts that the CDC and the U.S. Public Health Service had determined should be kept secret (R. F. Kennedy, Jr., 2005, 2006, 2007; Kirby, 2005; R. F. Kennedy & Kirby, 2009 ☉) would be discovered and made public. When Kirby published his 2005 book titled *Evidence of Harm,* he made use of public documents obtained through **legal discovery**—for example, by parent groups (including Putchildrenfirst.org ☉) and by independent researchers (e.g., M. R. Geier & D. A. Geier). Soon a plethora of documents came to light showing attempts by key officials (at the CDC, in particular) to obfuscate evidence suggesting that increased exposure to multivalent vaccines was strongly correlated with the increasing number of autism cases being diagnosed. That evidence would ultimately lead to an intense reexamination of the whole concept of vaccination.

The evidence suggested strongly that some involvement of vaccines was associated with the rising prevalence of autism and neurodevelopmental disorders. While acknowledging that the correlation might just be coincidental, concerned parents and independent researchers were encouraged to dig deeper by the CDC's attempts to suppress information about the association of the uptake of new vaccines with the concomitant upsurge in the diagnosis of autism. If there was no real causative relationship, why hide the evidence? Arguments that a bad outcome is not necessarily caused by a prior event generally work best when the prior event did not involve any harmful agents. Of course, the disease agents in vaccines (not to mention the toxins and adventitious agents they contain) would not work at all for their intended purposes if they were completely benign; thus vaccines must contain biochemically recognizable disease agents or parts of them, and they also contain toxins. It is not unreasonable to suppose that disease agents working synergistically with each other, with harmful toxins, and/or with adventitious agents might very well be involved in producing the autism epidemic.

EVIDENCE OF A CAUSE–EFFECT RELATION

One thing that can be said with confidence is that the growth in the number of children being diagnosed with autism (as shown in Figures 1-1 and 2-3), which consists of predominantly severe cases—is *certainly not uncaused*. Systematic (nonrandom) change does not just happen accidentally; it must have one or many real causes.

There is an interesting history associated with the inadequate explanations examined in Chapter 2. Those explanations—namely, the broadened definition theory, the public awareness theory, the diagnostic substitution theory, the giftedness theory, and the it's-all-genetics theory—were popularized by the CDC, FDA, and other stakeholders in the vaccine industry after a more plausible possibility had already been proposed. Because of the long history of studies in experimental biochemistry and the vast literature dealing with toxicology (see Chapters 5–7), the suggestion was made early on that vaccines and some of their components might well be involved in contributing to the upsurge of cases of autism and neurological disorders in early childhood.

During the period when the percentage of children being exposed to vaccines was increasing, with mandates for DTP, hepatitis B, and Hib vaccines being added in the mid-1980s, autism was also on the rise. This fact, along with the passage of the Vaccine Injury Act of 1986, led to new concerns about the possible impact of vaccines in producing neurological disorders. Those concerns were expressed in a sufficient number of lawsuits by parents to precipitate the passing of the Vaccine Injury Act by Congress in 1986 and were destined to be followed up eventually by the CDC at the federal level and by its state-level counterparts.

Because California is the most populous state, and because the growing prevalence of autism diagnoses there has been well documented since the 1980s, it is unsurprising that the CDC focused its attention first on data from California. What is surprising is that when key officials in both Atlanta (home of the CDC) at the federal level and in Sacramento (the California state capital) discovered evidence of a strong correlation between the rising incidence of autism and the concomitant use of vaccines, they reported to the public that they had found no evidence of any association.

To say that SIDS deaths or neurological problems developing after vaccinations are completely coincidental is about as plausible as saying that the cracks in many buildings' foundations after earthquakes are unrelated to the seismic events. Vaccines are known to introduce significant biological challenges in the form of disease agents, with the goal of stimulating the body's immune system. This process carries an inherent risk. Therefore, saying that vaccines cannot be related to SIDS or to neurological disorders is similar to saying that water damage in low-lying areas is unrelated to flooding. Naturally, the officials at the CDC, other federal agencies, medical practitioners, and vaccine industry representatives would hope that concerns about vaccines and their components were unjustified, and that the vaccines and all their components would ultimately be vindicated.

Even after careful examination showed that increased use of vaccines was strongly correlated with the rising number of diagnosed cases of autism, the CDC and its collaborators continued to claim that no such correlation existed (Andrews et al., 2004; L. K. Ball, R. Ball, & Pratt, 2001; Dales et al., 2001; Offit, 2007; Shattuck, 2006). We now know that the CDC had ample evidence that the growing use of vaccines was strongly correlated with the rising prevalence of autism in particular. Similarly, the American Dental Association continued to argue that the mercury in dental amalgam was perfectly safe for children and unrelated to neurological disorders (Bellinger et al., 2006; Needleman, 2006) in spite of excellent toxicological studies showing the exact opposite.

Published and Unpublished Data

During the 1990s, additional attention was directed to the potential role of vaccines in producing the epidemic of neurological diseases and disorders including autism. Because of known and suspected interactions, concerns had especially been expressed about multivalent vaccines. Among them were the measles/mumps/rubella (MMR) vaccine (Stott et al., 2004; Wakefield et al., 1998) and the DTP. The latter, especially, came under intense scrutiny in the 1980s, leading to the passage of the Vaccine Injury Act of 1986.

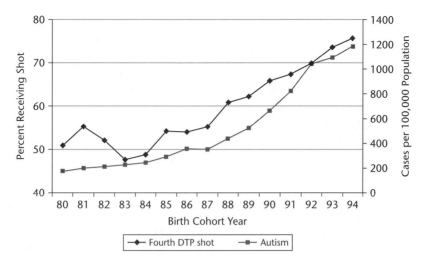

Figure 3-2 The correlation between the increasing uptake of the fourth DTP shot and the increasing diagnosis of autism in California, $r = .96$, $p < .0001$.

In 2001, a team of researchers associated with the CDC and the American Academy of Pediatrics published an article in the *Journal of the American Medical Association* (Dales et al., 2001) concluding that there was no association between rising rates of autism concomitant with increased rates of MMR vaccination. The authors argued that if autism rates had increased by 373% while coverage for the MMR at 24 months increased by only 14%, there could not be any correlation. As Richet's research had demonstrated, however, even a tiny increase in exposure to a toxin, especially one that is injected repeatedly, can produce disorder and even death, so the claim that the much greater increase in the rate of autism cannot have any association with the increased exposure to the MMR vaccine is based on faulty reasoning. The CDC appears to consider a 1:1 correlation of exposure to disease outcomes to be the standard of proof. In fact, that degree of correlation was nearly realized with the increasing use of various vaccines. Figure 3-2 shows the correlation between the diagnosis of autism per 100,000 persons with the increasing percentage of the U.S. children receiving the newly mandated fourth DTP shot. The correlation of .96 is so nearly perfect (1:1) that it is remarkable that CDC officials could claim that they had found no association between vaccines and the rising number of autism cases.

Of course, the DTP shots were not the only vaccines implicated. The discussion of the possible role of the MMR vaccination began to take shape with the discovery by Wakefield et al. in 1998 that the MMR vaccine was apparently associated with gut disease in individuals who had been diagnosed with autism. Next, we take another look at the MMR vaccine based on data published by Dales, Hammer, and Smith (2001).

Even as concerns were being raised about multivalent vaccines, especially MMR and DTP, new attention was being focused on the multidose vials of certain vaccines (DTP, HepB, and Hib, but not MMR) to which thimerosal, the ethyl mercury–containing preservative had been added from the beginning of their use. This mercury-laden component has been implicated by research in biochemistry and toxicology throughout its history as a factor in neurological disorders (see Chapters 5 and 6). It is also important to note that not only was the DTP shot the primary focus of the complaints leading up to the National Childhood Vaccine Injury Act of 1986, but it was also the first widely used multivalent vaccine containing thimerosal. In addition to scrutinizing the MMR vaccine, the CDC—not surprisingly—focused considerable attention on the DTP series, and the other vaccines, HepB and Hib, containing thimerosal.

In addition to the published study that disavowed any link between the MMR shots and the increased prevalence of neurological disorders (Dales et al., 2001), another study was performed simultaneously by the same CDC researchers focusing on the vaccines containing the mercury preservative, though they decided not to publish its findings. Figure 3-2 summarizes the unpublished portion of the data they collected. These data became publicly available as the result of a legal dispute; they had remained hidden until they were discovered by litigation through the Freedom of Information Act. The data are now available on the Putchildrenfirst.org Web site (2009 ●), which is sponsored by Lisa and J. B. Handley. To our knowledge, this evidence of the statistical correlation of vaccine uptake with the autism epidemic, and the reexamination of the Dales et al. (2001) data, is appearing in printed form for the first time in this book.

MMR versus DTP, HepB, and Hib

In 2001, Dr. Loring Dales, the primary author of the published study about the MMR shot and autism, and a key researcher working for the California Public Health Services and the CDC, provided data to his supervisors in a memo concerning the association of the DTP series with the rising rates of autism. Those data are graphed in Figure 3-2. The reason for looking at the fourth shot in the DTP series, along with two other vaccines (HepB and Hib) added to the mandated series in the 1980s, was the fact that multidose vials of these vaccines—during the time frame of interest—all contained thimerosal. Someone within the CDC hierarchy had asked for data on the thimerosal-laden shots. In a series of memos, Dales wrote on June 8, 2001:

> As requested, here are the data we have on (a) percentages of California children who had received 4 doses of DTP by their 2nd birthday (from annual statewide kindergarten retrospective surveys—same methods/data source as described in our March 7, 2001, *JAMA* paper on MMR and autism), and (b) numbers of autism cases in California's Department of Developmental Services regional service center system (also same data here as described in the same *JAMA* paper), for the birth years 1980–1994. ●

Some Interesting Unpublished Data

Figure 3-2 shows the plot of the data provided by Dales concerning the fourth shot in the thimerosal-containing DTP series. In this figure, the incidence of autism diagnosis among California birth cohorts of children from 1980 to 1994 is plotted against the percentage of children receiving the fourth shot in the DTP series containing thimerosal. Although Dales and colleagues have argued that there is no association between the two lines, in fact the correlation is a staggering .96. That is, the association is so strong that approximately 92% of the variance in the autism diagnosis for children in successive birth cohorts in California can be predicted by the concomitant change in the percentage of children in the same birth cohorts in California who received their fourth DTP shot.

Public health officials in California and at the CDC were hoping to find no association between the rising number of vaccines being used and the rising incidence of autism. In fact, the memo from Dales that worked its way up the chain of command at the national level found the opposite outcome. The correlation between the increasing uptake of vaccines and the rising incidence of the autism cases was obvious from the graph alone. Although the 2001 Dales-authored memo did not provide all of the data on which its graphs were based, those graphs did demonstrate that while the percentage of children receiving the thimerosal-containing vaccines—in particular, the DTP, HepB, and Hib shots—was rising nationally, the rate of autism in California was rising almost in perfect cadence for the years for which national data were available. Dales mentioned to his superiors that there were no data specific to California on the rising percentages of children receiving the HepB series and the Hib shots. For this reason he included a graph (Figure 3-3), where the

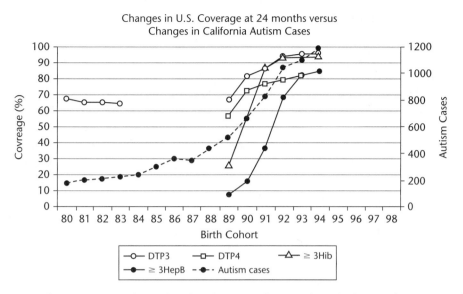

Figure 3-3 Data from memos exchanged within the CDC showing the correlation of rising use of vaccines nationally with the rising rate of the autism diagnosis in California.
Source: Retrieved July 1, 2008, from http://www.putchildrenfirst.org/intro.html). Government document in the Public Domain.

shots containing thimerosal came into focus, comparing the rising rate of the autism diagnosis in California against the rising percentage of children in distinct birth cohorts receiving those same shots nationally.

Data from the Most Populous State

The exchange of memos about the vaccines highlighted in Figure 3-3 took place because of their thimerosal content. Because he was not able to separate out the percentage of children in California who had received the thimerosal-containing shots from the national statistics, Dales used the national data set as the best available basis for estimating the percentage of California children receiving thimerosal-containing vaccines. This approach is reasonable given that California is the most populous state. It follows that the national statistics should, therefore, be fairly representative of the increasing use of those vaccines in California.

Although the original data on which the graph was based are not given in Dales's memo, we exploded the graph and carefully interpolated the vaccination rates, especially for the years 1989 to 1994. Then we calculated the correlations between the diagnosed cases of autism and the percentages of children receiving the thimerosal-containing vaccines for those years. For birth cohorts receiving all four of the recommended shots in the DTP series by their 24th month, the correlation with the diagnosis of autism is .97; for those getting only three of the DPT shots, the correlation is .90; for cohorts receiving up to three of the HepB series shots, the correlation is .99; for birth cohorts receiving up to three shots in the Hib series, the correlation is .92.

The correlation for any one of the series of shots taken by itself is substantial and cannot reasonably be attributed to chance. All of the correlations taken together suggest the inference that the likelihood of any given child in a cohort being diagnosed with autism increases with the uptake of a larger number of vaccinations by that child. With that fact in mind, we took another look at the data for the MMR series from the *Journal of the American Medical Association* article (Dales et al., 2001).

Another Look at the MMR Shots and Autism

The intense interest of the CDC in the MMR series—and the agency's apparent effort to show that vaccinations had no association with autism—began with the publication of Wakefield et al. (1998) showing a temporal association of exposure to the measles virus in 8 of 12 children with autism who also had inflammatory bowel disease. As noted earlier in this book, the fact that autism is commonly associated with gut problems had been noted but passed over by Kanner in as many as 9 of the 11 cases he diagnosed clear back in 1943. Similarly, Wakefield et al. (1998, p. 638) pointed out that bowel disease had been associated with autism by Asperger (1961). In Wakefield et al.'s study, in 8 of the 12 original cases he examined, parents reported that symptoms of autism were noted after the MMR vaccination. Needless to say, this report in *The Lancet* caused concern at the CDC and in professional medical organizations around the world. Of the 12 children reported on in Wakefield et al.'s study, 11 had chronic inflammation of the bowel. Most of the children showed an excess of "**methylmalonic-acid** . . . indicative of a functional vitamin B_{12} deficiency" (p. 639). There would be many follow-ups to the Wakefield et al. research and abundant additional evidence on both the presence of measles virus and the vitamin B_{12} deficiency they commented on.

With respect to the claim by Dales et al. (2001) that MMR has no association with autism, we did a follow-up analysis ourselves. Because these authors did not report the actual percentages of children receiving the vaccine in successive birth cohorts in the 2001 article, we interpolated from the published line graphs in that article and calculated the correlations between the percentage of children receiving the MMR vaccine by 17 or 24 months of age with the rate of autism diagnosed in the birth cohorts of the same years after they arrived in California schools. As with Figure 3-3, we exploded the graph and used perpendicular gridlines to interpolate and estimate the percentages in each series. The correlations between the use of the MMR vaccines by 17 and 24 months for the lines reported by Dales, Hammer, and Smith (2001) are .74 (see Figure 3-4) and .43 (see Figure 3-5), respectively. With sample sizes in the 600-plus range, as reported by Dales and colleagues for each data point in their published graph, both of these correlations are statistically significant ($p <$ .0001). Correlations of this strength would be expected to occur by chance in fewer than 1 sample per 10,000 of the same size.

THE DYNAMIC ROLE OF AGE AND MULTIPLE TOXINS

Research has shown that younger children are more vulnerable to injury and that, all else being held equal, multiple vaccines and toxins tend to interact, producing more injuries than if they were administered individually. Both these facts, as we will see in Chapter 6 especially, are well known to the CDC and to the drug manufacturers.

Younger Cohorts Are More Vulnerable to Injury

Given that older children have better-developed immune systems and are better able to cope with whatever challenges are inherent in the multivalent MMR vaccine, it is to be expected that the use of the MMR vaccines in younger children (i.e., the ones who received the MMR by their 17th month as contrasted with those who received it by their 24th month) would correlate more strongly with neurological conditions such as autism. In fact, the correlation with autism was higher among the children receiving the vaccine by the younger age, 17 months ($r = .74$; Figure 3-4), than among the children receiving the MMR shot up to five months later, by the age of 24 months ($r = .43$; Figure 3-5). The contrast in these correlations was significant ($t = 3.12$, $p < .001$). This is an interesting finding in itself, and one that is supported by research on the maturation of the immune system in infants. Older infants, as predicted, and as seen in the findings observed in the Dales et al. data, appear to be better able to tolerate and cope with the challenges presented by the injected disease

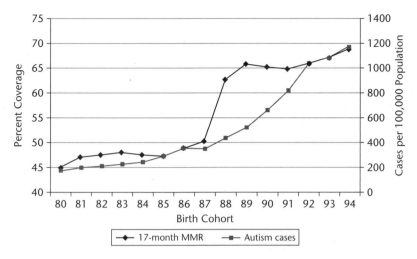

Figure 3-4 The correlation between the increasing uptake of the MMR shot, by month 17, and the increasing diagnosis of autism in California, $r = .74$, $p < .0001$.
Source: Adapted from Dales, Hammer, and Smith (2001).

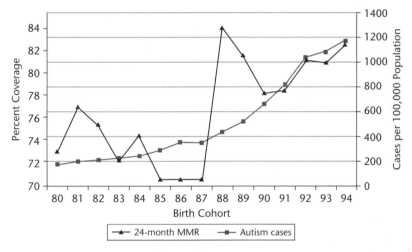

Figure 3-5 The correlation between the increasing uptake of the MMR shot, by month 24, and the increasing diagnosis of autism in California, $r = .43$, $p < .0001$.
Source: Adapted from Dales, Hammer, and Smith (2001).

agents and toxins. There is also evidence of a cumulative effect in the thimerosal-containing DTP series, where the correlation for the fourth shot in the series is .97 whereas that for the third shot in the series is .90.

Given that the MMR data and all the foregoing correlations for the thimerosal-containing vaccines are based on many data points for each birth year (with sample sizes ranging from a low of 600 to a high of 1900 children for each birth cohort, according to Dales et al., 2001), it follows that all of the correlations reported in the previous paragraphs are also statistically significant ($p < .0001$) and cannot reasonably be attributed to chance. Much less can all of them together be regarded as being produced by chance. That is, correlations of such strength cannot reasonably be regarded as uncaused. Given that we ruled out the alternative explanations for the rising incidence of autism cases in Chapter 2, we must conclude that some interaction between vaccines and the toxins they contain is, indeed, causally implicated with respect to the autism epidemic.

What is more important, in view of the amount of shared variance between the various measures, none of the correlations is negligible; even the least of them accounts for a substantial amount of the variability in the increasing number of autism cases in successive birth cohorts, and taken together they account for nearly all of it. The shared variance between the increasing number of diagnosed cases of autism and the increasing use of each vaccine ranges from a low of 18% (for MMR at 24 months) to a high of 98% (for the HepB series). It is true that the association is weaker for the MMR shots—18% for the MMR vaccine if received by 24 months and 55% for the MMR vaccine if received by 17 months—but these values also show a strong association of the MMR shots with the growth in the prevalence of autism cases.

Adjusting the Scale to See the Relation

The difference between our graphs in Figures 3-4 and 3-5 and the line graph originally published in Dales, Hammer, and Smith's (2001) article is that we set up the scales so as to make the correlation visible, which is the purpose of graphing such a relation. In creating such a visual representation, of course, the decision to use comparable scales for the graphing, as we have done in Figures 3-4 and 3-5, or very different ones, as Dales et al. did, as can easily be proved mathematically does not affect the actual value of the algebraic correlation at all. Rather, the correlation depends on the extent to which the respective measures—in this case, (A) the percentage of children receiving the MMR shots by 17 months of age, or (B) by 24 months of age, is associated algebraically with (C) the proportion of children later being diagnosed with autism when they enter school. Measures A, B, and C can be represented on any scale whatsoever for the visual representation, although some scales will be revealing whereas others will not.

A mathematical demonstration that the scale we use does not affect the correlation can be seen by considering that the correlation between scores 1, 2, and 3 on A, for example, with scores 70, 80, and 90 on B, for example, would remain exactly the same if we divided either scale by 100 or multiplied either one or both scales by 10 million. The correlation between the scales depends only on the distribution of scores within each of the scales relative to the distribution of scores in the other scale. If the proportional distance to the average score on A is kept the same by multiplying or dividing, it follows by the strictest mathematical reasoning that changing the scale by multiplication or division does not affect the correlation, but can alter its appearance in a graph.

By squishing the scale for the uptake of MMR vaccines, Dales, Hammer, and Smith (2001) made it appear that the correlation between MMR uptake and the growth in diagnosed cases of autism are hardly correlated at all. It is noteworthy that they did not report the numerical correlations in their published paper. But did the statisticians at the CDC actually neglect to compute such correlations?

It seems as if Dales and colleagues set up their scale to justify the claim that increasing uptake of MMR shots had no connection with autism. They used incomparable and separated scales to suggest there was no correlation when, in fact, the correlations for the MMR shot are both significant ($p < .0001$) with less than one chance in 10,000 that either of those correlations would be expected to occur by chance. Also, both correlations are substantial; that is, the increasing uptake of the MMR vaccine either by 17 months or by 24 months accounted for substantial proportions of the variance in the increasing diagnosis of autism (55% and 18%, respectively). From all of the foregoing evidence, it is reasonable to infer that the vaccines and their interactions are involved as causal factors in the autism epidemic.

Measles Virus and SSPE

It has been known for many years that the measles virus is a causal factor in the progressive, and usually fatal, disease condition called **subacute sclerosing panencephalitis** (**SSPE**). The symptoms of that disorder resemble those of "regressive" autism—cognitive decline, stereotyped tics sometimes accompanied by seizures, and deterioration of the central nervous system. In the past, the brain deterioration in any such case had to be determined by invasive tissue sampling, in the form of either a **biopsy** or an autopsy after death (Risk & Haddad, 1979). More recently, **magnetic resonance imaging** (**MRI**) has emerged as a viable technology for making this determination (Kastrup, Wanke, & Maschke, 2008). The prevailing CDC and WHO theory is that vaccination prevents infections by measles virus and that it does not cause SSPE (CDC, 2008g; H. Campbell, Andrews, K. E. Brown, & E. Miller, 2007; Onal et al., 2006).

However, some evidence indicates not only that SSPE occurs in persons who have been vaccinated (Brouns, Verlinde, Lagae, De Koster, Lemmens, & Van de Casseye, 2001), but also that the likelihood of its occurrence is greater in persons who have been vaccinated with measles virus than in persons who have not been vaccinated. The chance of unvaccinated persons contracting SSPE, in the study conducted by Onal et al. (2006), was actually greater for persons who had received the recommended vaccination. This finding, though not highlighted by Onal et al., was confirmed by Akram, Naz, Malik, and Hamid in 2008. The latter authors found that 86% of the 50 the patients whom they studied had been vaccinated for measles prior to the onset of SSPE. More than half of them (31 of the 50) had also had the measles prior to the onset of SSPE, and 77% of them had been vaccinated against measles. In these authors' sample, SSPE was 3.1 times more likely to occur in males than in females—a ratio similar to that observed in autism.

A Toxic Potpourri

If the rising percentages of children receiving the MMR vaccines are considered together with the increasing uptake of the thimerosal-containing vaccines for the years 1989 to 1994, the variance in the increasing incidence of autism is almost completely accounted for. Granted, even such a high correlation cannot be directly interpreted as a singular causal explanation for autism because genetic factors are also at play. Nevertheless, the correlations observed certainly suggest that vaccines are causally involved in producing the upsurge of autism diagnoses. To suppose that there is no association between the increased use of vaccines and the increased incidence of autism is analogous to supposing there is no association between thunder and lightning. We can see from many different angles that there is a relation.

Also, as the research discussed in Chapters 5 and 6 shows, the challenges presented by introducing toxins, disease agents, and adventitious contaminants into the body through vaccines and other medical procedures (e.g., dental amalgam) cannot reasonably be expected *not to produce biochemical interactions*. As the foregoing analyses have already suggested, some of the interactions seem to lead to neurological disorders and others, to death, as in SIDS. In Chapter 7, we consider the theoretical logic underlying the argument that vaccines in particular must be involved in producing neurological and related disorders. This logic focuses on balances at the atomic and molecular levels: To deny the virtual certainty of such interactions would be to deny that any medicines or vaccines might potentially produce any biochemical effects of any kind. But medicines, including vaccines, certainly can and do produce biochemical interactions.

The Unwanted Findings

The findings depicted in Figure 3-2 were so unwanted and potentially damaging to the vaccine industry (including members of the medical profession, the manufacturers of vaccines, and the CDC promoters of the vaccine schedule) that they decided to try to make them "go away." As early as December 17, 1999, a discussion was under way to try to find some other explanation for the evident correlation of vaccines with neurological disorders. In a memo written on that date by the Epidemic Intelligence Service Officer Thomas Verstraeten to his superior (Robert Davis and copied to Frank

DeStefano ●) at the CDC, it is evident that someone had suggested that Verstraeten find a way to minimize the evident impact in particular of the mercury-containing shots on the incidence of neurological disorders. His memo contained the words, "It just won't go away," in the subject line.

Verstraeten explained in an email dated December 17, 1999, that as he was examining

> the increase of mercury for the first three months divided by the average [infant's] body weight in the first, second and third month . . . except for epilepsy, all the harm is done in the first month. . . . these neurologic developmental conditions are very much related (odds of having one when also having the other go from 20 to 100!). . . . As you'll see some of the RRs [rate ratios—that is, dose-to-disorder relations] increase over the categories and I haven't yet found an alternative explanation. . . . Please let me know if you can think of one. Frank [DeStefano] proposes we discuss this on a call after New Year.

The Simpsonwood Conference

A few months later, in June 2000, the Simpsonwood Conference was convened to discuss the evident correlation of vaccines with neurological disorders in general and with autism in particular. Forty representatives from the CDC and pharmaceutical companies, plus 11 paid consultants, met to examine the relationship between thimerosal and neurological disorders, as reported to the Vaccine Safety Datalink. Walter Orenstein opened that conference by noting that

> concerns were raised last summer that mercury, as methyl mercury in vaccines [sic; "ethyl" mercury is probably intended here because there is no methyl mercury in vaccines as far as is known] might exceed safe levels. (Simpsonwood Conference, 2000, p. 1 ●)

The conference was expected to provide advice to the policy-making Advisory Committee on Immunization Practices concerning "options with regard to mercury in vaccines" (p. 2).

The data presented, which are at the end of the transcript, were marked "CONFIDENTIAL" and "DO NOT COPY OR RELEASE." In addition, multiple warnings were placed within the document itself, and various attempts were made to shield it from public view (R. F. Kennedy, Jr., 2005 ●). Frank DeStefano was a participant at Simpsonwood and introduced himself there as an employee of the CDC, identifying himself as "Medical Epidemiologist in the National Immunization Program and the Director of the Vaccine Safety Datalink" (Simpsonwood Conference, 2000, p. 4 ●). DeStefano continued to hold the view that there is no evidence of a link between vaccines and autism at least until 2007. He argued that there is "compelling scientific evidence against a causal association" (DeStefano, 2007, p. 756). As we will see, what he is referring to is CDC's alleged inability to see the association in their own data. The difficulty is comparable to failing to detect the elephant that is standing on your foot.

Legal Actions Follow

Under the Freedom of Information Act (1966–2007), the scientific findings that vaccines were strongly associated with neurological disorders were brought to light and subjected to public scrutiny. The research conducted for this book is part of a much larger ongoing process including legal actions that have led to the discovery of many secret documents, including the whole transcript of the Simpsonwood Conference (2000). Many of the key documents that were uncovered can be found at the Web site of Putchildrenfirst.org ●. The deliberate decision to hide the data showing the correlation between thimerosal and neurological disorders, including autism, is evident throughout that documentation. In the meantime, the number of children being diagnosed with autism was increasing at an accelerating pace (see Figures 1-1 and 2-3). No one associated with the vaccine industry wanted either result—the correlation with vaccines or the rising rate of autism diagnosis—to be true, and they hoped to avoid the growing public furor about the issue.

At the center of the controversy was the troubling question about the mercury found in the DTP, HepB, and Hib vaccines. That issue would lead members of the public to raise a lot of other questions about contaminants, interactive effects, and the harm that had already been done over several decades by the increasing use of injected and oral vaccines.

The Bad News (What They Didn't Want to Hear)

In its zeal to minimize the bad tidings—especially the undesirable findings that thimerosal was associated with an increasing rate of autism diagnosis in successive birth cohorts—the U.S. Public Health Service, acting mainly through its subagency, the CDC, issued a series of ambivalent statements. On the one hand, these missives denied or cast doubt on the idea that autism and neurological disorders were actually increasing; on the other hand, they denied that vaccines might have anything to do with whatever increase might be occurring. That ambivalent approach toward the evidence of an increasing rate of diagnosis of autism persists today. For instance, at its main Web site on May 11, 2009, the CDC still includes a disclaimer concerning the "Prevalence of ASDs [Autism Spectrum Disorders]":

> It is clear that more children than ever before are being classified as having autism spectrum disorders (ASDs). But, it is unclear how much of this increase is due to changes in how we identify and classify ASDs in people, and how much is due to a true increase in prevalence. By current standards, ASDs are the second most common serious developmental disability after mental retardation/intellectual impairment, but they are still less common than other conditions that affect children's development, such as speech and language impairments, learning disabilities, and attention deficit/hyperactivity disorder (ADHD). (CDC, 2008d 💿)

Thoughtful readers will recall that the various versions of the *DSM* from 1987 forward all acknowledged that about half the cases of autism (or more according to *DSM-III*) would also receive a diagnosis of mental retardation, thus potentially inflating the estimates in that category. Also, diagnostic substitution has supposedly been occurring (Shattuck, 2006), with cases being switched from both the mental retardation and the learning disability categories to the autism category, thereby depleting the former categories and inflating the category of ASDs. It is interesting that the CDC is using all of these supposed trends to explain growth in the ASDs—growth that, according to the same CDC, is not really occurring at all. In the meantime, the CDC is just as ill equipped to explain the increase in the ADHD category as to explain the increase in ASDs, and ADHD is just as likely to be associated with vaccine injuries.

Many officials, and the public at large, hoped that the alarming numbers being reported, especially under the requirements of the Individuals with Disabilities Education Act of 1990 (IDEA) and its revisions, were somehow mistaken, inflated, or just plain misleading. In their search for the hoped-for explanation that would make the problem go away, the CDC and the medical community at large would latch on to one theory after another, even when the several theories combined were mutually inconsistent and sometimes logically contradicted each other (e.g., see the five popular theories discussed in Chapter 2). In fact, concerning the evident autism epidemic, they would generally argue in favor of every theory except for the most plausible one—that we really are in the middle of an epidemic of serious neurological disorders, in which severe autism appears front and center.

DISCOVERIES OF INTEREST

Why did Dr. Tom Verstraeten write a memo to Dr. Robert Davis in 1999, while both were CDC employees investigating the role of the mercury in vaccines as a suspected causal factor in neurological conditions (including autism), saying, "It just won't go away"? In the memo, which was never intended for public viewing, Verstraeten (1999 🔊) noted that the neurological conditions associated with vaccine poisoning were closely related to each other and that most of the harm appeared to have been done in the first month after vaccination.

Three years after the Verstraeten memo, and two years after the Simpsonwood Conference, a peculiar series of provisions would be added to the Homeland Security Act of 2002, literally in the middle of the night. On November 25, 2002, that 484-page legislative act was signed into law with four paragraphs (Sections 1714–1717) specifically protecting drug manufacturers from civil litigation concerning injuries sustained from thimerosal. A few days earlier, Congressman Dan Burton, chairman of the House Committee on Government Reform, had written an open statement on "Facts and Fiction About Thimerosal in Vaccines" dated November 18, 2002 🔊, which called attention to injuries suspected to be caused by thimerosal. No doubt the public concerns about vaccines in general and thimerosal specifically precipitated the amendments, which especially protected the pharmaceutical company Eli Lilly on the thimerosal issue. Later, the amendments would be repealed, but the important fact to note, with respect to the back-and-forth in negotiating the public policy, was the intense involvement of big pharmaceutical interests, the U.S. Congress, vaccines, and thimerosal.

Bioweapons? Domestic Terror?

At the time the Homeland Security Act of 2002 (HSA, 2002) was being forged, there was some discussion of terrorist threats using beefed-up anthrax and smallpox disease agents as bioweapons. Interestingly, vaccines against those particular disease agents never included the preservative thimerosal. So why was it necessary for the HSA bill to protect Eli Lilly as the manufacturer of the neurotoxin thimerosal that was being placed in other vaccines? As we have already noted, this mercury compound was found in the DTP series, the HepB series, and Hib.

Meanwhile, in the background, a growing number of parents had filed suits under the 1986 Vaccine Injury Compensation Act claiming that their children were injured by vaccines, and in particular by thimerosal as manufactured by Eli Lilly. By July 2006, Edlich, Son, et al. (2007) reported the number of suits related to the role of thimerosal in autism had risen to 5030. Also, according to their figures, almost half the awards doled out by the U.S. Court of Federal Claims for vaccine injuries from 1988 to 2007 were paid in connection with injuries attributed to the thimerosal-containing DTP series.

If there were no evidence of harm from the mercury and/or other contaminants in vaccines, or from the vaccines themselves, why were late-night deals made to include the amendments in Sections 1714–1717 in HSA 2002? Interestingly, it was just that back-stage manipulation of the Homeland Security Act, according to medical journalist David Kirby, that led him to do the investigative work that would result in his award-winning book *Evidence of Harm* (2005). If thimerosal and other components of vaccines were not doing harm, why the last-minute effort to tack on special protection for the manufacturer of thimerosal, Eli Lilly, in the Homeland Security Act?

In fact, overwhelming evidence already existed showing that the mercury in thimerosal (see the data in Figures 3-2 and 3-3 and the discussion in Chapters 5 and 6) along with other components and contaminants in widely used vaccines were implicated in causing autism and a host of related disorders and disease conditions (e.g., see the research sources cited by Edlich, Son, et al., 2007; also Chapters 5 and 6). The last-minute effort to protect the drug companies—and, by extension, the government agencies charged with guarding the public from harm by medicines and vaccines in particular—was tantamount to an admission of guilty knowledge. That is, the drug lobbyists; the U.S. Public Health Service (now called the Department of Health and Human Services) and its subagencies, the CDC and the FDA; and certain politicians receiving support from pharmaceutical companies were demonstrating by their actions that they knew the vaccines were doing harm in many cases.

A Thin Disguise

The rationale cited for linking the protective amendments to the HSA 2002 legislation was the threat of a bioterrorist attack with anthrax or the smallpox virus. However, the vaccines developed to protect against those elements in particular have never contained thimerosal. Thus the question becomes, why attach special protections for Eli Lilly, the manufacturer of thimerosal, to the Homeland Security Act in such a secretive manner?

Barbara Loe Fisher, president of the National Vaccine Information Center, summed up the historic changes of the Homeland Security Act of 2002 in this way:

> Section 304 of the bill removed from the states their historic control over public health laws, including vaccination laws, and handed it over to federal health officials. Simultaneously, Sections 1714–1717 of the bill shielded the pharmaceutical industry from lawsuits for injuries caused by FDA-approved vaccines, such as mercury-containing pediatric vaccines associated with the development of autism in many children. (Fisher, 2002 ●)

The result of the amendments, if they had been allowed to stand—Sections 1714–1717 were subsequently repealed by the U.S. Congress Consolidated Appropriations Resolution P.L. 108–7 (2003)—would have been to provide an additional layer of insulation to vaccine manufacturers, protecting them from any legal liability for harm done by vaccines or their components. The Congressional Research Service (CRS) of the Library of Congress summed up the impact of the repealed sections 1714–1717 as being intended to

> limit the **tort liability** [wrongdoing usually caused by negligence rather than resulting from intentional harm] of manufacturers and administrators of the components and ingredients of various vaccines; these sections reportedly were designed to benefit pharmaceutical manufacturer Eli Lilly in suits against it concerning Thimerosal. (CRS, 2005 ●)

Why was thimerosal singled out for attention in an act of Congress in the first place, and why would Eli Lilly be especially in need of protection? The implication is that some power brokers and lobbyists in Congress knew in advance that the manufacturer of thimerosal had caused neurological injuries by recommending its use in vaccines. In attempting to disguise the protection of Eli Lilly from liability for thimerosal, the U.S. Congress—whether knowingly or not, we do not know—was made party to some interesting after dark activity.

The Vaccine Injury Compensation Act of 1986 had already effectively made the U.S. federal government liable for any vaccine injuries under the CDC immunization schedule. Thus, under existing law, vaccine manufacturers were well protected from civil suits before the amendments of Sections 1714–1717 were added to HSA 2002. So why did the sponsors of those amendments propose them in the first place? As we will see, the disappointing but necessary inference seems to be that the vaccine manufacturers and some of their collaborators with influence in the U.S. Congress knew they had done harm before the amendments were proposed, and they wanted to build an even more impenetrable bunker in which to hide from the coming firestorm of public outrage.

Did the CDC and FDA Really Intend to Remove Thimerosal in 1999?

Because of the Freedom of Information Act (1966–2007), it was possible for concerned citizens to gain access to the CDC's internal correspondence, which showed that in the same year that the CDC proposed to eliminate mercury from vaccines (1999), Merck and SmithKline Beecham, two of the largest manufacturers of vaccines, wrote privately to the CDC director, announcing that they could produce thimerosal-free vaccines immediately. The manufacturers offered to create a sufficient supply to remove all stockpiles of the mercury-loaded versions (the actual memos can be found on the Putchildrenfirst.org Web site; see Mahmoud, 1999; Jabarra, 1999; Kaplan, 1999 ●).

Dr. Jeffrey P. Koplan, then director of the CDC, on behalf of the CDC declined the offer to produce thimerosal-free vaccines immediately ●. This move ran counter to the U.S. Public Health Service's own September 1999 public statement that manufacturers should get the mercury out of the vaccines "as soon as possible" (American Academy of Pediatrics & Public Health Service, 1999 ●); the Public Health Service is the parent organization for the CDC. Instead, the CDC authorized the continued use of stockpiled vaccines, which still contained thimerosal.

Governmental Ambivalence

In June 2000, Dr. Roger Bernier, then the Associate Director for Science inthe National Immunization Program and one of the principal organizers of the Simpsonwood Conference sponsored by the CDC, noted that the policy makers at CDC had entertained second thoughts concerning their own recommendation to remove the mercury from vaccines "as soon as possible." In his opening remarks at Simpsonwood concerning the research on vaccines containing thimerosal, Bernier said:

> [I]n October of 1999 the ACIP [Advisory Committee on Immunization Practices] looked this situation over again and did not express a preference for any of the vaccines that were thimerosal free. They said the vaccines [with thimerosal] could be continued to be used, but reiterated the importance of the long term goal to try to remove thimerosal as soon as possible. (Simpsonwood Conference, 2000, p. 12 ●)

The reasoning was that honoring the published recommendation to remove mercury from vaccines too quickly would send the wrong message to the public—namely, that thimerosal had already done a lot of harm over its seven decades of use.

One of the conferees, Dr. Paul Offit (the patent holder for Merck's RotaTeq vaccine), critiqued the mixed message sent by the CDC concerning thimerosal. Commenting retrospectively on the 1999 joint statement of the American Academy of Pediatrics and the U.S. Public Health Service, which had recommended the removal of thimerosal from all vaccines, he wrote:

> Critics wondered how removing something that hadn't been found to be unsafe could make vaccines safer. But many parents, frightened by a sudden change in policy, reasoned that thimerosal was targeted because it was harmful—and their faith in the vaccine infrastructure was shaken. Doctors were also confused by the recommendation. (Offit, 2007, p. 1278)

Thimerosal Continues to Be Used

As a result of its ambivalent policy, and contrary to the recommendations in the 1999 public statement, the CDC continued to authorize the use of millions of doses of thimerosal-containing vaccines in the United States and abroad. As documented by Robert F. Kennedy, Jr., in a *Huffington Post* article in 2006 ●, the CDC delayed following its own published advice concerning thimerosal by not only using stockpiles of thimerosal-containing vaccines in the United States, but also shipping huge quantities to developing countries. Kennedy quoted an unnamed federal official who said that "an immediate withdrawal might discredit the international vaccine programs for which CDC is an important partner."

The WHO, the international counterpart to the CDC, has continued to advocate the use of thimerosal-containing vaccines abroad—an effort that is funded in part by U.S. dollars. Kennedy (2006) notes that WHO, as a subagency of the United Nations,

> is now injecting children in developing countries with the same amounts of thimerosal we were giving American kids at their highest exposures, but in a shorter period.

In the same article, Kennedy asserts that the real motivation for the CDC's delay in removing thimerosal from U.S. vaccines has to do with the costs to drug manufacturers.

Another motivation for the delay, as noted explicitly at the Simpsonwood Conference, was to avoid any sort of admission that the thimerosal used in medicines and vaccines from the 1930s forward had already done harm and that it had directly contributed to the creation of the autism epidemic. At the Simpsonwood Conference, one participant—Dr. William Weil, representing the Committee on Environmental Health at the American Academy of Pediatrics—made the following point:

> [The] dose related relationships [between mercury and autism] are linear and statistically significant. You can play with this all you want. They are linear. They are statistically significant. (Simpsonwood Conference, 2000, p. 207 ●)

Evidence of a dose-related relationship between thimerosal and autism is implicit in Figure 3-3 where the cumulative impact of multiple doses can be inferred from the coincidence of the rising use of thimerosal-containing vaccines with the upward trend in autism in the California data.

The fact that the CDC did not really intend to follow its own advice to "remove thimerosal as soon as possible" from all vaccines was made perfectly clear by Dr. John Clements, representative from the Expanded Program on Immunization at the World Health Organization in Geneva, at the Simpsonwood Conference. At the end of the conference, he told the other attendees:

> My mandate as I sit here in this group is to make sure at the end of the day that 100,000,000 are immunized with DTP, hepatitis B and if possible Hib, this year, next year, and for many years to come, and that will have to be with thimerosal-containing vaccines. (Simpsonwood Conference, 2000, p. 248)

A HOPELESS PROGNOSIS?

The idea that autism is caused by unknown genetic factors clearly hindered the discovery of the toxins and other factors involved in its etiology. Coupled with the fact that autism was defined and diagnosed from 1943 forward in terms of behavioral characteristics, with little or no reference to concomitant medical conditions such as chronic vomiting, bloody diarrhea, bowel disease, seizures, and the like, the genetic explanation was consistent with the claim that autism must remain a mystery until the genetic details could someday be worked out.

Meanwhile, the conclusion that "autism is a mystery, an unsolvable puzzle" would often be used to dismiss the idea proposed by many parents that toxins from vaccines, dental amalgam, viruses, bacteria, and fungi were involved in their children's autism. To describe this situation, David Kennedy (2007) proposed the phrase "manufactured uncertainty," which had formerly applied to the tobacco industry's defense that there was no known link between cancers, heart disease, and other ailments and tobacco use. The CDC, FDA, American Dental Association, and American Academy of Pediatrics maintain that research has not definitively demonstrated any association between the known toxins in vaccines and medicines and the etiology of neurological disorders in general and autism in particular. In adopting such a defensive posture, J. P. Baker (2008) ostensibly agrees with the CDC that the recommendation to remove thimerosal in 1999 was made in spite of the fact that "there was no evidence that the use of thimerosal as a vaccine preservative had caused any true harm" (p. 250).

A Lifelong Condition?

The uncertainty about the causes of autism is commonly used to defend the conclusion that the diagnosis is a lifelong sentence. If the causal basis is genetic, once autism has been discovered and diagnosed in any particular child, little more than behavioral therapy can be administered to alleviate its effects. The prognosis for actual recovery, according to the official diagnosis, is virtually hopeless. When Jon Shestack and Portia Iversen asked the doctor what could be done to help their son Dov, the doctor said, "Nothing." He told them to go home, have a good cry, and then get on with their lives because there was nothing they could do about autism. Medical doctor and researcher Brian Jepson took the same approach with his own wife, Laurie Jepson, when their son was diagnosed with autism: He told her that they would just have to accept the diagnosis and move on. Laurie, he said, needed to give up the notion that there might be a way for their son Aaron to recover. Brian Jepson was inclined to accept the neurologist's recommendation that Aaron would eventually need to be institutionalized and that his parents should "not to waste" their "time and money" on experimental treatments that were, according to the neurologist, "expensive and unproven" (Jepson & Johnson, 2007, p. 2).

Laurie Jepson, like many mothers of children who have been diagnosed with autism, found the hopeless prognosis unacceptable. She hoped somehow to recover her child, who seemed to have become lost inside the strange and mysterious world of autism. Similarly, Jenny McCarthy (2007a) would tell Oprah Winfrey that she knew her boy Evan was still in there and that she intended to rescue him.

Rounding Up Unusual Suspects

For McCarthy, the Jepsons, and thousands of other parents whose children were being diagnosed near the beginning of the new millennium, hope came from a few individuals who took a closer look at neglected symptoms of the disorder and inferred that some kind of poisoning had to be involved. As explained in Chapter 2, genetic factors cannot change as fast as the exponential growth in the number of cases would require. So, genetic factors could not be the whole explanation for autism. If there is no such thing as a genetic epidemic, the rising number of cases must have some other explanation. Among the obvious suspects were environmental toxins.

Because of the great confidence of the general public in vaccines, which were traditionally seen as bulwarks of safety against disease, there would be plenty of resistance to the hypothesis that vaccines might be part of the problem. The first clue suggesting the involvement of vaccines—and one that was there from 1943 forward—was the large number of severe cases of classic Kanner-type autism, in which a period of normal development is followed by a precipitous descent into socially unresponsive, nonverbal, stereotyped behavior. Was it merely coincidental that the descent often began almost immediately or soon after a series of vaccinations?

Researchers and Detectives Against Their Will

The parents who undertook this journey of discovery were ordinary people from a broad cross section of the world's population. None of them, as Shestack observed in 2003, wanted to know anything about autism. The necessity to find out about it was forced on them.

Some of these parents were highly educated professionals in medicine, law, and the sciences, and some had financial resources. Among the unlikely sleuths who were brought together by the devastating impact of autism was the team of medical researchers led by Sally Bernard. Her son was one of the many children diagnosed during the period of exponential growth in cases of autism. The sequence of events leading to her becoming (or at least being credited with being) the ring leader of a group later called the "mercury moms" is partially chronicled by Kirby (2005; also see J. P. Baker, 2008). Indeed, Bernard herself and her collaborators would often use that phrase to refer to themselves. Through their relentless advocacy, the members of this group helped to energize a growing think tank of independent researchers from around the world. Bernard and colleagues would begin to examine, consolidate, and publish the extensive research evidence pertaining to the role played by mercury in helping to create the current epidemic of neurological disorders, including autism at its center.

Shoot All the Messengers?

When it was revealed that mercury (Bernard et al., 2001), as well as other toxins and an impressive array of disease agents, were being placed in the bloodstreams of younger and younger infants through a dramatically increasing number of vaccinations (Cave, 2001), the reaction from vaccine manufacturers and promoters of the vaccination programs (especially the CDC, FDA, and pediatricians responsible for oversight of the use of vaccines) was absolutely predictable. The general public, including the authors of this book, had been convinced for many years that vaccines were good and that any questions raised concerning their safety had to be coming from left field, if not from the extreme lunatic fringe. No one was willing to believe that vaccines might be involved in causing something as devastating as severe autism. Likewise, no one dared to think that the toxic impact of vaccines in genetically susceptible families would soon be linked to a host of other diseases and disorders across a much wider range than the officially recognized autism spectrum.

In reality, as we will see in subsequent chapters, not only would the search for causes of the autism epidemic lead to the rounding up of some very unusual suspects (including vaccines and the silver fillings placed in our own mouths by our dentists), but the resulting explosion of knowledge available in the public domain would also catapult the health sciences in general and the medical profession in particular into a whole new era. The autism epidemic would lead to a long-needed paradigm shift toward a more holistic, systems-oriented, communication-based approach to medicine and the health sciences. We believe that we are witnessing and contributing to that shift at this very moment. Also, autism is playing a crucial role both in forcing the ongoing reconceptualization of interacting systems and in making healthcare professionals more accountable to patients and their families.

As a result, a very healthy thing is happening in the health sciences industry. Patients and their families are demanding that healthcare providers study the most up-to-date relevant research. Doctors who have slipped into the mode of serving as sales representatives for pharmaceutical companies (Fugh-Berman & Ahari, 2007; Whitney, 2005) are being required to actually consider information about drug interactions, side effects, special susceptibilities, and the like by better-informed patients (O'Connor et al., 2007). Goff et al. (2008) specifically note patient "concerns about the pharmaceutical industry's influence on doctors' prescribing practices" (p. 236). Does your doctor know what is in your medicines? (See Figure 3-6.) The research suggests that when doctors and patients have access and agree on the relevant information, everyone gets better results and costs go down as communication and knowledge increase (Epstein, Alper, & Quill, 2004). Better-informed patients mean better results in health care all around (E. S. Fisher, 2008). Is there any reason to suppose that things should be different with respect to vaccines, toxins, and autism?

WE'LL DO IT OURSELVES: PARENTS TAKE ACTION

The first step in realizing the hope that it might be possible to recover from severe autism was for a few persistent parents, especially the "mercury moms" (and a few dads), to identify and publish

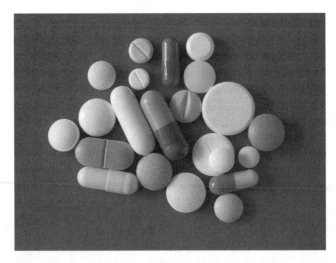

Figure 3-6 What's in your prescription? Does your doctor know?
Source: © ajt/ShutterStock, Inc.

information about the role of certain toxins delivered to patients through medical practices. Following on the heels of the Wakefield et al. (1998) research into the MMR vaccine and autism, probably the single most important event was the publication of the paper by Sally Bernard and her colleagues in *Medical Hypotheses* in 2001. In this article and a subsequent 2002 publication, they proposed that autism could be seen as a form of mercury poisoning (Bernard, Enayati, Redwood, Roger, & Binstock, 2001; Bernard, Enayati, Roger, Binstock, & Redwood, 2002). We examine that hypothesis carefully in the next two chapters of this book. For the moment, it is important to see it in its historical context.

Events Leading Up to the Mercury Hypothesis

In 1997, a New Jersey Congressman named Frank Pallone became concerned about the mercury levels in fish and the industrial pollution contributing to its accumulation in these food sources. Pallone pressed the government—the FDA, in particular—to take another look at mercury toxicity in licensed drugs and vaccines. The resulting data were published in 2001 in the vaccine-friendly journal of *Pediatrics*, in an article written by L. K. Ball, R. Ball, and Pratt. Their conclusion would become the CDC's public statement on the matter: Not to worry, no harm done. But in the background, alarm bells were sounding. Neal Halsey, then head of the Institute for Vaccine Safety at Johns Hopkins, would tell Arthur Allen, "From the beginning, I saw thimerosal as something different. . . . It was the first strong evidence of a causal association with neurological impairment. I was very concerned" (Allen, 2002, p. 1). Because the article appearing on a Sunday had used the word "autism" in its title, the follow-up by Halsey on the very next Friday clarified that "he was referring to developmental delay, not to autism" (Allen, 2002). Nevertheless, the beehives in Washington were already buzzing about Halsey's inadvertent admission.

When it became painfully clear that tens of millions of six-month-old American babies had received 187.5 micrograms of ethyl mercury in thimerosal from the middle 1980s forward, and some had gotten even more, Halsey was among those who began to worry. He told Arthur Allen:

> My first reaction was simply disbelief, which was the reaction of almost everybody involved in vaccines. . . . In most vaccine containers, thimerosal is listed as a mercury derivative, a hundredth of a percent. And what I believed, and what everybody else believed, was that it

was truly a trace, a biologically insignificant amount. My honest belief is that if the labels had had the mercury content in micrograms, this would have been uncovered years ago. But the fact is, no one did the calculation. (Allen, 2002, p. 2 ●)

In 1998, a world-renowned British medical researcher, Andrew Wakefield, published evidence of a link between the gut disease in severe autism and the measles virus administered in MMR shots. By then, the mercury levels in vaccines were already drawing international attention. In August 1998, the U.S. FDA raised concerns about the issue. Soon thereafter, on September 8, 1998, the Safety Working Party of the European Agency for the Evaluation of Medicinal Products issued a paper titled "Assessment of the Toxicity of Thimerosal in Relation to Its Use in Medicinal Products." Its authors concluded:

> There is ample evidence from the literature that thiomersal [thimerosal] may cause sensitiza-tion and subsequent allergic reactions . . . the use of thimerosal in vaccines given to infants in accordance with various national vaccine programs may in certain cases result in approxi-mately two times higher intake of ethyl mercury during the first year of life than what can be considered reasonably safe. Given the great uncertainty of the estimations of safe levels in young children, it is suggested to restrict the use of thimerosal in vaccines. (Quoted by Burton, 2002, pp. E1019–1020 ●)

The concern with ethyl mercury in vaccines would turn out to be grounded in a vast body of solid research. When the young Dr. Thomas Verstraeten began to find undeniable evidence of thi-merosal poisoning in the Vaccine Safety Datalink records at CDC, he went to the literature on mercury, with which he was, according to his own comments, unfamiliar beforehand. (We review the toxicology and its important theoretical consequences in Chapters 5 and 6.) When he became acquainted with that literature, Verstraeten was amazed. He said, "When . . . I went back through the literature, I was actually stunned by what I saw" (Simpsonwood Conference, 2000, p. 162). Interestingly, parents from a great diversity of professions, including medicine, were independently discovering for themselves what Halsey and others were just becoming alarmed about. Predictably, the promoters of the use of thimerosal, disease agents, and whatever other toxins may have crept into the vaccines during their production, were put on the defensive. The outcome would be referred to by Ashcraft and Gerel (n.d., ●) as a "public health disaster" from "toxic exposure [that] was entirely avoidable." In fact, the exposure was initially orchestrated, later repudiated (in 1999), and then repeatedly exonerated by the CDC.

Getting Organized and Informed

It is no wonder that the most aggressive, hopeful, and effective organizations pursuing the etiology and treatment of autism, as noted by the director of the National Institute of Mental Health in 2003, were formed by parents. However, it would be a mistake to suppose, as some have sug-gested or implied (e.g., Shattuck, 2006), that parents sought a diagnosis of autism to get insurance payoffs or federal funds. Although that idea has been suggested as one of the motivations for diagnostic substitution (i.e., preferring a diagnosis of autism over some other disorder), it could hardly be further from the truth. The universal reaction of parents to the diagnosis of autism is one of grief, in most cases followed by a period of despair. It is not a diagnosis that a parent would willfully choose.

The reaction of being overwhelmed with grief can be found in the many stories told in popular sources by the parents of children with autism. In a series of articles in *Redbook Magazine*, Nancy Rones tells about the Kalkowskis and their son Ryan (Rones, 2008a, 2008b). Ryan was developing normally up to about 17 months when he "began to backslide" into "regressive autism" (2008a, p. 172). Nicole Kalkowski tells how difficult it was to do ordinary things like grocery shopping:

> I didn't want people looking at Ryan acting up and thinking, *Wow, that's really awful,* . . . I'd have a family over for a barbecue and instead of socializing, I hid in my bedroom with Ryan. . . . (2008a, p. 173)

In Nicole's case, other parents who were also coping with autism helped her. She found the Talk About Curing Autism Web site and saw Jenny McCarthy's story of the recovery from autism for her own child and others. Nicole said,

> With tears running down my face, I watched a video on the site about kids who had regressed and were recovering, some to a point of being considered "typical" children again. . . . It made me believe recovery was possible for Ryan. (2008a, p. 176)

Without hope that causes could be discovered and dealt with, why would anyone ever search for a road to recovery? To look for a way out of a bad situation, we have to believe that it is possible to find a way out. There has to be a glimmer of hope.

Documenting Recovery

Among the first to document a complete recovery from severe autism was Stan Kurtz. He was a technology executive in the computing industry when his son Ethan, at the age of two years, descended into severe autism. It was a year before Ethan was diagnosed in 2003. For a year after that, in spite of multiple therapies, Ethan continued to show all the symptoms characteristic of severe autism. He was socially unresponsive, was largely nonverbal, and manifested stereotypical movements such as hand-flapping. In addition, Ethan had gut problems, mini-seizures, motor control issues, and "floppy child syndrome," in which large muscle groups lack normal tone. All of these symptoms are documented on the DVD accompanying this text. The video of *Ethan's Recovery* can be viewed there or on the Web (Kurtz, 2005–2008b, used by permission ◉).

When Stan Kurtz was told that his son was "too autistic to learn," he gave up his career and devoted himself full-time to helping his son. From the age of two until about the age of four, Ethan remained severely autistic. At Kurtz's Web site, his biographer, Laura Shanahan, explains that Stan was "unprepared for the resistance from doctors, specialists, family and friends." Kurtz reported, "I was told by prominent doctors that autism treatment was not science-based. . . . Parents couldn't change medicine" (Shanahan, 2005–2008).

But Kurtz refused to give up. He learned all he could about autism. One of his key resources was another parent of a child diagnosed with autism and a founder of three organizations devoted to autism: Dr. Bernard Rimland, who founded the Autism Research Institute. Another organization that Kurtz relied heavily on—also founded by Rimland and parents of children with autism—was Defeat Autism Now! Armed with his growing conviction that toxins and disease agents were causative factors in autism, Kurtz began to build a recovery program for his son. Before using any drug, supplement, or food source on his son, however, he first tried the treatment on himself.

In the course of developing a regimen to help his son, Kurtz found himself recovering from his own ADHD and irritable bowel syndrome. His own improvements would provide the basis for significant advances that Kurtz, who is not a medical doctor (as he notes in all his videos and in every presentation), would contribute to medical science. Kurtz is just a highly motivated parent willing to go the distance for the sake of his son. Along the way, he would make several breakthroughs that would benefit many children besides his own son and that would give hope to many parents.

The Fruits of Valid Hope

Among the parents who would be helped by Stan Kurtz's documentation of the recovery of his son Ethan from severe and protracted autism was none other than Jenny McCarthy. It is difficult to estimate the impact of her book, *Louder Than Words: A Mother's Journey in Healing Autism* (released September 17, 2007). The TACA Web site (2008 ●) summed up its message in one sentence: "We give families who have been handed a life-sentence a possibility of escape." Among the most important contributors to the possibility of escape was Stan Kurtz.

Perhaps Kurtz was able to make multiple advances in this area because he brought a fresh and unbiased approach to biomedical treatments of neurological and gut-related diseases, disorders, and toxicity. The fact that nonspecialists have often contributed to scientific advances, even revolutions, throughout history is well documented (Kuhn, 1962). Among the contributions of Stan Kurtz was the development of a nasal spray containing vitamin B_{12} that, for some individuals with neurological disorders such as autism, ADHD, and related conditions, seems to have a remarkable impact. It has been known at least since 1981 (Lowe, Cohen, S. Miller, & J. G. Young, 1981) that one form of vitamin B_{12}, known as **methylcobalimin**, is essential to certain neurological processes involved in autism and related disorders. Several years before Kurtz's nasal spray was introduced as a treatment for neurological problems, one of the renowned researchers on the treatment of autism, Dr. L. Y. Tsai (1999), had already noted that

preliminary studies of major neurotransmitters and other neurochemical agents strongly suggest that neurochemical factors play a major role in autism . . . new avenues of investigation . . . may lead to the development of more effective medication treatments in persons with autism. (p. 651)

After the development of the vitamin B_{12} nasal spray, Dr. Richard Deth, another important researcher in this area, observed that Kurtz seemed to have demonstrated a key element of human attention. Many individuals with various neurological diagnoses report remarkable improvements almost immediately after using the nasal spray (see the videos at Kurtz, 2005–2008a ●). Unwilling to profit from families affected by autism and related disorders, Kurtz published the design of the MB12 nasal spray and takes no profits from its sale.

Infections Reduce Ability to Clear Toxins

Kurtz also was the first researcher to demonstrate that undiagnosed viral, fungal, or bacterial infections can interfere with the body's ability to clear toxins. In connection with this discovery, he developed an antiviral/antifungal strategy, which enabled his own child's recovery, to be used in combination with the MB12 nasal spray. To overcome the resistance by the medical community to his findings, Kurtz followed an innovative approach: He documented recoveries and, with the permission of the individuals involved and funding from the Autism Research Institute, published the videos on the Internet. Kurtz's documented findings have had a significant impact and have led to

a formal study of the [MB12 nasal] spray on individuals with ADHD and drug addiction, [that] is now being conducted jointly with Stan, Dr. Richard Deth, and researchers at the University of California at Los Angeles (UCLA). (Kurtz, 2005–2008a ●)

Kurtz is an effective communicator, and his rational, simple, easy-to-understand explanations make sense to anyone willing to consider seriously his reasoning and the evidence in favor of it. In his videos, he explains, for instance, what he means by "recovery" in simple language. Kurtz uses the analogy of being hit by a bus to illustrate the difference between being cured and being recovered:

> You cannot be cured of being hit by a bus, but you can recover from it. You might even be able to recover enough that you do not need to park in special parking spaces when you go shopping. If you are fortunate enough, you might recover well enough that you gain back so much of your functioning such that no one would know you were ever in an accident. (Kurtz, 2007 ●)

He goes on to define three levels of recovery. The first level is when

> symptoms improve well enough that [children with autism] start functioning like neurotypical children. They are still autistic but they are making great strides. To me, this means, "greatly improved." (Kurtz, 2007)

A second level is achieved when

> symptoms lessen to the degree that they lose their diagnosis. They are no longer considered autistic. This is one degree of recovery. Typically you might see children like this having some residual symptoms of social, verbal, or learning nuances or ADHD-type symptoms that might alert a specialist to suspect that the child once had an autism diagnosis. For the most part they are free of their symptoms and will likely lead what many would consider a relatively normal life in society. (Kurtz, 2007)

The third level Stan describes is higher still. It is achieved when the symptoms can no longer be detected. This is the case when

> if you met the child in a room of his or her peers and did not know the child had a diagnosis, you would not be able to tell there ever was a diagnosis. When I refer to "recovery," I typically mean this level or maybe something arguably close. My son recovered from autism to this degree. (Kurtz, 2007 ●)

Readers can see for themselves that Ethan Kurtz actually did recover from severe autism by viewing the video (*Ethan's Recovery*). In the video documentation, we see Ethan regressing into autism at age two, when he was diagnosed with PDD (pervasive developmental disorder). We see him remaining in that condition for approximately two years. At the age of three, his diagnosis was changed to autism. We also see him 21 days after he began to recover from gut infections and also began to talk in full sentences. In the case of his son Ethan, Stan Kurtz has documented the third and highest level of recovery—the sort of recovery that is so complete that it becomes impossible to detect from present behaviors that Ethan had ever had all the major and defining symptoms of severe autism.

In working with his own son, and in studying and documenting many other recoveries since then, Kurtz has come to a belief about the nature of autism that is certainly worth considering:

> My current position based on my experience with my son and seeing anecdotal reports from parents is that an antiviral (often a prescription but sometimes natural products) in combination with an azole [Nizoral, Diflucan, Sporanox] antifungal and some other prescription antifungals, as well as dietary supplementation, dietary intervention, and, at times, metals detoxification, given simultaneously may improve the health and symptoms of a child with autism and related disorders. (Kurtz, 2007)

When new hypotheses suggested that autism should perhaps be thought of as a multiple-systems disorder caused in part or in whole by toxins, disease agents, and/or their interactions, the notion that it might be treated by changes in diet, reduction of exposure to toxins (or their removal from the body), or other medical interventions to kill or remove disease agents gave parents reasonable hope. For some, it has been enough to motivate the journey toward recovery.

SUMMING UP AND LOOKING AHEAD

This chapter presented evidence from multiple sources showing a strong correlation between the increasing incidence of autism (and of other neurological conditions) and the increasing use of mandated vaccines. The Vaccine Injury Act of 1986 was a legislative response to the escalating number of civil lawsuits involving DTP vaccines, which contained thimerosal. We documented here the series of ambivalent policy statements by the CDC concerning thimerosal, and how the CDC delayed enforcement of the 1999 joint recommendation against using thimerosal in vaccines in the United States. To this date, the CDC continues to defend the use of thimerosal-containing vaccines both abroad and in certain medicines and flu vaccines sold in the U.S. market.

In stark contrast to the lack of vigor that has marked the official response to the growing epidemic, parents of children with autism have sensibly taken matters into their own hands. They have committed substantial resources to the discovery of causes and effective treatments of autism. Some well-educated and deeply motivated parents—including some distinguished medical doctors and researchers—have demonstrated that certain toxins and disease agents are factors in causing autism. Because of their successes, other independent researchers have begun to re-examine the autism mystery with a view toward etiology and the possibility of full recoveries. The new perspective suggests that many individuals on the autism spectrum can be treated and that many—possibly a majority—of those individuals can be recovered.

As we will see in Chapter 4, as soon as the mercury hypothesis was plainly stated, individuals trained in medicine, toxicology, and many other fields of research began to take a closer look at autism. We count ourselves among those researchers. On the basis of solid research and irrefutable logic, we believe the research discussed here and in subsequent chapters has identified key factors that are causing the autism epidemic. The surprise is that many of the causal factors were hiding in plain sight.

STUDY AND DISCUSSION QUESTIONS

1. In 2003, the director of the National Institute of Mental Health credited parent-founded organizations with doing more research on autism than government-funded agencies such as the U.S. Public Health Service. Is this what we should expect? If not, why do we find it to be so? If it is expected, what is the role of the Public Health Service?

2. What were the main purposes of the Vaccine Injury Act of 1986?

3. What lessons were learned from the Simpsonwood Conference of 2000?

4. Discuss the foundation of medical ethics in relation to the watchdog role of the CDC, FDA, and the ethical statements of professional medical organizations such as the AAP. To what extent do you think they are honoring the Hippocratic Oath, for example, or the Golden Rule?

5. What do you suppose will be some of the likely effects of the continued use of thimerosal in vaccines that are being shipped to developing countries?

6. What do you make of the observed correlations between the percentage of children receiving the DTP4 (the fourth dose in a four-shot series), HepB, Hib, and the MMR shots and the prevalence of autism? Could these associations be coincidental?

7. Discuss the proposition that better-informed patients would mean better results in health care all around.

8. If the presence of disease agents in the gut can make children with autism more susceptible to injury from toxins, what are the implications for vaccines?

9. Why is it surprising that dietary adjustments might change the course of autism in many children? Should it be surprising?

10. Consider the documented cases of recovery from autism. If removing toxins, implementing dietary changes, and eliminating disease causing agents from vaccines can enable children to recover, what are the implications for theories of causation?

chapter four

The Mercury Hypothesis

OBJECTIVES

In this chapter, we

1. Consider why the CDC was particularly interested in certain vaccine combinations.

2. Discuss the hypothesis that autism, in many cases, is a manifestation of mercury poisoning.

3. Compare the symptoms of mercury poisoning and autism.

4. Summarize the research leading up to the mercury hypothesis.

5. Consider the reasons for putting mercury in vaccines.

6. Revisit the efforts of the CDC and other parties to minimize the threat posed by vaccines.

7. Discuss the erosion of public confidence in vaccines and why toxins in the vaccines have become the focus of current public concern.

In this chapter we sum up evidence that led certain parent/researchers to the hypothesis that the behavioral symptoms of severe autism suggest it may be due to mercury poisoning. The symptoms, in a large percentage of instances, are virtually identical. Unless the diagnosis of mercury poisoning is known in advance, it is virtually impossible to tell the difference between the cumulative impact of mercury poisoning and the behavioral features of autism. The resemblances first met with amazement and disbelief (or at least denial) by promoters of thimerosal (ethyl mercury). Denial would also come from users of the elemental mercury found in dental amalgam. Eventually, disbelief faded to dismay that the main sources of mercury in children were coming from medical procedures—vaccines, fillings with dental amalgam, and the like. Because babies are especially susceptible to damage from toxins, disease agents, and their interactions, parents would suspect vaccines.

The mercury hypothesis would reawaken interest in the theory proposed by Andrew Wakefield in 1998 that the measles virus was involved in many cases of autism. That article was just the beginning of the recent woes of the CDC with respect to interactions between the toxins and disease agents in various vaccines. What they have known all along is that combining many different toxins either in succession or at the same time makes things more dangerous. Wakefield's research helped to encourage the re-examination of toxins in general. Later, when the mercury hypothesis appeared in a respected peer-reviewed medical journal (see *Medical Hypotheses*, 2009 ◑), activity in the U.S. Public Health Service subagences, especially the CDC and FDA began to ramp up. When the CDC and various promoters of vaccines began to react against the array of research evidence brought to bear on the issues, the public concern about the possible role of vaccines in the autism epidemic, only began to escalate.

In this chapter, we document the progression of public understanding about the link between autism and toxins. When a plausible theory is backed up by decades of sound research and by irrefutable logic, the public becomes reasonably impatient with perfunctory bureaucratic denials. When the denials are accompanied by what are seen by some as attempts to conceal evidence, public disapproval shading into anger is predictable and reasonable.

POISONING BY ETHYL MERCURY COMPARED TO AUTISM

Among the most plausible reports suggesting a link between mercury poisoning and autism was a series of papers by Bernard and colleagues (Bernard, 2004; Bernard et al., 2001; Bernard et al., 2002; Bernard, Redwood, & Blaxill, 2004). They noticed that the clinical symptoms of mercury poisoning are indistinguishable in the way they present themselves to observers from the symptoms of autism in its more severe forms. That is, the behavioral manifestations of mercury poisoning are nearly **isomorphic** with those of severe autism.

The evidence of the extreme toxicity of ethyl mercury had been there all along. However, it took a team of "mercury moms" to bring it into the public view. They first published their idea in 2001 in the peer-reviewed, *Medical Hypotheses* (2009 ◑), a journal that has been publishing groundbreaking and frequently cited material since 1975. It took a group of determined mercury moms to show that it is implausible to argue that there is *not* a connection between mercury poisoning and the autism epidemic.

Correlation of Mercury Poisoning and Autism

Bernard et al. (2001) showed that the symptoms of autism and mercury poisoning are essentially the same. We sum up the symptoms here in terms of the sign systems involved in both autism and mercury poisoning. In doing so, we follow the developmental sequence for sign systems that we have laid out elsewhere in theoretical and practical research on early child development (J. W. Oller et al., 2006). We use the same system we have proposed for an across the board reclassification of communication disorders (J. W. Oller et al., 2010). Our summary condenses the one given by Bernard et al. (2001, Table 1, p. 463) and that of Cave (2001, pp. 67–69). Bernard and colleagues gave details up to the time their work went to press and cited a great deal of relevant research. Cave included a table summing up the symptoms of both mercury poisoning and autism. Both she and Bernard et al. presented the symptoms at issue in a somewhat different order than we use here. Our order conforms to the constructive relations within the whole hierarchy of sign systems as detailed in our work with Badon in 2006 and 2010.

The important point here, in this chapter, is that the symptoms in cases of severe autism and in actual known and well-documented events of mercury poisoning—some of which affected substantial populations—are profoundly similar. In the next section of this chapter, we list the symptoms shared by mercury poisoning and autism in order from the lowest to the highest affected representational systems. We begin with symptoms of damage to the autonomic systems (especially the signs showing that digestion is adversely affected), then we work upward through the symptoms associated with sensory, sensory–motor, and sensory–motor–linguistic systems. Each of the sets of symptoms described is well documented in scientific research cited by Bernard et al. (2001) in no fewer than 181 reports, many of them detailing research on mercury poisoning. Later, in Chapters 5 and 6, we present a detailed technical review of the toxicology of mercury poisoning, and in Chapter 7 we focus more specifically on the mercury, other toxins, and disease agents in vaccines.

Suffice it to say for the moment that mercury is not the whole story by a long shot, but it is a central part of the unraveling mystery of autism that we set out to solve. For now it is enough to note that the mercury hypothesis as put forward by Bernard and colleagues revealed a great deal of common ground between mercury poisoning and autism:

- *Physical symptoms* (in the body and autonomic systems) shared by severe autism and mercury poisoning include skin rashes, inflammation of the skin, itching, tremors and loss of balance, difficulty sitting, crawling, walking, loss of normal muscle tone (e.g., abnormally tense or abnormally lax muscles), unexplained grimacing and/or staring episodes, abnormal reflexes, unexplained and seemingly purposeless repetitive jerky movements, self-injurious behaviors such as head-banging (in extreme cases rendering the person unconscious), sleep disorders, problems chewing and/or swallowing, loss of control of urination or bowel movements, diarrhea, intense abdominal pain/discomfort in bowel movements, inflammation of the colon, loss of appetite, extreme narrowing of taste preferences, nausea, vomiting, lesions in the gut, and abnormal permeability of the colon.
- *Sensory symptoms* shared by severe autism and mercury poisoning include sensitivity in the mouth and extremities, sensitivity to certain sounds (e.g., the humming of a florescent light) and/or mild to profound hearing loss, sensitivity to touch possibly with extreme aversion to a gentle touch, oversensitivity to light, and/or blurred vision.
- Shared *motor symptoms* commonly observed in severe autism and mercury poisoning include circling, toe-walking, hand-flapping, head-banging, rocking or spinning motions, and unusual postures.
- *Linguistic, social, and behavioral symptoms* common to severe autism and mercury poisoning include loss of speech production and/or comprehension; social withdrawal; mood swings; impaired affective expressions and/or loss of facial recognition or comprehension of ordinary emotional signs (e.g., of joy, fear, sadness) in others; evidence of irrational fears; irritability; aggression and extreme panic/anger tantrums; failure to make eye contact or establish joint attention; apparent loss of words, comprehension, and intelligence; inability to concentrate or attend or respond normally (e.g., individuals may stop responding to their own names); regression to a babbling (echoic) repetition of surface forms without evidence of comprehension of meaning; loss of short-term verbal and/or auditory memory for meaning; loss of ability to comprehend a series of events shown in actions or pictures; loss of ability to imitate or produce a series of intentional movements; and loss of power to sequence, plan, or organize actions, or to comprehend complex commands, and carry them out.

Major Mercury Poisoning Incidents

Widespread poisoning occurred in Minamata, Japan, where many people ate fish contaminated with mercury, and in Iraq, where hundreds of people ate seed grain intended for planting that had been treated with a mercury preservative.

In Minamata, a manufacturing process led to the dumping of mercury from about 1932 until 1968. Much of it ended up in the bay, where it contaminated the fish and poisoned their consumers.

In 1956, cases of mercury poisoning began to turn up (see "Minamata Disease," 2009 ●; Tsuda, Yorifuji, Takao, Miyai, & Babazono, 2008). If those cases were being seen in U.S. schools today— without any knowledge concerning the source of the mercury poisoning—many of the affected individuals would be diagnosed with autism or a related neurodevelopmental disorder.

Another instance of widespread mercury poisoning of a large population occurred in Iraq in 1971–1972 (Cox, Marsh, Myers, & Clarkson, 1995). As in the Minamata cases, the symptoms of mercury poisoning were amazingly similar to those seen in severe autism.

Full Circle with Acrodynia

An even more relevant kind of mercury poisoning from ethyl mercury in teething powders that were widely used with babies from about four to eight months of age between 1950 and 1954 was recognized (Dally, 1997). The term for this particular kind of poisoning is **acrodynia**, based on the Greek roots meaning "high" or "extreme" and "pain." Before it was discovered that mercury was the root cause of the poisoning, researchers noted that the condition affected boys more commonly than girls (about a 4:1 ratio) and its symptoms included a pinkish rash, itching of palms and soles, hypersensitivity to light, irritability, tremors of the hands and fingers, sensitivity to touch, and slowed movements.

Acrodynia was also accompanied by hand-flapping, which is one of the characteristic and defining symptoms of autism. Only about 1 in 500–1000 children are believed to have been exposed to the mercury-loaded teething powder eventually developed the disease. This result is consistent with one of the key genetic characteristics of autism. Notably, a study by Matheson, Clarkson, and Gelfand (1980) found that "pink disease" could be caused by ethyl mercury—the chemical variety of mercury that is the active agent in thimerosal. The genetic susceptibility of certain individuals to acrodynia is also consistent with the results of studies of distinct genetic strains of mice by Hornig, Chian, and Lipkin (2004). In fact, with the research on pink disease, the circle connecting mercury poisoning, thimerosal, and autism is essentially completed. The evidence may be circumstantial, inferential, and theoretical, but the logical connections are so complete as to leave little doubt that mercury is involved in the causation of autism.

Changing the Paradigm

Until Sally Bernard and her collaborators expressed the mercury hypothesis—the idea that autism is a form of mercury poisoning—there was little public interest in seeing autism as having anything to do with toxicity. Prior to the introduction of this hypothesis, autism was treated as if it were strictly a behavioral condition resulting from medically untreatable genetic peculiarities. The publication by Bernard, Enayati, Redwood, Roger, and Binstock (2001) would change the medical landscape and the public and professional interest in autism.

We are reminded of the impact made by another parent, Augusto Odone, on the neurodevelopmental disorder known as **adrenoleukodystrophy** (ADL). Augusto and his wife Michaela are credited with developing an oil that halts the progress of that disease—a disease that, coincidentally, is certain to be exacerbated by mercury poisoning. In ADL, the nerves enabling movement at the periphery are gradually incapacitated until the person with the disease can no longer breathe. Augusto Odone, a banker, received an honorary doctorate for his research on ADL. He not only discovered critical epigenetic factors involved in the expression of this genetic disease, but also showed that parents can make significant contributions to medicine. The story of the opposition Odone and his family faced is told in the film *Lorenzo's Oil* (G. M. Miller & Enright, 1992 ●; also see Odone, 2007–2009 ●). Ordinary people with extraordinary love and commitment can do seemingly impossible feats. If the story of autism is told in the future, it is likely to feature some of the "mercury moms" such as Sally Bernard, Lyn Redwood, Stan Kurtz, Jenny McCarthy, and so on who persisted in the pursuit of causation while many experts in the medical profession continued to say the quest was hopeless.

Judging Causality

One of the critical factors in determining causation in general is the sequence of events. Which event comes first, and which event comes later? Researchers look for correlated sequences of events to identify cause-and-effect relationships. In dealing with autism, parents of affected individuals, doctors, clinicians, and researchers are all somewhat like detectives investigating a possible crime. To some extent, they need to think like cops investigating a crime scene: When many coincidences occur, chance is usually not a viable explanation. At a later stage, the investigators evolve into very large "juries" considering evidence and rendering a verdict.

It is often pointed out that correlation does not prove causation—for example, fire trucks do not cause fires any more than thunder causes lightning. Nevertheless, the events in these trivial examples *are* causally related. Fires do have a role in bringing about the presence of fire trucks, and lightning does cause thunder by dispersing air molecules that come back together with a bang. Reliable correlations do not arise by chance, so causation is always involved in some way in nonrandom events and relations. When it comes to mercury poisoning and the neurological symptoms that follow from it, because the mercury is introduced prior to the poisoning, we are justified in supposing that the mercury is causing the symptoms. At the very least, we may say with confidence that there is no leap of inference in supposing that mercury causes the symptoms of mercury poisoning.

But what about mercury and autism? Is there a great leap in supposing that if the symptoms of mercury poisoning and autism are virtually the same, that mercury poisoning might be among the causes of autism? Mutter, Naumann, Schneider, Walach, and Haley (2005), along with others, have noted that the observed increase in autism and related neurological disorders in the last several decades coincides with a parallel sequence of events ensuring increasing public exposure to mercury poisoning.

Since the 1950s, exposure to dental amalgam has increased in tandem with the rising standard of living and the greater accessibility of dental care. Similarly, the number of vaccines required by law in the United States, and as mandated by the CDC in the United States and by the WHO worldwide, has increased in step with the skyrocketing incidence of autism and related communication disorders. The incidence of mercury poisoning is up, and so are neurological disorders and diseases. The question then becomes, is there a causal relation here?

Coincidence or Causality?

Is it merely a coincidence that the first cases of severe childhood autism were documented by Leo Kanner (1943) just a few years after thimerosal was introduced as a preservative in multidose diphtheria vaccine (Cave, 2001)? Subsequently, the number of vaccines mandated for use in the United States (see Figure 4-1 adapted from McCarthy & Kartzinel, 2009, p. 310 with data from the 2009 CDC vaccine schedule), including those containing the mercury preservative, continued to rise along with autism and related neurological disorders. Although the FDA, CDC, and AAP, deny any causal link between the growing number of children with autism and the concomitant rise in mercury dosing from mandated vaccines, positive empirical evidence refutes their claim.

On this subject, the FDA cites studies that have found no significant results. The FDA/CBER Web site (2009) concerning the thimerosal controversy fails to include citations of the toxicology studies with rodents, sheep, pigs, dogs, monkeys, and humans that have found positive results of damage to nerves and organs. Specifically, studies with rodents and monkeys have shown that the mercury in thimerosal and in dental amalgam crosses the blood-brain barrier and persists in the central nervous system with a variable half-life depending on the type of mercury and the age of the organism poisoned by it (Burbacher et al., 2005).

CDC Vaccines in 2009										
	DTaP	Flu	HepB	HepA	Hib	IPV	PCV	MMR	Varicella	RV
Birth			✓							
1			✓							
2	✓				✓	✓	✓			✓
3										
4	✓				✓	✓	✓			✓
5										
6	✓	✓			✓		✓			✓
12										
15	✓		✓	✓	✓	✓	✓	✓	✓	
18		✓								
23 months				✓						
2 yrs		✓								
3 yrs		✓								
4 yrs								✓	✓	
5 yrs		✓								
6 yrs	✓	✓				✓				

CDC Vaccines in 1983			
	DTP	OP	MMR
2	✓	✓	
4	✓	✓	
6	✓		
15	✓	✓	
18	✓		
48 months	✓	✓	

DTaP = Diphtheria and tetanus toxoids and acellular pertussis
Flu = Influenza
HepB = Hepatitis B
HepA = Hepatitis A
Hib = *Haemophilus influenzae* type b
IPV = Inactivated poliovirus

PCV = Pneumococcal
MMR = Measles, mumps, rubella
Varicella = Chickenpox
RV = Rotavirus

Figure 4-1 CDC vaccine schedule in 1983 compared to 2009.
Source: Adapted from McCarthy & Kartzinel, 2009, p. 310, as updated with data from CDC 2009 schedule http://www.cdc.gov/vaccines/recs/schedules/downloads/child/2009/09_0-6yrs_schedule_pss.pdf

Both the ethyl mercury in thimerosal and the mercury vapors from dental amalgam are known to cross from the blood to the brain. With dental amalgam, the leakage into the bloodstream and vital organs occurs mainly as the liquid mercury contained within the amalgam is heated or disturbed by pressure (e.g., brushing the teeth, chewing gum or food, or drinking a cup of coffee), which causes the liquid mercury within the amalgam to release mercury vapor (D. Kennedy, 2007; or click on the "Smoking Teeth" link on the DVD ⬤). Leakage of mercury into the blood also occurs when body tissues come in contact with the liquid mercury in the amalgam; for example, if the filling is placed at the gum line or exposed to the tongue, cheeks, or to other tooth surfaces where the tissues come in contact with the toxin, noticeable inflammation often occurs. The inflammation can commonly be seen at the gum line by a nonspecialist.

As mentioned earlier, ethyl mercury is still incorporated into some vaccines in the United States—most notably the influenza vaccines produced by various manufacturers including Merck,

CSL Limited, GlaxoSmithKline, Novartis, and Sanofi-Pasteur (Institute for Vaccine Safety, 2009 ●). This substance is known to be highly neurotoxic even in concentrations containing parts per billion. In defense of using thimerosal in vaccines, the FDA in 2009 was still citing research claiming that it is safe in contact lens solutions. Actually, thimerosal was shown to be genetically toxic in lens solutions as early as 1982 (Lovely et al., 1982) and was later shown to destroy human corneas (Bodaghi, Weber, Arnoux, Jaulerry, Le Hoang, & Colin, 2005).

Recommended Removal of Mercury

In 2009, the FDA claimed that thimerosal was safe. Just 10 years earlier, the U.S. Public Health Service (its parent agency), the American Academy of Pediatrics, and the pharmaceutical companies that manufacture vaccines had recommended that mercury-containing vaccines should be discontinued or replaced as soon as possible by vaccines without the mercury. If there were no evidence of any harm ever having been done by mercury, why would the FDA/CBER (2009 ●) have agreed that removing thimerosal was "a prudent measure in support of the public health goal to reduce mercury exposure of infants and children as much as possible"?

If the mercury in vaccines is safe, why was it ever prudent and advisable to remove it immediately? The rational conclusion is that thimerosal is *not* safe and that political expediency may have driven the FDA's decision-making process. In fact, mercury is causally involved in a great many disorders, including autism. The toxicology of Chapters 5 and 6 remove any reasonable doubt about that relationship.

Empirically Proving a Null Hypothesis?

Those who have tried to prove that no connection exists between mercury poisoning and autism or other neurological disorders have undertaken a logically impossible task refuted by contrary logic and overwhelming empirical evidence. To claim that mercury has no effect in neurological conditions such as autism requires empirical proof of a null hypothesis. This is logically impossible because it requires testing and ruling out one by one all of the possible ways in all possible situations that mercury might cause neurodegenerative conditions.

No number of experiments in any combination would be sufficient to achieve this goal. *It is never possible to prove a null hypothesis by any number of empirical tests.* The most that can be hoped for is to *disprove* a null hypothesis—that is, we can disprove the null claim that there is no association between mercury poisoning and autism by just one demonstration that mercury does cause neurological disorders. In fact, there are hundreds of such empirical disproofs of the claim that mercury has no relation to neurological problems.

It has long been accepted that empirical science advances by empirical disproofs of general or universal claims (Platt, 1964; Popper, 1959). The Wright brothers disproved the universal claim that flight is impossible for humans. Edison disproved the claim that no metal could sustain a sufficient electrical current to produce an affordable light bulb. Henry Ford empirically disproved all of the general arguments against the possibility of horseless carriages. Roger Bannister showed a human could run a mile in less than four minutes. Likewise, it takes just one positive demonstration that mercury poisoning causes the symptoms of autism to prove that mercury is not safe in vaccines or in human teeth. Once a null hypothesis has been refuted by empirical evidence, it cannot be reestablished—yet that is exactly what the CDC, FDA, AAP, ADA, and pharmaceutical companies have attempted in referring to failed attempts to find a mercury–autism link.

Putting a toxin of known potency inside human bodies—particularly when the persons being harmed are defenseless infants—is irresponsible. Although some have claimed that additional empirical studies are required to show that mercury is harmful, it would make just as much sense to say that more research is necessary to show that human flight, affordable electric light bulbs, and the four-minute mile may someday be achieved. Put simply, the research evidence already shows that mercury injected, ingested, or implanted in teeth is neurotoxic.

The essential problem faced by the advocates of the "We can't find any evidence" position is hinted at by Clarkson and Magos in their 2006 review article: "[E]pidemiological studies, no matter how well conducted, can never prove the absence of risks" (p. 641). Actually, Clarkson and Magos understate the problem faced by those who would defend the practice of putting mercury directly inside the human body. For critiques of this line of defense, see the work of Herbert et al. (2006) and Mutter, Naumann, and Guethlin (2007). No amount of failed research can refute a single successful study linking mercury poisoning to neurotoxicity and to communication disorders such as autism.

In fact, as soon as the biochemistry of the toxins had been researched and demonstrated in rats, what could be the reason for repeating the poisoning on a large scale with humans? Does it make sense to suggest that we should wait another 50 years or so for epidemiologists to figure out how to show on a huge scale that mercury has caused vast, insidious, and long-lasting damage in human populations? We already have evidence of widespread mercury poisoning through the incidents in Japan, in Iraq, and in the industrialized nations of the West involving acrodynia. Instead, the more salient question is this: Why was the policy of injecting children with a known poison ever considered sensible?

WHY INJECT A POTENT NEUROTOXIN INTO THE BLOODSTREAM?

Thimerosal is a **disinfectant germicide** widely used for topical treatment of cuts and infections under the trade name Merthiolate; it was produced by drug giant Eli Lilly in 1927 (D. A. Geier, Sykes, & M. R. Geier, 2007) and was first patented in 1928 (Kharasch, 1928, 1932, 1935; also see J. P. Baker, 2008). The idea that it was ever harmless is immediately refuted by the fact that it was created to kill micro-organisms. Kharasch (1928 ◐) described thimerosal in U.S. Patent Number 1,672,615 as one of several substances "well-suited for intravenous injection" and also as "effective therapeutically as germicides." Thimerosal was included as a component in many vaccines and other medications used with humans from 1930 forward on the theory that it could kill infectious disease agents without harming the human consumers of the vaccines, medicines, cosmetics, and so forth.

According to J. P. Baker (2008), thimerosal was shown to be 40 to 50 times more effective than other disinfectants, notably **phenol**, against the bacterium *Staphylococcus aureus*. However, research published as early as 1935 showed it to be "35.3 times more toxic for embryonic chick heart tissue than for *Staphylococcus aureus*" (Salle & Lazarus, 1935). The upshot of that research and many other studies in toxicology that followed was that whatever preventive/curative qualities thimerosal might have in killing invaders were outweighed by the much greater damage done to the host. From the beginning, toxicology studies (including research funded by Eli Lilly) showed that the remedy in the case of thimerosal was, in many instances, worse than the diseases it was supposed to prevent.

How did such a potent neurotoxin end up in so many vaccines to be injected in human infants and young children? Unraveling this story is crucial to understanding the autism epidemic.

Why Focus on DTP, HepB, and Hib?

Why did the CDC focus so much attention on DTP, HepB, and Hib between 1999 and 2001? The one thing that these vaccines had in common was thimerosal. Although the CDC had joined with the AAP and the FDA in the public statement of 1999 proposing no longer to use thimerosal in vaccines, the 1999 statement had also denied any harm from the thimerosal in vaccines that were administered during the 1980s and 1990s. The denial also included the following claim concerning the safety of injecting thimerosal in vaccine recipients:

There is a significant safety margin incorporated into all the acceptable mercury exposure limits. Furthermore, there are no data or evidence of any harm caused by the level of exposure that some children may have encountered in following the existing immunization schedule [The data in Figure 3-3 contradict this statement, as did the Simpsonwood Conference of 2000]. Infants and children who have received thimerosal-containing vaccines do not need to be tested for mercury exposure. (American Academy of Pediatrics & Public Health Service, 1999, p. 568 ●)

It is interesting that the same principal author who published the defense of the MMR vaccine in 2001, Loring Dales, wrote an email with the subject title "DTP Coverage and Autism Caseload on Calif. Time Trend Data," on June 8, 2001, that laid the groundwork for the discussion leading up to the production of the data shown in Figure 3-3. The potential harm of mercury in vaccines was the apparent basis for the convening of the Simpsonwood Conference of 2000. It seems clear that the AAP, CDC, and FDA were concerned with showing that none of the shots in the vaccine schedule—particularly not the MMR (per Dales et al., 2001) and certainly not the thimerosal-containing shots—were causing autism or any neurological problems.

According to Robert F. Kennedy, Jr. (2005), just before the Simpsonwood Conference took place, an unpublished paper by Thomas Verstraeten, Robert Davis, and Frank DeStefano, titled "Risk of Neurologic and Renal Impairment Associated with Thimerosal-Containing Vaccines," was circulated on June 1, 2000. Kennedy has a copy of that paper, which

> was never published, but its findings were presented a week later at the Simpsonwood meetings in Georgia. The study examined cumulative mercury exposure at 1, 2, 3, and 6 months of age for more than 109,000 children born between 1992 and 1997 and found that the risks of language and speech delays, and developmental delays in general are increased by exposures to mercury from thimerosal containing vaccines during the first six months of life. (2005, footnote 48, p. 15)

The meeting to discuss this issue was held at the private Simpsonwood Retreat Center in Norcross, Georgia, without any public announcement. According to Kennedy (2005), the choice of the venue was made for the following purpose:

> to avoid the reach of the Freedom of Information laws which public health officials interpreted to cover only meetings at government offices. (pp. 15–16 ●)

The fact that the meetings were secret, however, did not prevent a congressional committee headed by Dan Burton and private organizations such as Safe Minds from gaining access to the transcript of the meetings that was also intended to be kept secret (Safeminds.org, 2009; also see Putchildrenfirst.org, 2009 ●).

Behind Closed Doors

The Simpsonwood transcript reveals that the point of the conference was to prevent the information about the toxicity of thimerosal from becoming public knowledge. Although most of the participants were willing to tell the public that they had found no evidence of any relation between thimerosal and neurodevelopmental disorders, they acknowledged that they knew something was going on as suggested by evidence that ethyl mercury was interacting with the various vaccines. After two days of reviewing Verstraeten's results from examinations of the Vaccine Safety Datalink (VSD), Dr. Bill Weil, a consultant to the American Academy of Pediatrics, concluded, "You can play with [the results] all you want—they are statistically significant" (Simpsonwood Conference, 2000, p. 207 ●).

After receiving a phone call on the second day of the Simpsonwood Conference informing him of the birth of a grandson, Dr. Richard Johnston, an immunologist and pediatrician from the University of Colorado, said, "I do not want [my] grandson to get a thimerosal-containing vaccine. . . . I want that grandson to only be given thimerosal-free vaccines" (p. 200). Dr. Robert Brent, a pediatrician at the Alfred I. du Pont Hospital for Children in Delaware, said:

> If an allegation was made that a child's neurobehavioral findings were caused by thimerosal containing vaccines, you could readily find a junk scientist who would support the claim with "a reasonable degree of certainty." But you will not find a scientist with any integrity who would say the refuse [sic—should probably read "reverse"] with the data that is available. And that is true. So we are in a bad position from the standpoint of defending any lawsuits if they were initiated, and I am concerned. (p. 229)

Dr. John Clements, an advisor to the Vaccines and Biologics division of the World Health Organization, said:

> [T]his study should not have been done at all, because the outcome of it could have, to some extent, been predicted [i.e., there was plenty of evidence already known from the toxicology research] and we have all reached this point now where we are left hanging, even though I hear the majority of the consultants say to the Board that they are not convinced there is a causality direct link between thimerosal and various neurological outcomes. . . . how we handle it from here is extremely problematic. . . . there is now the point at which the research results have to be handled, and even if this committee decides that there is no association and that information gets out, the work has been done; and through Freedom of Information, that will be taken by others and will be used in other ways beyond the control of this group. And I am very concerned about that as I suspect it is already too late. . . . (p. 248)

Keeping the Information from the Public

At the closing of the Simpsonwood Conference, Dr. Robert T. Chen, who was then the Chief of Vaccine Safety and Development at the National Immunization Program at CDC, said:

> We have been privileged so far that given the sensitivity of information, we have been able to manage to keep it out of, let's say, less responsible hands. (p. 256)

The group was admonished on the first day by Dr. Roger Bernier, the Associate Director for Science at the CDC National Immunization Program (NIP):

> [L]et me just reemphasize, if I could, the importance of trying to protect the information that we have been talking about. . . . We have asked you to keep this information confidential. We do have a plan for discussing these data at the upcoming meeting of the Advisory Committee on Immunization Practices [ACIP] on June 21 and June 22. At that time CDC plans to make a public release of this information. . . . (p. 113)

The promised public release would never occur. What was eventually published, three years later, was a watered-down version of the results presented at the Simpsonwood Conference (see Verstraeten et al., 2003). Nevertheless, the information that was reviewed at the conference was eventually pried out of the hands of the CDC through legal action.

At the meeting, Dr. Bernier continued:

> I think it would serve all of our interests best if we could continue to consider these data embargoed. . . . If we could consider these data in a certain protected environment. So we are asking people who have done a great job protecting this information up until now, to continue to do that until the time of the ACIP meeting. So to basically consider this embargoed information. (Simpsonwood Conference, 2000, p. 113 ●)

Vaccine Safety Datalink

The key study by Verstraeten et al., and the main focus of the Simpsonwood Conference, was never published; indeed, the CDC later would seek to prevent independent researchers from gaining access to the data he used. The Vaccine Safety Datalink (VSD), which was created in 1997 to ensure "adequacy of the surveillance for significant vaccine adverse events and the general safety of routine vaccine products" (R. T. Chen et al., 1997, p. 772), would be outsourced from a public agency to a private entity, thereby blocking access to it as well. Some have speculated that the outsourcing was a move to prevent independent researchers and the public from gaining access under the law. In effect, the outsourcing by the CDC voided the intentions of the Freedom of Information Act as applied to those data.

In 2002, the American Association of Health Plans (AAHP) was awarded a $190 million contract to take the information in the Vaccine Safety Datalink and effectively to hide it from public view (CDC, Procurements and Grants Office, 2002; also see R. F. Kennedy, Jr., 2005, p. 27). The advocates for preventing public access to the Vaccine Safety Datalink insisted that the data, now under the supervision of the AAHP, had to be kept from independent researchers to guard the identity of individuals represented in the database (see Institute of Medicine, 2005). However, one persistent team of researchers, David A. Geier and his father Mark R. Geier, after months of exhausting work—compared by Robert F. Kennedy, Jr. (2005, p. 53) to climbing a bureaucratic Mount Everest—finally got access to part of the data, though the CDC had told them that Verstraeten's original data were lost.

Preceding the Scramble at the CDC, FDA, and AAP

The data that began to emerge contradicted the claims made by all of the critically involved entities—the pediatricians who administered the shots; the CDC, which mandated use of the vaccines; and the FDA, which certified their safety for use with human patients. Clearly, these public watchdogs and the entities from which they were supposed to protect the public all had a great deal on the line. Of course, the children and families affected by autism and related disorders had even more at stake.

For at least two years prior to June 2001, when the California vaccine-related data were being discussed by CDC officials, activity was going on behind the scenes concerning thimerosal and its 49.55% ethyl mercury content. The paper titled "Autism: A Novel Form of Mercury Poisoning," had been under discussion and was about to appear in *Medical Hypotheses.* It showed mountains of research evidence (much of which we summarize and update in Chapter 5) pointing to the undeniable fact that the symptoms of autism and poisoning by mercury are so similar that they are often indistinguishable (Bernard et al., 2001).

That paper had been under review by editors of *Medical Hypotheses,* who were talking to their professional friends about its content. The hypothesis that mercury was one of—if not the main—causal factor in the autism epidemic was coming under scrutiny by the public. What was becoming apparent to informed parents, independent researchers, and a few doctors who were seeing increasing numbers of affected children was that an overwhelming body of research already supported the notion that mercury poisoning was involved in the etiology of autism, neurodevelopmental disorders, and a host of neurologically related disorders and chronic diseases.

THROUGH THE EYE OF THE NEEDLE

The truth can sometimes be suppressed for a while, but it seems to have a way of coming out eventually. Public knowledge of the ethyl mercury content in vaccines was increasing even before the 2001 paper by Bernard et al. appeared. The best approach for the CDC and those responsible for putting it in there would have been to come clean. It was a terrible mistake, but mistakes do happen. Unfortunately for health consumers, those entities took a different path.

2001: Mercury Going Public

In 2001, the same year that the mercury hypothesis appeared in print in *Medical Hypotheses*, Dr. Stephanie Cave published her book titled *What Your Doctor May Not Tell You about Children's Vaccination*. Given the amount of time required to write and publish a manuscript in book form, both the mercury hypothesis and Cave's book had to be under discussion prior to the private email exchanges at the CDC in June 2001 (see the email from D. Simpson, 2001 ☉). As Cave wrote:

> In our office we are currently seeing more than six hundred children with autism and several hundred with attention deficit hyperactivity disorder (ADHD). I believe these children have been poisoned by mercury from various sources including directly through injections of vaccines (hepatitis B, DTP, and Hib). . . . (2001, p. 78)

The data shown in Figure 3-3, which is based on the email exchange at the CDC in June 2001, were generated by the agency in an effort to refute the hypothesis that mercury was a causal factor in the autism epidemic. The actual data, however, showed the opposite result: Mercury-containing vaccines appeared to be among the factors involved in producing the autism epidemic.

In fact, the trend of association between the shots and the rising incidence of autism is so clear that two obvious questions are answered by it: First, why did the CDC and the California health authorities not publish these findings? (It would make them look bad.) Second, why would those officials want to hide the data from the public? (Because they were not really looking for evidence of a causal relationship of any sort, but rather hoping *not* to find evidence of any such link.)

In 1997, Dr. Robert T. Chen, the CDC leader of the Vaccine Safety Datalink team, predicted that the results from the system "may often be negative (i.e., may show no elevations in risks associated with vaccination)"; he also acknowledged that no such "negative" (actually null) findings could possibly "disprove an alleged reaction" (p. 772). Nevertheless, Chen's admission would not keep the CDC from claiming that it had disproved all possible associations of ethyl mercury with autism. The CDC would also dismiss the possibility of interactions with other vaccines and vaccine components. In reality, one of the earliest results of the VSD team was to show that combining the DTP vaccine (a thimerosal-containing vaccine) and the MMR vaccine increased the risk of a severe adverse reaction—a seizure within a narrow 30-day window—by 300% (Chen et al., 1997, p. 765).

CDC: "Looking and Looking—But We Just Can't Find Anything!"

It is clear from CDC internal email exchanges, especially the series attached to Diane Simpson's email of June 11, 2001, that the CDC's investigations of thimerosal had just one purpose: They were intended to rule out any possibility of a correlation between the rising incidence of autism and the various vaccine series containing thimerosal, especially the series of four DPT shots. The DTP series (see Figure 3-2) was of particular interest because of the cumulative amount of ethyl mercury resulting from four successive doses. The CDC and the Vaccine Safety Datalink team were also well aware of the huge number of lawsuits that had been filed in civil courts in the 1980s claiming vaccine injury from the DTP series. In fact, the litigation associated with the DTP series preceded the enactment of the Vaccine Injury Act of 1986. Thus, when the issue of thimerosal and its ethyl mercury content was raised, the CDC had plenty of prior evidence suggesting that something was going wrong in the DTP series.

Interestingly, the other shots discussed in the 2001 memos, along with the DTP series, just happened to be the ones containing ethyl mercury—namely, the hepatitis B (HepB) series and the *Haemophilus influenzae* type B (Hib) series. The common element among the data examined by the CDC (and summed up in Figures 3-2 and 3-3) was thimerosal and its 49.55% ethyl mercury content. The results show a remarkably strong association between autism and these vaccines, especially if the combined effects of the various series were taken into consideration. Previous research and sound theory have clearly shown that combined effects of multiple toxins and disease agents are, on the whole, logically certain to be worse than their separate effects. R. T. Chen and the VSD team had already demonstrated the combined power of the MMR and DTP vaccines in their 1997 paper, where they noted that the combination was associated with between 210% to 300% more injuries than either vaccine given separately. The maximal effect was observed when the DTP followed the MMR shot by 8 to 14 days. However, if both shots were given on the same day, there was an increased likelihood of a seizure within the defined 30-day period after the shots that was examined in the research reported by Chen et al.

Fast-forwarding to more recent events, on March 29, 2008, Julie Gerberding, director of the CDC, explained the official position to Dr. Sanjay Gupta on the CNN program *House Call*:

> What we can say absolutely for sure is that we don't really understand the causes of autism. . . . while the attention is focused on vaccines, in a sense, it means people are not looking for other causes. I mean, we've got to keep reminding ourselves that the vaccine story has been one that's been debated for many, many years now. We keep looking and looking and looking. And we really cannot turn up any information. (*House Call with Dr. Sanjay Gupta*, 2008 💿)

Gerberding's claim of "looking and looking" and not being able to find anything is remarkable given the extensive research support for the mercury hypothesis that had been published seven years before her remarks aired (see Bernard et al., 2001). Also, the CDC had commissioned, sponsored, and guided the outcomes of eight different panels at the Institute of Medicine to investigate the relationship between vaccines and neurological disorders, especially the autism spectrum. All the research goes against Gerberding's claim that the CDC had found nothing to support the mercury–autism link.

Evidence of Guilty Knowledge

When the ethyl mercury in vaccines began to attract public attention, it also began to generate a high level of public concern and many civil lawsuits. In response, the promoters of its use rallied to defend the vaccines. The efforts would involve the highest levels of our federal government and included an attempt to protect the manufacturer of thimerosal in language added at the last minute to the Homeland Security Act (HSA) of 2002. At first the source of the last-minute addition to the law was a mystery—but it would not remain a secret for long.

Just before the HSA was signed into law by President George W. Bush, additional text was—literally in the middle of the night—added to the bill to protect Eli Lilly in particular from being sued for manufacturing and promoting thimerosal as a preservative in vaccines. In addition to its wide use in vaccines mandated by the CDC, thimerosal has been used in many other medical applications. For example, it has been part of immunoglobulin preparations, especially **Rho(D)-immune globulin** preparations for pregnant Rh-negative women (D. A. Geier, Mumper, Gladfelter, Coleman, & M. R. Geier, 2008). It has been used in antiseptic ointments for treating cuts, nasal sprays, eye solutions, vaginal spermicides, diaper rash treatments, kidney dialysis machines, and rinsing solutions for blood and fluid treatments (Marn-Pernat, Buturovic-Ponikvar, Logar, Horvat, & Ponikvar, 2005). It has also been used as a preservative in many injectable biological products, including skin test antigens, **antivenins**, ophthalmic and nasal products, and tattoo inks (see D. A. Geier et al., 2007; also "Thiomersal," 2009 ●). Thimerosal has also been used in the vitamin K shot commonly given to newborns, and is incorporated in flu shots recommended by the CDC and WHO for infants (Bodaghi et al., 2005; Cave, 2001). As noted earlier, thimerosal is also a component in many flu shots used in the United States and in vaccines that are being used in developing nations.

The Midnight Addition

The midnight addition to the HSA 2002 bill consisted of a special protection for Eli Lilly against thimerosal suits. The discovery of this subterfuge spurred medical journalist David Kirby to begin researching his book *Evidence of Harm*, which would appear three years later ●. In the course of the discussion following the passage of the HSA, just who added the special protection for Eli Lilly came out in a series of revelations followed by a public proclamation of the source of the amendments.

On November 25, 2002, when President Bush signed the Homeland Security Act into law as H.R. 5005, he said, "I particularly want to pay homage to Dick Armey, who shepherded the bill to the floor of the House of Representatives." Later, in an interview with CBS News (2002 ●), Armey admitted that he added the amendments to protect Eli Lilly's liability as the manufacturer and distributor of thimerosal: "I did it and I'm proud of it. . . . It's a matter of national security. . . . We need their vaccines if the country is attacked with germ weapons." At the time, Armey was the House Majority Leader. He denied any input from Eli Lilly but said, "[T]hey asked me to do it at the White House."

According to the same CBS report, there were several interesting ties between high-ranking federal officials and Eli Lilly:

> President Bush's father [former President George H. W. Bush] . . . sat on the company's board in the 1970s; White House budget director Mitch Daniels [was] once an Eli Lilly executive; and Eli Lilly CEO Sidney Taurel, . . . serves on the President's Homeland Security Advisory Council. (CBS News, 2002 ●)

FOLLOW THE MONEY

From the early 1930s, the research supposedly showing thimerosal to be safe for use in human beings was funded by Eli Lilly. There is a lot of money in vaccines, and the industry has thrived on government support. According to Steve Mitchell (2007), senior medical correspondent for United Press International, Kalorama Information (a leading medical markets resource) the worldwide vaccine market was expected to top $23 billion in 2002. The largest share of that market focuses on vaccines for children. Is it any wonder that the drug companies are friends of power brokers in Washington, D.C.?

Big Donations to Influential Persons

Eli Lilly continues to be a generous friend to congressional supporters and paid consultants at the CDC and FDA:

Congressional consideration for Eli Lilly makes sense: In the 2002 election cycle, the company gave more than $1.5 million to federal candidates, with three quarters to Republicans, making it the fourth-biggest giver in the pharmaceutical industry, according to the Center for Responsive Politics. In the current election cycle, the company already has given close to $230,000 (67 percent to Republicans) to federal candidates. (Fuentes, 2003 ●)

It is no surprise that money can buy influence. The question is which of the "research" findings have really been based on unbiased examination of evidence and how much has reflected the funder's priorities?

The creator of thimerosal, Morris Selig Kharasch, was on a fellowship funded by Eli Lilly prior to filing several patents claiming thimerosal as his invention on behalf of the pharmaceutical company. The researchers who are often referred to by the CDC and FDA as having proved that thimerosal is safe for injection into human bloodstreams—H. M. Powell and W. A. Jamieson (1931)—were Lilly employees. The doctors who injected the first 22 human patients with thimerosal in an effort to kill the bacteria involved in **meningococcal meningitis**—H. C. Smithburn, G. F. Kempf, L. G. Zerfas, and L. H. Gilman—were employed at a Lilly clinic (Smithburn et al., 1930). Could the results of those early reports have been biased to meet the ambitions of the drug company rather than to benefit the patients? According to the report by Smithburn et al. (1930, pp. 779–780), 64% of those patients died. In fact, the injections may have caused "dangerous anaphylactic reactions" (p. 780) in some of those who received doses as large as 50 cm^3 with 1% thimerosal in solution (according to Powell & Jamieson, 1931, p. 306).

As detailed in the lawsuit brought by the Counter family against Eli Lilly in 2002, there has been a long history of "research results" that were bought and paid for in advance. The Counter family has charged Lilly with "products liability, negligence, misrepresentation, fraud, and conspiracy" (*Counter v. Lilly*, 2002 ●). Their argument is that Lilly had guilty knowledge that its product was extremely toxic from the beginning. As documents from both the pharmaceutical company and government sources show, seven of the humans treated with thimerosal by Smithburn and colleagues (1930) died within the first 24 hours, probably as a result of the medication. Others, judging from the table published later by Powell and Jamieson (1931, pp. 307–308), died after a few days. The longest reported survival period in the initial study of thimerosal was 62 days. In addition, Powell and Jamieson neglected to mention the fact—which was reported by Smithburn et al. (1930)—that they were putting the ethyl mercury toxin into the bloodstreams of very sick people who had meningitis. Two of the patients who lived 1 and 3 days, respectively, had tissue reactions, one of which was attributed to a prior heart condition, and another lasted 28 days with "infiltration phlebitis" (translation: blood clots), whose effects Powell and Jamieson said were "not definitely due to mercury" (p. 308).

Still Not Enough Evidence

Currently, 5300 cases are being pursued in the U.S. Court of Federal Claims by families who believe their children with autism were injured by the thimerosal found in vaccines, or by the MMR series, or by the combination (see Chapter 8 for more details). The position of Eli Lilly and the manufacturers of vaccines on this issue remains the same: There just isn't enough evidence to show that ethyl mercury or vaccines did any harm.

The CDC's own account of the major events related to thimerosal can be found at the agency's Web site under the title "Timeline: Thimerosal in Vaccines (1999–2008)." Here are some quotes:

1999: No evidence of harm.

2001: No evidence of harm from the use of thimerosal as a preservative, other than redness and swelling at the injection site.

2003: No consistent significant associations between exposure to thimerosal-containing vaccines and a variety of kidney, nervous system, and developmental problems; does not find a link between thimerosal-containing vaccines and autism in Denmark and Sweden.

2004: ACIP does not recommend using the thimerosal-free flu vaccine over the thimerosal-containing flu vaccine, and states that the benefits of flu vaccination outweigh any risk from thimerosal exposure; no association between thimerosal-containing vaccines and autism.

2006: FDA concludes that the evidence reviewed by the IOM in 2004 does not support an association between thimerosal-containing vaccines and autism.

2007: CDC study does not support an association between early exposure to thimerosal in vaccines and nervous system disorders in children between the ages of 7 and 10 years; evidence from several studies examining trends in vaccine use and changes in autism frequency does not support an association.

2008: CDC begins a thimerosal and autism study in three U.S. managed care organizations to find out if exposure to thimerosal in infancy is related to the development of autism. (CDC, 2008c 🌐)

According to the same Web site, a study in Italy is comparing "the prevalence of nervous system disorders among children who were exposed to different amounts of thimerosal in vaccines during infancy."

PREARRANGED OUTCOMES

The history of reviews by the CDC keeps coming back to the null hypothesis: Ethyl mercury is not at all harmful if it is placed in vaccines with other contaminants and disease agents. How do we know this? Because the CDC, FDA, and some consultants (whose work is funded by drug companies) cannot find any evidence of harm. However, when we look at the abundant research, we discover that literally hundreds of empirical studies with animals and humans refute the preferred null outcome. Meanwhile, the government sponsored reviews keep claiming to have proved one or another preferred null outcome. Surprisingly, the intention to prove that no vaccine-autism link exists has often been made known—even publicly—in advance.

Independent Institute of Medicine?

In September 2000, immediately following the Simpsonwood Conference, the CDC joined with the National Institutes of Health to provide a $2 million grant to the independent Institute of Medicine (IOM) to have a Vaccine Safety Review Panel look into the possible role of thimerosal in neurodevelopmental disorders (CDC, 2000).

The panel convened in January 2001 and noted that they were looking for a way out of a tight spot for the CDC. In fact, three issues were to be addressed: the controversy over thimerosal following the Simpsonwood Conference; the question raised even earlier about measles virus and autism in the research of Dr. Andrew Wakefield; and the known interaction between the thimerosal-containing DTP vaccine and the MMR vaccine, which had been noted in 1997 by Dr. Robert T. Chen, then chief of CDC/Immunization Safety Branch, to increase the chance of an adverse reaction by as much as 300% within a 30-day period after the shots.

Dr. Michael Kaback summed up the CDC's problem at the "closed meeting" of the Institute of Medicine's Immunization Safety Review Committee:

> We have got a dragon by the tail here. At the end of the line, what we know is—and I agree—that the more negative that presentation [the IOM report] is, the less likely people are to use vaccination, immunization, and we know what the results of that will be. We are

kind of caught in a trap. How we [the CDC] work our way out of the trap, I think is the charge. (Institute of Medicine, 2001a, pp. 32–33 🌑)

The chair of the Review Committee for CDC, Dr. Marie McCormick, was more blunt. According to the transcript of the meeting, she understood the meetings to be about

safety on a population basis, but it is also safety for the individual child. I am wondering if we take this dual perspective, we may address more of the parent concerns, perhaps developing a better message if we think what comes down the stream as opposed to CDC, which wants us to declare, well, these things are pretty safe on a population basis. I offer that as one strategy as we take this dual track. (p. 33)

She noted that the focus was first to be on the MMR issues raised by Wakefield et al. (1998) and then on thimerosal.

Who Decides Which Issues the IOM Addresses?

When Dr. Christopher Wilson asked, "Is it only MMR? We are also supposed to look at thimerosal."

McCormick replied, "Not on this round."

Wilson then objected:

. . . if we are going to look at autism and we have three candidates [MMR, thimerosal, and their interaction], can we really fundamentally look at them in isolation? In fact, in the real world, they don't occur in isolation. Individuals that got MMR also got vaccines with thimerosal. (p. 45)

In the ensuing discussion, detailed in the next several pages of the transcript, participants in the meeting focused on how the questions to be addressed by the IOM review panel would be limited. Dr. Al Berg finally asked:

What general methods are we going to use to prune the tree? How are we going to decide that issue X is more worthy of our time than issue Y? (p. 50)

Dr. Kathleen Stratton, a member of the IOM staff and study director of the Immunization Safety Review Committee, answered:

Actually, you don't have to make that decision. We don't have to make that decision. CDC will tell us which topic we will address when. (p. 50)

Was the Outcome of the Meeting Preordained?

Dr. Richard Johnston, the immunologist from the Simpsonwood Conference who didn't want his grandson to get thimerosal-containing vaccines, was also a participant in the Vaccine Safety Review Panel. Upon hearing Dr. Stratton's remark, he commented, "That's news to me" (p. 50). Johnston was evidently surprised at the fact that CDC was in such firm control. Stratton continued immediately to explain how the process would unfold:

. . . they have asked us to do MMR, to look at MMR and autism first. Then, they have asked us to do thimerosal and autism second. . . . how they are related, that is a separate issue. . . . Then they will decide what the third topic is . . . based on what is bugging them, what they are being attacked on. (p. 51)

Stratton also explained, in the same context, how issues are chosen at the CDC:

> . . . something new might come up that all of a sudden has erupted from a trial or from just a squeaky wheel or from *60 Minutes*. All of a sudden Jeff Copeland [director of the CDC] and Walt Orenstein [director of the National Immunization Program at the CDC] and the Surgeon General and everybody [are] being beat over their heads and they need to try to resolve something. . . . to be expedient, it is better that they determine it [what the IOM discusses and when]. (pp. 51–52)

Seeking Clarity

Dr. Gerald Medoff immediately added, "They [the CDC folks] are paying for it" (p. 52)—but that is not quite right. In reality, taxpayers pay the bills at the CDC and the IOM, including funding of all its expert panels and committees.

Stratton pointed out to Medoff that the money was not important, "just the boundaries." She asked Berg, "Does that make you feel any better?"

Berg, who was evidently a neophyte in regard to the IOM's dealings with the CDC, grumbled, "Now I am curious what other parts of the methods the CDC has figured out for us" (p. 51).

A short while later, reflecting on issues that had been raised to the CDC, Stratton seemed to experience a moment of clarity on the issue of the MMR vaccine and the thimerosal found in the DTP, HepB, and Hib vaccines. Explaining the real heart of the issues at stake, she said:

> In general they [the CDC folks] worry that if there is a big safety concern that people won't get immunized when they should. (pp. 52–53)

At the same time, she pointed out, some people were clearly reporting vaccine injuries:

> They say—and I believe them—that people are getting immunized when they really shouldn't. What if there really is a terrible hidden truth about one of these things? (pp. 52–53)

Anticipating Issues

As the morning wore on, with attendees making analogies about other problems faced by the CDC and dealt with by other IOM panels in the past (e.g., Agent Orange and Vietnam veterans who developed cancers), the members of the Vaccine Safety Review Panel seemed to lapse into a thoughtful mode. Lamenting that there was not a more forward-looking plan at the CDC about how to anticipate issues, McCormick returned to vaccines and autism, saying:

> If they had set up prospectively a mechanism for looking at some of these adverse events in a much more systematic way, it would have been more reassuring and at least acknowledging that they occurred, as opposed to now sitting there with this organization with 20 years' worth of case report[s] saying, "You have been doing harm to our kids and you have been shuffling on us and ignoring us!" (p. 54)

She was alluding to the session of January 11, 2001, when Congressional Representatives Burton and Weldon, officials from the CDC, and others had heard testimony from Barbara Loe Fisher, one of the parents who founded an organization to address the autism epidemic. Fisher (2001) is cofounder and president of the National Vaccine Information Center (NVIC). "Her oldest son was left with multiple learning disabilities and attention-deficit disorder after a severe reaction to his fourth DTP shot in 1980 when he was two and a half years old" (Fisher, 2009 ⬤).

After lunch, it was time for a dose of CDC reality again. A latecomer, Dr. Steven Goodman, raised the question of just what the IOM could and could not do. Stratton commented again on the boundaries set by the CDC:

> We said this before you got here, and I think we said this yesterday. The point of no return, the line we will not cross in public policy, is pull the vaccine, change the schedule. . . . We wouldn't say compensate, we wouldn't say pull the vaccine, we wouldn't say stop the program. (p. 74)

Bias within Sponsored Research

With the kinds of policies and practices at CDC in place to restrain and direct the Institute of Medicine whenever a new safety issue comes up, it is unsurprising that CDC creates research findings to suit its purposes. In fact, this was the complaint of Robert F. Kennedy, Jr. (2005), concerning the way the CDC handled the thimerosal issue in particular. After more data began to appear from reliable (albeit sometimes hostile) sources showing a clear association between vaccines and autism, the CDC used IOM reports to perform damage control and sponsored research of its own with predetermined outcomes—the "we looked and looked and just can't find a thing" type of outcomes.

In fact, the same basic maneuvering occurred in conjunction with the issue of the MMR vaccine and the relationship between autism, neurological disorders, and gut disease with both the measles virus and thimerosal. The CDC's strategy has been to focus on the issues one by one, treating them singly, as if they were unrelated. When the agency's own research—for example, that carried out by R. T. Chen et al. (1997)—showed dramatic interactions between the MMR and DTP vaccines (a 210% to 300% increase in seizures within a 30-day window), the CDC nevertheless denied the evidence of causation. As McCormick told the IOM panel on January 12, 2001, "We are not ever going to come down that [autism] is a true side effect of [vaccine exposure]" (p. 97). At the same meeting Berg, who is associated professionally with various universities and hospitals as well as drug manufacturer Merck, complained that the CDC sometimes wants the experts on the IOM panels to go beyond the data:

> . . . CDC is, in my view, one of the malefactors on this issue, because they are always pushing to go beyond the data and say, "Yes, but." (Institute of Medicine, 2001a, p. 125)

In addition to watering down the results reported at the Simpsonwood Conference by Verstraeten, the CDC evidently persuaded this researcher in 2003, along with a long list of additional CDC authors, to say that "no consistent significant associations" were found:

> No consistent significant associations were found between TCVs [thimerosal-containing vaccines] and neurodevelopmental outcomes. Conflicting results were found at different HMOs for certain outcomes. For resolving the conflicting findings, studies with uniform neurodevelopmental assessments of children with a range of cumulative thimerosal exposures are needed. (Verstraeten et al., 2003, p. 1039)

This conclusion was technically correct only because the researchers at CDC had included data from an unreliable HMO that was not part of the data set originally reported at the Simpsonwood Conference. It was also misleading to imply that the CDC did not have evidence concerning "cumulative thimerosal exposures"; the agency had available both data from California (based on thousands of cases) and reports from the Vaccine Safety Datalink (based on millions of cases).

CDC: Still Looking and Looking

The smoke and mirrors continued with a series of sponsored papers reaching the same foreordained conclusions. Dales, Hammer, and Smith (2001), for example, reported that there was no association between autism and MMR. At the time of their 2001 publication, both Dales and Hammer were employed by the Immunization Branch of the California Department of Health Services (the California counterpart of the CDC).

In May 2001, Dr. Gordon Douglas, Director of strategic planning for the Vaccine Research Center at the National Institutes of Health (NIH), told an audience at Princeton University in no uncertain terms that the purpose of the CDC-sponsored studies concerning thimerosal and MMR was to rule out any links between the vaccines and autism. According to Douglas, it was the research on the toxicity of thimerosal and of measles virus in gut disease that was "harmful," not the virus or thimerosal:

> Four current studies are taking place at the CDC in collaboration with the NIH to *rule out the proposed links between immunizations and autism, immunizations and possible developmental regression, inflammatory bowel disease and the MMR vaccine, and thimerosal and the risk of autism* [italics added]. In order to undo the harmful effects of research claiming to link the MMR vaccine to an elevated risk of autism, we need to conduct and publicize additional studies, strengthen the program to assure parents of MMR's safety, and further educate pediatricians and primary care physicians. (p. 3 ◐)

Robert F. Kennedy, Jr. (2005, p. 30), points out that "Dr. Douglas also works for the thimerosal vaccine producer Aventis and formerly served as president of Merck's vaccination program."

As a wealth of evidence shows, the CDC has funded, supervised, and then published its own defense of the MMR and thimerosal-containing vaccines (DTP, HepB, and Hib) at taxpayers' expense. According to the final report on this issue published by the Institute of Medicine, which was part of the ninth official meeting of that group and consisted of a public gathering on February 9, 2004:

> This eighth and final report of the Immunization Safety Review Committee examines the hypothesis that vaccines, specifically the measles–mumps–rubella (MMR) vaccine and thimerosal-containing vaccines, are causally associated with autism. . . . The committee . . . favors rejection of a causal relationship between the MMR vaccine and autism . . . rejection of a causal relationship between thimerosal-containing vaccines and autism. . . . does not recommend a policy review of the current schedule . . . for . . . the MMR vaccine or thimerosal-containing vaccines. . . . recommends that available funding for autism research be channeled to the most promising areas. (IOM, 2004 ◐)

That statement was issued in 2004. Apparently the CDC heeded its own advice, at least for the next several years. In 2008, Dr. Jeffrey P. Baker, writing for the *American Journal of Public Health* (a house publication of the U.S. Public Health Service), said:

> Despite the reassurance of no less than eight safety review panels conducted by the Institute of Medicine (IOM) since 2001, many parents continue to fear that childhood vaccines can cause a host of adverse effects ranging from immune dysfunction to attention deficit disorder and autism. (p. 244)

There have been no more Institute of Medicine panels set up to reassure the public that thimerosal is safe. Baker says:

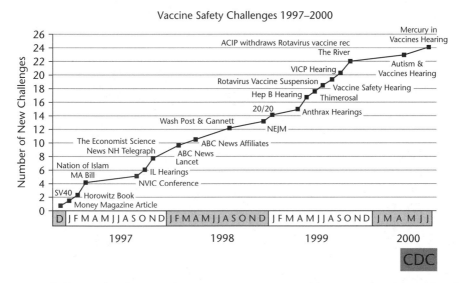

Figure 4-2 New challenges for the CDC from 1997–2000. Prepared by Dr. Walter Orenstein while he was still director of the National Immunization Program for the Centers for Disease Control and Prevention. *Source*: Courtesy of Nicolle Rager Fuller, National Science Foundation.

It is not my intent to answer whether mercury in vaccines explains the increasing prevalence of autism; the IOM has already determined over the course of two [*sic*; actually eight] reviews that available evidence fails to support such a conclusion. (p. 244)

Considering that all the reviews were sponsored and supervised by the CDC, and that the journals publishing defenses of thimerosal also receive funding from vested interests, it is not surprising that public concerns have not been assuaged. Accordingly, it might be predicted that the official CDC (2008c 🌐) Web site on vaccines and thimerosal reported in 2008 that the CDC was still looking and looking for the elusive relationship between the neurotoxin ethyl mercury and the mysterious condition known as autism—in the United States and in Italy, at least.

CDC Challenges Grow and Grow

Although government agencies have tried to put the issue of the vaccines–autism link to rest, it keeps coming up again. In 2001, with almost prophetic foresight, Dr. Walt Orenstein, the director of the National Immunization Program, not only anticipated why the IOM panels dealing with the issue would continue to be necessary, but also drew the picture presented as Figure 4-2. According to Orenstein, the panels were going to be necessary because "challenges" (translation: "really serious complaints") to the CDC's work were increasing.

Orenstein's (2001) diagram showed an increasing number of public challenges faced by the CDC in connection with its vaccine programs. The facts at the time of this writing show that the challenges the CDC would face after Dr. Orenstein's talk only became more intense. Things have changed little since he drew his diagram—except for the fact that a great many more people are taking an interest in the issues at stake.

As the long history of the extreme toxicity of the ethyl mercury in vaccines (Chapter 5) becomes better known, and as the interactions among disease agents and various toxins in the mandated vaccines become better recognized by the general public—events that are certain to occur owing to the increasing availability of information on the Internet—public interest in the CDC's inner workings will only intensify. Is it just a coincidence that the upsurge in diagnoses of autism seems to look a lot like the upsurge in "challenges" faced by the CDC depicted in Orenstein's diagram?

SUMMING UP AND LOOKING AHEAD

The mercury hypothesis was first put forward in 2001 by Bernard et al. The publication of evidence supporting this hypothesis, along with other reports focusing on vaccines—especially the work by Cave (2001) and Wakefield et al. (1998)—have made the public a great deal more aware about some of the undesirable components in vaccines. Although the CDC has sponsored a substantial body of research intended to rule out any association between vaccines and autism (including eight IOM investigations conducted between 2001 and 2004), the potential for bias in the IOM studies has made many people more wary of their reported findings. Toxins do interact with biological disease agents—that much is clear. As a consequence, the efforts of the CDC to allay the reasonable concerns of the public, as J. P. Baker (2008) acknowledged, have had the opposite effect. In fact, the scope of the growing public concern is implicit in the fact that the CDC continues to report searching for the alleged relation between thimerosal and autism.

The thimerosal issue has not gone away. When it was revealed that the CDC had been setting strict limits on the issues covered by IOM hearings and had been effectively shaping the recommendations of IOM committees, the interest in the vaccine components associated with autism and neurological disorders was bound to increase.

In the next chapter, we look intensively into the relevant toxicology with particular interest in thimerosal. We also consider the evidence that some interactions between toxins (e.g., ethyl mercury and aluminum, both of which are found in certain thimerosal-containing vaccines) are more potent than the same toxins acting separately.

STUDY AND DISCUSSION QUESTIONS

1. Given that the MMR shot did not contain thimerosal, why did questions raised about MMR come up again when the mercury hypothesis was published?

2. When you consider the research findings reported by the IOM panels and the CDC as part of their efforts to discover whether thimerosal can cause or exacerbate autism and other chronic disease conditions, how do you explain the constant recycling of the same conclusions? Did they reflect the truth, wishful thinking, or something else? Why did the government agencies come back in 2008 to what they had said eight times over is an unprofitable line of research—still looking for what they say cannot be found?

3. What are the various rationales for denying an association between a potent neurotoxin such as thimerosal and autism? Compare them with the arguments that such an association must exist. What is the basis for the latter argument? Compare and contrast the competing alternatives. Which is more logical? Less apt to be influenced by bias? Which alternative is simpler, more consistent, and more comprehensive as an explanation of empirical facts?

4. What is logically wrong with the claim that a dozen, or hundred, or any number of failed attempts to accomplish some objective, or to find some obscure relation, proves that the objective is impossible to achieve?

5. Discuss the reasons for putting thimerosal into vaccines.

6. What do you think the purpose of the Vaccine Safety Datalink was, is, and ought to be?

7. How do you think the CDC is spending most of its money—in defending itself against public inquiries about vaccine injuries or in protecting the public from injuries?

8. Which kind of watchdog agency could be set up to ensure that the watchdogs—especially the CDC and the FDA—actually watch out for the public interest?

9. Have you noticed a lot of public ads urging parents to vaccinate their children? If you were asked to qualify that spending of tax dollars, how would you classify it: As research spending to ensure vaccine safety? As an attempt to restore confidence in the CDC? As pharmaceutical marketing of vaccines? As lobbying by vaccine interests? Discuss and defend your position.

10. Have the findings by the IOM panels (eight of them between 2001 and 2004) reassured you that vaccines are unrelated to the autism epidemic? Why or why not?

chapter five

Toxins and the Research

OBJECTIVES

In this chapter, we

1. Introduce and explain the different varieties of mercury—that is, salts versus alkyls.

2. Introduce the concept of a free radical and its electrical charge.

3. Consider why organic forms of mercury (alkyls) are biochemically more active and, therefore, more toxic than inorganic (salt) varieties.

4. Summarize the history of research on the toxicity of mercury.

5. Review historical incidents of mercury poisoning.

6. Consider the effects of ethyl mercury as applied in medicines.

7. Review the most recent research concerning ethyl mercury and its causal impact on chronic neurological diseases and disorders such as autism.

There is a clichéd but true approach for the first lecture in biochemistry.[1] Because that subject, biochemistry, is the essential focus of this chapter, it may be interesting to keep the following introduction in mind. The biochemistry professor often constructs a chain of reasoning that goes something like this:

Mathematics may be dry and abstract, but
applied mathematics is physics, and
applied physics is chemistry, and
applied chemistry is biochemistry, and
biochemistry is interesting!

[1] Stephanie Grant is to be credited with pointing out this common statement about biochemistry in a seminar on the autism epidemic at the University of Louisiana in Lafayette.

At the risk of understatement, we can say that the biochemistry of toxins is really interesting. In fact, it is often a matter of life and death. Toxins are, in fact, interesting from every conceivable angle.

In this chapter we examine mercury, one of the toxins that is widely used in medicine, and some of its interactions. Mercury comes in a considerable variety of dynamic forms, some of which are more stable than others. For our purposes, we are most interested in the forms of mercury found in human bodies, especially the kind of mercury found in vaccines (thimerosal) and medical practices such as dentistry. These healthcare practices are not the only sources of the mercury found in human bodies, but they are the ones of greatest interest with respect to the autism epidemic and to chronic neurological disorders and diseases in general. As discussed in previous chapters, the forms of mercury commonly used in medicine, especially thimerosal and dental amalgam, are deeply implicated in the autism epidemic. This chapter examines the toxicology of the various forms of mercury and summarizes the research showing their impact on neurological disorders and diseases in general and autism spectrum disorders in particular.

ETHYL MERCURY AND NEURODEVELOPMENTAL DISORDERS

Research on the effects of ethyl mercury on animals and humans has always shown it to be extremely toxic, especially with respect to the brain, gut, and other vital organs. The form that this compound takes in thimerosal was not so much discovered as invented by Morris Selig Kharasch (1928). Thimerosal was intended to kill microbes (harmful bacteria and fungi) on or inside living plants, animals, and persons. Obviously, thimerosal had to be toxic to achieve its killing purpose. Thus it follows that thimerosal is and always was toxic. This characteristic was known from the work of Smithburn et al. (1930) as well as from Powell and Jamieson (1931) forward.

Likewise, the research on mercury in general, but especially the organic variety known as ethyl mercury (the kind found in thimerosal), has always shown that it is an extremely potent poison. The history of how mercury came to be used as an antiseptic preservative, an antimicrobial additive in medicines placed on or inside the body, is an amazing story. Ethyl mercury, the kind of mercury used in thimerosal, has a peculiarly unstable biochemistry. Sorting out its effects on human beings is the key purpose of this chapter.

Another kind of mercury that is widely used in medical practices, especially in dentistry, is the silvery metal known as elemental mercury. This form has the highly desirable physical property of being a liquid at room temperature. Elemental mercury combines readily with other metals, such as silver, copper, and zinc, to form mixtures known as dental amalgams. However, those mixtures are not stable alloys, as the American Dental Association (ADA, 1995–2009a 💿) claims, but rather give off mercury vapor when warmed or disturbed by normal chewing. For a dramatic visual demonstration of how the metallic mercury vaporizes from dental amalgam, see the "Smoking Teeth" video on the DVD; also visit the International Academy of Oral Medicine and Toxicology (IAOMT, 2008) Web site for a wealth of information about mercury vapor. 💿

Two Streams of "Findings": Which to Trust?

There have been two streams of literature on the toxicity of the forms of mercury used in medicine. On the one hand, there has been a stream of research funded by drug companies and the manufacturers of medical mercury. That line of research has been funded, for the most part, by companies and organizations that have a vested interest in its outcomes and applications. According to these sources, thimerosal and dental amalgam, both of which are approximately 50% mercury by weight, are harmless. On the other hand, a different stream of independent toxicology has shown that both forms of mercury are extremely toxic, especially to nerve cells and genes. Mercury in all its forms is neurotoxic and genotoxic. It is just plain toxic in general, and its interactions with other toxins and disease agents are of particular interest with respect to vaccines, medicines, and medical practices such as dentistry.

When mercury products were originally being developed for the medical market, the drug company Eli Lilly (in the case of thimerosal) and the professional association ADA (sponsoring the research with dental amalgam) also became involved either directly or indirectly in the patenting of the products. In the case of thimerosal, the patents were filed by an employee of Eli Lilly named Morris Selig Kharasch (1928, 1932, 1935). In the case of dental amalgam, two patents were filed by Richard M. Waterstrat on behalf of the American Dental Association Health Foundation (in April 1977 and March 1978). It is true that many other patents are held on the varieties and processes involved in the production of dental amalgam. On a practical level, this means that the ADA can absolve itself of most of the patent-related liability for its promotion of the many different varieties and uses of dental amalgam.

However, patents are not the only—or even the main—issue. The primary concerns relate to the corporate entities that have produced and promoted the use of mercury in medicines and that have actually caused the medicines to be placed in human bodies.

Chains and Whole Networks of Product Liability for Severe Injuries

What is at stake in civil courts is the potential liability for injuries to persons who claim the toxicity of the products was knowingly misrepresented by their manufacturer or creator and by other entities in the line leading down to the trusting consumers (e.g., see *Counter v. Lilly*, 2002, and Edlich, Son, et al., 2007). The monetary stakes are very high and in the case of neurological disorders and diseases, the alleged damages are devastating to the individuals and families affected. In fact, it was a CDC consultant, Dr. Christopher Wilson, who said at a closed meeting of an Institute of Medicine (IOM) panel working for the CDC:

> It doesn't take me very long to figure out that autism is a severe outcome. So, I am not going to spend more than a nanosecond thinking about whether to call this a severe outcome. (Institute of Medicine, 2001, p. 97 ●)

Because neurological diseases and disorders are typically severe, the potential liability for any misrepresentation of the products in question and the harm they have done in the past, or are doing in the present, causes genuine concern in all the entities in the chain of product liability. That chain of responsibility leads logically all the way from the manufacturer clear down to the final consumer who might be or have been injured (see the arguments in *Counter v. Lilly*, 2002).

In fact, the chain metaphor is not adequate unless it is thought of as an intermeshed network of chains covering essentially all of the entities and persons between the manufacturer and end users of the product(s). The product liability issues extend backward from the consumer not only to the original creators and patent holders, but also through the doctors who have placed the products in the bodies of their patients, the professional organizations that represent the doctors (e.g., the American Academy of Pediatrics and the American Dental Association), and the government entities (e.g., FDA and CDC) that said it was safe to use the products in question. In the case of thimerosal in vaccines, for the better part of seven decades the CDC has insisted that it was necessary for consumers to expose themselves and/or their children to these injections. The CDC mandated the thimerosal-containing vaccines in particular for more than half a century and continues to recommend their use in certain medical applications including its use as a preservative in multidose vials of certain vaccines. The chains of networked liability for any harm done, of course, extend outward to companies that have used the products to create additional derivatives, and so on.

Vested Interest and the Harmless Outcome

Because of the vastness of the potential liability for any harm done, many entities have a vested interest in showing that thimerosal and dental amalgam are safe. To that end, they have sponsored numerous studies the results of which (not surprisingly) were interpreted by their sponsors as revealing that these products are harmless. But did the sponsored reports measure up to the requirements of genuine research? Or did they merely aim for and reach a predetermined conclusion without subjecting the products to thorough experimental testing, or, worse yet, were the experimental studies designed or reported in ways that would prevent or conceal unfavorable results?

In addition to research sponsored by groups with a vested interest, there is another stream of work that has been produced by relatively independent investigators, laboratories, and sometimes competitors in the pharmaceutical industry that is less apt to be influenced by ownership, warranties of safety, or other vested interests that might cause the researchers to try to obtain a particular predetermined outcome. Entities with large vested interests predictably hope to minimize their liability by maximizing the safety of their products. In the case of the two products addressed in this chapter, the vested interests have grown to gigantic proportions since the 1930s. Likewise, the liability for potential injuries—given that thimerosal has been injected in millions of people and that dental amalgam has been placed in billions of teeth—is enormous.

The big difference between the independent researchers and the promoters of the medicinal products in question is that one group tends to agree on a certain message for the public (the sponsored research "outcomes"), whereas the other group makes every effort to make the message depend on sound theories and empirical facts. The difference in the end is about the same as that between propaganda and critical thinking. Put simply, independent researchers and people seeking the causes of diseases and disorders do not plan their research to obtain a predetermined outcome.

Known Lethality of Thimerosal from 1930

The evidence has been clear from the very beginning that thimerosal was dangerously toxic. Over time, the diversity and longevity of its toxic effects have only become clearer with accumulating knowledge about specific varieties of mercury. Managers at Eli Lilly were well aware of positive studies linking thimerosal to extreme harm and death in human beings from the first use of thimerosal in injections for human beings. For legal documentation demonstrating their awareness of the harm being done by thimerosal, see the report by Bothwell (2002b); also see *Counter v. Lilly*, 2002, for information about Lilly and thimerosal. ● At both of the foregoing Web sites, important milestones and documents obtained by Waters & Kraus, LLP, in connection with legal actions against Eli Lilly are laid out chronologically.

> The documents clearly demonstrate that Lilly's thimerosal product, the mercury-based vaccine preservative implicated in a number of recent lawsuits as causing neurological injury to infants, was known as early as April 1930 to be dangerous. (Bothwell, 2002a)

Although thimerosal was promoted for use in biological products for humans by Powell and Jamieson (1931), these researchers actually found that within a day to a week, a single dose of 20 milligrams per kilogram of body weight killed a significant percentage of the rabbits they were using as experimental lab animals. As the dosage was increased, thimerosal killed more and more rabbits, as can be seen in Table 5-1.

Figure 5-1 graphs the data from Table 5-1. This graph reveals that 50% of the rabbits in Powell and Jamieson's study died at a dose of approximately 27.9 milligrams of thimerosal per kilogram of body weight within a week. Thus 27.9 mg/kg/week would be the estimated **LD$_{50}$** for thimerosal in rabbits—that is, the dose that kills 50% of the recipients. Powell and Jamieson (both of whom were employees of Eli Lilly Company), however, stressed that many of their rabbits were unaffected, during a week's time, by relatively large doses of thimerosal and that experimental rats survived when they were given even larger doses (also see J. P. Baker, 2008, p. 245). As the dosage for rabbits

Table 5-1 Quantity of Thimerosal (Merthiolate) in Milligrams per Kilogram of Body Weight Administered Intravenously to Rabbits by Powell and Jamieson (1931)

Thimerosal	Deaths (%) After One Week
15	0%
20	3.2%
25	29.3%
30	64.6%
35	84.6%
40	91.7%

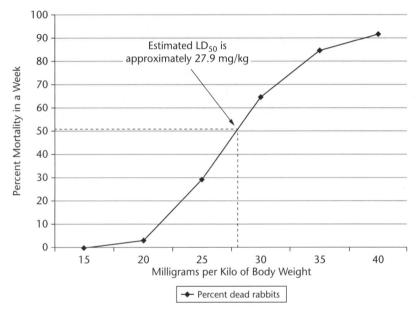

Figure 5-1 Estimated lethal dose of thimerosal for 50 percent of the rabbits in experiments reported by Marks, Powell, and Jamieson (1931).
Source: Marks, H. H., Powell, H. M., & Jamieson, W. A. (1931). Merthiolate as a skin disinfecting agent. *Journal of Laboratory and Clinical Medicine, 18.*

was increased up to 40 milligrams of thimerosal per kilogram of body weight, however, within a week or less 91% of the animals were dead (as can be seen in Figure 5-1). If the objective had been to kill all of the lab animals, thimerosal was fairly effective. Of course, that was not the purpose of the study. The purpose of using thimerosal, according to its inventor, Kharasch, was to kill invading microbes—not the tissues and organs of the host that was being invaded.

Ethyl Mercury (Organic) Compared to Mercury Salts (Inorganic)

Table 5-2 compares the relative toxicity of ethyl mercury, an organic variety, with the inorganic salts. This table is drawn from information made available by the U.S. Department of Energy, Office of Environmental Management, in its Risk Assessment Information System (RAIS—most recently updated on August 17, 2005).

The comparisons in Table 5-2 sum up the effects usually based on oral administration of the inorganic mercury salts listed. Generally speaking, it stands to reason that injecting a toxin into the

Table 5-2 Comparison of LD_{50} Values for Orally Administered Mercury Salts in Rats and Mice

Mercury Compound Administered	Species	LD_{50} (mg/kg at which 50% of the animals died)
Mercurous chloride (Hg2Cl2)	Rats	166
	Mice	1500
Mercuric cyanide (Hg(CN)2)	Rats	25
	Mice	33
Mercurous sulfate (Hg2SO4)	Rats	205
	Mice	152
Mercuric sulfate (HgSO4)	Rats	57
	Mice	25

Source: Adapted from von Burg, 1995. Reprinted from the public domain government document.

bloodstream is more dangerous than eating it or placing it on the surface of the body as an antiseptic. With oral consumption, some of the uptake can be reduced by excretion through the urine or bowel. With placement on the skin, even if the skin is broken by a cut, only some of the toxin can be expected to enter the bloodstream. By contrast, 100% of the ethyl mercury in thimerosal, which is typically administered through a direct injection, enters the body's tissues immediately. Such an injection should have a more potent impact than oral or topical administration; if this is so, the safety requirements for injections should be more stringent than those for foods, or even those for oral and topical medicines. Oddly, the FDA regulations have been stricter for topical applications of thimerosal than for injections in the form of vaccines (see Robert F. Kennedy, Jr., 2005, p. 23).

Comparing the data for the toxicity of mercury salt compounds from the Office of Environmental Management (2005), we discover that thimerosal—according to the data reported by Powell and Jamieson (1931)—is approximately twice as toxic as the most toxic form of **inorganic mercury**. The greater toxicity of thimerosal than inorganic mercury compounds is what should be expected in view of the instability of the mercury in thimerosal, as pointed out by Kharasch as early as 1932, but is not reflected in CDC recommendations or statements.

For this reason, the Office of Environmental Management (2009 ⬤) estimates the LD_{50} for lab animals and humans at the same levels for methyl mercury poisoning while carefully avoiding any mention of ethyl mercury. A search of that organization's Web site fails to turn up even a word about ethyl mercury, although research has long shown that this substance has roughly the same LD_{50} as methyl mercury.

As Clarkson (2002) points out, the biochemical processes of transforming ethyl mercury into the mercury salts that end up in the kidneys are somewhat different from the dynamics for transforming methyl mercury into some of the same salts. The main evidence of the difference, according to Clarkson, is that ethyl mercury also damages the kidneys. For this reason, Clarkson speculates that "inorganic mercury [transformed mercury in the shape of salts] released from ethyl mercury may be the proximate toxic agent for kidney damage" (p. 21). However, the organic mercury forms (ethyl and methyl mercury) are sufficiently similar that Clarkson concedes that "immediate tissue disposition of mercury following a dose of thimerosal appears to be both qualitatively and quantitatively similar to that of methyl mercury" (p. 21); he also admits that "damage to the nervous system is caused by the intact organomercurial radical, whether methyl or ethyl" (p. 21).

So why is the ubiquitous ethyl mercury not mentioned alongside methyl and phenyl in the government Web site warning of the dangers of methyl mercury? The answer seems to have something to do with the use of thimerosal (which contains ethyl mercury) in vaccines and other medicines. The government seems to be avoiding the association of the several alkyl forms of mercury with the one form of mercury it has approved for injections and other medical uses. Also, there seem to be efforts to suggest that the form of mercury found in dental amalgam is so different from the toxic vapors associated with it that mercury-containing amalgam is harmless as well.

Of course, all claims that mercury in any form is harmless are ultimately false. In fact, Clarkson and Magos (2006) acknowledge that mercury vapors—the kind that escape from dental amalgam— are, if anything, even more harmful than the mercury salts derived from organic forms such as ethyl and methyl. But the upshot of all the toxicology research is clear: Mercury does not have any nontoxic forms. Clarkson and Magos conclude:

> [I]norganic mercury is found in neuronal cells after methyl mercury exposure. It is especially high after ethyl mercury exposure, but the nature of the brain damage appears to be the same as with methyl mercury. (2006, p. 653)

The hypothesis that ethyl mercury must be more toxic than inorganic forms of mercury is a simple and logically necessary inference from the chemical nature of ethyl mercury as described by Kharasch (1932, 1935). Ethyl mercury is less stable and more apt to bond with bodily proteins, so it must be more toxic than more stable mercury salts. We can test this hypothesis by comparing the results reported by Powell and Jamieson (1931) with rabbits against the results reported for the toxicity of inorganic mercury in rats and mice as summarized by von Burg (1995; see also Agency for Toxic Substances and Disease Registry [ATSDR], 1989; Office of Environmental Management, Risk Assessment Information System, 2005). The von Burg summary of LD_{50} estimates for four mercury salt compounds appears in Table 5-2. The most lethal of the toxins is mercuric cyanide, with an LD_{50} for rats at 25 mg/kg and for mice at 33 mg/kg. Comparing the estimated LD_{50} for ethyl mercury (Figure 5-1) at 13.8 mg/kg, the hypothesis for rodents—supposing that the figures for rabbits, rats, and mice are reasonably comparable—is confirmed: Ethyl mercury is about twice as toxic as any of the inorganic mercury compounds listed in Table 5-2.

Toxicity for Humans

Having shown that ethyl mercury is more toxic than inorganic mercury compounds in rodents, we can take the question a step further with respect to humans by referring to the data sketchily reported by Smithburn et al. (1930) and repeated secondhand by Powell and Jamieson (1931). In the section of their report titled "Toxicity in Man," the latter pair indicated that they injected "merthiolate . . . intravenously into 22 persons in doses up to 50 cubic centimeters of 1% solution" (p. 306). Their tabled data (pp. 307–308) show that they almost certainly gave lethal doses of thimerosal to most, if not all, of their 22 patients.

The largest total dose administered was 1800 milligrams of thimerosal to a man who weighed 180 pounds (81.8 kg), or 22 milligrams of thimerosal per kilogram of body weight. Approximately half of this dose—10.9 milligrams per kilogram of body weight—consisted of ethyl mercury. However, the largest dose in terms of milligrams of ethyl mercury per kilogram of body weight was to a 14-year-old girl who appears to have survived for 16 days. She received 13.3 milligrams of ethyl mercury per kilogram of body weight. The next largest dose was to a 2-year-old boy weighing 30 pounds (13.6 kg), who received a dose of 12.7 mg ethyl mercury per kilogram and seems to have lived only 6 days afterward. On average, the 22 patients received 5.6 milligrams of ethyl mercury per kilogram of body weight.

The main trouble with the data reported by Powell and Jamieson (1931) is that these results are confounded by the unknown severity of the meningitis disease. For that reason, it is impossible to tell what impact the ethyl mercury might have had over and above the impact of the disease.

It appears that 7 of the patients died within one day of their last dose of ethyl mercury, while the average survival ("observation") rate was 20.4 days. The study included 9 patients younger than

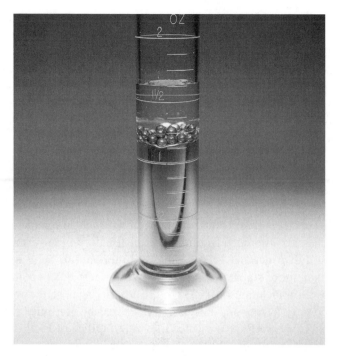

Figure 5-2 Elemental mercury floats metal BBs.
Source: © Charles D. Winters/Photo Researchers, Inc.

9 years of age and 3 patients older than age 50. The older patients all seem to have expired in 3 days or less. Of the 9 younger patients, 3 died within a day and 1 within 6 days. Only one patient was followed for 62 days, all the others having recovered enough to leave the hospital or having died by that point. Smithburn et al. (1930) do not single out the 22 patients who received thimerosal injections, but they do note that of the 144 persons who were hospitalized for meningitis, 64% died.

Taking account of the confounding factor of meningococcal meningitis, the upshot of the results of Powell and Jamieson (1931) is that ethyl mercury was extremely toxic for the 22 humans who received injections containing this substance. If we take the days of "observation" as the time for which the patients survived after the injections, the impact seems to have been lethal within 24 hours for slightly less than one-third of the cases.

The Office of Environmental Management's RAIS (2005 ●) acknowledges that "organic mercurials are more readily absorbed than are inorganic forms." As a result, the organic forms are necessarily, because of their chemical nature and electrical charge, more toxic to humans than the inorganic varieties.

Organic Forms Are More Toxic Than Inorganic Forms

The organic forms of mercury are derived from living organisms that ingest, breathe, or absorb either inorganic mercury or raw **elemental mercury**. The form of mercury referred to in the literature as "elemental" is the metal itself, which is liquid at room temperature (e.g., the shiny silvery metal floating brass BBs at the bottom of the tube of glass in Figure 5-2). Mercury was the metal concentrated inside the silvery tip of the old-style glass thermometers of which Fahrenheit's first is shown in Figure 5-3. Because of its silver color and its liquid form at room temperature, elemental mercury has also been called "quicksilver."

The fact that metallic mercury is liquid at room temperature enables dentists to mix it with certain other metals to form the silvery gray metal filling material known as dental amalgam.

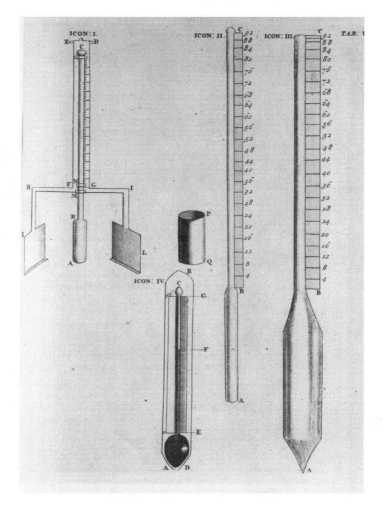

Figure 5-3 Design of the thermometer invented by Daniel Gabriel Fahrenheit.
Source: Courtesy of National Library of Medicine.

Elemental mercury is not very toxic so long as it is not breathed, ingested, or absorbed through the skin. In its metallic form, it is less toxic than its compounds. However, elemental mercury, if heated only slightly or disturbed in any way by movement, gives off mercury vapor that can easily be inhaled and is highly toxic. The Office of Environmental Management's RAIS (2005 ◕) says:

> Inhalation of mercury vapor may cause irritation of the respiratory tract, renal disorders, central nervous system effects characterized by neurobehavioral changes, peripheral nervous system toxicity, renal toxicity (**immunologic glomerular disease**), and death.

Glomerular disease has to do with the small blood vessels in the kidneys (the **glomeruli**). When these are damaged or destroyed in sufficient numbers, kidney dysfunction follows.

Toxicity of Dental Amalgam

The most common and largest source of mercury contamination in humans, and the largest industrial source worldwide, according to the World Health Organization, consists of the silvery material in dental amalgam. Dental amalgam fillings are a relatively unstable mixture of various metals that can be mixed mainly on account of the mercury in them and then they harden at room temperature. They contain anywhere from 45% to 55% mercury (WHO, 2005). Interestingly, the ADA continues to recommend dental amalgam as the preferred material for the vast majority of fillings (ADA, 1995–2009a 🌐; ADA, 2005). The argument is that mercury-based dental amalgam is hard, durable, and easy to work with.

Regarding the safety of putting elemental mercury mixtures in the mouths of human beings, the ADA points out that by 2002 approximately 70 million amalgam fillings were being placed each year in the United States alone (Bellinger et al., 2006). More recently, the estimated number of fillings placed annually has increased to about 100 million per year (ADA, 1995–2009a). Because so much mercury is used in fillings, the ADA contends that it must be safe. This argument is a little like saying that DDT must have been perfectly safe during the decades from 1940 to 1960 when it was most widely used all over the world—but see the discussion of DDT in Chapter 7, which proves otherwise. Today, the mercury used by dentists in "silver" fillings accounts for 55% of the world's mercury in manufactured products of any kind (Barr, 2004 🌐). According to Barr's report on behalf of the Environmental Protection Agency, dental amalgam accounted for approximately 1088 tons of mercury in 2004.

Environmental Contamination?

According to the official ADA Web site (1995–2009c 🌐), "less than one percent of the mercury released into the environment comes from amalgam." However, the WHO (2003 🌐) has reported that medical waste incinerators alone account for approximately "10% of all mercury air releases." Similarly, the Convention for the Protection of the Marine Environment of the North-East Atlantic (OSPAR) has estimated that in the United Kingdom alone 7.41 metric tons of mercury from dental amalgam is dumped in sewage, in air, or on the land, with an additional 11.5 metric tons being recycled or disposed of in clinical waste each year. Comparing this with the ADA estimate of 100 million amalgam fillings, dental mercury is clearly a major source of mercury contamination worldwide.

According to OSPAR, the "mercury contained in dental amalgam and in laboratory and medical devices accounts for about 53% of the total mercury emissions" (WHO, 2003). This estimate is fairly consistent with data from Barr (2004), making the EPA and OSPAR estimates of contamination from dental amalgam about 50 times greater than the estimates developed by the ADA.

Body Burden and Dental Amalgam

Research with human participants who have one or more amalgam fillings shows that approximately two-thirds of the mercury in their bodies originates in the amalgam (Aposhian, Bruce, Alter, Dart, Hurlbut, & Aposhian, 1992; Leong, Syed, & Lorscheider, 2001). Also, Owhadi and Boulos (2008) have described ways in which the body burden can accumulate over time until it reaches a critical level after which the toxicity manifests in disorders, malfunctions, and diseases. In neonates, body mercury levels are closely correlated with amalgam fillings either placed or removed during the pregnancy of their mothers (Counter & Buchanan, 2004; Counter, Buchanan, Ortega, & Laurell, 2002; Palkovicova, Ursinyova, Masanova, Yu, & Hertz-Picciotto, 2008; Razagui & Haswell, 2001). The research is also clear that the combined toxin levels in medicines can produce potent interactive effects in neonates (Slotkin, Oliver, & Seidler, 2005). Studies show that mercury damages the glial cells in the brains of neonates (Cedrola et al., 2003) and that it damages DNA by breaking it up into fragments (Parran, Barker, & Ehrich, 2005).

Some evidence suggests the same sort of gender bias in the handling of dental mercury as is seen in autism spectrum disorders. Woods and colleagues (Woods, Martin, Leroux, DeRouen, Bernardo, et al., 2008; Woods, Martin, Leroux, DeRouen, Leitão, et al., 2007) have shown a strong positive correlation between the number of dental amalgam surfaces leaking mercury vapors and urinary mercury in children. Evidently the children in this study were the same ones referred to in a defense of using dental amalgam in children by seven of the same authors published in *Journal of the American Medical Association* (*JAMA*) just one year earlier (see DeRouen et al., 2006). Amazingly, while reporting in *JAMA* that "amalgam should remain a viable dental restorative option for children" (p. 1784), these authors actually showed that mercury levels were greatly increased in children with mercury fillings. A year later, 7 of the original 11 authors who published the *JAMA* defense of dental mercury teamed with 3 additional authors to reach a conclusion with a rather different implication about safety:

> Urinary mercury concentrations are highly correlated with both number of amalgam fillings and time since placement in children. Girls excrete significantly higher concentrations of mercury in the urine than boys with comparable treatment, suggesting possible sex-related differences in mercury handling and susceptibility to mercury toxicity. (Woods, Martin, Leroux, DeRouen, Leitao et al., 2007, p. 1527)

It is interesting that the excretion of mercury from dental amalgam is higher in girls than in boys. This finding is consistent with the fact that neurological disorders in general and autism in particular are also more common in boys.

Dental Amalgam: Not the Only Maternal Source of Mercury

The research also shows that dental amalgam in children is not the only maternal source of mercury toxicity for them (Zahir, Rizwi, Haq, & Khan, 2005). Unborn and nursing babies can get mercury from their mothers through breast milk.

Dorea (2007) has argued that "maternal exposure to environmental Hg [mercury] during pregnancy can predispose nursing children to neurodevelopmental disorders" (p. 387). Marques, Dorea, Fonseca, Bastos, and Malm (2007) have confirmed that the mother's mercury levels fall during breastfeeding while the nursing infant's level rises. Certainly, it is known that methyl mercury in nursing mice is transmitted by the dams to their pups (Franco et al., 2006). Also, as Sundberg, Jonsson, Karlsson, and Oskarsson (1999) have shown, again with mice, using both inorganic and organic (methyl) mercury, "almost all mercury delivered via milk [is] absorbed" (p. 160). These researchers also found that the organic methyl mercury was more readily transmitted to the nursing pups than the inorganic mercury salt they studied.

In view of the fact that dental mercury is absorbed by the mother in a highly volatile vaporous form—according to Clarkson and Magos (2006), the most poisonous kind of all—it would seem reasonable to suppose that the developing fetus and the nursing baby are both highly susceptible to toxicity received from a toxic mother. If we ask which route of transfer of toxins is more dangerous—through the placenta into the unborn baby or through the mother's milk into the nursing infant—the research with mice by Nielsen and Andersen (1995) suggests, consistent with everything we know of developmental vulnerability, that the earlier period is characterized by greater vulnerability. These researchers were able to evaluate the exposures separately and found that transfer of methyl mercury before birth was more harmful than later transfer through mother's milk.

Considering how many amalgam fillings are being placed (100 million per year since 2007, according to the American Dental Association), remarkably few studies have been done to assess the harm done by dental mercury placed in a mother's teeth to her unborn child. However, Palkovicova, Ursinyova, Masanova, Yu, and Hertz-Picciotto (2008) have studied the dental mercury impact on unborn babies in 99 human mother–infant pairs. While claiming that no mercury "concentrations reached the level considered to be hazardous for neurodevelopmental effects in children," they found, nevertheless, that levels of the mercury in the unborn baby (based on samples of blood from the umbilical cord) were strongly correlated with levels in the mother and significantly correlated with the number of the mother's fillings and the length of time since the last one was placed in her mouth.

Making the connection for nursing human babies, Da Costa, Malm, and Dorea (2005), while noting that dental amalgam fillings are the "primary source of inorganic Hg contamination of humans," found that the level of mercury in the breast milk of nursing mothers during the first 7 to 30 days was strongly correlated with the number of amalgam surfaces leaking mercury vapors. In their study, the average concentration of mercury in the breast milk was 5.73 parts per million and was substantially and significantly correlated with the number of amalgam surfaces ($r = 0.61$, $p < 0.01$). An earlier study in Sweden of 30 women who were breastfeeding their babies (Oskarsson, Schutz, Skerfving, Hallen, & Lagerkvist, 1996) showed a strong correlation between inorganic mercury in blood and milk ($r = 0.961$, $p < 0.0001$). The authors concluded that "mercury from amalgam fillings was the main source of mercury in milk" (p. 234).

Other Medicines Containing Mercury

Although the mercury in dental amalgam is a primary source of contamination and a danger to unborn infants, there are still more toxic forms of mercury. One of them, ethyl mercury, is being transferred to many unborn babies through injections of Rho-gamma globulins administered to their Rh-negative mothers. Ethyl mercury is also being directly injected into millions of other infants and young children through thimerosal-containing vaccines.

THE RELATIVE INSTABILITY OF THIMEROSAL

Two basic types of mercury compounds are distinguished: the chemically stable kind referred to as **salts** and the chemically unstable type known as **alkyls**. A variety of relatively stable inorganic salts can be formed from elemental mercury. In addition, the more volatile organic alkyls include methyl and ethyl mercury. The salts are relatively stable chemically with respect to their electrical balance, whereas the alkyls are unstable. Unlike the salts, in which all electrons are paired up and bonded within the compound, the alkyls contain an electron that is not paired up with a bond; thus they are **free radicals**. The alkyls are like loose cannons looking for a place to bump into and stick momentarily, knocking loose other free radicals, which in turn damage additional molecular systems, and so on.

Because of their propensity to engage in reactions, the alkyls are a great deal more toxic and dangerous than the acutely toxic mercury salts. Both types of mercury—salts and alkyls—tend to disrupt all kinds of normal biochemical processes in living organisms. It is essential to note that it was the inventor of thimerosal himself, Kharasch, who helped to clarify the dangerous and special volatility and the biochemical reactivity of such free radicals as ethyl mercury (see Westheimer, 1960).

Kharasch's Warning About Thimerosal

At the time of his initial invention of thimerosal, Kharasch was supported on a fellowship from Eli Lilly (see *Counter v. Lilly*, 2002 ●). Later, as we will see in Chapter 6, his discovery and clarification of the function of free radicals would be important to developing the theory of *oxidative stress* and the currently most widely accepted theory of **mortality**. More recently, theoretical advances that Kharasch contributed have led to a better understanding of how the genetic inheritance of an organism, including the human genome itself, can be corrupted by genotoxins (see Sanford, 2005). As a consequence of its volatility, ethyl mercury is also highly damaging to genetic material. Put simply, it is a potent genotoxin.

Interestingly, Kharasch himself became concerned about the potential harm that thimerosal could do. He also noted how it could become virtually useless as a preservative: Thimerosal would lose its antiseptic qualities whenever its free-radical component (ethyl mercury) bonded with bodily enzymes and proteins in medicinal applications—as in vaccines, for instance. In other words, the killing power of mercury against undesirable microbes (e.g., bacteria and fungi) would be reduced by its tendency to link up ad libitum with whatever biological proteins might be handy. In doing so, it would be more apt to damage the abundant living tissues in the host than to kill the relatively available microbes that would be, if the organism is alive, fewer in number. Later research, as we will see in Chapter 6, would confirm Kharasch's expectation. In his third patent on thimerosal (Kharasch, 1935), he noted that the ethyl form of mercury has "medicinally undesirable properties" (also quoted by D. A. Geier et al., 2007, p. 278), such as doing more damage to the host than to the invading microbes.

(Mis)Representation of Mercury's Toxicology

Contrary to the widely publicized claims of the CDC that the ethyl mercury from thimerosal is less toxic than inorganic mercury salts, the research and biochemistry show the opposite. The original research that is commonly cited by the CDC and FDA in support of the use of thimerosal as an injectable preservative for vaccines and other products is that conducted by Powell and Jamieson (1931). As we have already seen, their research actually showed, using rabbits and rats as subjects, that ethyl mercury in thimerosal is *more toxic than mercury salts*. Ethyl mercury is also more toxic than methyl mercury to the extent that ethyl mercury causes damage to the kidneys in addition to the brain, gut, and other organs.

Nevertheless, the party line at the FDA and within the CDC, with respect to thimerosal in vaccines, tends to disavow knowledge of significant harm being done by ethyl mercury:

> The only known side effects of receiving low doses of thimerosal in vaccines have been minor reactions such as redness and swelling at the injection site. (National Institute of Allergy and Infectious Diseases [NIAID], 2008 ◉)

Convoluted Policy at FDA

It is noteworthy that the FDA has taken a strikingly different position on the toxicity of thimerosal used in topical applications. The FDA withdrew its approval of mercury-containing over-the-counter (OTC) topical disinfectants and medications in a "Final Rule" published in the *Federal Register* on Wednesday, April 22, 1998—16 years after the change was first recommended in an "advance notice of proposed rulemaking (ANPRM)" on January 5, 1982 ◉. The blanket change declared that the following mercury-containing OTC drugs were being removed: "Ammoniated mercury; calomel (mercurous chloride); merbromin (mercurochrome); mercuric chloride (bichloride of mercury, mercury chloride); mercufenol chloride (ortho-chloromercuriphenol, orthohydroxyphenylmercuric chloride); mercuric salicylate; mercuric sulfide (red mercuric sulfide); mercuric oxide, yellow; mercury; mercury chloride; mercury oleate; nitromersol; parachloromercuriphenol; phenylmercuric nitrate; thimerosal; vitromersol; and zyloxin" (1998, p. 19799). These products were being removed because the FDA ruled "they have not been shown to be generally recognized as safe and effective for their intended use" (p. 19799). It was further required that "these ingredients should be eliminated from OTC drug products 6 months after the date of publication in the *Federal Register* of this final rule regardless of whether further testing is undertaken to justify future use" (p. 19799).

Before the withdrawal of FDA approval for Merthiolate and Mercurichrome, they, along with thimerosal, and merbromin, were all common topical antiseptics stocked in most households. These darkened bottles with glass or plastic applicators for daubing the liquid on cuts, scratches, and abrasions were a staple in first aid kits. Yet, is it not curious that the FDA continued to hold from 1982 through 1999 that thimerosal, one of the forbidden topical antiseptics, was safe to inject after the same agency had judged it unsafe for humans to put on the surface of their skin?

The withdrawal of FDA approval for the topical products (Merthiolate and Mercurichrome) is indicative of an extraordinary history. Robert F. Kennedy, Jr. (2005, pp. 4–6), sums it up with extensive references and documentation. In 1974, an FDA panel report concluded that organic mercury—thimerosal, in particular—was not safe to use in topical medicines and that it is not effective as an antiseptic (Subcommittee on Human Rights and Wellness, Government Reform Committee, 2003). The reasons turned out to be exactly as Kharasch (1935) had predicted: Thimerosal caused allergic reactions in a high percentage of cases, caused cell damage, and lost its power to kill microbes because of its tendency to attach itself to proteins within the host tissue.

In 1977, 10 newborn babies in Canada were killed by application of topical thimerosal to their umbilical cords (Fagan, Pritchard, Clarkson, & Greenwood, 1977). In 1982, the FDA proposed a new rule that would "classify over-the-counter (OTC) mercury-containing drugs for topical antimicrobial use as not generally recognized as safe and effective and as being misbranded" (quoted from the *Federal Register*; Food and Drug Administration, Department of Health and Human Services, 1998, pp. 19799–19800 ●). When the new rule did go into effect, it only branded as unsafe the *topical* mercury-containing drugs. In the meantime, although topical thimerosal was designated as unsafe for humans and reportedly (Rock, 2004) had been already banned from animal vaccines, the FDA continued to allow it to be used in an increasing number of injectable vaccines mandated for younger and younger human babies.

Injectable for Babies?

As the case brought against Eli Lilly by the Counter family shows, that pharmaceutical company was allowed to represent the injectable form of thimerosal to the public as "nontoxic" for decades; at the same time, the government required the topical form to be labeled as "poison" and marked it accordingly with the familiar skull and crossbones (see *Counter v. Lilly*, 2002 ●).

Meanwhile, as the warnings concerning the toxicity of topical uses of thimerosal grew more intense, proponents of the use of thimerosal in vaccines continued to argue publicly (as Offit, 2008, and others continue to do) that thimerosal is harmless when injected into the bloodstream. What is more, they have continued to advocate and defend its use in younger and younger babies. Although thimerosal has theoretically been banned from use in the United States in any newly licensed products since 2002, medical stockpiles containing thimerosal are still being used (D. A. Geier et al., 2007):

> Ironically, while thimerosal was being eliminated from topicals, it was becoming more ubiquitous in the immunization schedule for infants and pregnant women. . . . today thimerosal remains in numerous prescription and over-the-counter pharmaceutical products (Subcommittee on Human Rights and Wellness, 2003) and the influenza vaccine, now routinely recommended for administration to infants and pregnant women (Advisory Committee on Immunization Practices, 2006). (Geier et al., 2007, p. 575)

The CDC and FDA continue to hold to the theory that thimerosal is harmless in vaccines. Recall the quotes from both agencies concerning "minor reactions such as redness and swelling at the injection site" from the NIAID source cited earlier. Hence, the U.S. Public Health Service agrees with the WHO, and the pharmaceutical manufacturers, which continue to use and promote the use of thimerosal abroad.

Francois et al. (2005), representing the WHO and the CDC, have claimed:

> Thimerosal has been used for 60 years in infant vaccines and in other applications and has not been associated with adverse health effects in the general population. . . . Hence there is no stringent reason to stop the use of thimerosal-containing vaccines in current immunization programs worldwide. The balance of risks and benefits of these vaccines is very clearly positive. (pp. 954–955)

At present, U.S. agencies not only permit the use of thimerosal in influenza vaccines, but continue to recommend its use in vaccines given to infants and pregnant mothers in this country (CDC Advisory Committee on Immunization Practices, 2006; also see FDA/CBER, 2009 ●). The FDA and CDC also continue to argue that it is safe to use thimerosal without any restrictions in children outside the United States. Although most of the developed nations of Europe and some in Asia have banned thimerosal—and some have banned the mercury in dental amalgam as well—the ethyl mercury product is still being used widely in vaccines distributed to developing nations around the world.

Children abroad are receiving a larger dose of thimerosal in vaccines provided by the United States through the WHO than American children ever received under the CDC's recommended vaccination schedule (R. F. Kennedy, Jr., 2006 ●). Should we not at least consider the fact that babies are more susceptible to toxic injuries than adults, as has been repeatedly demonstrated in toxicology research concerned with mercury poisoning? Mercury is more poisonous to the developing forms of all the species that have been studied, right down to the larval stage of insects and other nonvertebrates. Von Burg (1995 ●), for instance, notes that, in general, "organic mercury compounds [e.g., methyl mercury, ethyl mercury] are more toxic than inorganic mercury compounds and larval stages are more sensitive than adult stages" (p. 489). These last points are crucial.

General Toxicity of Ethyl Mercury

A letter sent to W. A. Jamieson, director of the Biological Division at Eli Lilly, on July 22, 1935, from the director of Biological Laboratories at Pitman-Moore Company described an experimental use of thimerosal with dogs:

> [There was a] reaction in about 50% of the dogs injected with serum containing dilutions of Merthiolate, varying in 1 in 40,000 to 1 in 5,000, and we have demonstrated conclusively that there is no connection between the lot of serum and the reaction. In other words, Merthiolate is unsatisfactory as a preservative for serum intended for use on dogs. (Cited by D. A. Geier et al., 2007, p. 578)

Comparing phenyl and iodine preservatives, Welch (1939) showed that thimerosal was more toxic by several orders of magnitude than the other two chemicals. In trying to determine whether thimerosal might be used in chemotherapy, Welch and Hunter (1940) found that it was more toxic to the body's own white blood cells that fight infections than it was to infectious bacteria in human blood cultures. When 13 human patients with bacterial infections in the lining of their heart valves were treated with thimerosal, all of them died; autopsies done on several showed that ethyl mercury caused their deaths (Kinsella, 1941). On account of Merthiolate's (thimerosal's) toxicity, Ellis (1943, 1947) advocated withdrawing the product from the market and proposed prohibiting its use in injectable medicines.

Because of its toxicity and its tendency to become attached to proteins and other biochemicals in the body, during World War II (specifically in 1940 and 1941), the U.S. Army ruled out thimerosal as an unsuitable preservative for blood plasma or blood-related serum products (Kendrick, 1989). Among its other undesirable properties, as noted by Kharasch in his second and third patents of the product, was its documented tendency to produce extreme allergic reactions in some individuals. Cogswell and Shown (1948) pointed out, for instance, that not only did thimerosal tend to produce allergic reactions in multiple instances, but the common response in hospitals, unfortunately, was to apply more of the product even in cases where the allergy was already evident. That is, instead of discontinuing the use of the product containing ethyl mercury, the remedy for a skin rash caused by the ethyl mercury in thimerosal, for example, was to apply more of it in an attempt to treat the rash.

By 1948, H. E. Morton, North, and Engley had experimentally studied three forms of mercury alkyls used as antiseptics—phenyl, ethyl, and **merbromin**. The last of these three was used as an antiseptic marketed under the name **Mercurichrome** in the United States until the FDA removed it from the list of safe products in 1998. Its color, packaging, and applicator resembled those associated with the topical Merthiolate, which was also removed from the market at the same time. Both drugs were removed from the market because of the known toxicity of their organic mercury content.

Kharasch's Other Fear: Thimerosal's Ineffectiveness as a Preservative

In 1948, H. E. Morton and colleagues confirmed experimentally Kharasch's fears that thimerosal (Merthiolate) might not be effective against bacteria in many situations and that it might have "undesirable medicinal properties." According to these researchers, thimerosal was "not highly germicidal . . . in the presence of serum and other protein mediums" but it was "35 times more toxic for embryonic cells than for *Staphylococcus aureus*" (p. 41). In other words, thimerosal killed more of the host's cells than the invader's cells. H. E. Morton et al. also reported that the organomercurials were more toxic for white blood cells than for the bacteria they were supposed to kill.

Furthermore, Morton and colleagues noted the possibility that the organomercurial compounds could produce severe allergic reactions in some individuals. Recall Richet's work with anaphylactic encephalopathy, which clearly showed that a much smaller—many times smaller—second or third dose of a toxin to which a person has already developed a hypersensitivity could easily be fatal. Is it any wonder that the fourth shot in the DTP series (refer back to Figure 3-3) would cause concern in terms of its toxicology? Verstraeten reported that he was "stunned" when he began to consult the relevant literature. It is no surprise that the fourth shot in the DTP series seems to be remarkably closely related to the rising incidence of autism.

From the 1940s forward, the research on allergens showed that some individuals are far more apt to develop hypersensitivities than others. In addition, Engley (1950, 1956) found that thimerosal was toxic to human tissue cells even in the extremely low concentration of 10 parts per billion (ppb). Also, its greater affinity for the bodily proteins of the host's tissues rather than any microbes in those tissues rendered it ineffective against infectious bacteria and fungi. Because of its biochemistry, ethyl mercury tends to be a "loose cannon" of a free radical, attacking the host more often than the invaders.

At least since the 1970s, it has been known that the salts derived biochemically from the alkyl forms of mercury—including ethyl and methyl mercury—are similar in animals and humans both in their chemistry and in their toxic impact. Suzuki, Takemoto, Kashiwazaki, and Miyama (1973), for instance, showed that mercury salts had similar effects in humans and in experimental animals to such an extent that the lethal dose for 50% of the animals in a sample (LD_{50}) could be generalized from methyl mercury to ethyl:

[E]thyl mercury has an LD_{50} similar to that of methyl mercury salts and a high neurotoxicity similar to that of methyl mercury. (pp. 209–210 ◐)

CDC Says Research Is "Sparse" on Thimerosal

In view of the many studies on thimerosal dating from the 1930s forward to the present, it seems amazing that CDC-paid experts would come to the conclusion that the research on thimerosal is "sparse." As Robert F. Kennedy, Jr., has observed:

> Peer-reviewed studies demonstrating thimerosal's devastating toxicity to children, adults and animals could have filled a small library. (2005, p. 4)

Nevertheless, CDC-sponsored researchers insist that we just don't know what the effects of ethyl mercury might be or how it compares to methyl and other forms. Their profession of ignorance on such an important matter is troubling: The obligation of medical practitioners to help, rather than to harm, is not fulfilled adequately by ignorance. It is not the responsibility of the public to protect the CDC, but the reverse.

In one study paid for by the CDC, Parker, Schwartz, Todd, and Pickering (2004), after doing a highly selective review of research, suggested that even research with animals on the toxicity of thimerosal is sparse:

> Surprising, animal data on thimerosal **pharmacokinetics** [drug actions and effects] are sparse. (p. 802)

This claim is not correct. A Web of Science search for thimerosal (as well as thiomersal, or merthiolate, or ethyl mercury) from 1973 to the present, turned up 1148 references on May 19, 2009. In fact, a search on just the term "ethyl mercury" garnered 445 results on the same date. There are, in fact, hundreds of studies showing the toxicity of ethyl mercury with animals and humans. If we count experimental applications of thimerosal to humans in injectable products such as vaccines, the number of experiments becomes astronomical, and the data are mainly from human infants. Technical accounts of the thimerosal research literature are provided by Counter and Buchanan (2004), Mutter, Naumann, Schneider, Walach, and Haley (2005), D. A. Geier, et al. (2007), and H. A. Young, D. A. Geier, and M. R. Geier (2008). The most recent of these reviews shows a specific dose-related relation of thimerosal to neurodevelopmental disorders and autism based on the Vaccine Safety Datalink reports of 278,624 children receiving thimerosal-containing vaccines between 1991 and 1996. To say there has not been enough research to show that ethyl mercury is extremely toxic is nonsense.

The Sponsored Outcome

The journal *Pediatrics*, in which Parker, Schwartz, Todd, and Pickering published their paper (one of many papers sponsored by the CDC and drug manufacturers), is itself underwritten by drug companies. *Pediatrics* is the official journal of the American Academy of Pediatrics, which has advocated the use of thimerosal on behalf of the largest of the vaccine companies and has participated in getting the public to accept it. The AAP is also supported by Merck, Sanofi-Aventis, and others (see American Academy of Pediatrics, n.d.). Two of the authors of that study, claiming that the research on thimerosal is sparse, and that what little research there is shows the mercury additive to be perfectly safe for injection into infants, are CDC employees (Pickering and Schwarz). The research by Parker, and the assistant Todd, was supported on a federal grant from the National Institutes of Health. Collectively, the four authors conclude that the "sparse" research already done is sufficient to reach a firm conclusion:

> [T]here is no association between thimerosal-containing vaccines and NDDs [neurodevelopmental disorders], including autism. . . . (Parker et al., 2004, p. 802)

They go on to suggest that further research on the role played by ethyl mercury in neurodevelopmental disorders would be pointless:

> In the case of thimerosal and autism, a growing body of scientifically credible evidence suggests that there may be little to be gained from large additional research investments and, at a minimum, that it is time that additional significant investments in scientific or medical research related to thimerosal and autism be based on credible grounds that would lead one to believe that such investigations will contribute to understanding mechanisms that cause ASD. (p. 802)

The claim that there is no link between thimerosal and neurodevelopmental disorders has been promoted by the drug companies and the CDC to the extent that it is difficult not to view it, and the related research these parties have sponsored, as propaganda.

A plethora of independent research has reached just the opposite conclusion: Thimerosal is associated with neurodevelopmental disorders and it is logically impossible for it not to be in view of its active ingredient consisting of the highly neurotoxic ethyl mercury. The claims that it is safe to inject thimerosal into humans are patently false. If there is an argument against doing more research on the harmfulness of thimerosal, it would be that there is already abundant evidence confirming that the active ingredient in thimerosal is toxic and harmful. Therefore, further research in that respect would be redundant. In contrast, the CDC's argument for halting further investigations in this area seems to be that new research might contradict its sponsored papers reassuring the public that thimerosal in vaccines is safe. J. P. Baker (2008), for example, after a cursory review that concentrates on research sponsored by the CDC, concludes that thimerosal in particular is "far more benign than earlier mercurials" (p. 245). In fact, Baker nearly quotes a study published by the Eli Lilly chemists Marks, Powell, and Jamieson (1932), who said:

> Merthiolate has a low degree of toxicity for animals and human beings, does not **hemolyze** [rupture] red blood cells, and does not injure sensitive bacterial antigens [disease agents intended to provide immunity] and antibodies. It has been found to stimulate tissue cell growth and healing. (p. 443)

According to this view, thimerosal has almost magical healing properties and is completely harmless. These assessments, however, are false, as we have already seen from the toxicology research and as explained in greater detail in the following sections of this chapter.

Why the Ethyl Mercury in Thimerosal Is Especially Toxic

The reason that thimerosal is one of the causes—if not the principal cause—of the upsurge in neurodevelopmental disorders is because of its dynamic biochemical structure, which has bad effects when it gets involved with the rapidly changing biochemical systems of an infant. The dynamics of the ethyl mercury toxin interact with the changes going on during the unpacking of genetic material and the building of proteins necessary for early development to proceed from conception to birth and on to maturity. The dynamics of genetic development from before conception and on up to the age of six—the period during which developmental disorders are most likely to become symptomatic and during which mandated vaccines have their greatest impact—is especially susceptible to disruption by toxins. Ethyl mercury, it turns out, interferes with many dynamic developmental processes and acts synergistically with other toxins and disease agents.

The first reason for its extreme capacity to do harm is that ethyl mercury is an unstable free radical. This high reactivity presents a special dynamic to the biochemistry of any organism but especially to one engaged in rapid growth. The thimerosal in injectable medicines and vaccines typically goes directly into the bodily tissues of a rapidly developing baby. We will have a good deal more to say about the toxicity of free radicals in Chapter 6. For now, in addition to the unstable nature of ethyl mercury, it is important to keep in mind the age and body mass of the recipient when this chemical is typically being introduced through medicines and vaccines into the bodies of very small and immature human beings.

The "mercury moms" (see Chapter 4) followed a trail that was strewn not with bread crumbs of critical research findings, but rather with trainloads of toxicological data. It was supposedly a trail that the CDC could not find. Toxicologist Dr. Boyd Haley has marveled at the collective inability of the CDC, the FDA, and the American Academy of Pediatrics to notice the negative impact of thimerosal in the toxicology research. The analogy that comes to mind based on his comments is something like a crowd of researchers who cannot detect a train wreck that is occurring in their own front yard (Haley, 2006 ●).

Toxic for Animals, Toxic for Humans

Every known form of mercury, without exception, is highly toxic. Inorganic mercury, according to the Office of Environmental Management's RAIS (2005 ●), has "acute toxicity . . . in animals" that "*is similar to that observed in humans* [italics added]. . . . Neurological effects and death have been reported for various animal species receiving inorganic mercury orally." Curiously, sponsored research done by employees of the CDC, in collaboration with the American Academy of Pediatrics, has repeatedly failed to turn up any evidence of the toxicity of ethyl mercury and claims that the results of animal research do not generalize to humans.

The Office of Environmental Management's RAIS cites the Agency for Toxic Substances and Disease Registry as the source for its estimates (ATSDR, 1989; the Web site also refers to von Burg, 1995). It points out that lethal doses for 50% of the animals exposed in experimental studies—the standardized measure known as LD_{50}—for inorganic mercury "range from 10 to 40 mg/kg [milligrams of mercury per kilogram of body weight]." Of course, as Richet's research showed with anaphylactic encephalopathy (Richet, 1913), even much tinier doses can be lethal or extremely harmful in individuals who are hypersensitive. An authoritative source for this information—Suzuki, Takemoto, Kashiwazaki, and Miyama (1973), writing in the book on this subject edited by M. W. Miller and Clarkson—notes that the LD_{50} values for humans for both ethyl and methyl mercury are about the same: "ethyl mercury has an LD_{50} similar to that of methyl mercury salts and a high neurotoxicity similar to that of methyl mercury" (pp. 209–210).

According to the Office of Environmental Management's RAIS (2005 ●), "Generally, any form of mercury in high acute doses may cause tissue damage resulting from the ability of mercury to denature [i.e., modify, destroy, or incapacitate essential bodily] proteins, thereby disrupting cellular processes (WHO, 1976)." The same source notes that "lethal doses in humans range from . . . 10 to 42 mg Hg [mercury]/kg for a 70 kg adult . . . for inorganic mercuric salts (ATSDR, 1989)." Recall that the range for the lethal dose for humans as specified by the WHO includes the full range of quantities injected in patients suffering from meningococcal meningitis by Powell and Jamieson (1931). Three of their human patients received a dose expected to be lethal, and the average dosage for all the patients in that study was halfway to the lethal range. Also, the persons receiving the additional toxic burden were already sick enough to be hospitalized with a disease that, in the 1930s, was commonly fatal. Even so, the FDA insists that the Powell and Jamieson study of 1931 shows thimerosal safe for injection into infants.

MERCURY: MORE TOXIC THAN ESTIMATED

Estimates of harmful levels of ethyl mercury (not to mention the LD_{50}) based on experimental studies are undoubtedly too high. They are generally expressed in terms of milligrams per kilogram, where 10 to 42 one-thousandths of 1000 grams would be 10 to 42 parts per million, the estimated LD_{50}

for ethyl mercury for humans. However, vastly smaller quantities are known to have harmful cumulative effects, and even very small quantities can be lethal. The LD_{50} is merely the point at which 50% of the subjects are not just injured, but actually killed. Some individuals will die at much smaller exposure levels, and permanent damage can be done by smaller doses still.

Research by Parran, Barker, and Ehrich (2005) showed that as little as one-hundredth of a part per billion of thimerosal (or half as much, if it is pure ethyl mercury) can cause fragmentation of DNA in the **nerve growth factor** (**NGF**) in a developing human brain. The same investigators also found that even one part per billion can cause the death of nerve cells. Not only is thimerosal more toxic than published estimates of LD_{50} suggest, but those estimates rarely take account of cumulative effects over multiple doses, nor do they consider the effects of developing allergies and special sensitivities of individuals and genetically susceptible subgroups. For the latter groups, the estimates of a lethal or harmful quantity based on a single swallow or shot (a single **bolus**) are undoubtedly too high. The current research and known biochemistry require the inference that a much smaller quantity of thimerosal can cause critical harm and can induce disorders, especially if it is administered in repeated doses. The lethal or harmful dose on a second, third, or fourth exposure for sensitive individuals can be orders of magnitude smaller than the quantity that initiates the allergic response.

There are four reasons that we know the harmful/lethal dose of ethyl mercury is smaller than the same dose for mercury salts. Let us consider them one by one.

Unstable Free Radicals

Although the LD_{50} for thimerosal administered to humans has not yet been reported by RAIS, ATDSR, WHO, or the FDA, shortly after its invention it became known that thimerosal was considerably more chemically active and unstable than ordinary forms of inorganic mercury. In fact, Kharasch was immortalized in chemistry mainly because of his original demonstrations, stemming largely from his work with thimerosal, concerning the theory and behavior of "free radicals" (Westheimer, 1960).

In brief, free radicals are highly unstable, usually short-lived ions that are extremely reactive with other biochemicals, such as the proteins crucial to the body's cell structures, metabolism, and immune defenses. Central to the research leading Kharasch to understand and elucidate the nature of free radicals was his work with the ethyl mercury in thimerosal. As we will see in Chapter 6, Kharasch's work with free radicals was important to the development of the most widely accepted present-day understanding of mortality as well as the elucidation of chemically induced genetic mutations. For his ground-breaking work, he was praised highly by his fellow chemist and biographer, Frank Westheimer (1960). In addition, Kharasch received many accolades and a few awards before his death in 1957. For example, he received the Presidential Merit Award in 1948 for his services to the Chemical Warfare Service during World War II (Westheimer, 1960, p. 132). Owing to the unstable and transitory nature of the free radicals that are released from thimerosal, Kharasch expressed reservations about the use of thimerosal in humans soon after his initial patent application was made in 1928 (see D. A. Geier et al., 2007).

The key issues, as Kharasch (1932, 1935) would spell out in later U.S. patent applications (numbers 1,862,896 and 2,012,820), had to do precisely with the tendency of thimerosal to form unstable free radicals. There were two problems that he pointed out: the tendency for ethyl mercury to do harm to the person receiving an injection and the fact that the free radicals of ethyl mercury lost their disinfectant potency. As Kharasch warned in his third patent application for thimerosal in 1935,

[Its] compounds . . . tend to form disassociation products and to thereby both lose their effectiveness as antiseptic germicides and to develop certain medicinally undesirable properties. (Also cited by Geier et al., 2007, p. 578)

Even in his earlier 1932 application, Kharasch had referred to "burning properties" produced by the free radicals released from a stagnant solution of thimerosal (D. A. Geier et al., 2007, p. 577). The organic ethyl mercury by-product in particular was known to disrupt neurological and other biological processes in all of the organisms studied. Kharasch explained in his 1935 patent application how "thimerosal would break down" and how "the ethyl mercury breakdown product was the one mediating thimerosal toxicity" (p. 577).

Thus the claim that the volatile nature of ethyl mercury was known in the early 1930s is substantiated. Eli Lilly had to know about the danger from the report made by Smithburn et al. (1930), and the company was reminded of these risks by Kharasch's second and third patent applications in 1932 and 1935.

The Impact of Ethyl Mercury on a Developing Organism

Another reason that estimates of injurious or lethal ethyl mercury are too high is that the estimates are typically based on studies with adult organisms. However, the uses sanctioned by the FDA, CDC, WHO, and other organizations most commonly involve infants or children younger than age six. The aggressive vaccination schedules recommended by the CDC have increasingly called for more numerous doses to be delivered to ever-younger children. At the Simpsonwood Conference in 2000, it is curious that the 11 experts assembled by the CDC, plus the 40 other experts from drug companies and vaccine manufacturers, seemed unaware of the long history of research showing the greater impact of toxins on developing infants. In fact, the research showing that both unborn babies and newborns are far more susceptible to injury than adults is pervasive and unequivocal. It is not debatable.

Oddly, while urging removal of thimerosal in its topical over-the-counter form, the CDC and FDA have continued to license and condone the use of thimerosal in vaccines and in medicines for pregnant women. Because the thimerosal in vaccines and in immunoglobulin preparations administered to pregnant women goes directly into the blood of the unborn baby, it is certain that the estimates of the potential injurious or lethal effects of ethyl mercury, which are based on studies in adult organisms, are far too high. When a given quantity of thimerosal is used in medicines that are injected into pregnant women or into the bloodstreams of rapidly developing infants and young children, the ethyl mercury is certain to be more harmful than it would be, all else being equal, in an adult.

Younger organisms are more susceptible to toxic damage for two reasons. First, they are more apt to be injured or killed by the toxin on account of the rapid growth processes that are under way in their bodies. Second, if the same dosage given to an adult is administered to an infant, the relative impact must be enormously greater owing to the child's smaller body mass. Even if the body mass difference is compensated for by a proportionate reduction of the dose, the earlier the age of exposure to thimerosal, the more severe its toxic impact can be expected to be. All of the relevant research in toxicology shows these predictions to be correct; they are uncontroversial and well known.

THE LONG HISTORY OF MERCURY AND ITS TOXICITY

In this section, we review some of the critical history leading up to the introduction of the mercury hypothesis as a source of autism. The idea that a group of overzealous, frantic parents just pulled the hypothesis that mercury is related to the autism epidemic out of the clear blue sky is false—yet that is the view often suggested by representatives of the CDC and FDA.

Silly Parents and a Few Naive Physicians

Dr. Paul Offit, a member of the CDC Advisory Committee on Immunization Practices and co-inventor of a rotavirus vaccine recommended by the CDC for universal use in infants, has made the following statement:

> Attention by the news media has caused some parents to fear that thimerosal contained in vaccines might harm their children. . . . Some parents, alerted by stories in the news media or on the World Wide Web, are concerned that substances such as thimerosal, formaldehyde, aluminum, antibiotics, and gelatin are harmful. . . . the removal of thimerosal from vaccines caused some parents and physicians to believe that vaccines that contain thimerosal were harmful, *independent of dose or age of administration* [italics added]. (Offit & Jew, 2003, pp. 1394–1396)

We do not know of any parents anywhere who believe what Offit says in the italicized portion of the preceding quote. Of course, pediatricians administering vaccines—DTP, HepB, and Hib—from their inception until about 2002 almost universally gave the same dose of 12.5 micrograms of thimerosal in each dose irrespective of the child's weight or age. It is the pediatricians who seem to ignore the age and size of the child and to play fast and loose with the number of doses given on a single "well-baby visit." Consider the 20 pathogens plus contaminants administered to four-month-old Vance Walker just 56 hours before his death.

It is also interesting that the CDC officials blame news media and the World Wide Web for the criticism of vaccines when, as we will see, it was research published in reputable peer-reviewed medical and other research journals that finally prodded the FDA into its action in 1999, when it proposed banning thimerosal. It was empirical evidence—actual firsthand observations of injuries—that led parents to look askance at the components contained in vaccines, especially organic mercury. After observing injuries, they began to look to the toxicology data and soon found that the research in support of the theory that mercury is harmful is ubiquitous. Nevertheless, the CDC continues to take the view that naive parents, and some uninformed physicians, influenced by the media and especially by sources on the untrustworthy World Wide Web, have come to believe that ethyl mercury and other contaminants injected into the bloodstream of infants might be harmful.

Another claim made by CDC officials to defend the ethyl mercury in thimerosal, not to mention the other toxins, is that ethyl mercury is a lot less harmful than methyl mercury; ergo, ethyl mercury is safe for human use. Offit (2007) presents the standard party line at CDC by insisting:

> Ethyl mercury is excreted from the body much more quickly than methyl mercury and is therefore much less likely to accumulate. For this reason, the safety guidelines that had been established for methyl mercury weren't likely to be predictive of the safety of ethyl mercury. (p. 1278)

It would be more sensible to argue that drunk drivers don't cause traffic fatalities and, as R. F. Kennedy, Jr., has noted (2005), that tobacco smoke is not linked to cancers. There is no reasonable doubt or debate that organic mercury is more toxic than the inorganic variety. True, information in support of the mercury hypothesis is becoming more widely available on the World Wide Web and in the news media—but both sources are also saturated with information provided by the CDC, FDA, and vaccine manufacturers.

The real sources of the knowledge that the ethyl mercury in thimerosal-containing vaccines is extremely toxic are biochemistry, rational theory, empirical evidence, and a great deal of published research. Conversely, the CDC's actions, which suggest the agency is trying to conceal evidence, have done a great deal to convince the public that we all need to take a much closer look at vaccines. At the same time, the public has become more aware of the tens of thousands of parents who believe that their children were injured by vaccines, and has begun to heed their calls for action.

Both the methyl and ethyl varieties of organic mercury are extremely toxic, as thoroughly demonstrated by biochemistry and research evidence and contrary to what the CDC has been saying about the greater potency of methyl mercury. In some respects, the research shows the two main forms of organic mercury (methyl mercury and ethyl mercury, though other varieties exist) used in fungicides, bactericides, and pesticides are more toxic to living organisms than raw elemental mercury or its inorganic compounds.

Poisoning by Organic Mercury in Japan

During the mercury poisoning that occurred in Minamata, Japan, which became known as early as 1956, the source was eventually traced to dumping of mercuric sulfate in the industrial wastewater from the Chisso Corporation's chemical factory. A partially documented article about Minamata disease is available on Wikipedia ("Minamata Disease," 2009 ◉), and various scholarly treatments concerning the toxicology are linked there and on the DVD with this book (see especially Clarkson & Magos, 2006; Clarkson & Strain, 2003; Clarkson, Smith, & Doherty, 1973; D. A. Geier et al., 2007).

In an effort to get rid of its industrial waste, Chisso Corporation dumped mercuric sulfate, one of the highly toxic mercury salt compounds (see Table 5-2), into its wastewater. The salt was then transported by drainage into Minamata Bay, where it was transformed into an organic toxin, methyl mercury, by aquatic organisms and fish. The biochemistry is complex but the theory is that water organisms eat or absorb the mercuric sulfate and then convert it from a salt to an alkyl—that is, methyl mercury (Clarkson & Magos, 2006). In Japan, the methyl mercury eventually worked its way up the food chain until the people around Minamata Bay ate enough of the poisoned fish to be poisoned themselves by methyl mercury. Clarkson and Strain (2003) note that "the central nervous system is the prime target" (p. 1539S). By the early 1960s, the alarm had been sounded in Japan about special damage to unborn babies (Tokuomi et al., 1962); soon thereafter, Matsumoto and Takeuchi (1965) would tell the awful tale in English in the United States. The poisoning would continue to affect babies born during the period for years to come; Tomoko Uemura, for example, died of methyl mercury poisoning from Minamata disease in 1971.

We had hoped to show here the well-known photo of her by W. Eugene Smith; in that famous photograph, Tomoko's mother cradles her teen-age daughter's stunted, cramped, and twisted body. The photo is usually referred to as "Tomoko Uemura in Her Bath, Minamata, 1972." Another photo shows just one of Tomoko's twisted hands. The story of what happened in Minamata and of why the Uemuras no longer grant permission to reprint the photograph can be found at the Web site maintained by W. Eugene Smith's surviving wife, Aileen Mieko Smith (2001; also see A. M. Smith, 2004, both linked on the *Autism DVD* and the book by E. W. Smith & A. M. Smith, 1975). The pictures at Aileen's Web site also tell the story of Minamata poisoning in black and white pictures by W. Eugene Smith with a voice over narrative. They do not, however, include the most famous picture of that period, which was the one of Tomoko's bath.

Although the impact of methyl mercury poisoning was evident in pets and adults in Japan, its most dramatic effects were seen in unborn babies whose mothers were poisoned. Tomoko Uemura was among them. As Clarkson and Strain note, "Methyl mercury poisoning is characterized by a long latent period between exposure and the appearance of signs and symptoms" (2003, p. 1540S; also see Nierenberg et al., 1998; Weiss, Clarkson, & Simon, 2002). It was found that unborn babies were especially susceptible to methyl mercury poisoning during the Minamata outbreak, a result that was later confirmed with data from earlier poisonings and from the subsequent Iraqi incidents. The symptoms were mainly neurological in nature, including paralysis (as can be seen in some of the pictures at Aileen Mieko Smith's Web site, 2004), loss of motor control, insomnia, and digestive problems. In adults, and throughout the population in the vicinity of Minamata, symptoms of memory loss, psychological depression, numbness in the extremities, overall muscle weakness, narrowing of the field of vision, and loss of speech and hearing abilities were also reported.

Incidents by Methyl Mercury and Ethyl Mercury in Iraq

In the best-known instance of Iraqi mercury poisoning, which occurred in 1971, grain treated with methyl mercury fungicide was intended for planting rather than making bread. However, this was not the first instance of mercury poisoning in Iraq—just the best known because it involved so many people. Ethyl mercury poisonings had occurred in Iraq on several previous occasions (Al-Kassab & Saigh, 1962; Dahhan & Orfaly, 1962; Damlugi, 1962; Jalili & Abbasi, 1961).

All of these incidents happened because ethyl mercury and methyl mercury were used as fungicides for seed grains meant for planting. Clarkson and Strain (2003) explain how these disasters were unintentionally set up:

> In the early 20th century, the potent fungicidal properties of both methyl and ethyl mercury compounds were discovered. This led to the wide application of methyl and ethyl mercury as seed dressing. Cereal grains such as wheat are highly susceptible to a fungal infection when planted in soil. The resulting disease, which is commonly referred to as "blunt disease," can cause wide devastation and substantial reduction in the crop yield. The short-chain alkyl (methyl and ethyl) mercury compounds kill the fungus while the seed is in the soil and are not accumulated into the growing plant. (p. 1539S)

In 1971, widespread poisoning by methyl mercury occurred in part because of the failure of the Iraqi grain crop of 1970, and perhaps in part because the Iraqis either did not understand the warnings in English not to eat the orange/pink-colored methyl mercury–treated grain or chose not to heed the warnings. People were hungry; as a result, some of the 90,000 tons of the mercury-treated grain shipped from the United States and Mexico (Engler, 1985, p. 489) was used for making the traditional Iraqi bread. The outcome was widespread poisoning by methyl mercury (Bakir et al., 1973; Clarkson et al., 1973). Infants born to poisoned mothers during this time not only had high levels of mercury, but also showed the same symptoms as individuals affected in the Minamata incident.

In a follow-up study of Iraqi women exposed in 1971, Marsh et al. (1987) noted developmental delays and mild neurological changes in children of women with low exposure as judged by mercury concentrations in their hair. As found in subsequent studies, and especially the work of Holmes, Blaxill, and Haley (2003), the hair is one of the dumping grounds the body uses to get rid of mercury. The Office of Environmental Management's RAIS (2005) asserts that "in Japan and Iraq . . . ingestion of methyl mercury contaminated food resulted in severe toxicity and death in adults and severe central nervous system effects in infants." Following that same line of reasoning, Clarkson and Strain (2003) mention that "a milder form of prenatal poisoning . . . was characterized by a history of delayed achievement of developmental milestones and abnormal reflexes" (p. 1540S). These are also characteristic symptoms of autism, as pointed out by Bernard et al. (2001).

In addition to assessing the methyl mercury poisoning of 1971, researchers have been able to examine data from other Iraqi mercury poisoning episodes and from the Minamata incident. All of these data show that "the prenatal stage of the life cycle is the most vulnerable" (Clarkson & Strain, 2003, p. 1539S). More importantly, several incidents involving poisoning with the ethyl mercury variety of fungicides yielded data relevant to the ongoing discussion.

Poisoning with Ethyl Mercury

After facts began to accumulate on methyl mercury poisoning in the Iraq incident of 1971–1972, it came out that ethyl mercury used in fungicides for the same purposes had resulted in similar (though less widespread) poisonings in the 1950s and 1960s. Although Clarkson (2002, p. 14) had suggested that "about the thimerosal molecule . . . in the form of ethyl mercury . . . there is limited toxicologic information" he and Strain would themselves note that after the fungicidal properties of organic mercury were discovered, there was "wide application of methyl and ethyl mercury as seed dressing" (2003, p. 1539S; also mentioned by Clarkson & Magos, p. 624).Together with Strain, Clarkson acknowledges that within a couple of decades of these applications, there were some ominous poisoning incidents with both types of mercury and a peculiar difference was noted in the toxic effects of ethyl mercury:

> several massive outbreaks of poisoning . . . reported from developing countries in the 1950s–1970s period. The signs and symptoms were identical to those reported after occupational exposure to methyl mercury, except *in the case of ethyl mercury, kidney damage was also manifested* [italics added]. (Clarkson & Strain, 2003, p. 1540S)

Jalili and Abbasi (1961) make it clear that it was specifically an ethyl mercury derivative that caused some of the known poisoning events and deaths:

> Poisoning by a fungicide used for seed-borne diseases of cereals, **ethyl mercury *p*-toluene sulfonanilide** (Granoson M, DuPont) is described. It affected a large number of farmers and their families who used the dressed seed in the preparation of home-made bread. Many systems were involved, including the kidneys, the gastrointestinal tract, the skin, the heart, and the muscles, but involvement of the nervous system was the most constant with disturbance of speech, **cerebellar ataxia**, and **spasticity**. Mental abnormalities were occasionally observed. (p. 303)

Obviously, the symptoms described here are specific to neurodevelopmental disorders in the autism spectrum. Jalili and Abbasi went on to note that 100 patients with ethyl mercury poisoning were treated at a hospital in Mosul in 1956, of whom 14 died, and that 221 cases were admitted to a single hospital in Baghdad in 1960.

Generalizing Research Results from Animals to Humans

Interest in ethyl mercury as a toxin was greatly increased after the various poisonings with fungicides began to come to light. In 1972, Mukai obtained funding from the National Institutes of Health to study an animal model. He demonstrated that ethyl mercury produced the typical neurologic symptoms of mercury poisoning in mice in injections containing less than 6 parts per million of ethyl mercury. Tryphona and Nielsen (1973) showed that ethyl mercury fed to pigs at a rate of less than one part per million per day damaged not only the nerve cells in young pigs, but also the blood vessels supplying those cells with oxygen and nutrients. They also showed general systemic damage to the kidneys and in the gut from the esophagus to the colon. Subsequently, as documented by D. A. Geier, Sykes, and M. R. Geier (2007), similar results were observed with cattle, sheep, and monkeys. In all those cases, mercury in various forms could be found in the brain, blood, kidney, liver, and muscle for a long time after the exposure to ethyl mercury.

These results generally extend to humans on account of the similar biochemistry across all these mammals. In fact, as Clarkson, Vyas, and Ballatorl (2007) have argued, and as extensive research across different species shows, organic mercury of the ethyl variety crosses the blood-brain barrier and is distributed by the blood throughout the body. Because of its special affinity for the sulfur compounds in nerve tissues, a lot of it ends up in the neurological system. It is no wonder that significant levels of mercury in the brains of the young pigs studied by Tryphona and Nielsen (1973) still showed up in measurable quantities 140 days after consuming their last dose of less than one part per million of ethyl mercury as part of their diet. In another study in which pigs received ethyl mercury in their feed, significant levels of the toxin could still be detected eight months after the last dose (Saley, 1970).

This result shows that the LD_{50} based on a single bolus administration is insufficient; because mercury accumulates in the body, total exposure to this agent must be considered.

The generalization of results to humans is also supported by accidental exposures to ethyl mercury by swallowing quantities of it and by occupational exposures. A surprising number of such cases are well documented. With human poisonings of this type, we have the benefit (if it can be considered that) of having detailed reports by the affected individuals of their symptoms as they develop over time. Early signs include muscular weakness, lack of energy, achiness, rapid heartbeat, and headaches. These symptoms worsen to include nausea; loss of appetite; diarrhea; sleeplessness; memory loss; tremors in the fingers, hands, and feet; and, in extreme cases, death (Bakulina, 1968; Derban, 1974; Mukhtarova, 1977; Nizov & Shestakov, 1971; Shustov & Syganova, 1970; Zhang, 1984).

Mukhtarova (1977), in particular, showed that humans poisoned by ethyl mercury showed some of the same abnormalities in brain tissues that were observed earlier by Tryphona and Nielsen (1973) in young pigs. They observed gross changes in blood vessels supplying the brain and nervous system. Zhang (1984) reported on 41 patients in China who ate rice contaminated by ethyl mercury chloride and found that the severity of symptoms was related to body size and the amount of the tainted rice consumed. Symptoms had not abated after five months from the time of poisoning. Derban (1974) gave details about the impact on speech functions in children poisoned by ethyl mercury in Ghana, describing a child with "incontinence of urine and feces and complete loss of speech" (p. 50).

Generalizing Mercury-Related Results to Thimerosal

As with the more widespread methyl mercury poisoning that would occur later in Iraq, Bakulina documented the poisoning of unborn human babies in 1968 by ethyl mercury consumed by their mothers. His report showed that the ethyl mercury consumed by the mother entered the developing fetus. Also, there was evidence that breastfeeding was a means of conveying the poison from poisoned mothers to their nursing infants. A critical finding, as noted by D. A. Geier, Sykes, and M. R. Geier (2007), was that the children showed symptoms three and four years after the poisoning of their mothers (Bakulina, 1968, p. 63).

Later studies of the incident in Iraq especially showed that epilepsy was a common outcome of the poisoning of the unborn and nursing children. This disorder was observed to occur for at least two years after the chronic exposure had ended and was found in approximately 10% of the cases. Except for the loss of speech or failure to develop language normally, the human infants and children affected showed the same symptoms observed in animal poisoning with ethyl mercury: nerve damage as evidenced by body movements, rapid and irregular heart rhythms, the blueness described as **cyanosis** (Figure 5-4), abnormal fluctuations of blood pressure, and general damage to the nervous system. Secondary symptoms occurred in the liver, kidneys, and gut as well. In his account of ethyl mercury poisoning in children, some of whom were subsequently autopsied, Mal'tsev (1972) showed inflammation and bleeding in the brain and spinal cord as well as in the kidneys, liver, heart, and intestines. He commented that his observations suggested that the third and fourth months of fetal development were the most vulnerable to damage from ethyl mercury.

Could the results of ethyl mercury poisoning in animals and humans be generalized to thimerosal? That is, would the results have been similar if thimerosal had been the toxic agent rather than some other form of ethyl mercury? An interesting, though tragic case reported by Rohyans, Walson, G. A. Wood, and Macdonald (1984) suggests that even if the toxic agent being ingested were thimerosal itself, similar results would follow. At least, that is what happened in the case of a little boy whose ears were irrigated with merthiolate (thimerosal) in an effort to treat his middle ear infection. Because the child had a broken eardrum, some of the thimerosal was swallowed, and he was poisoned. Before his death, he showed symptoms very much similar to those described in other instances of ethyl mercury poisoning.

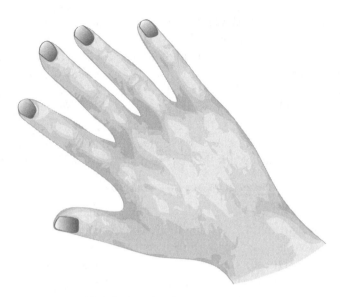

Figure 5-4 Cyanosis of the nail beds in a human being.

Other instances of thimerosal poisoning in humans have been documented in the peer-reviewed literature. M. Koch and Trapp (2006) reported that after a 38-year-old woman was poisoned by accidental exposure to 2.25 parts per million of ethyl mercury in thimerosal, she was chelated as a treatment to save her. Later, the authorities at that hospital, according to W. F. Koch and Trapp, "replaced thimerosal with a commercially available mercury-free disinfectant" and recommended against using thimerosal in the future (p. e31).

Safe for Infants?

Although Clarkson and Strain (2003) say that the symptoms of methyl mercury and ethyl mercury poisoning are "identical" except that ethyl mercury also damages the kidneys, they seem to think ethyl mercury is nonetheless safe to use in vaccines in small quantities in injectable form. In this regard, they subscribe to the basic CDC doctrine:

> the risks associated with not vaccinating children far outweigh the theoretical risk of exposure to thimerosal in vaccines. (Clarkson & Strain, 2003, p. 645)

If CDC researchers acknowledge that ethyl mercury has toxicity comparable to that of methyl mercury, except for additional damage to kidneys, why do they think it is safe to inject ethyl mercury into the bloodstream of humans?

On the one hand, ethyl mercury is extremely toxic; on the other hand, as a component in thimerosal, it is supposedly safe enough to inject into infants. All of the known research shows that the alkyl mercury forms—methyl, ethyl, phenyl, and so on—are more damaging to younger organisms than to adults. However, at the Simpsonwood Conference, when asked whether thimerosal exposure before birth, at birth, or six months later would make a difference, Clarkson said:

> As far as I know the literature, there just isn't that much evidence one way or the other as to whether exposure shortly after birth or exposure at six months would make a difference. In theory it could, but I don't know of any studies that have actually tested that. (Simpsonwood Conference, 2000, p. 21)

In view of Clarkson's own reviews of the vast literature on the toxicology of ethyl and methyl mercury (e.g., Clarkson & Magos, 2005; Clarkson & Strain, 2003) and the fact that both varieties tend to harm unborn babies and newborns more than adults, it is clear—even without presenting any additional evidence—that thimerosal must be relatively more harmful in younger infants.

Nevertheless, participants at the Simpsonwood Conference affirmed that no difference is recommended in the dose size for shots containing thimerosal based on the weight of the infants. With this observation, it became clear that it is the CDC—not the parents of children with autism—who fail to take full account of the literature on dose-related effects of toxins. The smaller the infant is, the greater the toxic effect will be, even if the dose remains the same. It is a matter of simple math.

Thimerosal Still Approved by CDC and WHO Worldwide

The theory concerning the continued use of thimerosal in vaccines and medicines is that the risk of preventable diseases outweighs the risk of using thimerosal (Clements & McIntyre, 2006), especially in developing countries (Clarkson & Magos, 2006). For example, Munoz et al. (2007) speak for the Chilean Society of Infectious Diseases and the Consultive [*sic*] Committee of Immunizations, saying that Chile will continue to use thimerosal-containing vaccines, presumably on the WHO recommended schedule. Except for the absence of the Hib vaccine, many countries continue to follow the vaccination schedule employed in the United States during the 1980s and 1990s.

With reference to the program recommended by the Ministry of Health of Brazil, Marques, Dorea, Fonseca, Bastos, and Malm (2007) point out that children normally receive doses of HepB at birth, 1 month, and 6 months and DTP at 2, 4, and 6 months. The exposure to ethyl mercury in this schedule would consist of 25 micrograms in each of six doses, giving a total of 150 micrograms over the baby's first six months of life. The authors studied 82 normal infants who were breastfed with the intention of assessing the interaction of breastfeeding with ethyl mercury exposure. They estimated that the babies would receive even more mercury exposure from their mother's milk during their first month of life, with 40% of the total expected exposure coming over the 6 months of breastfeeding. Marques et al. then adjusted for the body weight of infants, but found on the day of vaccination that the amount of ethyl mercury from the vaccine was many times greater (5.7 to 11.3 parts per billion, adjusted for the baby's weight) than the amount of mercury attributed to the mother's milk from breastfeeding (0.266 part per billion). Interestingly, the mothers excreted less mercury in their own hair while breastfeeding, as their mercury was presumably going to the baby. In tandem, during the six months of breastfeeding, the mercury excreted in the infant's hair increased by 446%. The authors speculated that the size of the dose and the fact that the ethyl mercury in thimerosal was injected into the infants accounted for the amount of mercury in the babies' hair at six months of age.

Although proponents of the continued use of thimerosal often mention upfront that its use was discontinued in the United States in 1999 (e.g., McMahon, Iskander, Haber, Braun, & R. Ball, 2008), we know that this is not correct. This supposition is especially misleading with respect to the CDC's continued promotion of the use of thimerosal in U.S. medicines and vaccines and even more so with respect to the WHO's recommended use of thimerosal-containing vaccines abroad.

One Dose Size for All Babies?

The CDC's and WHO's recommendations related to thimerosal-containing vaccines are based on the theory that "one size fits all" when it comes to children from birth to the age of six years—smaller, younger, bigger, older, no matter. Yet the toxicology research is unequivocal in showing that smaller and younger babies are more vulnerable to toxic injuries from every kind of toxin, especially ethyl mercury and methyl mercury. This relationship was clearly seen in the poisonings reviewed earlier in this chapter. The knowledge that younger and smaller babies are certain to be more vulnerable, assuming that all else is held equal, is algebraically certain. In addition, this relationship is confirmed and amplified in recent and richly documented reviews of the toxicology literature (see D. A. Geier et al., 2008; D. A. Geier et al., 2007).

What is the impact of the ratio of the dose of the toxin to the size of the organism? The simple answer is, as the size of the organism decreases or as the size of the dose increases, the ratio changes unfavorably, such that the adverse impact increases to the limit of killing the organism. The research on this relationship is clear as Clarkson stressed to the lead author of this book in an email (personal communication, December 9, 2006). For instance, Blair et al. (1975) dosed squirrel monkeys with either saline solution or thiomersal [British usage for "thimerosal"] in quantities ranging from 418 parts per billion (in the low-dose group) to 2280 parts per billion in the high-dose group. They found that "accumulation of mercury from chronic use of thiomersal-preserved medicines is viewed as a potential health hazard for man" (p. 171). Van Horn et al. (1977) studied the toxicity of thimerosal on human cells in a culture. An exposure of the cornea to a solution of 5 ten-thousandths of 1% thimerosal for 5 hours was damaging and higher concentrations at even one-thousandth of 1% thimerosal caused damage to the cornea within 2 hours and virtual destruction in 5 hours. At one-hundredth of 1% thimerosal, the cornea was damaged and cells were destroyed in an hour.

Kharasch's fears from 1932 and 1935 were confirmed. The unstable ethyl mercury free radicals attach themselves to bodily proteins with devastating effect (Kharasch & Mayo, 1933; Kharasch, McBay, & Urry, 1945). Also, the toxic effects are clearly related to the size of the dose. The greater affinity of the ethyl mercury for the proteins of the human cells as contrasted with any potential bacterium in those cells makes thimerosal relatively ineffective as an antiseptic, even as it becomes harmful and in many instances lethal to cells of the host.

KNOWN TOXICITY OF THIMEROSAL

We have noted that thimerosal would never have been proposed as an antimicrobial unless it had substantial killing power. It is true that the idea of putting it in vaccines was motivated by public safety (Baker, 2008). Multidose vials of vaccine proved to be unsafe because of their contamination by invading microbes. For example, tainted vaccine lots caused disease and death in well-documented incidents in 1916 and 1928 (p. 244). A straightforward solution would have been to repackage the vaccines in single doses. The vaccine manufacturers, however, did not prefer that approach so the search began for a preservative that could support the multidose packaging. That approach was motivated by both convenience and cost: It is easier to give a single injection than multiple shots and it is less expensive to package vaccines in multidose vials.

As a result, a search was begun for a preservative that could be used in multidose vaccines and other medicines intended for injection. The hope of Kharasch and his employer Eli Lilly was to release the killing power of some additive against undesirable microbes but to chemically restrain it with respect to the host. Vaccinologists also wanted a preservative that would not neutralize the disease agents in the vaccine so much that they would fail to engender a sufficient reaction to cause antibody production.

J. P. Baker (2008) supposes, based mainly on the research of Powell and Jamieson (1931), that essentially all of the objectives were fulfilled with the discovery of thimerosal. He claims that thimerosal had greater bacterial killing power, produced less damage than other preservatives to the disease agents in vaccines (which were believed necessary to produce immunity), and did no real harm to the host. Trusting the statements of the eight CDC-sponsored, Institute of Medicine panels of experts convened between 2001 and 2004, Baker sets aside the question of how toxic thimerosal is for humans: "Instead, I examine the historical questions that have been raised in the debate" (p. 244). For our own part, we think the history of the toxicology, and especially the growing understanding of how thimerosal works from a biochemical perspective, is the most important part of that ongoing discussion.

In the following section, for all of the foregoing reasons, it is important to examine the toxicology of thimerosal in greater detail than is common to proponents who look back to superficial summaries rather than the actual biochemistry. The active component in thimerosal is a potent general toxin as well as a severe neurotoxin. Also, contrary to the common sponsored reports, the genotoxic properties of thimerosal have been documented from the 1930s forward.

General Toxicity of Thimerosal

The general toxicity of thimerosal is established theoretically from its biochemistry as well as by empirical evidence from its first applications in medicine. The primary sites of bodily damage done by ethyl mercury poisoning are found in the brain and spinal cord. Also, research has shown that the brain and the gut of animals (including humans) are the primary targets in cases involving ethyl mercury poisoning. From the early 1930s, there have been many studies whose results demonstrate the extreme toxicity of thimerosal.

The results obtained by Salle and Lazarus (1935) with baby chicks were confirmed in humans in 1941, when Kinsella reported on 13 human patients treated for a bacterial infection of the heart with thimerosal. All of those patients died, and subsequent autopsies confirmed that thimerosal caused their deaths. Study after study, as thoroughly documented by D. A. Geier, Sykes, and M. R. Geier (2007) would appear throughout the 1940s, 1950s, and 1960s confirming the toxicity of thimerosal. During the period in question, thimerosal was repeatedly shown to be ineffective against harmful bacteria but lethal to hosts.

An important study by Trakhtenberg (1950) studied the toxicity of ethyl mercury—the kind found in thimerosal—in a vaporous form when it was inhaled by mice. The mice showed disrupted breathing and paralysis of their hind legs as well as "cyanosis" (blue coloring) of the nose, tail, and ears. All of the lab animals died within 6 to 15 hours. Later, in a study where the exposures were incremental over time, the brain and spinal cord were mainly affected. Again, hind limb paralysis spread to the front limbs and was followed by death within a little more than a month (pp. 13–17). This study confirms and explains the injuries sustained from thimerosal by human subjects when treated by Smithburn et al. (1930) when they put merthiolate directly into the infected noses of their patients. The "symptomatic" responses were not described by Smithburn and colleagues, but we can infer that they were similar to those of the mice poisoned by ethyl mercury vapors in the study by Trakhtenberg in 1950.

During World War II, thimerosal was evaluated as a preservative for blood plasma and was found unsatisfactory for this application for the very reasons cited by Kharasch (1932, 1935). The problem making thimerosal unsuitable as a preservative in plasma preparations was that it damaged bodily proteins and was ineffective in eliminating any contaminating microbes. Some of those findings would be elaborated by Engley (1956), who was the first to show thimerosal to be toxic to human tissues in concentrations as tiny as 10 parts per billion, though more recent research pushes the harmful concentration to a still lower level. It is noteworthy that the threshold for injury indicated by Engley's work in 1956 was already 2000 times smaller than the estimated LD_{50} for methyl mercury (and ethyl) exposure for humans according to the Office of Environmental Management.

In the 1960s, mass poisonings of pigs with ethyl mercury from tainted feed confirmed much of what was already known from studies of thimerosal in mice. Also, when people ate the meat of the poisoned pigs, the humans experienced similar symptoms, showing that the research results obtained in mice, pigs, and other mammals are relevant to human beings. In the case of the poisoned pigs, symptoms included extreme problems in the brain, indicated by paralysis of the hind limbs, and in the gut, indicated by bloating and the "belly flop" posture of the animals. The pigs would lie on their bellies, bloated and obviously in pain. (This is a familiar posture often occurring in nonverbal children with autism: bending double over the arm or back of a chair.)

The generalization from ethyl mercury poisoning to thimerosal poisoning is justified by research with vaccines using mice. Nelson and Gottshall (1967) showed that the vaccine for whooping cough (the "P"—pertussis—in DTP) was more toxic for mice when it contained thimerosal than the same preparation when it omitted thimerosal. The main indicator in their study was an increase in deaths. In 1972, Axton reported an accidental exposure of six human patients to a dose of thimerosal that was 1000 greater than intended. Five of them died. In this case, the local manufacturer of a thimerosal-containing medicine read the intended concentration as 0.51 gram rather than the intended 0.51 milligram. The result was an accidental exposure—showing that thimerosal can be deadly to human beings.

In 1973, in a letter published in the *British Medical Journal*, A. G. Nash noted that thimerosal in combination with an aluminum plate used in a surgical procedure produced heat and burned a patient. He cited two other sources reporting similar burns caused by the same combination of chemicals. The fact that thimerosal and aluminum are both found in DTP vaccines today (see RxList, 2009 ●), particularly in the pertussis portion, is reasonable cause for concern.

As mentioned earlier, Fagan et al. (1977) published a report of 10 infants who died when thimerosal was used as a disinfectant on their umbilical cords. In this incident, 13 babies were treated for a defective development of the stomach wall where the intestines protrude into the cord; 10 of them died as a result of the thimerosal treatment. In the same year, van Horn et al. (1977) demonstrated that thimerosal has devastating effects on the human cornea and surrounding tissue.

In 1979, Anundi, Hogberg, and Stead published an explanation of how thimerosal exposure could interact with other toxins to deplete the body's main detoxifier, **glutathione (GSH)**, which is essential to protect cells against toxic damage. Later, the proposal of Anundi and colleagues would be confirmed in a variety of ways. By 1979, however, Anundi and colleagues had already shown how thimerosal in combination with other biochemicals could do even more damage than thimerosal by itself.

In 1982, the FDA's Advisory Review Panel on over-the-counter (OTC) Miscellaneous External Drug Products delivered its report to the FDA on mercury-related products (as referred to in Food and Drug Administration, 1998, p. 19800). It found 18 products containing mercury either unsafe or ineffective, or both. As explained later in Congress by Representative Dan Burton, "mercury compounds [Merthiolate and Mercurichrome among them] as a class are of dubious value for antimicrobial use" (Subcommittee on Human Rights and Wellness, 2003, p. 61). The panel members noted that while the mercury in such compounds slows the growth of bacteria, it does not kill those pathogens (p. 61). The organic mercurials were also found to be highly allergenic. The panel cited a Swedish study showing that 10% of the school children tested, 16% of the military recruits, 18% of the twins, and 26% of medical students tested were allergic to thimerosal.

In 1992, Rosenblum, Nishimura, Ellis, and Nelson demonstrated with mice some of the details of how thimerosal causes damage to tiny blood vessels and to blood cells, as had already been observed in human subjects during eye surgeries. Contrary to assertion made by Marks, Powell, and Jamieson (1932), thimerosal can hemolyze (rupture the cell wall and effectively destroy) red blood cells both in animals and in humans. (See Figure 5-5.)

Although Kharasch was trying to create an organic compound that would be less toxic than the salt known as mercury bichloride, he actually succeeded in producing one that was more toxic (Subcommittee on Human Rights and Wellness, 2003, p. 61). It is true that a recommendation was made in 1982 by the FDA, but the agency would not actually withdraw its approval for OTC topical merthiolate until 1998. Concern had been raised much earlier about the potential for methyl mercury poisoning from fish and the results of studies showing that the impact of such poisoning was greater in younger and smaller individuals. In 2004, Counter and Buchanan developed a clear and

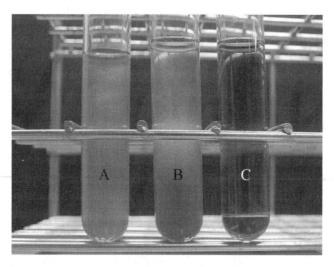

Figure 5-5 A, normal, non-hemolyzed (in tact) red blood cells from a sheep in 0.5% saline solution; B, sedimented after one hour; and C, hemolyzed (ruptured by toxic hemolysis).
Source: Courtesy of Yukihiro Tambe, PhD.

well-supported argument about why children are especially susceptible to poisoning by various forms of mercury, including the ethyl variety found in thimerosal. Mainly their argument focused on the dynamic changes taking place in unborn children and newborn infants at the biochemical level.

Herdman, Marcelo, Huang, Niles, Dhar, and Kiningham (2006) explored the way in which thimerosal kills developing nerve cells. Their research confirmed that this agent acts by affecting the signaling pathway by which cells communicate with one another. S. K. Ghosh, Chaudhuri, Gachhui, Mandal, and S. Ghosh (2007) investigated how some yeast cells resist inorganic mercury poisoning. They noted, however, that cells which can resist ordinary inorganic mercury poisoning are still susceptible to poisoning by organic mercury, including the ethyl mercury in thimerosal; many of those cells will ultimately die. Yole, Wickstrom, and Blakley (2007) found that thimerosal was lethal to cells at concentrations of 25.8 to 48.4 parts per billion after one minute to four hours of exposure. Although the different forms of mercury caused cell death and disrupted processes involved in neuronal growth in different ways, the research shows that both thimerosal and inorganic mercury are highly neurotoxic in extremely small quantities.

Minami, Oda, and Yamazaki (2007) took the question about thimerosal and autism a couple of steps further by testing whether damage to the **blood–brain barrier** (**BBB**) would cause a very small quantity of thimerosal to be significantly more toxic to brain tissue. They showed that thimerosal crosses the BBB in mice following an injection of 60 parts per billion. Brain mercury was significantly higher 48 hours later, reaching a maximum after 72 hours. It was still higher in the injected mice than in non-injected controls one week later. However, when the researchers chemically damaged the BBB in experimental mice and then injected only one-fifth as much thimerosal (12 ppb, a bit less than the dose used in the Hib vaccine throughout the 1980s and 1990s, or half what was used in the DTP and HepB vaccines, for instance), the brain mercury levels were higher at 24 and 72 hours in the injected mice than in the non-injected controls. Without the damaging agent, a dose of 12 parts per billion of thimerosal did not increase brain mercury measurably, however, in experimental mice. This finding is important in showing that the interactions of vaccine components probably play a role in the harm done by thimerosal.

Later, the same group of researchers administered two different chemicals—**dimercaprol** and **D-penicillamine**—in an attempt to remove brain mercury once daily from days three to six. These chemicals, which literally claw out the mercury from its chemical associations with bodily proteins, are known as **chelators**; the removal process is termed **chelation**. Both dimercaprol and D-penicillamine proved effective in lowering brain mercury in the experimental mice.

Thimerosal as Genotoxic

In 1937, it had already been demonstrated that ethyl mercury changes the dynamics of genetic material in plants. The implication of research by Sass (1937) with grain seeds treated with ethyl mercury was that this additive produced "malformation of the seedlings of corn and other cereals" (p. 95). The plants that grew from the treated seeds tended to be deformed in certain ways. The nature of the deformities also had an ethyl mercury signature; that is, they were predictable. Sass described them as causing the stems, leaves, and internal nuclei of the seed cells to be grossly distorted. In animal research, the kind of toxins producing such malformations are referred to as **teratogens** (derived from the Greek root for "monster"). It was already predictable from the work of Sass (1937) that the genotoxicity of thimerosal would be extreme enough to produce gross malformations.

Today, with advances in the understanding of the biochemical dynamics of atoms and molecules in the liquids and tissues of living organisms, it is common to speak of **toxicokinetics** on account of the movement that is constantly taking place within the ethyl mercury compound of interest and to speak of **toxicodynamics** with reference to interactions within cells, tissues, and organ systems (Dorea & Marques, 2008, p. 414). Kharasch (1932, 1935) had already warned that the ethyl mercury in thimerosal in particular was a heavy metal and, therefore, could attach itself to bodily proteins. More recently, Sharma, Goloubinoff, and Kristen (2008) have shown in greater detail just how the ethyl mercury can interfere with bodily proteins, especially in the rapidly developing systems to produce "prenatal and developmental defects." For bodily proteins to do their work within the dynamic systems of cells, tissues, and organs, they have to assume certain shapes that involve folding and unfolding of rapidly moving three-dimensional dynamic systems.

Glimpsing the Systems Disrupted by Thimerosal

Much more can be said along this line with respect to the immune systems and the body's systems for detoxification (which we discuss in more detail in Chapter 10). The dynamic processes of detoxification, immune responses, and ordinary metabolism involve a great deal of unpacking, rearranging, and sometimes repacking of proteins. "Heavy metal ions" of lead, mercury, and cadmium are known to interfere with these processes. Sharma and colleagues assert that the "toxic scope of heavy metals seems to be substantially larger than assumed so far" (2008, p. 214).

To get a glimpse of the complexities at stake, just a superficial one into the tiny worlds of our inner beings, see the animated excursion into the bloodstream created by Viel, Lue, and Liebler (2007 ◯), titled "Inner Life of the Cell." When viewing that video, notice the remarkable parts played by neural fibrils formed from the protein called **actin**. It turns out that both actin and **tubulin** (another bioprotein) are major ingredients in the myelin sheath that insulates the major nerves of the body. Next, to get an idea of just how damaging mercury can be, consider its destructive role as seen in the research animation produced by Leong, Syed, and Lorscheider (2001 ◯), titled "How Mercury Damages Neurofibrils." With the foregoing animations in mind, and realizing that they are oversimplifications of the complexities at stake, consider the damage we are invariably doing by injecting ethyl mercury into the bloodstream of humans, both children and adults.

GENETIC ABNORMALITIES

The effects of mercury on genetics have been well documented in animal models. Oharazawa (1968) showed how ethyl mercury could cause chromosome abnormalities and birth defects in mice. Goncharuk (1971) revealed the deleterious effects of ethyl mercury in rats. In this study, the toxin interfered with the mating cycle, fertility, and ability of offspring to reproduce in successive generations of rats. Also, there was evidence of poisoning of nursing babies through their mother's milk, and the offspring of poisoned rats were smaller, prone to deformed bones, and early death. Itoi, Ishii, and Konek (1972) studied the genotoxicity of thimerosal in rabbits. Doses of 0.02% to 0.2% solutions in pregnant rabbits resulted in more dead and deformed baby rabbits (up to 18% dead fetuses and 9.1% deformed, respectively).

By 1977, Parry had developed a test for the mutagenic properties of different chemicals using yeast cells. His procedure showed that thimerosal is genotoxic in quantities as small as 1 ten-thousandth of a part per billion (i.e., 0.0001 microgram per milliliter). Compare the genotoxicity by Parry's measure with its toxicity for human tissues as estimated by Engley (1986) at 10 parts per million. Thus Parry's test for the genotoxicity of thimerosal showed it to be 10,000 times more toxic than Engley had estimated in 1956.

Also released in 1977, along with Parry's test for mutagenicity, was a large-scale study carried out by the National Institute of Neurological and Communicative Disorders and Stroke in collaboration with the FDA focusing on the risks of thimerosal exposure during pregnancy. The study of more than 50,000 pregnancies showed that thimerosal exposure increased the risk of birth defects by 269% (Heinonen, Sloan, & Shapiro, 1977). In the 1980s, in addition to showing that thimerosal was extremely destructive to human corneas and the surrounding tissues, Lovely, Levin, and Klekowski (1982) revealed that the thimerosal in commercial contact-lens solutions being sold at that time was highly genotoxic.

Humphrey, Cole, Pendergrass, and Kiningham (2005) showed how thimerosal causes cell death in neurons. The ethyl mercury in thimerosal affects the communication between cells by altering the **mitochondria** (genetic material) in the cell's cytoplasm. In their study, after just two hours of thimerosal exposure at a level of 5 parts per billion, membrane damage and cell shrinkage were observable signs of lost viability. There was a dose- and time-dependent increase in cell death with thimerosal exposure. Cells exposed for 24 hours showed the kinds of deformations common to the beginning stages of cancers.

Additional proof of the genotoxicity of thimerosal specifically was provided by Wu, Liang, O'Hara, Yalowich, and Hasinoff (2008). They used **mass spectroscopy** to detect reactions of the ethyl mercury in thimerosal with proteins and DNA. Along the way, these researchers confirmed that glutathione helps to protect cells from thimerosal damage, but does not prevent the toxin from fragmenting DNA. The upshot, once again, is that thimerosal is highly genotoxic.

Eke and Celik (2008) showed genotoxic effects of thimerosal in cultured human white blood cells (**lymphocytes**; see Figure 5-6) at concentrations between 0.2 and 0.6 parts per million of thimerosal compared with untreated controls. Their results with lymphocyte cultures showed damage to the cells themselves and to their genetic viability at the tested levels of exposure to thimerosal.

SUMMING UP AND LOOKING AHEAD

An independent stream of research has thoroughly demonstrated the general toxicity of ethyl mercury to humans. Mercury in essentially all of its forms—both elemental and as salts and alkyls—is an extreme xenobiotic with neurotoxic and genotoxic properties.

Thimerosal, which contains ethyl mercury, was invented by Kharasch, who intended it to be placed in injectable medicines and vaccines. Kharasch, however, was wary of the additive's potential to do harm in medicines and showed how thimerosal could become ineffective as an antimicrobial preservative as a result of its chemical dynamics—a prediction that proved correct. Subsequent

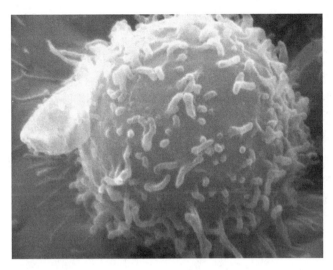

Figure 5-6 Electron microscope image of a human white blood cell (lymphocyte).
Source: Courtesy of Dr. Triche/National Cancer Institute (September 20, 1976).

research, across many different experimental contexts, has confirmed the extreme toxicity of ethyl mercury. These positive results are consistent with our growing knowledge of nanotechnologies and the dynamics of how systems interact in biochemistry.

In the next chapter, we take a broader and more general view of the ways free radicals of all kinds interact to create a generalized form of toxic stress, the condition loosely referred to as "oxidative stress." In later chapters, we will strike a more hopeful note in regard to research in this area: In such a climate of need as has been created by the autism epidemic, it is becoming increasingly clear that a deeper, wider, and more coherent view of the crucial role of communication systems is emerging. To understand the abnormalities of diseases and disorders, we need to know how normal, healthy systems work when all is going well. For this reason, as we will argue in subsequent chapters, the autism epidemic is actually producing a wholesome paradigm shift in the health sciences.

STUDY AND DISCUSSION QUESTIONS

1. Why should biochemistry be important to autism and neurological disorders?

2. What is the meaning of LD_{50} for the components in vaccines? Why should a more stringent standard be applied to them than to other potential and real toxic exposures?

3. According to the toxicology research, what kinds of mercury are the safest to handle? The least safe? Which ones are safe to put inside the bloodstream or the mouth? Which is more toxic—lead, mercury, aluminum, cadmium, manganese, copper, iron, or zinc?

4. Why would different agencies disagree so much on the amount of mercury being dumped in rivers and oceans from dental amalgam?

5. What chemical properties were the drug manufacturers hoping to find in thimerosal? Why do you suppose Kharasch was so explicit in warnings included in his second and third applications for patents on thimerosal?

6. Why are "organic" forms of mercury more absorbable and potentially more dangerous than "inorganic" forms?

7. Why would the study of free radicals, toxins, and biochemistry, earn Kharasch recognition from the Chemical Warfare Service during World War II? Are you surprised to discover an association between vaccine research and chemical warfare? Why or why not?

8. What do poisoning episodes in Iraq and Japan have to do with the ingredients in vaccines?

9. Why are cyanosis and hemolysis significant issues in mercury poisoning?

10. What are the distinctive requirements of genotoxins as contrasted with other kinds of toxins?

chapter six

Oxidative Stress

OBJECTIVES

In this chapter, we

1. Discuss the theory of free radicals and oxidative stress.

2. Consider the cascading effects, domino model of disorders and diseases.

3. Review the theory of oxidative stress in autism and the autism epidemic.

4. Examine the research associating mercury poisoning with encephalopathies, Alzheimer's disease, Parkinson's disease, scleroses, dystrophies, allergies, and asthma.

5. Discuss the role of epigenetic factors in families and the evidence that common genetic factors play a key role in susceptibilities to hypersensitivities.

6. Consider measures of oxidative stress and show that they are elevated in autism.

During the later 1980s and throughout the 1990s, it could be argued that the toxicology of thimerosal was hidden in the looming shadows thrown by vaccine injuries. This phenomenon was well documented in 2002 by Walter Orenstein, then director of the U.S. National Immunization Program (refer back to Figure 4-2). The role played by organic mercury in combination with genetic tendencies, disease agents, and other toxins would be explored in more depth later, mostly after the beginning of the twenty-first century. For the relationships between vaccine injuries, toxins, and oxidative stress to come to light, several lines of thought would have to converge. In particular, the role of free radicals in creating oxidative stress would have to be elaborated and better understood. Also, in spite of considerable controversy over the existence of the autism epidemic, the role of oxidative stress, immune system dysfunction, and generalized inflammation of the gut and brain in autism along with its growing incidence would be demonstrated and would become increasingly well known.

CONVERGING THEORIES, TRUE STORIES, AND INCONSISTENT DENIALS

In the decades leading up to the beginning of the new millennium, no one seemed to know how or why vaccines, especially the DTP series, could be involved in so many injuries. However, the Vaccine Injury Act of 1986 had not just fallen out of the sky. Near the end of the twentieth century, though disputed by vested interests, research would invariably link the MMR with autism, encephalopathy, and gut disease (Wakefield, 2000, 2005, 2006, 2007, 2008; Wakefield et al., 2000; Wakefield, Ashwood, Limb, & Anthony, 2005; Wakefield et al., 1998). In addition, evidence would continue to accrue showing that the four DTP shots, in combination with the MMR shots and the new HepB and Hib series, were collectively having an interactive—and injurious—effect.

More Vaccines, More Toxins, and More Denials

As new vaccines were added into the recommended vaccination schedule, children were not only getting more ethyl mercury, but were also being injected with additional disease agents and other toxins. Contrary to implied and explicit attempts to prove the null hypotheses that autism is not on the rise and that it is certainly not related to any specific factors in vaccines or dental amalgam, it was becoming increasingly obvious that more children were being injured—and parents wanted to know why and how.

As the number of disease agents to which children around the world were being exposed through a hypodermic needle was increasing (Figure 6-1), not surprisingly the public chorus demanding a closer examination of those injections would consequently grow in intensity. The current vaccination schedule, which calls for a total of 36 loaded needles in the behind, arm, or thigh, would give anyone pause. As legal issues about the role of vaccines in neurodevelopmental disorders intensified, near the end of the twentieth century various lines of thought began to converge (J. P. Baker, 2008).

On the one hand, plenty of evidence indicated that heavy metals were playing havoc with human neurology and there were also growing concerns about industrial toxins and agricultural pollution on a large scale (Basel Action Network, 2004). On the other hand, several theories, disparate research streams, empirical findings, and the CDC denials were also converging on the same "mystery." What was causing all the neurological problems? The CDC was deeply puzzled and just

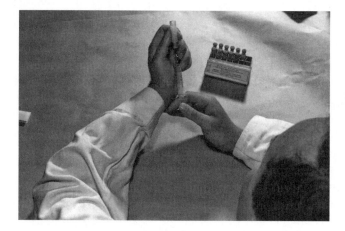

Figure 6-1 Doctor draws a dose of rabies vaccine into a hypodermic syringe.
Source: Courtesy of CDC. Modified from image 8311 retrieved February 19, 2009, at http://phil.cdc.gov/phil/details.asp. Public domain.

could not figure it all out. Many agencies continued to hear reliable testimony from parents whose children were being diagnosed with autism in ever growing numbers, and in many cases with what pediatricians and specialists thought were unrelated disease conditions such as chronic vomiting, allergies, and immune dysfunctions. Were all these issues unrelated? Meanwhile, the growing epidemic of autism would increasingly either be denied or would be set aside as an inevitable, perhaps unsolvable, mystery.

The Case of Wesley Sykes

With the research backing her up, it was impossible to dismiss the testimony of a parent such as Karen Sykes. She testified before the Institute of Medicine's Immunization Safety Review Committee (July 16, 2001) concerning her son, Wesley. She told how Wesley regressed (more accurately, fell and crashed) from a normal childhood into autism, and how getting rid of toxic stress released him from it. After a series of vaccinations, Wesley developed classic severe autism with "chronic diarrhea that lasted for more than a year, loss of speech, loss of receptive language, and hand flapping and hand biting" (IOM, 2001b, p. 218).

In her testimony, Sykes systematically checked off one after another of the symptoms of oxidative stress and poisoning documented in the research on autism that were also displayed by her son Wesley. It all began one morning when she found Wesley with blue lips (cyanosis) and teeth chattering on a warm day in July. Karen Sykes would later learn more than she ever wanted to know about yeast and bacterial infections accompanying mercury toxicity. She would learn about how calcium uptake is disrupted in the blood and about Wesley's abdominal pain from gut disease. She would learn the hard way about Wakefield's research on the measles virus and would observe first-hand as Wesley was subsequently diagnosed with measles, even though his only exposure came from his MMR vaccination at 17 months.

Sykes's testimony also described how Wesley's chelation therapy under the supervision of pediatrician Dr. Mary Megson had produced enormous quantities of mercury and how Wesley began to improve after the treatment. She was already ahead of the curve concerning the research on the role of mercury toxicity in autism, but when the inflamed patch of thickened skin on Wesley's thigh, where he had received several vaccine injections finally began to disappear, Sykes was convinced that the vaccines were involved in his autism. Wesley was five years old at the time of his mother's testimony during the public meeting of the CDC's 2001 Institute of Medicine Immunization Safety Review Committee on thimerosal.

Epidemiologists—notably Dr. Eric Fombonne and colleagues—commonly argue that single cases such as Wesley's situation cannot be used as any basis for decision making or policy building. But Fombonne's argument can be refuted by a moment's thought: No epidemiological study can claim any validity except to the extent that it connects true statements about diseases and disorders with actual individual cases such as that of Wesley Sykes. The individuals have to be accounted for. It seems, however, that the CDC response has consistently been either to deny that individual injuries have been caused by vaccines or to claim that in the rare instances where vaccines do cause injuries, arguments about the greater "public good" should prevail. The latter argument, however, skims over the fact that the public consists of individuals like Wesley Sykes and his mother. Without individuals like Wesley and his mom, the epidemiological arguments are empty.

Is Money Really the Issue?

Occasionally, the CDC has pointed to money as a motivating factor for the supposed autism epidemic. Spokespersons defending the CDC and FDA sometimes have said outright, or strongly implied (Shattuck, 2006), that parent groups were just seeking juicy federal handouts. They would more often subtly imply that the autism epidemic was being greatly exaggerated and that critics of the official policy sought to be rewarded with federal dollars. In an editorial commentary published by the *Journal of the American Medical Association*, Fombonne would complain:

> [T]he current social context seems to exert a stronger influence on the debate than the scientific arguments. Although claims about an epidemic of autism have the most weak [*sic*] empirical support, . . . children with autism, their families, and professionals involved in their care and in research have seen welcome and legitimate increases in public funding. Yet, ironically, what has triggered substantial social policy changes in autism appears to have little connection with the state of the science. . . . further consideration should be given to how and to why the least evidence-based claims have achieved such impressive changes in funding policy. (2003b, pp. 88–89)

Is Fombonne saying that too much public money has been spent on research into the causes of the autism epidemic of which he has denied the existence? The internal contradictions in his statement are almost too many to process. Actually, the research to which Fombonne has persistently objected has generally not been funded by the CDC, FDA, or NIH—or indeed, by any federal sources. The funding for research on the toxins and disease agents involved in causing the autism epidemic has come largely from private resources (e.g., the "mercury moms" and private individuals including Barbara Loe Fisher, Lisa and J. B. Handley, Jon Shestack and Portia Iversen, Bob and Suzanne Wright, Jenny McCarthy, and Jim Carrey).

Believing Many Impossible Things Before Breakfast

No one has been more vocal or effective in denying every aspect of the autism epidemic than Fombonne. He appears to be able to find epidemiological or other negative evidence to prove any null hypothesis that might be favorable to the CDC, FDA, and WHO vaccine policies. Since 1996, he has disputed everything from the existence of the autism epidemic to all of its known and suspected causes, with the possible exception of genetics (Fombonne, 1996, 2001, 2003a, 2003b, 2008).

For example, Fombonne and colleagues insist that the nonexistent autism epidemic cannot be caused by the measles virus because they could not find any evidence of such viruses in 54 children with autism (D'Souza et al., 2006). In their report of the search for measles virus they conducted with reference to 54 children with autism, they imply having proved the null hypothesis that measles virus is not associated with the autism epidemic: "There is no evidence of measles virus persistence in the peripheral blood mononuclear cells of children with autism spectrum disorder" (p. 1664). In effect they generalize from their method to other methods that might have been applied to their sample of 54 cases supposing that those individuals are unaffected by measles virus because their method did not turn up any evidence and further that their method allows them to extend the null hypothesis to "children with autism spectrum disorder" in general. Such reasoning is illogical, erroneous, and always unjustified. We cannot reason from a specific failed search to the nonexistence of whatever we were searching for.

The search method used by D'Souza and colleagues is reasonable enough in its own right and possibly relevant (perhaps it could work), but even so, these facts cannot justify their leap of inference to a general null hypothesis. Just because no measles virus could be found in the 54 cases at hand by their method does not prove that it could not be found by some different one, or that measles virus is not associated with autism at all. Their results do not justify any general inference at all except possibly that their method may be generally inadequate. To claim that they have demonstrated a general null hypothesis, as they do, is to commit a profound logical error. A thousand studies of the type they conducted could not justify the null conclusion they have reached, but just one contrary result would be sufficient to disprove it. What is more, there are many empirical results that disprove the null hypothesis they seem to think they have "proved."

In contrast, Wakefield et al. (1998) demonstrated that measles virus was associated with gut disease in 8 of 11 individuals they studied by examining tissue taken from within the intestinal wall and/or from spinal fluid. More importantly, the association of measles virus with autism has a long empirical history and has never been in any reasonable doubt. On the contrary, the very discovery of the rubella virus, the generally accepted proximate cause of measles (after an incubation period of about eight days to two weeks; Richardson, Elliman, Maguire, Simpson, & Nicoll, 2001), was linked with an epidemic that occurred in the early 1960s (Siegel, Fuerst, & Guinee, 1971). That epidemic resulted in a higher than usual number of miscarriages and/or birth defects in pregnancies that came to term during the period. The measles epidemic was known to be associated with a significant upturn in cases of mental retardation, and the virus would later be associated with encephalopathies and autism (Akram, Naz, Malik, & Hamid, 2008; Brouns et al., 2001; Onal et al., 2006; Risk & Haddad, 1979).

Meanwhile, in addition to arguing that measles virus is unassociated with autism, Fombonne and colleagues, for example, Micali, Chakrabarti, and Fombonne (2004), also insist that autism cannot be associated with autoimmunity. The latter group surveyed relatives of 79 individuals with autism (and 61 controls) and could not find any association between autism and autoimmune diseases. According to these authors, "Medical and autoimmune disorders in both groups were endorsed [presumably they mean that both were reported] by few relatives" (p. 21). Thus this group of researchers appears to believe that their failure to find evidence of autoimmunity in the survey of relatives of the 79 cases entitles them to rule out autoimmunity as a possible factor in all cases of autism, thereby proving another null hypothesis.

Similarly, Fombonne and colleagues believe they have ruled out the possibility that vaccines could be associated with the autism epidemic (the epidemic that they say does not exist). Fombonne, Zakarian, Bennett, Meng, and McLean-Heywood (2006) reported that they could not find any evidence of links between autism and vaccines in general—again, proving a null hypothesis. They suggest that all possible claims about involvement of vaccines in causing autism must be false. In fact, according to Shevell and Fombonne (2006), all the arguments about ethyl mercury poisoning, vaccine-linked measles viruses, autoimmunity, and vaccine-based toxicity in general should be regarded as "urban legends."

To bolster his argument that ethyl mercury cannot have played a role in causing the autism epidemic, Fombonne (2008) contradicts his long-standing claim that there is no autism epidemic by arguing, in effect, that the increase in autism diagnoses has continued since thimerosal was banned. The title of his 2008 article neatly summarizes his position: "Thimerosal Disappears But Autism Remains" (p. 15). He does not seem to think that the continued use of thimerosal in vaccines in the United States until 2002 and its ongoing use in flu shots recommended for pregnant women, infants, and children (something he claims ended in 1999) has had any impact on the cohorts of children who have continued to be diagnosed throughout the new millennium.

The foregoing denials of the roots of the autism epidemic are problematic because of their internal inconsistencies. Of course, the many repeated denials only serve to focus additional public attention on the causative agents that independent researchers are consistently pointing to as the most likely causes of the autism epidemic. One is reminded of Lewis Carroll's (1871) *Through the Looking Glass*, where the Red Queen tells Alice, "Why sometimes I've believed as many as six impossible things before breakfast" (p. 609).

Three Problems in Denials about Known and Suspected Causal Factors

Three problems in this line of thinking show why independent researchers and parent groups are unlikely to be convinced by such denials.

First, the failed efforts to find causative factors in the epidemic of which they deny the existence are flawed in the same way that it would be irrelevant to try to refute, say, Edison's invention of the light bulb by showing 54 ways plus another 79 different ways that Edison might have failed if he hadn't been a money-hungry exaggerator. As students of elementary courses in the logic of scientific measurement understand, null hypotheses cannot be *proved* by failed efforts to *dis*prove them. However, they *can* be ruled out by successful and coherent designs showing significant positive results. For example, Chapter 5 summarizes the many studies that have disproved the null hypothesis that thimerosal is not linked to neurological disorders; in other words, thimerosal has been shown to be linked to such disorders and diseases in general and to be linked to autism in particular. Similarly, Wakefield's research, along with that of others showing an association of measles virus, gut disease, and autism rules out the null hypothesis that the MMR vaccine has nothing to do with the sort of brain and gut abnormalities commonly seen with the diagnosis of autism. In this chapter we rule out many other null hypotheses, including the one that Fombonne has promoted concerning autoimmunity and autism. In addition, we show that toxicity in general, as well as causal factors such as thimerosal and the measles virus, are linked to neurological disorders, gut disease, and autoimmunity, and to autism in particular.

A second problem with denials of the existence of the autism epidemic, and of its known and suspected causal roots, is that the designs on which the denials have been based are quite generally inappropriate as tests of the issues at stake. The designs are commonly set up so that they cannot possibly uncover what the sponsored research is supposedly looking for. Why, for instance, would anyone expect a survey of relatives of 79 children with autism to definitively answer the question of whether autoimmune disorders are involved in autism? Such a design could not possibly provide a definitive answer to such a question. In fact, it is reminiscent of the question that Hugh Grant puts to Sandra Bullock in the 2002 movie, *Two Weeks Notice* (M. Lawrence, 2002). When she tells him (at about 1 : 52 into the clip) that he is "the most selfish human being on the planet," he responds: "Well that's just silly. Have you met everyone on the planet?" Has the CDC or its affiliated researchers actually investigated *all* the ways that autoimmunity might be involved in autism or, for that matter, in the 79 families in question? Could any failure to discover a relationship from a survey of the type conducted generalize to all cases of autism investigated by all possible methods? Can any number of failed searches rule out the positive evidence turned up in even one well-designed study carried out by other researchers?

The third problem is the insistence that there really is no autism epidemic. Why bother with the research in that case? The most devastating refutations of arguments formed in defense of the toxins, disease agents, and the interactions known to be associated with neurological disorders and diseases are to be found in the internal inconsistencies those arguments contain. The argument by Fombonne (2008) that the continued upsurge in diagnoses of autism shows that thimerosal could not have been a causal factor is inconsistent with the claim that no such upsurge has taken place. Also, the claim that thimerosal ceased to be a factor in 1999 is incorrect (see D. A. Geier et al., 2007). In fact, cohorts of children exposed to thimerosal in the United States were still entering first grade in 2008, so Fombonne's assessment is inconsistent and premature concerning the supposed facts on which it was based.

Could Vaccines Be Involved?

In 1986, Congress became involved in this issue through its passage of the Vaccine Injury Act. Nevertheless, there was no real consensus on just *how* the vaccines—the DTP series in particular—were causing the problems addressed by this legislation. A few years later, the fact that topical medicines (not to mention vaccines) contained organic mercury began to attract attention from thoughtful researchers and a few individuals in Congress—in particular, Representative Frank

Pallone of New Jersey and later Representatives Dan Burton and Dave Weldon. FDA personnel also realized that mercury was one of the obvious suspects in the rising number of vaccine injuries being reported.

During the same time frame, while the incidence of autism and neurodevelopmental disorders was following what appeared to be an exponential growth curve, some curious contradictions in policy were being belatedly enacted and enforced by the FDA. Specifically, even as the FDA recommended the banning of organic mercury (thimerosal and merbromin) from topical medicines in 1982 (a ban that was officially implemented in 1998), the same agency continued to turn a blind eye to the ethyl mercury being injected into millions of children through the mandatory sequence of vaccines. The FDA also continued to allow the use of thimerosal-containing injections for Rh-negative pregnant mothers throughout the same time frame.

As concerns were growing that dental mercury in pregnant and nursing mothers had to be involved in neurodevelopmental disorders, the FDA stood by the American Dental Association and the American Academy of Pediatrics, not to mention other professional medical organizations, in denying the theory that medical mercury had any role in the autism epidemic. Many dentists would tell their patients that they get more exposure from a tuna fish sandwich than from a dental filling—a patently false statement (though one apparently believed by many dentists).

Similarly, the American Academy of Pediatrics would stand shoulder to shoulder with the CDC, FDA, and the vaccine manufacturers in maintaining that the tiny exposure to mercury in vaccines, or dental mercury for that matter, was nothing to worry about. Most certainly, they claimed, it could not be involved in producing any neurodevelopmental disorders.

A Hollow Defense Spurs Action

The long-term defense of vaccines containing ethyl mercury by the CDC and its international counterpart, the WHO, continues apace. These organizations argue that the cost of a few vaccine injuries is a small (and necessary) price to pay to prevent worldwide outbreaks of more serious diseases. But are those injuries so rare? By 2001, about 10 in every 1500 children born in the United States were being diagnosed with autism, and parents generally were becoming increasingly reluctant to accept the idea that chickenpox, mumps, childhood measles, flu, or a stomach virus would be worse than autism. Is the threat of severe autism—with its chronic vomiting, bloody diarrhea with nonverbal hand-flapping, head-banging, social withdrawal, or even sudden infant death syndrome—to be preferred over the chance of a childhood disease such as the chickenpox or the mumps? Such an idea can be quickly dismissed, and parents did not waste much time on the idea that autism is preferable to the stomach flu.

When the CDC went from 10 mandated vaccinations before the age of six years in 1986 to 36 mandated vaccines in 2008, parents of children with neurological diagnoses began to ask serious questions about what was being put in their children's bloodstreams. The reasonable concerns of parents and their reports to doctors and clinicians also spurred independent researchers (Cave, 2001; D. A. Geier et al., 2007; Wakefield et al., 1998) to examine the interactions of toxins and disease agents across the multitude of bodily systems, the neurological and digestive systems, the detoxification systems, and disease defense systems (Jepson & J. Johnson, 2007).

MORE THAN GENETICS

In the ensuing discussion, as independent researchers and people whose own children and grandchildren were increasingly at risk of a neurodevelopment disorder began to give more intense scrutiny to the autism issue, multiple lines of thought began to point to the same conclusion. The need to supplement the genetic explanation of autism became increasingly evident. When researchers in different disciplines began to talk to one another and to read reports concerning the interrelatedness of the bodily systems affected by severe autism in particular, it became clear that they were dealing with a great deal more than genetically determined behavioral problems. The digestive issues were serious, extensive, and common. In many instances, children seemed to be progressing perfectly well until about the time of their third or fourth well-baby visit to the pediatrician. The vaccines seemed to be involved in their descent into autism.

Interactions Are Critical

Something had to be interacting with the genes. Also, as researchers and theoreticians began to contemplate the meaning of the genetic explanation, it became obvious that genetic mutations them-selves are not spontaneous. They, too, must be caused by something. Some of the causes have been known for a long time, such as cumulative physical damage from radiation, toxins, disease agents, and physical forces (e.g., electromagnetic fields).

To invoke genetics as the sole explanation of the rising incidence of autism and neurological diseases and disorders is like invoking the existence of air to explain plane crashes. Can air be the sole factor involved in causing plane crashes? Hardly. Other factors, such as physical equipment failures from wear and tear, weather conditions, knowledge and training of the crew, and especially communication between the pilot in the air and controllers on the ground, come into play. In fact, the research shows that communication breakdowns are the main factor in air traffic accidents (Yan, 2009). Similarly, communication breakdowns are the key factors in genetic disorders as well (Sanford, 2005).

The genetic material that dynamically enables and guides the process of growth and development through interaction with the bodily proteins, cells, tissues, organs, and the world within and outside the body is very important but does not by itself produce any diseases or disorders. Certainly, it is not the sole cause of autism or any other neurological conditions or diseases. Over time, it has become certain that genetic factors alone—important though they might be—are not the whole story.

The sort of interactions that must occur for diseases and disorders of any kind to be manifested can be envisioned in terms of the domino model illustrated in Figure 6-2. The idea is that systems inside the living body interact and communicate with one another. This fact is not disputed, yet it is neglected in the piecemeal, fragmented, partial theories that are commonly employed to explain the origins of autism. When the eight Institute of Medicine panels were convened to examine how some component in a vaccine (thimerosal, the measles virus, aluminum, or whatever) related to autism, they were specifically directed by the CDC to steer clear of any interactions between differ-ent vaccines (see Chapter 4). For instance, panel members were directed explicitly to avoid the interaction between the MMR vaccine and the thimerosal vaccines. At one panel meeting, Dr. Chris-topher Wilson had asked if it was even reasonable to look at those issues "in isolation" because, as he pointed out to the Institute of Medicine's Immunization Safety Review Committee (2001a), "in the real world, they don't occur in isolation. Individuals that got the MMR vaccine also received vaccines with thimerosal" (pp. 45–46 ●).

Drugs Cannot Work Without Interactions

The one thing that is probably most clear from clinical trials of vaccines and other drugs is that the interactions are essential. This is obvious in the reports of adverse events to the Vaccine Adverse Event Reporting System (VAERS) and in vaccine injuries recorded in the Vaccine Safety Datalink. As the CDC research team headed by Dr. Robert T. Chen (1997) showed in the first publication concerning the Vaccine Safety Datalink, the DTP vaccine, in particular, was 300% more likely to produce seizures if given 8 to 14 days after the MMR vaccine. Interestingly, this is just about exactly the estimated incubation period for the measles virus (Richardson et al., 2001). The risk of a seizure if the MMR and DTP shots were administered on the same day was also higher (by a factor of 210%)

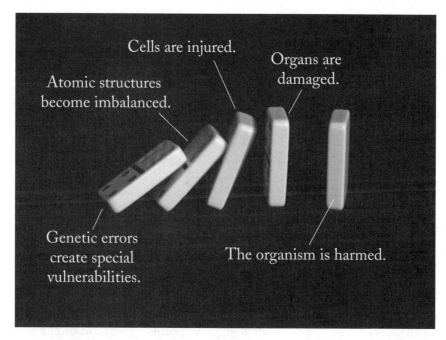

Figure 6-2 The domino model (cascading effects model) applied from genetics upward through cells, organs, and interactions involving the whole organism.
Source: © Jones and Bartlett Publishers. Photographed by Kimberly Potvin.

than if they were administered separately. Considering that the number of cases in the data sample for DTP was 549,488 and the number in the MMR sample was 310,618, these results cannot be taken lightly. The 1997 study by Chen and colleagues was not only the first one published by the CDC showing conclusively that vaccine interactions, especially those involving the MMR and DTP vaccines, produce injuries, but also probably the last. The agency has since taken the position that all approved vaccines have always been very safe and could never cause anything so serious as autism.

Nevertheless, the results of Chen and colleagues (1997), showing an interaction between the MMR and DTP vaccines, agree with ordinary logic. More toxins and more disease agents thrown together in the bloodstream of a vulnerable infant will produce more harm to the child. The DTP and MMR vaccines have to be more dangerous when they are given together than when they are administered separately. Chen et al.'s results also demonstrated that the disease agents and their components were clearly interacting—leading to the unsurprising conclusion that they interact to increase the burden on the body's systems. Instead of fighting a battle only with the disease agents and toxic components injected in the DTP vaccine, the infant's system is being simultaneously challenged to fight off both the disease agents in the MMR vaccine and any other toxins that shot may contain. Logically, fighting off 20 opponents simultaneously is more difficult than fighting one at a time.

More importantly, the work of Chen et al. (1997) revealed that the danger of a seizure if the DTP vaccine is given 8 to 14 days after the MMR vaccine is increased by some action of one or more of the disease agents in the MMR injection. Thus the internal battle going on with components of the MMR vaccine is actually more intense after a week or two than it was on the day when the injection was first administered. In view of the fact that each shot contains multiple disease agents and multiple toxins in addition to its disease agents, is it any surprise that giving both vaccinations in close temporal proximity increases the risk of a serious reaction? Also, is it irrelevant that the

DTP shot, during the period of interest covered in the Chen et al. (1997) report (1991 to 1996), contained a full load of thimerosal in many cases?

It is obvious from a strictly logical perspective, and also from vast numbers of studies of clinical applications of drugs and vaccines, that interactions are absolutely critical. If disease agents can only produce immunity (as we will see in greater detail in Chapter 7) when they are sufficiently potent to trigger an immune response (e.g., the production of antibodies against one or more disease agents), it follows that interactions are where the drug manufacturers earn their money. To ignore the interactions between drugs and the body's own chemistry would be to ignore the most essential factors of importance to medicine and the health sciences in general.

Required: A More Comprehensive Perspective

The interactions between drugs, toxins, disease agents, and the body's own systems for excretion of wastes, ordinary digestion and elimination, detoxification, and defenses against invading microbes are essential factors that must be considered when addressing the roots of autism. The piecemeal theories cited to support such untenable notions as the idea that "one dose-size fits all" never really made any sense, and they have become more obviously inadequate in the face of the growing understanding of the body's multilayered systems of communication. One thing that has been made obvious through the study of autism is that communication across the systems—from the genetics of individuals and families all the way up to social systems, policy making, and international relations—is crucial. Successful and accurate communication is essential at every level of human existence. Communication is crucial from genes to proteins, to cells, to bodily tissues, to organs, to the body as a whole, to the family unit, and to the largest social entities including governments.

To understand something as complex as the autism epidemic, theories of the health sciences and medicine in general require a major shift. They must become more comprehensive and more profound, yet simpler. Focusing exclusively on the intricate complexities of some narrow specialization has become increasingly suspect. Fragmented approaches to health must be replaced by models taking account of the fact that the brain, gut, and bloodstream are connected. Similarly, just as certainly as a viable union between sperm and egg depends on successful communications at many levels, just as certainly as the umbilical cord connects an unborn baby to its mother, and just as certainly as the bloodstream connects the gut and the brain, genes are connected through a multi-layered system of communication with the developing body of the human baby. The success of a baby's development and growth to maturity depends not only on the child's genetic endowment from the parents, but also on nurturing and on communications from others. As is becoming increasingly obvious, the success of the child's own development also depends in many cases on how well pediatricians, dentists, and vast bureaucracies understand the processes of development from before birth all the way to maturity. The success of the whole complex ultimately depends on effective communication from start to finish and all the way in between.

To the extent that the transmission of messages from one system to the next is successful, the entire process of growth and development will thrive. To the extent that messages go awry, disorders and diseases will result. Challenges to successful communication from genes to proteins, and on up the various levels to maturity, do come from disease agents, toxins, and higher level conflicts. However, it is upon successful communication that everything else depends.

The Domino (Cascading Effects) Model

The body's systems are related. When something goes wrong in the genetic systems it can have an upward cascading effect on essentially all aspects of development. With respect to diseases and disorders, the direction of movement is generally one-way, reflected in development over time, and the negative impact is usually irreversible. The problems can arise at any level, but the earlier they enter the picture, the more apt they are to have long-lasting and severe effects. As Figure 6-2 suggests, when genetic errors occur, they may cause atomic and molecular systems to be thrown off, leading to cell injuries, organ damage, and subsequent problems up the hierarchy.

Interestingly, the biochemical theory that would show how cumulative injuries at the atomic and molecular levels could cause greater susceptibility to disease, virtually guaranteeing aging and ultimately the death of the individual organism, was postulated by Morris Selig Kharasch. During the process of inventing thimerosal, Kharasch came to realize that the unpaired electron in the outer ring of ethyl mercury made it a "free radical" and gave it the natural propensity to connect with bodily proteins in a way that would lead to extreme toxicity. According to the renowned University of Cambridge historian of science and medicine C. A. Russell, Kharasch discovered in 1929 that a free radical such as is found in ethyl mercury can break the hydrogen bonds holding a living protein together and can cause two additional free radicals to be released from the protein (Kharasch & Mayo, 1933; Kharasch et al., 1945; Russell, 2004; Westheimer, 1960). According to Russell (p. 24), the recognition of this "additive" reaction between very different molecular components led to the development of what would properly be termed **organic chemistry**, the study of the dynamics of chemistry inside living organisms.

It was precisely because of the potential impact of free radicals on bodily proteins that Kharasch warned of the "undesirable" qualities of ethyl mercury (1932, 1935). Even just one free radical could interact with a protein in such a way as to liberate two more with an exceedingly disruptive cascading impact on organic processes. The protein affected directly by the ethyl mercury would be damaged, and it in turn would potentially damage at least two more, and so on. Where the damage would end was unpredictable, but the fact that it would occur was not in doubt. Interestingly, it was his own discovery of the "additive" power of free radicals that made Kharasch wary of the potential harm that would eventually be done by the ethyl mercury in thimerosal.

FREE RADICALS CAUSE OXIDATIVE STRESS

The contribution of Kharasch in demonstrating the so-called **heterolytic reactions** of free radicals in modern biochemistry would lead not only to the development of organic chemistry as it is known today, but also to current theories of oxidative stress. Today, it is widely accepted that oxidative stress causes some diseases outright and makes others worse. Oxidative stress, according to the theory proposed by Denham Harman (1956, 2003), is critically involved in aging and mortality. Also, as will be shown in following sections, oxidative stress plays a role in disrupting communications between the body's cells and its own immune systems, and it appears to be causally involved in producing the autism epidemic.

How Free Radicals Work

The fact that free radicals cause oxidative stress is widely accepted, although D. Harman's theory about how oxidative stress works in aging appears to be incomplete. For instance, this theory of aging cannot explain why regular vigorous exercise, which ought to increase oxidative stress through increased uptake of oxygen, actually seems to increase general health and longevity. However, Harman's theory of oxidative stress and aging does account for the action of certain vitamins (notably, E, A, D, and B_{12}, among others) that help to scavenge free radicals. It explains why vitamin E, for instance, has notable healing powers (if used in moderation).

Although toxins can operate at much higher levels of the biochemistry (e.g., at the level of the brain and whole nervous system; see Pabello & Lawrence, 2006), cumulative injuries can begin with an imbalance of something as small as an **electron**. An electron can be thought of as a negatively charged particle or wave. In an atomic system, an electron is attracted by the positive electrical charge of a larger particle known as a **proton**. When the negative and positive charges

Figure 6-3   An imaginary proton.

come into balance, the result is what is called a stable though dynamic *atomic system* (Carpi, 1999 ⚫).

As Carpi shows at his award-winning Web site, the chemical stability of the elements beginning with hydrogen and working upward through helium, lithium, and so forth, largely depends on the balance between electrons and protons. When the atomic system of a given chemical element contains an equal number of protons and electrons, the system is relatively stable and not chemically reactive. However, when the balance of electrons to protons is thrown off by as little as plus or minus a single electron, the chemistry gets interesting. If an atom or molecule has an excess of just one electron more than its protons can hold onto, it becomes a ready donor of that extra electron— making it an **oxidizer**. In the reverse situation, if an atom or molecule has a shortage of just one electron (i.e., one fewer electron than it has protons), it is in an unstable state seeking to fill the void, and making it a **reducer**.

What Is Oxidative Stress?

The theory of oxidative stress is actually an atomic conception of how toxins work when they are released inside a living organism. In theory free radicals have one or more electrons to donate, with heavy metals being the richest donors in terms of all the elements of the periodic table. Thus the theory of free radicals shows how toxins throw biochemical systems out of balance at the level of something as small and seemingly insignificant as an electron.

To get an idea just how small an electron is, consider an example given by Carpi (1999): A hyphen such as the one between the quotes "-" is approximately 1 millimeter in length, yet occupies enough space to contain about 20 million hydrogen atoms. Suppose we represented a proton as the ball approximately 1 centimeter in diameter as in Figure 6-3. If it were the center of a stable hydrogen atom, its electron would occupy a spherical volume approximately a quarter of a mile in radius and could be found at any given moment anywhere within that sphere roughly a half mile across (according to Carpi, the size of the Meadowlands Stadium in New Jersey). The electron in that area would be hard to find because it is approximately 1000 times smaller than the proton. If we could shrink the entire model of the proton with its tiny electron orbiting it until 20 million of those models would fit on a single hyphen, the electron would still be many orders of magnitude smaller than just one of the 20 million hydrogen atoms that can theoretically fit on a single hyphen only a millimeter in length. The differences to be contemplated are so large that it is virtually impossible to imagine them, much less visualize them in terms of a model drawn to scale: there just is no sheet of paper that is big enough to contain that model. Besides, if it were big enough, we would get lost on it looking for the electron.

As the theory of **quantum physics** suggests, the electron behaves in such a way as to be anywhere within its **orbital** space 90% of the time; during the other 10% of the time, its location is unknown. Because of its peculiar quantum properties, an electron is typically depicted as a cloud-like entity occupying a space—thus it is more like a wave than it is like a particle or ball.

It is interesting that something so small and seemingly insignificant as an electron could be so important to the theory of oxidative stress. The term "oxidative" is loosely associated with oxygen, which has an **oxidative number** of –2. This oxidative number means that oxygen can capture up to two electrons from an oxidizing agent; because its oxidative number is negative, oxygen is a reducer.

The process of **chemical oxidation** is balanced by the counterprocess called **chemical reduction**, so the number and weight of the interacting chemicals tend to equalize. The interactive balancing processes are referred to by the term **redox** (short for "reduction–oxidation"), which suggests both halves of the balancing reactions with reduction being one half and oxidation the other. The inside of a living cell is normally a reducing environment in which highly active enzymes (special proteins) release energy by converting sugars into energy through the normal process of metabolism. Toxins—especially positively charged metal compounds such as organic mercury in any form (e.g., ethyl, methyl, phenyl)—disrupt the normal redox cycle within the cell. For this reason, oxidation inside living cells is tantamount to toxicity.

In addition to the electron-releasing free radical of the ethyl mercury in thimerosal, for example, the process of oxidation, as demonstrated by Kharasch, releases double-bonded oxygen molecules called **peroxides**. According to Russell (2004), Kharasch discovered that when free radicals were involved, the "addition reactions" didn't balance out as expected. It was this discovery in 1928, according to Russell, that marked the true beginning of modern organic chemistry. The peroxide molecules can easily form additional free radicals, along with whatever other toxins are already bouncing around. The resulting reactions can damage essentially everything inside the cell—its proteins, its energy-storing fatty acids, and its DNA, especially the DNA in the mitochondria that enables the cell to communicate within itself and with other cells outside of itself. Most importantly, the damage done by oxidative stress makes it difficult or even impossible for the cell to communicate with other bodily systems, especially the body's own immune systems. When those communication systems break down within a cell, the body's immune systems are apt to attack and destroy it as if it were a foreign substance or a disease agent.

Standard Theory of Mortality

The out-of-balance free radicals damage the organism within which they are released. It follows that if free radicals are involved in essentially all of the body's degenerative conditions, disorders, and diseases, as Denham Harman inferred, they are also primary agents in producing the cumulative damage called aging—and thus serve as the guarantee of mortality (Harman, 1956). (For an interview with Harman, see Loren and D. B. Harris, 1998. ☻)

In an effort to counteract the actions of free radicals (the general descriptor used for oxidizing agents), Harman began to search for **antioxidants**—that is, chemicals and compounds that would bind the free radicals and render them harmless, thereby increasing the health and life span of the organism. By 1969, his work had begun to attract the interest of other researchers and the general public. When it was demonstrated that the life span of mice, rats, fruit flies, and microorganisms could be increased by certain vitamins acting as antioxidants, Harman's theory of free radicals, at least from 1981 forward, became the dominant explanation of aging and mortality. The research showed that **vitamin E** (found in wheat-germ oil; see "Tocopherol," 2009 ☻), **vitamin C** (found in citrus fruits and especially kiwi; see "Vitamin C," 2009 ☻), and **beta-carotene** (a source from which the liver manufactures **vitamin A**, which is important to vision and is found in carrots and sweet potatoes; see University of Maryland Medical Center, 2008 ☻) were all effective antioxidants.

What is becoming better understood is that the redox cycle is assisted by certain antioxidants that help to maintain its communication with the body's immune systems. Among the most important of those antioxidants is glutathione (GSH).

The Glutathione Cycle

A peroxide form of the glutathione molecule was discovered in 1957 by G. C. Mills and was shown to prevent oxidative breakdown of **hemoglobin**. This particular form is **glutathione peroxidase**

(**GPx**). As we will see, it plays an important role in autism spectrum disorders and in immune systems diseases.

Various forms of glutathione are known to be involved in antioxidant activity and in maintaining communication with the immune systems of the body. The most basic form of glutathione (GSH) consists of three amino acids: cysteine, glutamate, and glycine. It is manufactured by most cells of the body, but especially by the liver. The great antioxidant power of glutathione depends on a cycle by which glutathione moves from its reduced form, GSH, to an oxidized form, GSSG, standing for glutathione disulfide, and back again to GSH. Normally, the reduced form, GSH, which has the power to donate an electron to a free radical, thereby detoxifying it and preventing it from disrupting other proteins within the cell, is about nine times more abundant than the oxidized form (see "Glutathione," 2009; "Glutathione Peroxidase," 2009 ●).

When two of the oxidized forms of glutathione, abbreviated as GS, meet up, they combine to form a harmless, non-oxidative variant of glutathione known as GSSG. In the process they give up two positively charged hydrogen atoms that readily combine with oxygen to form the highly toxic hydrogen peroxide (H_2O_2). However, the GPx discovered by Mills is involved in converting hydrogen peroxide to water (H_2O). The required reactions are likely because of the normal abundance of glutathione within the cell. When the glutathione cycle is working well, toxins are efficiently neutralized and communications between the cell and the body's immune systems continue as normal. However, when glutathione supplies are overwhelmed, or are missing for want of the genes involved in their construction, or when the amino acids that enable the construction of the needed glutathione are missing, the health of individual proteins is at risk from toxins. In this circumstance, a cascade of cumulative small disasters can grow into disorder, disease, and even death (see Figure 6-3). If the capacity to generate glutathione is reduced because of a genetic defect, then toxins—for instance, from vaccines (Rossignol, 2007), dental amalgam (Palkovicova et al., 2008), or pesticides (Giordano, Afsharinejad, Guizzetti, Vitalone, Kavanagh, & Costa, 2007)—may deplete glutathione leading to oxidative stress and causing cyanosis and the host of cumulative dysfunctions that lead to disruption of nerve functions and subsequently to such disorders as autism.

Damaged Bits and Pieces

Oxidative stress accompanies developmental and degenerative disorders. Not only autism, but essentially all of the neurological disorders affecting speech, language, and hearing are implicated. Among the disorders and diseases that have been shown to be linked to stress caused by toxins, especially mercury poisoning, are Alzheimer's disease (Nishida et al., 2007), Parkinson's disease (Pearce et al., 1997), **multiple sclerosis**, rheumatoid arthritis, and many types of autoimmune and metabolic imbalances. To see what may be going on in autism, therefore, it is important to consider how damaged bits and pieces of biochemicals can end up doing widespread cumulative harm.

Segura-Aguilar and Kostrzewa (2006) observe that toxins, such as mercury, interfere with important combinations of proteins and are "indigenous to Alzheimer disease [and] Parkinson's disease" (p. 263). They go on to point out that a new variety of neurological disorders has emerged that is being referred to as *neuroAIDS*. In this disorder we see interaction between the **microglia**, the cells that police and clean the brain among other functions, and the **macrophages**, the main immune attack cells of the body at large. The macrophages are among the most important cells in the body's defenses against diseases. Their name in Greek means "big" (*macro-*) "eaters" (*-phages*). Macrophages do a great deal of work in defense of the body and in disposal of waste, picking up the trash.

In neuroAIDS, the body's immune cells attack its own nerves, creating inflammation that is part of the neurodegenerative process in Alzheimer's disease, Parkinson's disease, and a host of neurological disorders. Accordingly, Segura-Aguilar and Kostrzewa conclude that we can now say that "the entire spectrum of neuroscience is within the purview of neurotoxins and neurotoxicity mechanisms" (p. 263). Of course, that scope also includes the autism spectrum disorders.

A Common Problem in Autism and Alzheimer's Disease?

It is interesting that oxidative stress and metals known to cause it are factors in autism and in degenerative diseases such as Alzheimer's disease. Autoimmunity and toxic injury are both involved in these disorders. Alzheimer's disease has been known since 1906, when Alois Alzheimer [1864–1915], a German psychiatrist, published a report of a 50-year-old woman who had died with the condition just five years after he began to treat her. Her condition appeared to be an advancing **senile dementia**, a condition of deterioration associated with advancing old age. Because Alzheimer's disease commonly affects older persons, it has sometimes been referred to as "old-timer's disease," but there is no doubt that this condition is affected by toxins that damage cortical tissues.

Among the elements that are diminished in Alzheimer's disease is the neurotransmitter **acetylcholine** ("Alzheimer's Disease," 2009; also see Domingo, 2006; Ferreira, Vieira, & de Felice, 2007 ⊚). The fact that abilities fluctuate within the same person in a 24-hour period, or over even shorter time spans, has led Palop, Chin, and Mucke (2006) to speculate that conditions such as Alzheimer's disease cannot be exclusively caused by neuronal damage, but rather must involve elements of toxicity that can be intermittently overcome. Nerve cells cannot suddenly be regenerated, so the changing levels must be owed to something else: Perhaps ups and downs in the toxic impact of "abnormal proteins" (Palop et al., 2006, p. 768) could explain the observed ups and downs in abilities.

The current consensus is that certain proteins—in particular, the **beta amyloids**, which are important to normal neuronal functions—literally get bent out of shape and broken in pieces by toxins. Among the known offending toxins are heavy metals, especially mercury (Leong et al., 2001). Once this happens, the twisted proteins form the **plaques** that are characteristic of Alzheimer's disease (Ferreira et al., 2007). As shown in Figure 6-4, a series of circular formations define the plaques. Another hallmark of Alzheimer's disease is a sort of **neurofibrillary tangle**; it is not shown in Figure 6-4, but can be viewed in Leong, Syed, and Lorscheider (2001), which shows the neurotoxic impact of minute quantities of mercury (on the DVD, click "How Mercury Damages

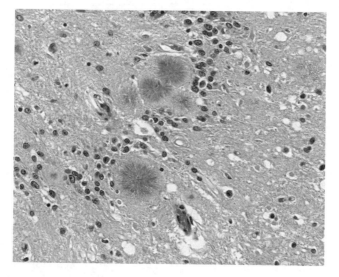

Figure 6-4   Amyloid plaques in the cortex of a patient with Alzheimer's disease.
Source: © Science Source/Photo Researchers, Inc.

Neurofibrils" 👁). Also, a diagram of both plaques and tangles is available from the American Health Assistance Foundation (2000–2008).

Metals such as iron, zinc, potassium, magnesium, selenium, and the like are required by the body for certain metabolic purposes. However, when these metals are not properly linked to other elements for their normal constructive uses in proteins, they need to be reduced and/or disposed of; otherwise, they will produce toxic stress. Some metals, even in extremely small quantities, are much more damaging than others. Of course, essentially any chemical, protein, or biological substance in sufficient quantity can produce toxic effects, but heavy metals such as mercury, lead, nickel, cadmium, manganese, and aluminum are toxic in relatively small quantities. The most neurotoxic of those metals, by a fairly large margin, is mercury. Interestingly, it is the metal most clearly implicated as a principal cause of oxidative stress in autism spectrum disorders. Mercury is also evidently a principal toxin in either precipitating or exacerbating autoimmune disorders in general.

Toxicity: Associated with Self-Immune Diseases and Autism

If oxidative stress exceeds a relatively low limit—a limit that may differ depending on the genetics of the individual—the detoxification systems may become overloaded. In such a case, the immune systems will take over and attack the damaged cells as if they were disease agents.

When the body begins to attack itself because of oxidative stress, the condition crosses over from mere toxicity to self-immunity and thus into the class of **autoimmune diseases**. Among the various autoimmune diseases that critically involve the brain and gut as in many cases of severe autism are multiple sclerosis (D. A. Geier & M. R. Geier, 2005) and **celiac disease** (Wakefield et al., 1998). Both of these classes of disease conditions are associated with mercury poisoning as well as autism. Another autoimmune disease that is directly associated with mercury poisoning is **glomerular kidney disease** (Guzzi et al., 2008). In multiple sclerosis, the immune system attacks the central nervous system. The result is the stripping of myelin from nerves in the brain and spinal column. Because mercury in essentially all of its forms (inorganic as well as organic) attacks the brain and nervous system more than any other internal target, it is unsurprising that mercury poisoning is a causative factor in the expression of multiple sclerosis.

Although the link is denied by the American Dental Association (Zentz, 2006), the American Academy of Family Practitioners (Kimmel, 2002), and the WHO (Francois et al., 2005), evidence shows that mercury poisoning can exacerbate multiple sclerosis and, in fact, any demyelinating disease condition (M. J. Carson, 2002; D. A. Geier & M. R. Geier, 2005; Girard, 2007; Mutter, Naumann, Walach, & Daschner, 2005). In celiac disease, and various other diseases of the gut, the lining of the intestines is attacked; oxidative stress, and mercury poisoning in particular, makes this condition worse. As discussed in Chapter 5, the toxicology clearly links gut disease and glomerular kidney disease to mercury poisoning (Clarkson & Magos, 2006). Recent research by Mouridsen, Rich, Isager, and Nedergaard (2007) also shows that parents of children diagnosed with autism are more likely to have parents with autoimmune diseases—**ulcerative colitis** on the side of the mother and **type 1 diabetes** (the autoimmune kind) on the side of the father. This single result refutes the null hypothesis proposed by Fombonne and colleagues denying that autism is associated with autoimmune disorders.

Oxidative stress leading to autoimmune diseases, as demonstrated by D. A. Geier and M. R. Geier (2005) through data gleaned from the Vaccine Adverse Event Reporting System, can be brought on by vaccines. For instance, Geier and Geier showed that the HepB vaccine increases the likelihood of autoimmune attacks on the nervous system and the vascular system. In addition to a 520% increased likelihood of a multiple sclerosis diagnosis after receiving the HepB vaccine (compared to a control group who did not receive the HepB vaccine but did receive a tetanus vaccine), patients had an increased risk of autoimmune attacks on the central nervous system, the optic nerve, and the blood and vascular systems following hepatitis B vaccination. Diagnosed autoimmune diseases included an 1800% increase in the diagnosis of **rheumatoid arthritis**; a 910% increase in the diagnosis of **lupus erythmatosus**, a condition in which the immune system intermittently attacks the nervous system, heart, lungs, and other organs; and a 210% increase in **thrombocytopenia**, a condition in which blood platelets become abnormally scarce.

Data gathered (but then suppressed) by the CDC reveal that the increasing use of the HepB vaccine from 1989 through 1994 was strongly correlated ($r = 0.99$, $p < 0.0001$) with the rising incidence of autism spectrum disorders during the same period (see Figure 3-3). Complaints about the HepB vaccine have also arisen in Europe (Girard, 2007). For example, the childhood onset of multiple sclerosis became known in Europe only after the widespread use of the HepB vaccine (Girard, 2007).

HLA Identifiers and Autism

Clinching the case for an association between autism and autoimmune diseases, L. C. Lee et al. (2006) found that mothers of children with autism were more likely to have a certain class of genes on chromosome 6 that distinguishes them both from the general population and from persons in families that do not have a child diagnosed with autism. The **human leukocyte antigen (HLA) system** was discovered through experimental work with tissue grafting and organ transplanting ("Human Leukocyte Antigen," 2009 ●). It involves a large number of genes that produce a complex of proteins involved in identifying cells that belong to the self as opposed to foreign cells. There are very short proteins that are involved in self-identification within the cell, as well as longer ones that are displayed on the surface of the cell to identify it as self to the body's immune systems. The HLA proteins in all cases are so varied and so numerous that the difficulty of finding suitable tissue and/or organ donors is exceedingly problematic except among very close relatives—and even then it poses a serious challenge.

Within the complex of genes involved in the HLA system, L. C. Lee and colleagues found a combination of particular genes and proteins in the HLA system designated as **serotype** DR4 that is much more common in mothers of a son with autism (by 554%) than in the general population. The DR4 serotype is also more common to boys diagnosed with autism (by 420%) than to male children in the general population. More importantly, certain genes associated with this serotype are also specific to certain autoimmune disorders that share important symptoms with autism spectrum disorders. The DR4 serotype is commonly encountered in multiple sclerosis, for example; like autism, multiple sclerosis principally involves the brain. This serotype also is commonly found in celiac disease, which involves the sort of lesions in the gut that are, in many cases, associated with autism. Finally, the DR4 serotype is often found in conjunction with glomerulonephritis, which affects the kidneys in a manner similar to ethyl mercury poisoning ("HLA-DR4," 2009 ●). It is noteworthy that this troika of autoimmune diseases shares common ground in terms of symptoms with both severe autism and ethyl mercury poisoning.

Orderly Dismantling: Apoptosis

Even if oxidative stress is relatively mild, it can interfere with communication between the cell's mitochondria (the DNA outside of its cell nucleus) and the body's basic constructive processes as governed by the **nuclear DNA** (the DNA within the cell nucleus). As Cannino, Di Liegro, and Rinaldi (2007) have shown, it is essential for the two types of DNA to communicate with each other during development. Disrupting the signaling systems within the cell, however, can cause the cell itself to misinterpret its own internal communications as well as foul its communications with the body's immune systems. As a result the cell may begin to dismantle itself in a process of "programmed cell death" called **apoptosis** ("Apoptosis," 2009 ●). This process of self-dismantling is often described somewhat inappropriately as "cell suicide," but it is known to be controlled under normal circumstances by a protein in the outer membrane of the mitochondria known as **apoptosis-inducing factor** (**AIF**). When that membrane is ruptured by mercury poisoning, for example, the AIF is released and cell dismantling is initiated prematurely.

In embryonic development, the division of fingers and toes, for example, is believed to depend on controlled apoptosis. Based on the research of Cannino and colleagues, it seems that the governance of that process critically depends on communication between the mitochondrial DNA and the nuclear DNA. During early development of the baby in the womb, cells contained in the tissue between the fingers and toes must be disassembled for the separation of the distinct digits to be completed. The process of normal growth crucially involves the disassembling of cells between the fingers and toes. The means by which the body controls which cells to build up and which ones to disassemble must be guided by the overall blueprint for the shape of the body, which is contained in the two kinds of DNA, but especially the nuclear kind.

The normal process of development, however, also depends critically on an *interaction* between both types of DNA. For the body to differentiate its left and right hands and feet, and the fingers and toes on each hand and foot, the individual cells and groups of cells must know their position in the body. The dynamic plan for the building up of tissues is contained within the DNA but must be communicated within and between the cells. As shown by Cannino and colleagues, cells communicate their position in the body both to themselves and to each other through interactions within different components of their nuclear and mitochondrial DNA.

The building up of some cells is sustained while others are assembled temporarily only to be systematically dismantled in the process of apoptosis. When the body is growing and developing, it is estimated that the equivalent of tens of billions of cells are systematically dismantled by apoptosis in an orderly way every day. For a child between the ages of 8 and 14 years, the number of cells dismantled amounts to replacement of the entire weight of the body in about one year ("Apoptosis," 2009 ●). When the process of internal communication governing normal apoptosis within the cell is sufficiently disrupted by oxidative stress, disease and disorder result. If apoptosis occurs too rapidly, growth in the affected organs and body parts is stunted. In contrast, if apoptosis occurs too infrequently, cells can proliferate to the point that they produce abnormal growths including cancers.

Premature Apoptosis Contrasted with Toxic Necrosis

In the case of apoptosis triggered by a toxin, such as ethyl mercury, the process can be described as premature cell dismantling. This kind of malfunction is believed to be caused by miscommunication between the cell within itself and with the immune systems that disassemble and redistribute the parts of dismantled cells. Parran, Barker, and Erlich (2005), for instance, have shown that as little as one-tenth of one part per billion of thimerosal can cause apoptosis. As early as 2002, Makani, Gollapudi, Yel, Chiplunkar, and Gupta suggested that thimerosal might trigger premature apoptosis. In their research, they examined effects on the mitochondrial pathway of apoptosis in certain immune killer cells. They found that the ethyl mercury in thimerosal—as distinct from **thiosalcylic acid** (its nonmercury component)—depending on the size of the dose caused release of free radicals and, by depleting the glutathione within and outside the cell, damaged the mitochondrial pathway.

Parran, Barker, and Erlich (2005) showed that an increase in the exposure to thimerosal at slightly less than one part per billion of ethyl mercury can cause the even more damaging (less controlled) sort of cell death known as **necrosis**. The difference between the orderly process of apoptosis and the disorderly process of necrosis is dramatic. It is analogous to the difference between a construction site where workers carefully take scaffolding down, piece by piece, and the sudden destruction wrought by the terrorist attacks in New York on September 11, 2001. The unexpected attacks demolished seven huge buildings, spewing toxins and debris in all directions. In the case of necrosis, as contrasted with apoptosis, the disintegration involves relatively complete and unordered destruction of the cell components on the inside, followed by swelling and bursting of the cell wall. The disorderly cell death in necrosis increases toxicity in the surrounding tissue.

In necrosis, the parts of the cell are not disassembled in an orderly way. As a result, any toxins, viruses, or bacteria inside the cell are released and scattered into the surrounding tissues. Because of the scattering of cell debris, the cleanup by the body's immune systems also tends to be messy and can involve collateral damage. The cleanup itself, as in the removal of debris from the World Trade Center site after September 11, 2001, results in the release of additional toxins into the surrounding area. The released toxins poison the cleanup crews themselves in much the way that uniformed personnel were poisoned at Ground Zero by breathing noxious gases and by inhaling and swallowing dust particles.

As a result of necrosis, surrounding tissues become inflamed and poisoned. Just as the puncturing of the colon can release toxins, bacteria, and viruses into the blood and into other cavities outside the colon, so the bursting of any cell wall can release undesirable elements that were formerly safely contained within the cell's wall or within its formerly sealed components. The kind of damage that results in the rupturing of cellular membranes is like what happens in the bruising of tissues of the brain, for example. The release of toxins by such bursting of cells, which is often referred to as **secondary trauma**, is often more severe than the primary impact on account of the toxins released.

Xiong, C. P. Lee, and Peterson (2001) have argued that the main factor in secondary injuries—those caused by bursting of cells and the concomitant release of toxins that follows—result from breakdowns in communication between the injured tissue and the immune system. Because the necrosis is not controlled by normal communication processes within and between cells, it is more difficult for the immune system to find and recycle components of the destroyed cell(s). This situation is very different from the one that occurs when a cell undergoes apoptosis. The evident solution of the immune system is to attack and destroy every remaining damaged cell that cannot properly identify itself as friendly (i.e., as part of the self). As a result, the cleanup of the area affected by the exploded necrotic cells commonly does more damage than the initial necrosis.

Autoimmunity Specific to Autism

There is a long history of the study of autoimmunity in autism spectrum disorders going back at least to Money, Bobrow, and Clarke (1971). More recently, positive evidence of the role played by autoimmunity in autism has continued to accumulate from many sources (Comi, Zimmerman, Frye, Law, & Peeden, 1999; Jyonouchi, Sun, & Le, 2001; Sweeten, Bowyer, Posey, Halberstadt, & McDougle, 2003). The most convincing evidence comes from studies showing specific self-immune antibodies in the blood of individuals diagnosed with autism (Jyonouchi et al., 2001; L. C. Lee et al., 2006; A. Vojdani, A. W. Campbell, Anyanwu, Kashanian, Bock, & E. Vojdani, 2002; A. Vojdani, Pangborn, E. Vojdani, & Cooper, 2003).

In particular, research has shown how certain individuals with autism may develop self-immune antibodies from disease agents combined with ethyl mercury and certain peptides in their diet (Vojdani et al., 2003, p. 189). Prior to this work, a series of studies had established that specific nerve-attacking, self-immune antibodies are common in individuals diagnosed with autism or a closely related neurological disorder (Connolly et al., 1999; Jyonouchi et al., 2001; E. Vojdani et al., 2002). It is also well known that the processes by which self-immunity is produced involve oxidative stress. Therefore, it is reasonable to predict that many indicators of oxidative stress will be found to be elevated in autism.

OXIDATIVE STRESS, AUTISM, AND NEUROLOGICAL DISORDERS

Stan Kurtz, the father who helped his son to recover from severe autism and the inventor of the nasal spray formula for vitamin B_{12} (methylcobalamin), has suggested a simple idea about the relationship between toxins and disease agents. He argues that the body generally prioritizes live, reproducing disease agents over toxins. Imagine you are the commander of an army being attacked by an army of ninjas—that is, measles viruses from an MMR vaccine—that can rapidly multiply themselves. At the same time, suppose you know your troops have just been sprayed with DDT, say, or injected with thimerosal. Which threat will you deal with first, the toxins or the rapidly multiplying ninjas? The best judgment, in most cases, will be to prioritize the active army of attackers and to deal with the toxin after the live attackers have been crushed.

SENSIBLE PRIORITIES

Kurtz supposes that if an infection coexists with toxicity, the body's immune system will generally deal with the infection as the highest priority and address the toxin only later, if and when the disease issues have been resolved. For example, in the case of Ethan Kurtz, it was only after the fungal infection in his gut was cleared up that he began to dump large quantities of mercury.

Kurtz's theory is that the disease condition is prioritized and must be cleared before the body will have sufficient resources to clear the toxin. Keeping in mind that the body's systems for immunity and detoxification normally work together in harmony, it follows that toxic disruptions that are sufficient to interfere with genetically controlled processes within the immune and detoxification systems will tend to be quite general. Therefore, we should hypothesize that the same processes that cause autoimmune disorders in autism will tend to cause them in general. In fact, the research supports this hypothesis.

As we have already seen, families in which a child is diagnosed with autism will also tend to have relatives diagnosed with autoimmune diseases such as ulcerative colitis (celiac disease) and type 1 diabetes as shown by Mouridsen, Rich, Isager, and Nedergaard (2007); this idea has been generalized to additional self-immune diseases such as Alzheimer's disease, multiple sclerosis, and rheumatoid arthritis by L. C. Lee et al. (2006). All of these disorders and diseases, along with **amyotrophic lateral sclerosis** (**ALS**; Moumen, Nouvelot, Duval, Lechevalier, & Viader, 1997), involve high levels of oxidative stress. It has also been suggested that ALS, in particular, may be causally associated with mercury poisoning (A. Costa, Branca, Pigatto, & Guzzi, 2008). T. A. Evans et al. (2008) point out that besides autoimmune diseases with extraordinarily high levels of oxidative stress, this list may include Parkinson's disease, cancers (in general), **atherosclerosis** (a chronic inflammation in the walls of arteries due to buildup of damaged proteins and fatty acids that are not being removed by white blood cells), age-related **macular degeneration** (**AMD**); a similar buildup of plaques inside the eye, and aging.

Are general levels of oxidative stress raised well above the average in autism spectrum disorders, as might be predicted? In fact, studies show that they are.

Elevated Oxidative Stress in Autism

We know some of the factors that cause oxidative stress, and we have already shown that certain of these factors—namely, the toxins and disease agents in vaccines—are clearly linked to the rising incidence of autism spectrum disorders. Research has also elucidated the impact of oxidative stress on apoptosis and necrosis; anyway we look at it, oxidative stress is generally a bad thing.

One way to rule out the null hypothesis that autism does not involve elevated oxidative stress is to measure it in persons with autism spectrum disorders. Logically, if oxidative stress is involved in the causation of the condition, it has to be generally elevated in autism. Assuming that oxidative stress must be generally elevated in persons with autism, the next step is to look for a particular measure that would not only show the elevation, but actually link it to specific causal factors such as (1) genetic damage producing a particular serotype susceptible to autoimmune diseases in general (e.g., HLA DR4)—a link that has already been made by L. C. Lee et al. (2006) and S. Lee et al.

(2006); (2) heavy metal poisoning—a link that was established by the many sources cited in Chapter 5; and (3) evidence of oxidative stress that is specific to persons with autism.

Reduced Glutathione and Glutathione Peroxidase

Among predictable measures of oxidative stress are reduced levels of glutathione (GSH) and glutathione peroxidase (GPx) in persons with autism. In fact, both of these predictions—which would be exceedingly unlikely guesses if we knew nothing of the biochemistry involved in autism spectrum disorders—are resoundingly confirmed in the research literature.

Golse, Debray-Ritzen, Durosay, Puget, and Michelson (1978) found that GPx was greatly reduced, by about 44.4%, in the red blood cells of 45 individuals diagnosed with autism compared against 41 matched controls without autism. From such results, we can reject the null hypothesis that oxidative stress is not a factor in autism (also see Yorbik, Sayal, Akay, Akbiyik, & Sohmen, 2002). We must conclude that oxidative stress is a highly significant factor and, therefore, reject the null hypothesis that oxidative stress is no different for persons with and without autism. In doing so, we reject the null hypothesis on the basis of a significant positive result (as predicted). When we get this type of result, the more unlikely, abstract, complicated, difficult-to-achieve, and theoretically plausible the predicted outcome may be, the more convincing is the rejection of the null hypothesis. In this case, because the contrast is significant, substantial, and in the predicted direction, the more certain we are in saying that oxidative stress—measured, for instance, in terms of elevated levels of GSH and GPx—in persons with autism is higher than in healthy persons who do not have autism. We are very confident in rejecting the null hypothesis.

Now compare the claim that oxidative stress is elevated in autism with that of someone who tries by a failed experiment—that is, an experiment that did not achieve any of the expected contrasts predicted by a reasonable theory—to argue for a null hypothesis. Consider how few ways there are for the positive result to be obtained by chance, as contrasted with how many ways there are to fail to get a predicted outcome. Typically, the chance of success in producing evidence of a positive and significant contrast (in GSH or GPx levels, for instance) if there really is no contrast between oxidative stress in healthy controls and persons diagnosed with autism is very slight. It gets smaller and smaller to a vanishing point as the experiments required for the demonstration, and the theory behind them, become more elaborate, abstract, and coherent.

What about a failed experiment that produces no contrast where rational theory shows that we should find one? Think about all the ways that a nonsignificant outcome, a null outcome, could be achieved. Perhaps the experimenters were simply not careful in collecting the data. They may have used an inappropriate measure; alternatively, they may have used an appropriate measure, but applied it badly or inappropriately. They may have simply recorded the wrong results. They may have used an erroneous scale or a faulty time frame, or committed some combination of errors that kept them from achieving success. Failures are so easy to get, in so many different ways, that they prove next to nothing and are amazingly uninformative. All they show is a failed effort.

Success, by contrast, especially if it is hard to achieve, and if the measures are complex, abstract, and based on a coherent and well-developed theory, is far more informative. Imagine a person who is lost at sea. Which will we weigh more heavily a thousand failed searches or the single search that finds and rescues the lost person? The more unlikely the outcome, the more informative is a significant positive result. By contrast, null results in failed searches are useless.

Publishing significant results makes sense, whereas publishing failures is usually not even recommended, although peer-review editorial boards do not always follow their own good rules. In addition, with successful experiments, if the design, measures, theory, and interpretations are valid, the results will be replicable, usually in many different ways. Such is the case with the prediction that oxidative stress is positively associated with autism spectrum disorders. The most widely accepted evidence in the sciences that a successful experiment was interpreted correctly, and that a null hypothesis can be ruled out with virtual certainty, is **replication** of results. If different researchers can repeat all or part of an experimental (measurement) procedure and obtain the same results, or ones with similar implications, we gain confidence that the theory underlying the prediction of the successful outcomes is on the right track. We gain confidence in ruling out the null hypothesis. By contrast, no number of failed searches can truly justify a null hypothesis—in this case, the claim that no relationship can be found between oxidative stress and autism. That sort of link has been demonstrated many times over.

This is what has been done with the use of GSH and GPx as measures of elevated oxidative stress in autism. James et al. (2004, 2005, 2006, 2009) effectively replicated the results obtained by earlier researchers (Golse et al., 1978; Yorbik et al., 2002). James and colleagues, however, used somewhat different methods and a richer theoretical perspective. Later, Ming et al. (2005) again replicated the results of Golse et al., Yorbik et al., and James et al. Ming and colleagues obtained the same results with 33 individuals with autism contrasted with 29 healthy individuals. Pasca et al. (2006) replicated the results of essentially all the former studies with respect to elevated levels of oxidative stress as indicated by depleted GSH and GPx. These researchers studied 12 individuals diagnosed with autism and 9 healthy controls. Pasca and colleagues also found, in agreement with Wakefield et al. (1998), that individuals with autism have reduced levels of vitamin B_{12} (methylcobalamin). As in other studies, there was greater variability in the individuals with autism than in healthy persons.

Karamouzi et al. (2007) replicated the foregoing results concerning reduced levels of GPx with a less invasive procedure using saliva from 18 individuals diagnosed with autism and 21 healthy age-matched controls. As in all of the foregoing replications, elevated levels of oxidative stress were found, as predicted on highly specific biochemicals, in individuals with autism.

Porphyrins in Urine and Oxidative Stress in Autism

Ming et al. (2005) also pointed out that because individuals with autism have reduced levels of GSH and especially GPx, they can be expected to have difficulty in ridding their bodies of the highly toxic hydrogen peroxide (H_2O_2) and related free radical products in damaged cells. It follows that the complex metal binding biochemicals known as **porphyrins** should, therefore, be elevated in the urine of persons with autism. (The term "porphyrin" is derived from the Greek root and cognate of the English word "purple.")

In Figure 6-5, Richard Wheeler has diagramed a healthy porphyrin known as **heme**; heme is the kind of porphyrin found in hemoglobin. The porphyrin in Figure 6-5 is the spiky-looking structure enclosing the embedded red sphere at the center of the picture. That sphere represents an **iron ion** of the sort found in hemoglobin. In Figure 6-5, Wheeler gives a scientist-artist's conception of the healthy porphyrin within the mitochondria—that critical part of the cell's DNA that comes especially from mother's chromosomes and that is crucial to the cell's communication within itself and with the immune system. Heme, in particular, is one of the crucial proteins that is damaged in the **erythrocytes** of individuals with autism (T. A. Evans et al., 2008; Pasca et al., 2006).

Heme can be seriously damaged by methyl mercury poisoning (Eisele et al., 2006). In addition, thimerosal, even in parts per billion concentrations, can cause hemolysis (see Figure 5-5), cytopenia (scarcity of red blood cells), and apoptosis (Rampersad et al., 2005). Because of the systematic cascade of cyclic relations in the biochemistry of our bodies, it follows that persons with autism should have some serious (diagnostic) irregularities in the porphyrins they excrete in their urine. Urine samples, like saliva samples, can be captured without invading the body of the individual. As a result, any biomarker that can be found in urine will be particularly convenient for the purposes of hypothesis testing and, therefore, for diagnosing disorders as well as for testing theories about

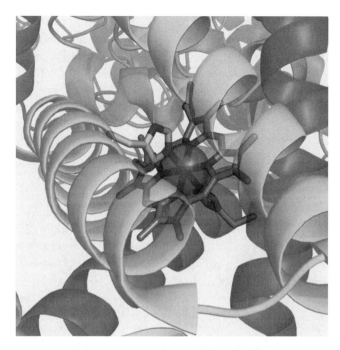

Figure 6-5 A conception of a metal (iron ion, the central sphere) captured inside porphyrin (heme) molecule within the cell's mitochondria.
Source: Courtesy of Richard Wheeler.

causation. We must predict, on the basis of all that is already known, that porphyrins excreted in the urine will be especially indicative of oxidative stress in persons with severe autism spectrum disorder. They will be indicative, in particular, of heavy metal toxicity.

Porphyrinuria in Autism

Nataf et al. (2006) showed that porphyrins in the urine of individuals with autism are a sensitive indicator of oxidative stress and of heavy metal (especially mercury) toxicity. If a general condition of **porphyrinuria** exists, the person in question has oxidative stress. In Nataf et al.'s study, several kinds of porphyrins in the urine were elevated in children diagnosed with autism as compared to controls. Taking age into account, the heme-derived uroporphyrin was significantly higher in children with autism ($n = 106$, $p < 0.001$) than in a comparable sample of children who did not have that diagnosis ($n = 107$).

It is interesting that there was no contrast in porphyrin levels between controls and individuals diagnosed with Asperger's disorder. This finding suggests that perhaps porphyrin measures of oxidative stress will be sufficiently sensitive to make a distinction between high-functioning autism and Asperger syndrome. However, that comparison was not made by Nataf and colleagues. Their design only permitted a comparison of the 106 cases diagnosed with "autistic disorder" according to criteria from *DSM-IV* (APA, 1994) and *ICD-10* (WHO, 1996–2009), the 11 cases diagnosed with Asperger syndrome, and the 107 children who did not have autism or Asperger syndrome. Nataf et al. also found that the indicator of heavy metal toxicity, precoproporphyrin, was higher in the children diagnosed with autistic disorder ($p < 0.001$) but not in the Asperger's group.

Following up on the work of Nataf et al., D. A. Geier and M. R. Geier (2006e, 2007b) have urged that "urinary porphyrin testing is clinically available, relatively inexpensive, and noninvasive" and that "porphyrins need to be routinely measured in ASDs to establish if mercury toxicity is a causative factor and to evaluate the effectiveness of chelation therapy" (2007b, p. 1723).

Owhadi and Boulos (2008) have carried the issue of oxidative stress to a slightly higher level of complexity. They have shown how it is possible for very small amounts of mercury, when administered in a short period of time in susceptible individuals, to inhibit the synthesis of glutathione and thus to make detoxification virtually impossible. Their findings show how mercury, which "interferes with the production of heme in the porphyrin pathway," is necessary to remove organic toxins (p. 1723). As a result, the response of the body to an input of toxins may be affected by feedback wherein the toxin itself (mercury, for example), when present at a relatively low but critical level, dramatically reduces the power of the body to detoxify itself. As a result, after a debilitating event occurs, even though the body may not yet appear to be suffering from toxic buildup, the accumulation can be occurring and may be expressed symptomatically later on.

Although a small increase in mercury burden—say, from multiple vaccines or from some combination of sources—may not be sufficient to trigger observable neurotoxic effects immediately, it may have already turned the switch to cause a sufficient accumulation of toxins so that extreme toxicity will be manifested at a later point in time. The model proposed by Owhadi and Boulos suggests that we cannot regard the body, or any of its organ systems, as static, deterministic, one-size-fits-all entities. Rather, the body consists of multiple dynamic interacting systems, such that well-being (health) involves holistic interactions between the dynamic organ systems inside the body and with the environment as well as the social systems outside the body.

Understanding Causation Brings Reasonable Hope

The research results summarized in this chapter point to a simple conclusion: Oxidative stress is involved in causing autism. We have learned from research with glutathione and porphyrins what some of the biochemical details are. The definitive evidence, however, has come more recently through the study of the terrible impact of oxidative stress on the brains of individuals with autism who have died.

T. A. Evans et al. (2008) have demonstrated conclusively through detailed examination of the biochemistry of free radical–induced oxidation in the brains of 27 living individuals with autism and 6 deceased patients with autism that the hallmark abnormalities are universally associated with oxidative stress. They postulate that "oxidative stress plays a role in the brain abnormalities in autism" (p. 62) and have been able to show impaired mitochondrial function and damage to cells, proteins, and DNA from oxidative stress. They contend that oxidative stress in brain tissues disrupts the normal "synchronization . . . between the various participating cortical areas, . . . in executing tasks involving reasoning, language, and social judgment," which are "the major symptom domains that define the syndrome of autism" (p. 68). In their report, these authors discuss the roles of glutathione (GSH), glutathione peroxidase (GPx), and heme in the porphyrin pathway leading to the excretion of heavy metals such as mercury.

During their work, Evans and colleagues found unequivocal evidence of oxidative injury in the brains of all the individuals diagnosed with autism whom they studied; they did not find similar damage in the brains of age-matched normal, healthy controls that they examined:

> [Oxidative damage] in the white matter and often extending well into the grey matter of axons was found in every case of autism examined. (p. 61)

They continued:

> Our finding suggests that oxidative damage to white matter may potentially contribute to the underfunctioning or disorganization of white matter tracts which could underlie the underfunctioning of the inter-regional communication process that make use of these tracts and result in functional underconnectivity. (p. 69)

Evans et al. found auto-antibodies specific to particular proteins in the brain tissue of the individuals with autism that they studied: "To our knowledge, this is the first direct evidence of increased oxidative stress in the autistic brain" (p. 69).

When the causes of oxidative stress are known, it is reasonable to expect that reducing the impact of those causal factors might have a curative—or should at least have an ameliorative—effect on autism. Indeed, this was the finding of Dr. Mary Megson in the case of Wesley Sykes. Her results are also well supported by the research literature showing improved symptoms in children with autism who have undergone dietary, medicinal, and, in some cases, chelation treatments (Owhadi & Boulos, 2008). In some notable cases, such as that of Ethan Kurtz, clearing up gut problems has been the key to detoxification and restoration of normal brain functions 🔵.

SUMMING UP AND LOOKING AHEAD

The theory of oxidative stress is presently the most widely accepted theory of mortality and is widely acknowledged as a plausible explanation for the causation of many diseases that involve toxins and self-immunity. Oxidative stress is substantially elevated in persons diagnosed with autism spectrum disorders.

The glutathione cycle plays a key role in neutralizing the impact of toxins while enabling their transport out of the body. In particular, the specialized glutathione peroxidase is involved in reducing hydrogen peroxide to water; the glutathione cycle, when it is functioning normally, replenishes the supply of this important antioxidant. Glutathione depletion is a necessary measure of oxidative stress, and the toxicity associated with it can account for the extreme neurological damage associated with the severe type of autism spectrum disorders. In addition, porphyrins such as the heme of hemoglobin, are involved in capturing and excreting heavy metals.

In the next chapter, we explore in greater detail the history of vaccines and their increasingly obvious involvement in causing the autism epidemic. Although vaccines are not the only culprits, they are playing a critical role in producing the autism epidemic. To see how we have come to this point in history, it is necessary to appreciate first and foremost how the mystique of miraculous powers came to be associated with vaccines. It's an amazing story in its own right, and we explore it in detail in Chapter 7.

STUDY AND DISCUSSION QUESTIONS

1. Discuss the converging themes of interest that have helped to focus worldwide attention on the autism epidemic.

2. Take a look at the discussion between Hugh Grant and Sandra Bullock in *Two Weeks Notice*, and compare it to attempts to prove any null hypothesis about toxins, disease agents, oxidative stress, and autism.

3. Why can't drugs work without interactions?

4. Discuss the term "additive" as applied to the power of one free radical to generate two more free radicals.

5. Why is glutathione so important to the body's functioning?

6. What's the difference between apoptosis and necrosis? Why are both processes important in understanding the autism epidemic and other chronic disease conditions?

7. Discuss crucial indicators and experimental evidence showing that oxidative stress is elevated in autism.

8. Why is a systems approach to be preferred over piecemeal explanations of the symptoms of autism?

9. Given what we know from the research concerning the indicators of disease conditions associated with autism, what do you think of the claim that persons diagnosed with autism will live about as long as persons who do not have this disorder?

10. Why would it be surprising not to find brain inflammation in persons diagnosed with autism? What evidence has been cited to support the null hypothesis that there is no brain inflammation in autism? Can you conceive of a study or series of them that might produce a sufficient amount of negative evidence to overturn the results reported by T. A. Evans et al. (2008)? Are the positive indicators and evidence of gut disease in persons with autism any easier to overturn?

chapter seven

Vaccines and Diseases

OBJECTIVES

In this chapter, we

1. Discuss the history of vaccines as well as the theory and research behind them.

2. Review the amazing success story of the supposed eradication of smallpox.

3. Consider the changes in hygiene, food processing, and waste disposal concurrent with the rise of vaccinations.

4. Discuss the reasons why vaccines have always generated some controversy and why they are never completely without risk.

5. Review the empirical evidences for exposure to undesirable viruses, toxins, and contaminants through vaccines.

6. Discuss the crisis in confidence that seems to be leading to a paradigm shift in medicine.

The notion that vaccines provide protection against deadly diseases has an interesting history. It is a story of which the public knows only a few bits and pieces. Most of us were taught about the victory over smallpox, and we heard the tale of the humble British doctor who discovered that exposure to the relatively harmless cowpox could prevent a much more deadly attack of smallpox. However, we are generally less aware of the amount of money currently invested in the vaccine industry, much less its sources. It is hardly a surprise to hear that there is big money in the vaccine industry, whose sales are expected to grow from $10 billion in 2007 to $23 billion in 2012 (S. Mitchell, 2007 ◕). It does interest the general public, however, to discover the extent to which the vaccine industry executives work hand-in-hand with the tax-supported agencies of the U.S. federal government, such as the CDC. Susan J. Landers (2008) at amednews.com, an official online news source of the American Medical Association, wrote:

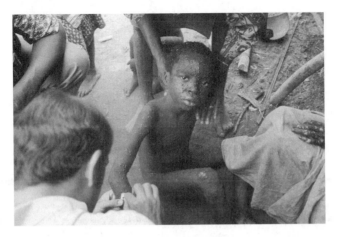

Figure 7-1 Small pox: disfiguring, debilitating, and deadly.
Source: Courtesy of Jean Roy/CDC.

Vaccines are hot. "The global vaccine market is set to double by the year 2016, fueled by unprecedented product innovations and global recognition of the benefits of immunization," said Michael D. Decker, MD, MPH, vice president for scientific and medical affairs at vaccine manufacturer Sanofi Pasteur, USA.

"This is one of the very best times to be involved in immunization because of all the excitement," noted Lance Rodewald, MD, Director of the Centers for Disease Control and Prevention's Immunization Services Division.

Like many aspects of history, some of the highlights about vaccines are well known. Nevertheless, many of the details—not to mention the worldwide dynamics of the moving picture—are relatively unknown to Americans and probably even less so to the worldwide population, for whom vaccines are only now becoming increasingly available thanks for the most part to the generosity of U.S. initiatives underwritten by taxpayers. In this chapter, we consider the vaccine story and its relationship to the autism epidemic.

RELIEF IN A NEEDLE

As anyone who has ever had a shot of an opium derivative such as Demorol can attest, powerful injected medications can quickly relieve pain or, for that matter, alleviate stress or anxiety. From such an experience, it is easy to see how someone could get hooked on drugs—even the kind that come through the stick of a hollow needle.

By contrast, when the subject is vaccination, the relief provided is more theoretical. We have to know something of the horror of a disease such as smallpox—for instance, see the child in Figure 7-1 who is infected with it—to appreciate the relief promised by an effective vaccination. When we consider that smallpox can be lethal in approximately 35% of adults and 80% of children, that it permanently scars all of its survivors while blinding 3.5% of them, it is unsurprising that the eradication of smallpox through vaccinations would help to create confidence in vaccines in general. What is generally not realized, however, is that the smallpox story seems to be unique. Bazin (2000) claims that the eradication of smallpox in 1980 was not only the first such event in the history of the world, but to date remains the only one of its kind. No other human disease, he argues, has been eradicated by vaccination. Nevertheless, the idea that vaccines bring miraculous protection from diseases has raised human confidence in medical practices to a higher level than any other event in history. For that reason, the story of the smallpox vaccine is the logical starting place for this chapter.

Smallpox: The Humble Beginnings of Vaccination

The first widely used vaccine in the Western world was based on a series of somewhat risky experiments—ones that would not be allowed today under the guidelines followed by current institutional review boards (IRBs). The test that made the British doctor Edward Jenner famous in 1796 was performed not on himself, but rather on an eight-year-old boy. According to Bazin (2000), Jenner had undergone a very risky and costly medical procedure to immunize himself against smallpox by exposure to a weakened form of the smallpox virus. This procedure, which was called **variolation,** involved exposure to the live smallpox virus and could lead to death (in about 1 in 50 cases) or transmission of the disease to others. However, having undergone the experiment himself, and based on his beliefs about disease transmission, when Jenner learned from milkmaids that cowpox evidently made them immune to smallpox, he formed the hypothesis that he could infect someone deliberately with the cowpox, thereby protecting that person from infection by smallpox.

With that background information in mind, Jenner deliberately infected an eight-year-old boy with cowpox—technically known by the Latin terms *Variolae* (meaning "pox" or "pustules") *vaccinae* (meaning "cow")—and then he exposed the same child to the potentially deadly smallpox virus, *Variolae verae* (meaning "true pox" = smallpox). The fact that the virus used by Jenner to inoculate the boy was associated with infections coming from cattle is the source of our modern English word *vaccine,* which is a direct derivative of the Latin word for "cow," *vacca*. The association with cows, however, has been all but forgotten in the generalized use of the word to refer to any disease agent or derivative used in vaccine exposures. Like the generalization of the brand name *Coke* for essentially any carbonated beverage, the word *vaccine* is universally applied to any preparation used to produce (or even believed to produce) immunity to any disease. The hideous and disfiguring look of the smallpox disease was well illustrated by Bazin (2000) in his book about the life and times of Edward Jenner.

Today, if Jenner were to ask permission to perform the experiment that would eventually lead to the development of the smallpox vaccine, any IRB in the modern world would probably deny it without a second thought. Jenner proposed to take fluid and tissue from the pustule of a woman infected with cowpox and use it to deliberately infect an eight-year-old boy with the known disease agent while also exposing him to proteins and infected tissue from the woman. It was Jenner's plan, after the boy had contracted and recovered from the disease of cowpox (now attributed to *vaccinia virus*; see Figure 7-2), to infect him deliberately with the much more virulent and potentially deadly smallpox virus, *Variolae verae*. The demonstration, which would be seen as questionable in many ways by today's standards (including the fact that Jenner used only one case from which to generalize his conclusion that cowpox makes its victims immune to smallpox), was nevertheless accepted as empirical proof that the relatively mild disease known as cowpox could inoculate human beings against the much more serious smallpox disease.

Widespread Acceptance and Proliferation

Because smallpox was a deadly disease and because outbreaks were relatively common at the time of Jenner's highly questionable demonstration, often affecting large populations, the news and public acceptance of his experiment spread rapidly. According to the CDC (1999a), the United States recommended universal vaccination of children in this country for smallpox from 1798—though 1898 is probably the correct year. In any case, according to the *Illustrated London News* (1853), the British Parliament did make smallpox vaccinations compulsory for the whole of the United Kingdom that same year. It is uncertain just when smallpox vaccinations were universally recommended to U.S. citizens, but according to numerous authorities they were commonly administered

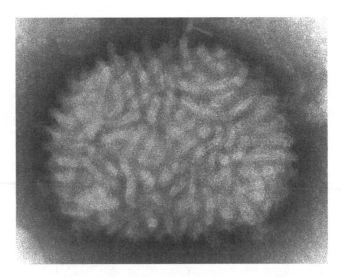

Figure 7-2 An electron micrograph of a vaccinia virus.
Source: Courtesy of Cynthia Goldsmith/CDC.

from the middle 1800s in the United States, England, and the rest of Europe (J. P. Baker & Katz, 2004; Chapin, 1913).

Vaccines aiming to generate immunity against other diseases followed at a rate that would continue to accelerate up to the present day, with vaccine production now at an all-time high and vaccines having become a multi-billion-dollar industry affecting the whole world. A few highlights of this history suggest an interesting progression. The first step was always to identify the supposed causative agent producing the disease, and then to isolate it. Subsequently, after studying the disease agent in a controlled setting, a less lethal, usually weakened form of the wild disease agent would be cultured or treated in some way, and then presented in the form of a vaccine.

The idea behind this process was implicit in the variolation procedure whereby Jenner subjected himself to a weakened form of the smallpox virus. When he came to believe that cowpox, which is produced (as now believed) by a virus similar to the smallpox virus, could provide immunity to smallpox, Jenner conceived his idea of a smallpox vaccine. Both of the disease agents in this case were "wild" forms (i.e., ones occurring naturally outside of laboratories), but Jenner's experiments on a single boy brought his contemporaries to the brink of the discovery of ways to culture and deliver all kinds of other disease agents, both wild and cultured, in what would come to be known universally as vaccines. The term "domesticated" might be preferred because it suggests that the culturing of disease agents would follow a path analogous to that by which animals were taken from their wild habitats and tamed to become beasts of burden and sources of food. However, the more aggressive breeding of disease agents that would soon occur was lurking in the shadows; for that reason, "domestication" seems too tame a term for the evolution that would occur in the next century and a half of vaccine production. In any case, peaceful purposes for vaccines would nevertheless advance in a series of faltering steps, before individuals associated with the growing military–industrial complex would begin work on unfriendly uses for vaccine research.

For a time after the beginning of smallpox vaccinations, peaceful uses of Jenner's idea would prevail. By 1885, Louis Pasteur had developed a vaccine for rabies. By 1897, the use of smallpox vaccine had spread so far throughout the Western world, at least according to the popular press, that the disease was substantially under control in the United Kingdom and in the former British colonies that had become the United States (J. P. Baker & Katz, 2004). In reality, however, the story was somewhat different. For example, the CDC (1999b) contradicts the claims of worldwide success with the smallpox vaccine made by J. P. Baker and Katz, as do records from Japan, Germany, Italy, the Philippines, and around the world, as we will see later in this chapter. In an article attributing success in combating infectious diseases mainly to vaccines, the CDC said the following about smallpox in particular:

> At the beginning of the 20th century, infectious diseases were widely prevalent in the United States and exacted an enormous toll on the population. For example, in 1900, 21,064 small-pox cases were reported, and 894 patients died. (1999b, p. 243 🌐)

Putting the death toll from infectious diseases in perspective, according to data from the U.S. Census Bureau (2000), in 1900 the U.S. population (rounded to the nearest thousand) totaled approximately 76,094,000. Doing the calculations, it becomes apparent that the "enormous toll" of the smallpox epidemic affecting the U.S. population in 1900 involved fewer than 3 persons per 10,000 and proved fatal to fewer than 1.2 persons per 100,000 in the whole population. Comparing the incidence of smallpox in 1900 to the estimated prevalence of autism now, if the rate of autism then were as it is now, there would have been 22 persons with autism for every one with smallpox. Also, for every person dying of smallpox, there should have been 556 with autism; over half with the severe non-verbal kind. The likelihood of severe autism should have been 144 times greater than contracting smallpox and 359 times greater than dying of it.

Here is another way of putting the smallpox threat of 1900 into perspective: Out of 10,000 exposures, we could expect fewer than 3 people to get smallpox in 1900; if 100,000 persons had been infected, 99,998 of them would have survived the disease. In 1999, the same source estimated the U.S. population at 272,690,813 people who were subject to 6,289,000 car accidents, of which 41,611 involved fatalities. Thus the chance of being killed in a car wreck in 1999 was 15 in 100,000, or 12.5 times greater than the chance of dying of smallpox in 1900.

Postponing consideration of claims about the effectiveness of vaccines in combating diseases, we now move on with the history as it is usually laid out by proponents of the increasingly intense CDC schedule. They almost universally argue that vaccines are the primary means by which deaths from infectious diseases were reduced in the twentieth century. We will have more to say about that issue a little later on.

By 1906, Jules Bordet, founder of the Pasteur Institute in Paris, together with a colleague, Octave Gengou, had isolated the whooping cough bacterium ("Pertussis," 2009; also see the references there 🌐). A vaccine for whooping cough would be produced soon afterward.

According to the brief history provided by the World Health Organization (2008a), the diphtheria vaccine was first used in the United States in 1923. Its introduction was followed closely by a vaccine for pertussis (whooping cough) in 1926, and by a vaccine for tetanus in 1927 (these dates concur with ones given by the CDC, 1999a, Table 1). For anyone who had seen the ravages of a disease such as tetanus, it is understandable that the vaccine was regarded as a blessing and any risks associated with it were generally welcomed as a slight inconvenience to be borne in hopes of being protected from a fate that some would describe as worse than death (see Figure 7-3).

The "Eradication" of Smallpox

As early as 1897, according to the CDC and proponents of vaccines, smallpox was effectively under control in much of the Western world (J. P. Baker & Katz, 2004). By 1936, the wild variant of smallpox had supposedly been practically eradicated from the Soviet Union (Tucker & Zilinskas, 2002). The smallpox vaccine was used through 1971 in the United States, but was—publicly at least—discontinued worldwide in 1980 after the last known case of smallpox was said to have been

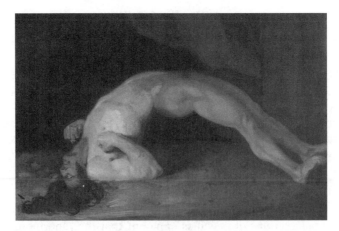

Figure 7-3 A man suffering from tetanus spasms as drawn by Sir Charles Bell, 1809.
Source: Courtesy of Royal College of Surgeons of Edinburgh.

treated in Somalia in 1977. The supposed eradication of that dreaded disease (see Figure 7-1) has been widely spoken of as one of the greatest triumphs of modern medicine. As the CDC often reminds the public, the case of the smallpox vaccine is supposed to represent the high water mark of the life-saving power of vaccines in general.

For instance, Kevin de Cock, a representative of the CDC in Nairobi and director of the department of HIV/AIDS at the World Health Organization, gives some sense of the reverence toward what vaccine proponents, such as Bazin, refer to as *The Eradication of Smallpox: Edward Jenner and the First and Only Eradication of a Human Infectious Disease*. That, at any rate, is the title of the book Bazin published in 2000 praising Edward Jenner. The reviewer of the book, Kevin de Cock, wanted to see even more enthusiasm. He lauded the book for its details concerning Jenner himself in the British journal *Nature Medicine* (2001), but lamented what he described as a failure "to capture the reality and vibrancy of disease eradication and elimination in the modern era."

De Cock's review makes it sound as though there are scores of similar vaccine success stories to be told. In fact, there are not. There are no such stories at all. Even the account of the eradication of smallpox based on an extensive history of the use of the smallpox vaccine all over the world, as we are about to see, appears to have been naive and premature.

As would become painfully evident in 2001, a series of highly secret vaccine programs had long been running in the background, out of the view of the public. The apparent mastery over the smallpox virus was just the public side of deeper and darker secret programs, especially in Russia and the former Soviet Union, implemented to develop super strains of smallpox, anthrax, plague, and other genetically engineered disease agents. The Russian effort to develop a super strain of the smallpox virus, one that would resist inoculation with the vaccinia virus, would become known from multiple sources, including a widely discussed accident involving a weaponized variant of smallpox that occurred in 1971 (Enserink, 2002). That incident and evidence associated with it would come out at about the turn of the millennium and would account for a huge effort by the Western world to protect itself anew from the threat of smallpox.

Smallpox: Almost Forgotten, but Not Gone

Only smallpox, among all the diseases of the world, has supposedly been eradicated by vaccination. We say "supposedly" for two reasons: First, as is well known, the smallpox disease—though almost forgotten by the general public—has never been truly destroyed. It is certainly not gone. Although the World Health Organization (2008b) set out to destroy all 400 or so of the known stockpiles of *Variolae verae* (the smallpox virus) in 1996, Western authorities were soon informed that it would be a bad idea for the peace-seeking nations of the world to destroy the last of the existing smallpox viruses in view of the certain knowledge that some nations were determined to use the smallpox virus, along with other disease agents, for the nefarious purposes of biological warfare. The other reason that we use the word "supposedly" in reference to the alleged eradication of smallpox by Jenner's cowpox solution is that the empirical evidence points to a very different explanation. We will come to that other alternative a little later in this chapter.

First, however, we address the point that the smallpox virus is still around and, according to many reports, exists in very great quantities in alleged bioweapons storehouses. A series of events that occurred late in the twentieth century and early in the twenty-first century forced the persons in the background at the CDC and WHO to reconsider the idea that smallpox was gone for good. For one, there was the defection and testimony to a congressional committee by Dr. Kantjan Alibekov, a high-ranking Russian bioweapons expert. Alibekov allegedly defected to the United States in 1992. We say "allegedly" because Alibekov's secret background began to be presented to the public through an appearance before a congressional committee in 1998 and then through a series of interviews with the press. According to his remarkable account—a sort of spy legend still being critically examined—he is a former enemy of civilization who helped to develop some of the most insanely criminal devices on the face of the earth. Thinking individuals everywhere will no doubt wonder what to believe or not to believe in his account. As students of the history of espionage and defections will readily appreciate, defectors are not always what they profess to be, so we take what Alibekov has said as subject to further examination.

Alibekov told U.S. authorities a great deal about the Russian bioweapons program in which he, by his own reporting, was a principal participant for 20 years prior to his defection. For the four years immediately preceding his defection to the West, he claimed to have served as the deputy director at Biopreparat, a key branch of the Russian bioweapons program. In 1998, in testimony before a congressional committee that has since been made public, and in various interviews, Alibekov, described potent **weaponized variants** of the smallpox virus. Within three years of his testimony, three additional events would spur public concern and extreme congressional interest in the information from Alibekov: One of the three tide-turning events would corroborate Alibekov's reports that the smallpox virus had already been weaponized by the former Soviet Union as early as 1971 and that ongoing research was taking great advantage of peacetime publications concerning both *Vaccinia* virus (the smallpox vaccine) and *Variola vera* (the smallpox virus itself). In particular, the Russian program was concentrating on genetic sequencing of both these viruses, and others, with a view toward making them more virulent and resistant to existing stockpiles of vaccines through genetic engineering.

"Disasters Come in Threes"

The first events to awaken the United States and the rest of the world to the very real threat of terrorism would occur on September 11, 2001, in New York City and Washington, D.C., and in Pennsylvania. On the heels of those terrorist attacks, just one week later (according to the postmark of September 18, 2001), there would be a bioterrorism wake-up call in the form of anthrax-laced mailings (see Figure 7-4). On October 9, 2001, letters with potent anthrax spores would hit the U.S. post office at Hamilton Township in Trenton, New Jersey, and the Brentwood office in Washington, D.C., that handles U.S. government mail. The highly lethal anthrax spores in a powdered form would eventually be traced to the biodefense labs at Fort Detrick in Frederick, Maryland. Before that trail could be established, however, anthrax infections would kill two postal workers—Joseph Curseen, Jr., and Thomas Morris, Jr.—and would infect 17 other individuals.

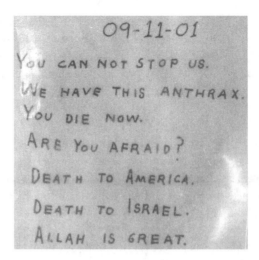

Figure 7-4 Anthrax letter to Thomas Daschle allegedly sent by Bruce E. Ivins. Photograph supplied by Richard Taylor.
Source: Courtesy of the FBI.

According to the report released on August 7, 2008, from the U.S. Federal Bureau of Investigation, the anthrax spores were handled and mailed exclusively by one individual: Bruce Edwards Ivins. He was a senior scientific researcher who had been working in the U.S. biodefense program at Fort Detrick and who had access to anthrax spores of a peculiar undisclosed quality. It seems likely that the spores in question had to do with ongoing research (hopefully of a defensive nature) into bioweapons at the laboratory. According to the public story, the FBI determined that Ivins was working alone and that after he learned of impending prosecution for his crimes he committed suicide by taking a large overdose of Tylenol and codeine (Willman, 2008b). The story that the government had a case against Ivins has since been removed from the *Los Angeles Times* Web site. Only a few weeks before it appeared, the suspect whom the FBI had supposedly paid Ivins to investigate, Dr. Steven Hatfill, had been vindicated at a cost of almost $5.82 million to taxpayers (Willman 2008a).

THE PLOT THICKENS

At about the time of the terrorist attack on September 11, 2001, and the anthrax attack that followed, a series of events would seemingly confirm the claim of Alibekov that Russia had in its possession, at least since 1971, a weaponized variant of the smallpox virus. Several questions come up in connection with the espionage-like revelations of weaponized viruses in the twenty-first century. They are not all new questions because, as is well known, biochemical warfare is not an entirely new concept. World War I was commonly referred to as the "chemists' war" owing to the use of various forms of poison gas during that conflict. Figure 7-5 is an image of allied troops in the western trenches in Europe during that war. Many similar images of World War I can be found on the Internet.

At a meeting in Geneva, Switzerland, on September 7, 1929, poisoned gas was supposedly banned forever from future wars because of the horrible cases of blindness and painful deaths it caused during World War I. That occasion was not the first time that chemical weapons had been banned, however. An earlier ban had been agreed to by multiple nations on August 27, 1874, in a pact known as the Brussels Declaration Concerning the Laws and Customs of War. It specifically made illegal the "employment of poison or poisoned weapons" in wars among the signatories. Later, more than a few additional international conferences and treaties would ban chemical weapons. On June 1, 1990, U.S. President George H. W. Bush and Soviet Premier Mikhail Gorbachev would sign

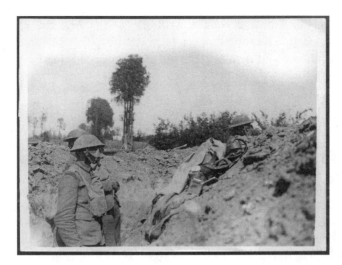

Figure 7-5 In World War I, commonly known as the "chemists' war," allied soldiers donned gas masks. *Source*: Courtesy of Trustees of the National Library of Scotland.

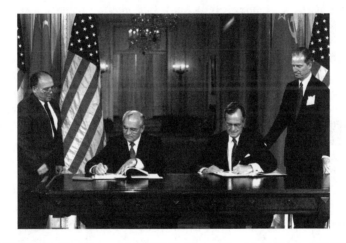

Figure 7-6 June 1, 1990, in the East Room of the White House, President George. H. W. Bush (viewer's right) and M. Gorbachev (left) sign an agreement to end chemical weapon production and to destroy stockpiles. *Source*: Courtesy of George Bush Presidential Library and Museum.

yet another such agreement banning chemical weapons and agreeing to begin destroying stockpiles in both the Soviet Union and in the United States (see Figure 7-6).

Later, Alibekov's testimony in 1998 would suggest that the anthrax scare of 2001, and the events that would follow up to the time of this writing in 2009, (including all the public meetings) were just for show. In the background, the Russians were, according to Alibekov, developing bioweapons all along. Likewise, the death of Bruce Edward Ivins on July 29, 2008 (the man credited with the anthrax poisonings of September and October of 2001), would demonstrate to the world that both the United States and Russia had ongoing programs dealing with bioweapons. Moreover, vaccine research would evidently be playing a key role in the shadowy background.

The Third Element: Weaponized Smallpox

In November 2001, General and Dr. Pyotr Burgasov, a former chief sanitary physician of the Soviet Union, gave an interview to *Moscow News* (Kvito, 2001) in which he acknowledged publicly for the first time an incident in Aralsk, a small town north of the Aral Sea in Kazakhstan, where a weaponized variant of smallpox supposedly infected 10 people. In their extensive documentary monograph with aerial photos and detailed analysis of the alleged infections, Tucker and Zilinskas made the following claims:

> The 1971 smallpox outbreak in Aralsk was unusual because the Soviet Union had eradicated endemic smallpox from its territory in 1936 [this claim may not be true] . . . the last previous outbreak of "imported" [wild] smallpox on Soviet soil had occurred a decade earlier, in 1961. Soviet health authorities kept the Aralsk outbreak secret and did not report it to the World Health Organization (WHO), as required under international agreement. Epidemics in the Union of Soviet Socialist Republics (USSR) often went unreported, because they undermined the propaganda image of the "socialist workers' paradise." In this case, however, there may have been another reason for keeping the smallpox outbreak under wraps—the Aralsk outbreak could have originated in a field test of weaponized smallpox virus at the nearby Soviet biological warfare (BW) testing grounds on Vozrozhdeniye Island in the Aral Sea. (2002, p. 1 ●)

In his interview with the *Moscow News,* Burgasov identified the incident, the time frame, and the weaponized smallpox vaccine allegedly being tested at the facility on Vozrozhdeniye Island in the Aral Sea. Burgasov told the *Moscow News* reporter:

> A research ship of the Aral fleet came 15 kilometers away from the island (it was forbidden to come any closer than 40 kilometers). The laboratory technician of this ship took samples of plankton twice a day from the top deck. The smallpox formulation, 400 grams of which was exploded on the island, "got her" and she became infected. After returning home to Aralsk, she infected several people, including children. All of them died. . . . I called Andropov, who at that time was chief of the KGB, and informed him of the exclusive recipe of smallpox in use on Vozrozhdeniye Island. He ordered that not another word be said about it. (Tucker & Zilinskas, 2002, pp. 20–21 ●)

It is interesting to wonder why Burgasov would come forward with this information concerning a highly secret program that had been unveiled in part by Kanatjan Alibekov, a traitor to Burgasov's Russia, just when he did. What could possibly have motivated him to do so? With that question unanswered but not forgotten, we proceed.

Further Documentation: Compliments of Private Research?

The documentation of this incident, which includes the aerial photos of the facility on Vozrozhdeniye Island and interviews with survivors (per Tucker & Zilinskas, 2002), confirms that the individuals involved had already been vaccinated against smallpox. Thus their infection by a wild form of the virus (according to the CDC claim that smallpox vaccine is effective) was supposedly unlikely. At any rate, soon after the anthrax attack of 2001, U.S. troops would be deployed on Vozrozhdeniye Island in the Aral Sea to prevent anthrax and other bioweapons from getting into the hands of terrorists.

According to Hogan (2002), it was the anthrax attack in the fall of 2001 that helped to speed up U.S. action in Vozrozhdeniye Island. Hogan says nothing about smallpox, but there seems to be little reason to doubt that a weaponized variant of smallpox virus was researched, if not produced, there. Taken together with the information from the interviews of Alibekov, the evidence produced by the Monterey Institute of International Studies in the monograph edited by Tucker and Zilinskas was sufficient to persuade the CDC and the WHO to do a midcourse correction on the plan to destroy all vestiges of the smallpox virus.

That information, and no doubt other information that has not been made public, was also sufficient to persuade the U.S. government to invest approximately half a billion dollars in stockpiling more than 195 million doses of smallpox vaccine produced by the British manufacturer, Acambis, between 2002 and 2008. According to a Reuter's news release on April 23, 2008, the British pharmaceutical company was awarded (in 2008) an additional contract for $425 million to produce 9 million doses of smallpox vaccine per year over the 10-year period between 2009 and 2019. The contract allows the CDC to bump up the production to 39 million doses in the fifth year if desired. In fact, the 195 million doses previously purchased beginning in 2002, according to the Reuters article, were obtained before the vaccine was approved by the FDA. Clearly, some of the folks at the CDC think the threat of weaponized smallpox is real and that something in the neighborhood of 300 million doses of vaccinia (the cowpox virus) will protect the U.S. population, numbered at about that many persons, against weaponized smallpox virus.

An Acknowledgment of the Smallpox Threat

In 2008, the WHO obliquely suggested the danger of weaponized smallpox in reiterating the policy that only the United States and Russia are permitted to keep the smallpox virus and to have knowledge of its DNA:

> The WHO Orthopoxvirus Committees meeting in 1994 and 1999 have recommended that no one other than the two WHO collaborating centres in the United States and the Russian Federation may have in possession at one time more than 20% of the viral DNA for variola virus. (WHO, 2008b ◉)

The WHO and CDC were urged to keep supplies of the virus on hand in the CDC labs in Atlanta and in the Russian counterpart in Novosibirsk so as not to tip the balance in favor of terrorists who might obtain it. Behind the scenes, at least since the information from Alibekov has been confirmed by additional sources (especially Burgasov), the United States has been diligently vaccinating its own troops.

In spite of the public claims that smallpox was completely eradicated in 1980 by the highly successful use of cultured forms of the cowpox (see Figure 7-2), some folks in the United States had to know that the Russian government was supporting extensive programs bent on developing biological weapons. It is known (or strongly believed by some) that the Russians and at least three other nations have stockpiles of smallpox virus and are believed or known to have weaponized variants of it (MSNBC.com News Services, 2007; U.N. Wire, 2002 ◉).

Public Evidence: No Longer Secret Knowledge

It is so strongly believed that enemies of the United States have developed weaponized variants of the smallpox virus (and other disease agents, especially anthrax) that huge stockpiles of vaccines (particularly vaccinia) have already been laid in store in the United States and members of the U.S. military have been routinely vaccinated against smallpox for several years. Knowledge of the smallpox program went public on March 7, 2007, when the 28-month-old child of a U.S. service member became sick with an infection caused by vaccinia, the disease agent in the smallpox vaccine. The vaccine had been administered to the little boy's father before dad was to be deployed overseas. Because the deployment was delayed, the father ended up spending time hugging, wrestling, sleeping with, and bathing the two-year-old boy, who subsequently became infected. The take-home message is that the United States has been routinely treating weaponized smallpox as a real threat to military personnel.

In fact, it is known that the United States had an official program for developing countermeasures against biological weapons, although it was supposedly a much less extensive program than the offensive one in the former Soviet Union. However, the U.S. bioweapons program was officially shut down by President Richard Nixon in 1969 (Alibek [alias Alibekov], 1998). In his testimony before the U.S. congressional committee in 1998 👁, Alibekov explained the process of weaponization in nontechnical terms. It is not necessary to be a specialist in vaccinology to see just how closely related the process of weaponization is to the sort of research done in developing vaccines. The first several steps are the same: They include isolating and culturing the disease agent, concentrating it, stabilizing it for long-term maintenance, and delivery. In weaponization, however, several additional processes may be carried out where the research knowledge required is the same or very similar, but the purposes for obtaining it are very different. In biodefense programs, the intention is to figure out how to counter bioweapon threats. In offensive weaponization research, the purpose is to kill, maim, and incapacitate a great many people, according to Alibekov. A key step is rendering the disease agent more virulent by genetic engineering.

In his official statement about biological weapons and terrorism, Alibekov claimed that it is possible to insert genes from a particularly robust and rapidly reproducing virus or bacterium into a weaponized variant of a highly lethal virus or bacterium. He said it is possible—at least in theory—to produce a variant of the smallpox virus through genetic engineering that would be far more resistant to vaccinia (i.e., cowpox vaccine). According to Alibekov and Burgasov, if the persons who died in Aralsk were exposed to weaponized smallpox, a vaccine-resistant smallpox virus may have been produced by the Russian scientists as early as 1970. However, as we will see in subsequent research with data from smallpox vaccination programs, an infection rate by smallpox at 3 in 10 or 30% is not uncommon in persons who received multiple injections of vaccinia. At any rate, the story released to the public about the Aralsk incident, mainly because of the efforts of Alibekov and Burgasov, appears to have been effective in motivating the CDC to commit almost a half billion dollars of U.S. funds to purchase enough smallpox vaccine from Acambis to vaccinate approximately the whole of the U.S. population.

If the story coming from the Russians is true, it is not difficult to understand why the CDC, in collaboration with other nations and the WHO, has been stockpiling millions of doses of what many hope is a more effective version of vaccinia. Meanwhile, the shocking picture of the two-year-old child infected by his father taken by Dr. John Marcinak (published by the CDC, 2007a 👁) gives us reason to suppose that the vaccinia virus itself—specifically, the cowpox used in inoculating troops—may also have been made more virulent. In any event, the standard theory of vaccines would lead us to suppose that an effective countermeasure to a weaponized form of smallpox would be a beefed-up version of cowpox, so to speak.

The Sinister Side of Published Vaccine Research

The history of vaccines, including the intensive research necessary for their development and proliferation, shows that there is a dark side to the research itself that has hardly come under public scrutiny until the present decade. Although research into vaccines and vaccinology in general is not intrinsically good or bad, as Alibekov pointed out, it is certainly possible to promote the interests of a weaponization program while pretending to do, or possibly actually doing, legitimate peaceful research that ends up being published in mainstream peer-reviewed public medical journals. Examples of reported research in the scientific literature pointed to by Alibekov include the analysis of the complete genome of the smallpox virus, which, he said, has been systematically compared to the genome of vaccinia by Russian bioweapons experts.

The fact that WHO has tried to legislatively limit accessibility to the genome information suggests that this information could be dangerous if it should fall into the wrong hands—as Alibekov suggests it already has. In the long run, however, how will knowledge of DNA sequences be kept secret? And what sanctions can the WHO take against violators? How effective was the WHO requirement that the Soviet Union report the epidemic of smallpox at Aralsk in 1971—or any other epidemic for that matter? The public learned about the Aralsk outbreak only some 32 years after it occurred.

Vaccinia: Also Weaponized?

According to a PBS (1995) interview with Alibekov, the vaccinia virus itself has been weaponized by at least four countries and there is a serious danger that one of the nations holding weaponized material might be willing to sell it to a terrorist organization. Alibekov has pointed out that research had already been published by 1998 commenting on the locus in the vaccinia genome where foreign genes from the **Ebolavirus**, for instance, could be inserted without loss of viral virulence. But why would virulence be sought in vaccinia if it were to be used in human inoculations, he wondered. It is reasonable to suppose that researchers at Acambis (maker of the smallpox vaccine) or some other research allies of Western governments are also striving to stay ahead of programs that have weaponized the smallpox virus and other disease agents. This thought brings yet another question: Why is it that all of this discussion has come out so publicly concerning programs that the Russians tried to keep secret for so long? Which part of the stories being told is true?

When it comes to quandaries pertaining to allegations made by potential enemies, a common rule of thumb is to draw inferences about motives. Commonly, it is recommended that we should "follow the money" by asking, Who has something to gain? We have already seen evidence in the form of some huge exchanges of cash, but our approach is to look for factual evidence in experimental studies that can be checked and rechecked where possible. With that caveat in mind, we argue that the most important tests of claims being made on behalf of countermeasures to bioweapons—measures being offered to the public at great expense by vaccine manufacturers and their collaborators—are not to be found by espionage and counterespionage. Instead, we need to look at the experimental evidence. Just how effective are vaccines in preventing targeted diseases? All the rest of the discussion hangs on that question, and it cannot be answered by opinion polls, voting, or force. This crucial question can only be answered empirically. So what do the data tell us on that score?

EXPERIMENTAL EVIDENCE OF VACCINE EFFICACY

Throughout the history of vaccinations, including the period prior to Jenner's supposed discovery, when the procedure called variolation was used to try to produce immunity to smallpox, concomitant factors affecting the incidence of infectious diseases, such as communal hygiene and sanitation were also coming under scrutiny and would change rapidly during the period when vaccination was becoming more and more common. Also, as discussed in prior chapters, vaccination has evolved into the most widely used means of transmission of toxins, disease agents, and their interactions directly into the bodies of human beings. When the practice of variolation was instituted in England in the first part of the eighteenth century, it is noteworthy that about 1 person in 50 would die from the smallpox infection produced by the procedure. The chance of dying from an outbreak of smallpox was considerably lower, even during major epidemics, but the variolation procedure nevertheless became well known and was practiced by the well-to-do. Today, we know that vaccines can cause seizures, neurological disorders, gut disease, and autism. Given these risks, it is reasonable and necessary to ask: To what extent can reductions in death and in the incidence of infectious diseases—for instance, smallpox—be attributed to vaccines as contrasted with other factors such as improved hygiene?

Because the smallpox vaccine is supposedly the most effective of all vaccines in the history of modern medicine, it is a logical starting point and the best test case for promoters of vaccines to show the efficacy of vaccines in disease prevention. What evidence is there that vaccinia actually reduces the likelihood of infection, or death, by smallpox? First, we consider a few of the many substantial population experiments with smallpox vaccine during the nineteenth and twentieth centuries comparing people who were vaccinated against people who were not. Then, we look to the case of polio vaccine, which has been used only in the latter half of the twentieth century and into the twenty-first century.

Why Look Back?

It is interesting that we must look back in time for the relevant experimental data concerning the efficacy of vaccinia in preventing smallpox for three reasons. First, few large-scale studies of smallpox vaccine were carried out after the middle of the twentieth century because the vaccine was almost universally applied from about 1897 forward. Also, all except military uses of the smallpox vaccine were discontinued from 1980 forward until the anthrax scare of September and October of 2001, at which time the CDC scrambled to stockpile hundreds of millions of doses against the threat of a bioterrorist attack with the smallpox virus. As a result, there are no comparative experimental data on the efficacy of vaccinia (versus no vaccinia) in preventing smallpox in the latter half of the twentieth century.

A second reason for the paucity of studies of the efficacy of smallpox vaccine is that authorities claimed from the middle 1800s forward that vaccines are good for the whole population of the world. Though sources differ, according to Sinclair (1992–1993), it was in 1852 that smallpox vaccinations were made mandatory in England. According to the proponents of vaccination, it would have been unconscionable, except in rare individual cases, not to vaccinate any group or segment of the population. For that reason, no intentional experimental comparisons of vaccinated against unvaccinated groups would be undertaken by agencies already committed to the idea that vaccination was necessary to prevent smallpox epidemics.

A third and final reason for the absence of experimental studies comparing matched groups of vaccinated versus unvaccinated individuals was that after about 1930 it was difficult in the industrialized world to find substantial numbers of unvaccinated persons.

If we look to the medical resources for efficacy studies, about all we find are references to the "amazing work of Dr. Jenner," who infected a single eight-year-old boy with cowpox, later attempted to infect him with smallpox, and claimed that the first infection prevented the second. The "miraculous" success of vaccines and the almost worshipful regard for Jenner largely hang on a single anecdote about an individual child. In fact, if the story is examined, it fails to meet the most basic requirements of experimental design. From 1796 to the present, it appears that Jenner's "success" was just taken on faith by doctors everywhere and was examined critically by very few of those who repeated the familiar story.

If we look for additional evidence, the bulk of it consists of references to milkmaids who avoided smallpox by being exposed to cowpox. From there, the trail leads very quickly to the almost universal use of vaccinia (cowpox virus), which, according to the tales told of Jenner's success, supposedly prevents smallpox. In 2008, the U.S. government alone committed more than a half billion dollars to stockpile 300 million doses of vaccinia in response to potential bioterrorism with weaponized smallpox vaccine. With that massive funding in mind, it is reasonable to ask for experimental evidence concerning the effectiveness of vaccinia as a preventative measure against smallpox.

In fact, no vaccine has a remotely comparable history. Vaccinia has been used in huge quantities to vaccinate millions of people from just a few decades after Jenner's "experiment" reported in 1796 until the present time. In 1980, the use of vaccinia in the general population was officially discontinued, though the vaccine has continued to be used periodically by the U.S. military and its allies as a countermeasure against the threat of bioterrorism, and is currently being stockpiled at a higher rate than at any time in the prior history of the world.

Given these facts, data on the experimental efficacy of smallpox vaccine ought to be in high demand at the present time. Such data are also extremely relevant to the questions currently under consideration with reference to the autism epidemic. If it is accepted that vaccines may sometimes cause severe reactions, including neurological disorders, autism, and even death, to what extent can the known risks be justified by the argument that vaccines save millions of lives every year? Smallpox is a critical case to examine because it is supposed to represent the most miraculously effective vaccine in the history of the world. Surely, if any vaccine is trustworthy, the vaccine for smallpox must be the one. If the claims of efficacy for the smallpox vaccine are shown to be false, then the arguments for vaccination in general become doubtful at best. The smallpox vaccine is universally pointed to as proof positive that vaccines have produced miraculous reductions in death by infectious diseases. If we cannot trust this vaccine, which of the many different vaccines that have followed can we trust? With that question in mind, the smallpox vaccine affords an extremely important test case for vaccine theory in general.

Comparing Highly Vaccinated with Virtually Unvaccinated Populations

In England, there is a well-documented period during which the people of Leicester rebelled against the national authority that was at that time requiring smallpox vaccinations of all British citizens. Through their action, the people of Leicester provided, at their own trouble and expense, some of the most important efficacy data and public records in the history of the smallpox vaccine.

From roughly 1849, according to the public records of Leicester, approximately 74% of the inhabitants of this town were vaccinated for smallpox, with the vaccination rate increasing to 93% in 1854 and to 94% in 1867, when the national government put certain fines in place for families that had formerly refused to vaccinate their children (Sinclair, 1992–1993). In 1873, during an epidemic of smallpox affecting the whole of England and much of Europe, in the heavily vaccinated Leicester community an estimated 13,320 persons per million became sick, and 360 of those infected individuals in Leicester died of smallpox.

Given that nearly all of the people who were infected, and nearly all of those who died, had been vaccinated for smallpox, confidence in the vaccination program reached a low ebb in Leicester. As a result, the township decided to permit the people residing in Leicester to refuse smallpox vaccinations, in defiance of the national authorities. This practice of refusing smallpox vaccinations in Leicester began with a legislative act of the local governing body so that from 1873 forward until 1904 fewer and fewer of the children in each new birth cohort were vaccinated. By 1904, the community was essentially unvaccinated. Leicester had gone from a high point in 1872, when 100% of the population received more than one vaccination for smallpox, to a low from 1888 until 1901, when fewer than 10% of the citizens of Leicester were vaccinated.

During this time the national government made many unsuccessful attempts to force vaccination on the people of Leicester. However, the fact that more people died during epidemics that occurred when vaccinations were at their peak than when vaccinations were refused by the majority of the population (see Figure 7-7) caused a general discontent with the government's policy. In his extensive statistical studies of the efficacy of the smallpox vaccine, J. T. Biggs (1912) showed that deaths from smallpox were higher in the years when the largest proportion of the population was being vaccinated. This is clearly evident from a comparison of the black line with diamonds in Figure 7-7, which shows the number of persons vaccinated per each birth cohort of 7500, as contrasted with the gray line with triangles, which shows smallpox-related deaths per million. Biggs also found from comparisons with the military in England at the time, that Leicester, with a smallpox vaccination rate

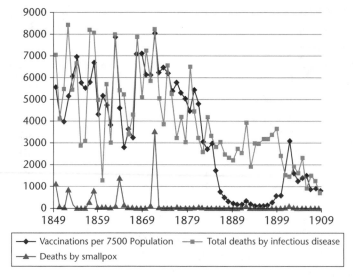

Figure 7-7 Data from J. T. Biggs, 1912, showing total vaccinations for smallpox per 7,500 recorded births in Leicester, England (black line with diamonds), plotted against recorded deaths per million persons from infectious diseases (gray line with squares) and deaths per million persons from smallpox (gray line with triangles).
Source: Data from J. T. Briggs, 1912.

of less than 43.3% averaged over the years 1860–1904, had a mortality rate from smallpox that was approximately half of the mortality rate among the 100% vaccinated and often re-vaccinated British military personnel for the same years.

Why would Leicester, with a population that was only 43.3% vaccinated during the time frame in question, have a rate of mortality from smallpox that was less than half of the mortality from smallpox in the army and navy, where 100% of the personnel were vaccinated? Biggs (1912) wrote:

> The town of Leicester is, and has been for the last twenty years, the least vaccinated town in the kingdom. Its average population from 1873 to 1894 was about two-thirds that of the Army during the same period. Yet the smallpox deaths in the Army and Navy were thirty-seven per million, those of Leicester under fifteen per million ●.

More Disease and Death Among the Vaccinated Populations

Interestingly, Biggs was commenting on the rate of smallpox mortalities relative to the percentage of persons vaccinated in Leicester versus the military. This is certainly a meaningful and reasonable comparison, and he made a number of other comparisons of the same kind between the relatively less vaccinated people of Leicester and the more heavily smallpox-vaccinated populations in Japan, London, Glasgow, Sheffield, in addition to the British army and navy. From 1880 through 1908, when Leicester was vaccinating less than half of its population, the town had a total of 1206 cases of smallpox and 61 deaths, giving a mortality rate from smallpox of 5.06%. During the same period, when Japan was vaccinating and revaccinating 100% of its population, Japan reported 288,779 cases and 77,415 deaths from smallpox, giving an average rate of death from smallpox of 26.81% in the more heavily vaccinated Japanese population, thus the smallpox mortality rate in Japan, where people were vaccinated at least twice for smallpox, was 5.30 times higher than the rate in Leicester. During similar time periods when London, Glasgow, and Sheffield were vaccinating approximately 90% of their populations, Leicester was vaccinating 43% of its population. However, deaths from smallpox on a percentage basis were more than twice as numerous in each of the heavily vaccinated cities.

In the graph presented in Figure 7-7, which was created from data published by Biggs (1910 👁), it appears that peaks in the percentage of persons vaccinated in a given year (expressed as persons vaccinated for samples of 7500 persons, depicted as the black line with diamonds) correspond to peaks in deaths from smallpox (shown as the gray line with triangles). Vaccine proponents might argue that the rise in percentage of persons vaccinated would reflect the population's greater confidence that vaccines could prevent smallpox. However, would people also seek a smallpox vaccination on account of an infection of measles, scarlet fever, whooping cough, diphtheria, or any other disease condition? If not, why would the number of total deaths from infectious diseases in general also peak in the years when the percentage of smallpox vaccinations also rose sharply? Examining the data graphed in Figure 7-7, it is evident that as smallpox vaccinations increased, so did deaths from infectious diseases in general. Not only was smallpox more lethal in years when vaccination was most depended on, but there were more deaths from infectious diseases in general during the years with the highest percentage of vaccinations.

We know that vaccination can cause disease in family members, as occurred in the case in which vaccinia infected the two-year-old son of a soldier who received a smallpox vaccination in 2007 (CDC, 2007a). However, it appears from Figure 7-7 that families and neighbors of persons vaccinated for smallpox are more apt to contract other infectious diseases as well. In fact, the graph shows unequivocally that vaccinated persons were not only more apt to have smallpox infections and deaths from smallpox after being vaccinated, but were even more likely to contract and die from other infectious illnesses. To get an idea of why so many people in Leicester would refuse vaccination in the face of fines and coercion from the central government, the report of a 73-year-old doctor named Spencer T. Hall is relevant. When the local governing body approved a policy of allowing the citizens of Leicester to refuse smallpox vaccinations, Dr. Hall said that his tears on that occasion

> were tears of joy and gratitude in having lived to see the vaccination question attain its present position. He had been vaccinated at two years of age, and very seriously injured; but at fourteen he had a severe attack of smallpox, which was followed by improved health. Far rather would he have smallpox than be vaccinated. He had paid fines for all his children [to prevent their being vaccinated and he said that] . . . in his long and wide experience he had never seen such evil results from smallpox as he had seen from vaccination. (Biggs, 1912 👁)

Smallpox Vaccination Correlated with Smallpox and Infectious Diseases

It is not the statistics concerning smallpox itself that are the most interesting facts of Figure 7-7, but rather the pattern of deaths from the combined infectious (Biggs called them "zymotic"—a now-archaic term that was the favored descriptor at that time) diseases including measles, scarlet fever, whooping cough, diphtheria, fevers, and diarrhea; the latter trend is shown as the gray line with squares in Figure 7-7. Each time a rising slope occurs in Figure 7-7, showing an increase in the percentage of the population being vaccinated for smallpox, there is a corresponding peak in deaths from infectious diseases.

In fact, the correlation between the number of deaths from infectious diseases and the percentage of the new birth cohort being vaccinated is 0.722 ($p < 0.0001$), whereas the correlation between the number of deaths from smallpox and the percentage of children being vaccinated for smallpox is 0.335 ($p < 0.005$). Both of these correlations are highly significant. If the vaccinations given were actually reducing the number of fatalities by providing protection from smallpox, the correlations in both cases should be negative. Instead, the reverse is true: The correlations are positive.

The implication is that the higher the percentage of persons being vaccinated, the more likely are deaths from smallpox. This result is highly significant. The correlation of vaccinations against smallpox with the number of deaths by smallpox would be expected to occur by chance in fewer than 5 instances out of 1000 trials. However, the association between the percentage of persons being vaccinated for smallpox and the likelihood of death from any one of the several infectious diseases being recorded (e.g., smallpox, measles, scarlet fever, whooping cough, diphtheria) was much stronger. The likelihood of a correlation of such strength (0.722) occurring by chance is less than 1 instance in 10,000 trials.

To compare the strength of these correlations, we must square the values; we then discover that the percentage of persons being vaccinated for smallpox accounts for 11.22% of the variance in deaths by smallpox on average, while the percentage of persons being vaccinated for smallpox accounts for 52.13% of the variance in deaths by infectious diseases in general. Thus it appears that a higher rate of smallpox vaccination among successive birth cohorts accounts for almost five times as much variance in deaths by all infectious diseases as for deaths by smallpox itself. Not only does the vaccine for cowpox *not* protect people against smallpox, but it actually appears to make them more vulnerable to smallpox, and to a host of other diseases. The vaccine makes individuals significantly more likely to contract smallpox and to die from it and, more importantly, makes it much more likely that a vaccinated individual will contract any one of several infectious diseases and be likely to die of that infection.

The Leicester data absolutely refute the claim that smallpox vaccination provides protection against smallpox. We say "absolutely" here because it takes only one such case to refute the null hypothesis that there is no association between vaccination and an increase in disease. That null hypothesis can be strongly rejected because there obviously is a positive association between greater use of the smallpox vaccine and increased occurrence of death by smallpox. More importantly, there is an even larger increase in the risk of death by infectious diseases in general after a smallpox vaccination than if a person were to just pass on the opportunity to be vaccinated.

Other Large-Scale Studies of the Effectiveness of Smallpox Vaccinations

Data from Germany

In 1896, Dr. Walter Hadwen gave a report concerning the compulsory vaccination for smallpox of children in Germany. He first observed that the Germans had kept better records than any country in Europe, except perhaps Sweden. From 1834 (nearly 20 years before England passed its Compulsory Vaccination Act), the German authorities required that,

> in addition to primary vaccination, every child had to be vaccinated over again when he started upon his school life; he had to be re-vaccinated on going from college to college; and re-vaccinated over again when he entered the Army, which meant every healthy male out of the whole of Prussia [Germany]. And so severe was the Act that if any man refused to be vaccinated he was ordered to be held down and vaccinated by force; and so thoroughly was it done that he was vaccinated in ten places on each arm. . . . thirty-five years after this Compulsory Vaccination Act. . . . small pox carried off [in 1869] no less than 124,978 of her vaccinated and re-vaccinated citizens . . . (Hadwen, 1896 ◉)

Statistics showing that smallpox vaccinations actually increased the incidence of smallpox are well documented not only for Germany, but for other countries as well.

Table 7-1 Data from the Italian Smallpox Epidemics of 1887, 1888, 1889

Epidemic Year	1887		1888		1889	
Smallpox deaths	Men	Women	Men	Women	Men	Women
Younger than age 20 years	5997	5983	7349	7353	5020	5031
Older than age 20 years	2459	1810	1990	1418	1290	803

Source: Data assembled by Dr. Carlo Ruata, Professor of Materia Medica, for a public talk in November 1898, at the University of Perugia, Italy. Retrieved February 6, 2009, from http://www.whale.to/vaccines/ruata_h.html.

Data from Italy

In Italy, with reference to smallpox deaths in 1887, 1888, and 1889, it occurred to Dr. Carlo Ruata that men older than the age of 20, by virtue of the fact that they were required to perform military service, during which time 100% of them would be vaccinated for smallpox, should have a lower death rate from smallpox than women older than age 20. The men and women younger than 20, by contrast, would be equally likely to be vaccinated or not. Therefore, men and women younger than the age of 20 should have been equally susceptible to smallpox mortality because they had an equal likelihood of being vaccinated or not.

These hypotheses were testable from data that were readily accessible and that are presented in Table 7-1. The first hypothesis to be tested is that men and women younger than 20 years of age should not differ with respect to vaccination and, therefore, should not show any dissimilarities with respect to number of deaths from smallpox. The second hypothesis to be tested is that men and women older than age 20 should differ with respect to vaccination, with men being 100% vaccinated (and some of them being vaccinated twice) while a significantly smaller proportion of women would receive vaccinations. Therefore, men older than age 20 should have lower smallpox mortality, reflecting the effectiveness of vaccination if it truly helps to prevent smallpox.

Using Ruata's original data, we calculated some additional statistics. We did two simple paired-means tests (t-tests) for men younger than age 20 versus women younger than age 20, and for men older than age 20 versus women older than age 20. The results were as follows: No differences in smallpox mortality rates were found between the equally vaccinated versus unvaccinated men and women in the under-20 group. The probability that the contrasts between the men and women in this group could arise by chance was very high ($p > 0.968$; that is, 968 times in 1000 studies, contrasts of the level found would be expected to occur strictly by chance). However, Ruata's hypothesis that the 100% vaccination of the men older than 20 (some of them being vaccinated for a second time) should afford them greater protection against smallpox must be rejected. In fact, men older than age 20 were, as can be seen from Table 7-1, considerably more apt to die of smallpox than the relatively less vaccinated women over 20 ($p < 0.01$; that is, there is less than one chance in 100 that differences as great as those observed would occur by chance).

The upshot of the comparison as reported by Ruata in a letter on May 10, 1899, is that smallpox vaccine evidently made the men older than age 20 more—rather than less—susceptible to death by smallpox. In his discussion of these data, Ruata reported that he had checked every year up to the most recent data available at the time of his talk (which was given in 1898). He reported in his later letter that the contrasts were the same across the entire decade beginning in 1887 and ending in 1897: The individuals who were vaccinated for smallpox were more apt to succumb to it.

Data from Japan

No country in the world seems to have had a more stringent policy for smallpox vaccination than Japan did in the latter part of the nineteenth century. U.S. Public Health Reports for September 2,

1910, however, reported that the population of Japan was approximately 48 million in 1910. Looking back over the decade (1898–1908), the same report gave the morbidity and mortality statistics on smallpox for three key years:

- 1898: 149,012 cases of smallpox, with 40,971 deaths—a mortality rate of 27.50%
- 1905: 10,704 cases of smallpox, with 3388 deaths—a mortality rate of 31.65%
- 1908: 18,075 cases of smallpox, with 5835 deaths—a mortality rate of 32.28% (see Higgins, 1920)

We saw earlier through a comparison between the morbidity and mortality rates for smallpox in Leicester, England, that when vaccination rates were less than 10%, there was a far lower mortality rate than in Japan, which had a vaccination rate of more than 100% (some people being vaccinated three times). Although the incidence of smallpox appeared to decline in the three successive years for which data were reported for Japan, why did the rate of death from smallpox—for vaccinated persons—appear to be rising? Also, why would the average mortality rate per smallpox infection for the heavily vaccinated persons in Japan—where people were being vaccinated, revaccinated, and revaccinated again (three times)—be about six times higher per smallpox infection than the mortality rate in Leicester (5.1%), where even one vaccination was refused by more than 90% of the population during a comparable time frame? In considering these questions, we must also bear in mind that the sample sizes in these experimental instances are huge—vastly greater than the meager enrollment in clinical trials (often numbering only a few hundred cases) for drugs and vaccines that must be carried out prior to licensing by the FDA, for instance.

Data from the Philippines

In 1896, the Philippines won its independence from Spain, though after a brief military conflict in 1901, it became a "protectorate" of the United States. In our discussion here, we concentrate on the years following these events, from 1905 until 1920. During that period, the United States began a vigorous campaign of vaccinating the island peoples throughout the Philippine archipelago. Many were required to submit to as many as two or three smallpox vaccinations; ultimately, the estimated population of 10 million people received 25 million vaccinations. According to W. F. Koch (1961), prior to the U.S. takeover of the Philippines, case mortality from smallpox was about 10%. By contrast, in 1918 and 1919 (when more than 95% of Filipinos had been vaccinated, including some as many as three times), the Philippines experienced the worst epidemic of smallpox ever recorded, with a mortality rate of about 60%.

Interestingly, according to the same source, the highest mortality rate occurred in Manila, where the most intense vaccination programs had been carried out by U.S. authorities. There, the mortality from smallpox was approximately 65%. The lowest mortality rate was observed in Mindanao, where, because of religious objections, fewer people submitted to vaccination. It is also worth noting that the rate of mortality in the Philippines was double what it had been in Japan during the prior decade and was approximately 13 times the rate in Leicester during the period when smallpox vaccinations were being refused by 90% of that city's population. In the Philippines, Dr. Victor de Jesus, Director of Health, reported 60,855 deaths from smallpox in the two-year period of 1918–1919:

> ... hundreds after hundreds of thousands of people were yearly vaccinated with the most unfortunate result that the 1918 epidemic looks prima facie as a flagrant failure. (As quoted by Sinclair, 1992–1993 ●)

On December 21, 1937, as recorded in the *Congressional Record*, Dr. William Howard Hay testified to the U.S. Congress about the severity of the Filipino outbreak. According to Hay, in 1918 and 1919,

> the Philippines suffered the worst attack of smallpox, the worst epidemic three times over, that had ever occurred in the history of the islands, and it was almost three times as fatal. The death rate ran as high as 60 percent in certain areas, where formerly it had been 10 and 15 percent. (Hay, 1937 ●)

Why would such a severe epidemic happen in a place that was so thoroughly vaccinated against smallpox? It seemed that the use of the vaccine was the means of either spreading the disease or making individuals a great deal more susceptible to infection by it. Recall the results discussed from Leicester and presented in Figure 7-7. In that city, susceptibility to infectious diseases in general was coincident year by year with vaccination for smallpox, with a correlation of 0.722 (producing a variance overlap of deaths from infectious diseases and percentage of persons vaccinated at 52%, $p < 0.0001$).

Observations by Expert Practitioners

A few months earlier, on June 25, 1937, Hay had given a report to the Medical Freedom Society that was also read into the *Congressional Record* of December 21, 1937. In that address he said:

> It is now 30 years since I have been confining myself to the treatment of chronic diseases. During those 30 years I have run against so many histories of little children who had never seen a sick day until they were vaccinated and who, in the several years that have followed, have never seen a well day since. I couldn't put my finger on the disease they have. They just weren't strong. Their resistance was gone. They were perfectly well before they were vaccinated. They have never been well since. ●

He went on then to talk about the practice of injecting pus from an infected animal or person into a child. His question was how this approach could possibly improve anyone's health.

As Ruata had observed some 40 years prior to Hay's testimony:

> Whereas the aim of therapeutics is to cure sickness in our bodies, and that of hygiene to maintain them in health by a salubrious environment, vaccination undertakes to modify our robust, healthy bodies in order to adapt them to an insalubrious environment. It belongs neither to therapeutics, nor to hygiene; it belongs to that fatal, fanciful, spurious science which, rejecting the teachings of experience, rests on dogma and creed, which in other departments of sociology have produced as many evils as vaccination has produced in medicine. (Ruata, 1898 ●)

Clinically exposing a person to disease agents, toxins, animal proteins, and whatever else a vaccine may contain does seem profoundly contrary to the foundational purposes of medicine. No one would propose mildly burning children to enable them to tolerate fire, yet exposure to many different disease agents, along with various known poisons and unknown other factors (animal proteins), is effectively being practiced as the means to enable infants to avoid infectious diseases.

Having reviewed the case of smallpox vaccine in particular, it appears that the practice of vaccination could hardly be the causal basis for the reduction in this disease's incidence worldwide over the last two centuries. On the contrary, it appears that the world's worst smallpox epidemics—

for example, in the Philippines in 1918 and 1919—were made worse by vaccination, if not actually caused by it. With these facts in mind, it is unsurprising that thoughtful individuals would be inclined to ask what was really responsible for the reduction in infectious diseases if not vaccination. Clearly, it was not smallpox vaccination that led to worldwide reduction in the incidence of infectious diseases. On the contrary, as Figure 7-7 plainly shows, vaccination had the opposite effect. Vaccination for smallpox on a dose-response basis was proportionately associated with an increase in deaths from all recorded infectious diseases. As the rate of vaccination increased, so did the rate of death from infectious disease. Also, as the number of exposures to smallpox vaccine increased (as in Japan and the Philippines), the mortality rate from smallpox likewise increased.

ASKING AND ANSWERING THE HARD QUESTIONS

It is evident from the foregoing experimental comparisons between vaccinated and unvaccinated populations that the smallpox vaccine clearly was not the cause of any reduction in either the incidence or the death rate from that disease. This fact did not go unnoticed by thoughtful doctors who had participated in the process of vaccination—people like Drs. Hall, Hadwen, Ruata, and Hay. It did not go unnoticed by huge populations of people, either. The residents in Leicester, England, right in the very heart and center of the United Kingdom, did not lightly reject smallpox vaccination. They did it with their eyes wide open and in punishable defiance against sanctions imposed on them by the central British government. Hall reported that he gladly paid the fines and very deliberately refused to vaccinate his children. He was not alone, and neither did he act on the basis of ignorance and superstition. Hall had been vaccinated and harmed by that vaccination, and had been infected by smallpox and survived it; he made his decision to refuse to vaccinate his own children on the basis of his experience and rational judgment as a physician.

Dr. Parry in the *British Medical Journal*

It was inevitable that some hard questions would be asked by medical practitioners about the smallpox vaccines. Consider the interesting letter published in the *British Medical Journal* by an orthodox practicing vaccinator, Dr. L. Parry. On January 21, 1928, in asking some pointed questions, he recounted certain facts about smallpox and vaccination. The editorial staff of the journal added the following comment:

> We think that Dr. Parry, in his desire for enlightenment, would have been wiser not to introduce assumptions of fact into the framework of his questions. ☻

In doing so, the editors implied that Parry's "assumptions of fact" were just assumptions. But Parry's arguments were not merely assumptions—they were well-grounded facts. Here are some of the details of facts supporting Parry's questions.

For one, Parry wondered why smallpox is "five times as likely to be fatal in the vaccinated as in the unvaccinated" (Parry, 1928, p. 116). We know this was true in the comparisons, for instance, recounted earlier between Leicester and Japan during the years 1886 to 1908 (Biggs, 1910). The contrast was even greater between vaccinated versus unvaccinated persons in the Philippines than in the Leicester data: The rate of mortality among the doubly and triply vaccinated individuals of Manila (more than 95% of whom were likely to be vaccinated more than once) was approximately 13 times greater than in Leicester where the one-time vaccination rate was less than 10%.

Parry also asked, "How is it that in some of our most highly vaccinated towns, for example, Bombay and Calcutta, smallpox is rife, whilst in some of our most poorly vaccinated towns, such as Leicester, it is almost unknown?" The statement of fact contained here is already supported by the statistics for Leicester and can easily be checked for India, where mortality rates for smallpox epidemics were commonly in the range of 25% to 30% during the nineteenth century (Banthia & Dyson, 1999).

In his letter, Parry asked, "How is it that something like 80 percent of the cases admitted into the Metropolitan Asylums Board smallpox hospitals have been vaccinated, whilst only 20 percent have not been vaccinated?" He also asked, "How is it that in Germany, the best-vaccinated country in the world [right at the top along with Japan, according to the sources cited previously], there are more deaths in proportion to the population than in England?" These claims were established earlier in this chapter.

Parry was probably attempting to gently lead his colleagues in the medical profession to the obvious contribution of sanitation and hygiene. He asked:

> How is it that as the percentage of people vaccinated has steadily fallen (from about 85 in 1870 to about 40 in 1925) the number of people attacked with variola [smallpox] has declined . . . and the case mortality percentage has progressively lessened? . . . What is the explanation? (Parry, 1928, p. 116)

In one word: sanitation. The industrialized world became a lot cleaner and the rates of infectious diseases of all kinds declined, including the rate of smallpox.

Sanitation: Avoiding Sources of Infection

In his talk in 1896 concerning the Gloucester epidemic then still raging, Dr. Hadwen referred to the failure of multiple smallpox vaccinations in Germany and then explained how the rising rate of smallpox infections was finally squelched. The Germans had, sensibly, not added still more smallpox vaccinations into the schedule, but did take some rather sensible sanitation measures. They cleaned up their drinking water, developed better drainage systems, got rid of slums in their cities, and built better housing for their soldiers—and the number of smallpox cases diminished.

According to Hadwen, what 35 years worth of vaccinations could not accomplish, better sanitation delivered. He went on to tell a charming tale about attitudes of the children in Germany (actually the whole world) to vaccinations. No one of them really likes to get stuck with a needle:

> Even the very children in Germany know well enough how it is hated, and in proof of this I may relate to you an amusing incident, A school inspector went to one of the schools the other day and asked the question of the class, "Why was Moses hidden by his mother in the bulrushes?" Very soon a little fellow put up his hand and replied, "Please sir, she did not want him to be vaccinated."

Over the two centuries while the now multi-billion-dollar vaccine industry was gearing up, many other changes were also occurring. Among those changes, especially in the developing world, were improvements in sanitation of all sorts that helped to prevent and lessen the spread of infectious diseases. It is not surprising, if all else is held equal, that infectious diseases are more widespread in areas with poor sanitation. Especially if we compare nineteenth-century Calcutta and Bombay with cleaner cities, it is no surprise that disease conditions were worse in India on the whole. Much the same can be said about conditions in present-day refugee camps, for instance, in those of the Sudan as shown in Figure 7-8 in comparison with the more hygienic conditions found in most parts of the industrialized world.

Is it any wonder that infectious diseases of all sorts are worse when people lack clean drinking water, healthy food, and sanitary ways to dispose of sewage? Figure 7-8 shows a refugee camp near the Darfur region of western Sudan, where many thousands of displaced people reside (Elbajir, 2008;

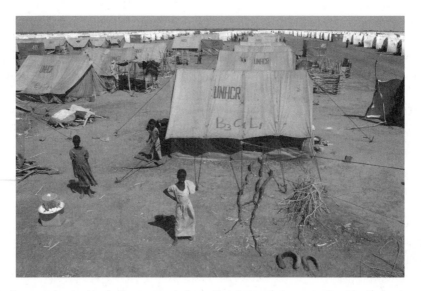

Figure 7-8 Refugee camp in Chad where people have fled from civil war in the Darfur region. *Source*: © Reuters/Stephanie Hancock/Landov.

Slavin, 2004; also see BBC News Channel, n. d.). Conditions were hardly different in Zaire in 1994 when refugee camps there were populated by people fleeing genocide in Rwanda during the First Congo War (J. F. Clark, 2002). Would it surprise anyone to find significant infectious diseases in these camps? Does anyone actually think that vaccination would save the people who reside in these conditions from death by infectious diseases owed to unclean drinking water, inadequate sewage disposal, and insufficient and often unsanitary nutrition? Or is there any doubt that such unhealthy conditions also provide a breeding ground for behavioral, social, and political problems of higher orders (see the video documentary from Smallshop Africa News, 2009 ⊙)?

The Central Role of Hygiene

As Dr. Miguel A. Faria, Jr. (2002), a contemporary neurosurgeon, has observed, the increasing life expectancy after 1930 was due in large measure to "widespread usage of antibiotics and the much improved standards in cleanliness, hygiene, and sanitation" (also see Faria, 2007a, 2007b). The CDC (1999b) itself has acknowledged the role of hygiene and sanitation in the reduction of infectious diseases that has occurred throughout the twentieth century. In the article titled "Achievements in Public Health, 1900–1999: Control of Infectious Diseases," even the CDC publication *Morbidity and Mortality Weekly Report* (*MMWR*) lists sanitation and hygiene as the most important factors in disease reduction. Such measures before 1900 resulted in cleaning up the sorts of conditions that still exist today in the most disease-ridden parts of the world, especially in refugee camps characterized by overcrowding, inadequate supplies of clean water and food, contact with raw sewage, and little or no opportunity to practice any sort of hygiene. These are exactly the sorts of conditions noted by the CDC (1999b) to be chiefly responsible for the spread of infectious diseases prior to 1900. In that article about controlling such public problems, the CDC, of course, was referring to historical epidemics prior to 1900, but their description of the conditions leading to such disasters is well suited to modern refugee camps as noted previously. The CDC report specified such causal factors as

> overcrowding in poor housing served by inadequate or nonexistent public water supplies and waste-disposal systems. These conditions resulted in repeated outbreaks of cholera, dysentery, TB [tuberculosis], typhoid fever, influenza, yellow fever, and malaria.

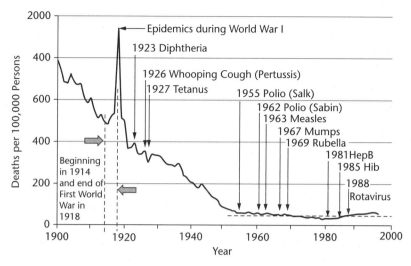

Figure 7-9 Data showing deaths (per 100,000 persons) by infectious diseases from 1900 to 1996 in the United States including the introduction of universal use of the named vaccines. Consolidated by the authors from the two different CDC reports of 1999a and 1999b.
Source: Statistics from CDC (July 30, 1999b, p. 243) and introduction of universal use of the named vaccines (from CDC, April 2, 1999a, p. 247).

By 1900, however, the incidence of many of these diseases had begun to decline because of public health improvements, implementation of which continued into the 20th century. Local, state, and federal efforts to improve sanitation and hygiene reinforced the concept of collective "public health" action (e.g., to prevent infection by providing clean drinking water). By 1900, 40 of the 45 states had established health departments. The first county health departments were established in 1908. From the 1930s through the 1950s, state and local health departments made substantial progress in disease prevention activities, including sewage disposal, water treatment, food safety, organized solid waste disposal, and public education about hygienic practices (e.g., food handling and handwashing). (CDC, 1999b, p. 621) 🌐

Although vaccines often get credit for the remarkable downturn in deaths from infectious diseases during the twentieth century, the facts show that sanitation was clearly the greater causal factor.

As can be seen from the graph of deaths per 100,000 persons from infectious diseases in Figure 7-9 (CDC, 1999b), the downward trend does not seem to have been affected much by the introduction of the 11 major vaccines that were licensed and recommended for universal use in the United States in the years indicated. The data in the graph are instructive and worth studying closely. The major upsurge in mortality that peaked in 1918 began shortly after the onset of World War I. The war began in Europe in 1914, but the United States did not enter the conflict until April 6, 1917 (Today in History, 1917). At roughly the same time, the number of deaths from infectious diseases in the United States began to climb upward, reaching its zenith in 1918. Of course, the mortality associated with the flu epidemic—pointed to by the CDC (1999b) as accounting for the upsurge in deaths from infectious disease from about 1917 to 1918—must have been accompanied by deaths from diseases other than the flu.

A huge factor in that period was the war itself. It is easy to see why epidemics of infectious disease tend to surge during times of war. As explained by Smallman-Raynor and Cliff (2004) in their book titled *War Epidemics,* "the geographical dispersal of highly concentrated (urban) populations, like the geographical concentration of widely dispersed (rural) populations, serves as an efficient mechanism for the historical propagation of war epidemics in civil populations" (p. 254). The reasons for this phenomenon are not hard to find, as explained by Marr (2005). World War I, for example, brought global involvement and countless opportunities for interaction between injured troops returning to hospitals back home. Smallman-Raynor and Cliff (2004) commented specifically on the flu epidemic of 1918, noting that returning Australian troops were quarantined aboard ship to avoid exposing the civilian population to the flu. At the same time, a raging smallpox epidemic in the Philippines occurred coincident with the peak in deaths from infectious disease, as shown in the graph of Figure 7-9.

If we look at the way crowding of war refugees takes place in any major conflict, it is not surprising that deaths from infectious diseases surge during wartime. The virtual graphic proof that World War I was a huge factor in the epidemic of infectious disease that culminated in 1918 is the fact that the peak of the epidemic is precisely defined at the time of the war's end. After 1918, the epidemic began to subside and deaths from infectious diseases in the United States dropped to their lowest point up to that time in the twentieth century, about four years after the war ended.

In 1923, there seems to have been a brief upturn in deaths from infectious disease at the time of the introduction of the diphtheria vaccine. The dates marked on the line thereafter (Figure 7-9) show the years in which other vaccines were universally recommended by the U.S. government. With the introduction of the whooping cough vaccine in 1926, there appears to have been an upturn in deaths, followed by a fairly sharp downturn in mortality with the introduction of the tetanus vaccine in 1927. Deaths by infectious disease continued to fall until the polio vaccines were introduced by Salk in 1955 (dead polio virus injected into the bloodstream) and by Sabin in 1962 (weakened but live virus taken orally in a sugar cube). If we draw a flat line from 1955 through 1996 (see the dotted line in Figure 7-9), it is relatively easy to see that the introduction of eight additional vaccines did nothing substantial to change the rate of death attributable to infectious diseases during nearly the whole latter half of the twentieth century. If anything, it appears toward the end of the century, as noted by the CDC (1999b), with the onset of the AIDS epidemic, that death from infectious diseases began in fact to rise again after the HepB, Hib, and rotavirus vaccines were added into the universal vaccination schedule for children. Did the vaccines reduce deaths by infectious diseases?

The main message to be taken from Figure 7-9 is that something other than vaccines caused the reduction in death rates attributable to infectious diseases. Diseases of that kind—smallpox being the only one that is seemingly extinct—have not, in fact, been eradicated by vaccines, but rather by hygiene and sanitation. Also, in some cases, the targeted virus supposed to cause a particular disease may not be the primary cause.

The Case of Polio Revisited

As neurosurgeon Dr. Russell Blaylock (2008–2009) points out with reference to the polio vaccine, a concomitant factor in the reduction of polio worldwide, but especially in the United States, was the diminishing use of the insecticide **DDT (dichloro-diphenyl-trichloroethane)**. The chemical formula for DDT was discovered in 1874, but the chemical was not used widely as an insecticide until it went into mass production in about 1939. The use of DDT, in particular, rose sharply during World War II. By the mid-1940s, DDT was a household commodity that was advertised as safe for animals, humans, and even foodstuffs, as can be seen in the materials gleaned by West (1999; also see Zimmerman & Lavine, 1946). For instance, there is an advertisement on West's Web site typical of the period appearing in an unnamed source around 1954 recommending DDT for all kinds of household, agricultural, and industrial uses. The substantial printed portion of the full-page ad says:

The great expectations held for DDT have been realized. During 1946, exhaustive scientific data have shown that, when properly used, DDT kills a host of destructive insect pests and is a benefactor of all humanity. (West, 1999 🔊)

The colorful illustration accompanying the advertisement from Killing Salt Chemicals shows a cartoon style chorus line of a dancing dog, a happy tomato, a housewife in her apron, a milk cow with her bell, a cheery peanut, and a rooster all receiving the DDT spray with smiles and singing the jingle, "DDT is good for me!" On the same page there are pictures with captions claiming in bold capital letters that DDT is good for fruits, steers, dairy products, all kinds of crops, home, and industry. For his work in developing the insecticide application of DDT, Paul Hermann Müller of Geigy Pharmaceutical received the Nobel Prize in Physiology or Medicine in 1948 (Müller, 1948 🔊).

The most important thing about DDT, as noted by Blaylock (2008), is that it affects the central nervous system, just as the polio virus is alleged to do. Other pesticides besides DDT are also known to attack the central nervous system, especially **benzene hexachloride (BHC)**, a related pesticide that is more lethal than DDT. For instance, Hayes and Laws (1991), as cited by West (1999, 2003), noted that the killing agents in BHC are "among the most toxic and environmentally persistent pesticides known." The two pesticides together have an extreme correlation with the incidence of polio.

Neurotoxic Pesticides and Polio

The linking of DDT in particular with polio, was first done by Morton S. Biskind in a series of publications in the scientific literature beginning in 1949. In that year he published four important papers about DDT poisoning and its impact on the central nervous system of animals and human beings. Biskind and Bieber (1949), writing for the *American Journal of Psychotherapy*, described DDT as the

> organic compound, first synthesized in 1874 and resurrected from decent interment in chemical archives in 1938, [that] has since attained world renown as the "miracle" insecticide. Beyond question, no other substance known to man was ever before developed so rapidly and spread indiscriminately over so large a portion of the earth in so short a time. (p. 261)

They continued:

> In previous reports (Biskind, 1949a–d) one of us . . . has pointed out the similarity between the known indications of DDT poisoning and the new and highly debilitating syndrome in the human being commonly attributed to a hypothetical "virus X." An identical relationship has also been found to exist between the new and highly fatal "X disease" . . . of cattle and intoxication with this pesticide (Biskind, 1949b, as quoted by Biskind & Bieber, 1949, p. 261)

The X disease of the central nervous system, Biskind argued, only incidentally involved the polio virus, which was then being called "X-virus" in the multiple publications he cited. As we know, the polio virus was subsequently isolated, killed, and rendered into the vaccine that would bear the name of its inventor, Jonas Salk. That vaccine would generally be credited with the near-disappearance of polio according to the standard CDC and WHO literature by about 1970:

[T]he licensing of Salk-type killed or inactivated poliovirus vaccine (IPV) in the United States in 1955 was accompanied by a dramatic reduction in disease incidence. But it was the introduction and mass administration of Sabin-type live (attenuated) oral poliovirus vaccine (OPV) in the early 1960s [1962, in fact] that was to break the chain of wild polio-virus transmission. (Trevelyan, Smallman-Raynor, & Cliff, 2005 ●)

But to what extent did the vaccines actually contribute to the reduced incidence of polio? Trevelyan, Smallman-Raynor, and Cliff acknowledge that sanitation played a large role. According to these authors, the evidence shows that the Sabin oral polio vaccine caused 94% of the 133 confirmed cases (CDC, 1998). These authors also say:

[I]nfection with poliovirus is overwhelmingly subclinical, with the estimated ratio of inapparent [nonsymptomatic] to severe (paralytic) infections ranging up to 850:1. (Trevelyan, Smallman-Raynor, & Cliff, 2005, p. 4)

This information raises a question: Given that so many persons carry the polio virus, why are so few infected with the disease? Evidently, the virus is unlikely to be the causal agent on account of the fact that nearly everyone tested has it, but hardly anyone who has the virus gets poliomyelitis in any of its forms. Some other causal factor must be at work.

Another explanation is that the disease is being caused by something else—for example, neurotoxicity that incidentally leads to a proliferation of the virus. To explain how the live Sabin virus sometimes produces polio in vaccinated individuals, the same hypothesis can be applied. There is no doubt that the Sabin vaccine introduces foreign material into the body that is associated with neurotoxic stress and disease. Symptoms of the three levels of polio described by Trevelyan and colleagues include:

[First level, abortive poliomyelitis:] a range of nonspecific symptoms including headache, sore throat, fever, and vomiting. Nonparalytic poliomyelitis [level two:] . . . those of the minor illness (though, typically, in a more severe form), along with stiffness of the neck, back, and legs. Hyperesthesia (heightened sensitivity of the body to sensory stimuli) and paresthesia (abnormal skin sensations, usually arising from peripheral nerve damage) may also be observed. Finally, in paralytic poliomyelitis [level three], paralysis (commonly of the lower limbs but potentially of all major muscle groups). . . . (Trevelyan, Smallman-Raynor, & Cliff, 2005, p. 4 ●)

According to the standard vaccine theory, each of the three levels of polio disease is caused by a different virus. However, if we compare the symptoms of insecticide poisoning by DDT, as described by Biskind and Bieber (1949), then neurotoxic poisoning, depending on its severity, produces the symptoms of poliomyelitis in all its forms:

Acute gastro-enteritis occurs, with nausea, vomiting, abdominal pain, and diarrhea usually associated with extreme tenesmus [unproductive straining to defecate—like vomiting when nothing is left to come out]. Coryza, cough, and persistent sore throat are common, often followed by a persistent or recurrent feeling of constriction or of a lump in the throat; occasionally the sensation of constriction extends substernally and to the back and may be associated with severe pain in either arm. In some cases the hyoid bone becomes acutely painful to pressure for a few days. Pain in the joints, generalized muscle weakness, and exhausting fatigue are usual; the latter are often so severe in the acute stage as to be described by some patients as paralysis. Pain and stiffness in the back of the neck is a

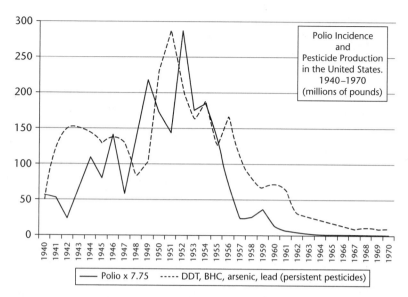

Figure 7-10 Polio incidence (solid line) plotted against the production in millions of pounds of neurotoxic insecticides (DDT, BHC, and those containing lead and arsenic) in the United States from 1940–1970. *Source*: Created by Jim West, (1999, 2003). Retrieved June 15, 2009, from http://www.wellwithin1.com/overview.htm. Used by permission.

frequent complaint. Sometimes the initial attack is ushered in by vertigo and syncope [sudden loss of consciousness]. Intractable headache . . . (Biskind & Bieber, 1949, pp. 262–263 ●)

In Figure 7-10, West graphed the incidence of polio as compiled by the U.S. Office of Vital Statistics for the years 1940 through 1967 (the solid line in the figure) against the millions of pounds of BHC, DDT, and insecticides containing lead and arsenic that were produced from 1940 to 1970 (see the dotted line in Figure 7-10 plotting data from Hayes & Laws, 1991). The clear implication of the graph is that poliomyelitis incidence appears to be related to the introduction of such neurotoxins into the food chain. Throughout the epidemic years of polio, not only was DDT applied liberally to food crops and animals, including dairy cattle, but it was also used liberally inside homes in spray cans and in close proximity to human beings. Officially, DDT was banned on December 31, 1972 (EPA, 2007 ●). In reality, the use of DDT and the other neurotoxic pesticides in Figure 7-10 began to decline in the United States from 1951 forward. After that time, production continued, as noted by West (2003), but supplies were increasingly shipped abroad for use outside the United States (also see Hayes & Laws, 1991).

Meanwhile, the incidence of polio was already falling sharply prior to the introduction of the first polio vaccine—the Salk vaccine, consisting of dead polio virus materials injected into the body tissues—which did not occur until 1955. The downward trend of polio incidence was, according to the statistics plotted in Figure 7-10, unaffected by the Salk vaccine, unless the increase in polio incidence that is apparent between 1956 and 1958 is an effect of the Salk vaccine. Otherwise, that vaccine appears to have had no independent effect on the downward trend line from 1954 forward. As for the Sabin vaccine, as the solid line in Figure 7-10 shows, polio had virtually disappeared entirely from the United States before its introduction in 1962. It seems exceedingly unlikely, therefore, that the isolated viruses attributed to the three "types" (degrees of severity) of polio are actually its primary causes. It is even less likely that the introduction of the polio vaccines had any significant impact on its diminishing incidence in the United States. Rather, it appears more likely that poliomyelitis is a secondary condition caused by neurotoxicity and that reduction of exposure to the toxins is the explanation for the near-disappearance of polio in the United States.

The most persuasive pieces of evidence for the Biskind hypothesis—that neurotoxins such as DDT can cause poliomyelitis—as elaborated by West (2003) and endorsed by Blaylock (2008), are the fact that the ups and downs in the use of the toxin correspond to changes in the incidence of polio and the fact that as the toxins ceased to be used in the United States or were increasingly shipped overseas for use elsewhere in the world, the disease disappeared in the United States (Blaylock, 2008–2009; West, 2008 ●). Such a strong correlation is not likely to be a product of chance. It also provides an explanation for the claim that the near-disappearance of polio from the industrialized world has very little to do with the introduction of the two polio vaccines, but has a great deal to do with the reduced exposure to neurotoxic insecticides.

SUMMING UP AND LOOKING AHEAD

In this chapter, we examined the legendary efficacy of the smallpox vaccine. According to empirical studies comparing heavily vaccinated populations—groups numbering in the hundreds of thousands and even up to 10 million or more—with relatively less vaccinated populations, it is evident that the cowpox vaccine had little to do with the alleged "eradication" of smallpox. On the contrary, the more heavily vaccinated populations of Japan, Germany, and the Philippines—where individuals received not one vaccination, but two or three smallpox vaccinations—experienced higher incidences of death from smallpox. The worst epidemics occurred in the populations that were subjected to the most intensive vaccination programs. Smallpox vaccinations were also correlated with increased deaths from infectious diseases in nineteenth-century Leicester, England. When the vaccinations were virtually halted there, deaths from smallpox nearly ended, and deaths from other infectious diseases also fell off dramatically. By contrast, sanitation without vaccination had a wholesome impact.

In the twentieth century, the general decline in epidemics of infectious diseases had a great deal more to do with hygiene and sanitation—reduction of crowding, the stress of wars, and direct exposure to toxins and disease agents—than with use of vaccines. Polio incidence appears to have risen and fallen with the introduction and removal of neurotoxins, especially DDT and BHC, along with the lead and arsenic insecticides.

As we look to the future, there remains the question of how best to defend against the potential threat of bioweapons based on infectious diseases. Vaccine proponents are committed to building stockpiles of vaccines specifically targeting particular disease agents. However, it seems reasonable to ask that if the Russians, in particular, did hold stockpiles of weaponized smallpox tested at Vozrozhdeniye Island in 1971, why would they go public about that fact in 2001 at the same time that the anthrax scare was initiated in the United States?

In an age of defection and disinformation, we may well wonder why we should (1) trust such information and (2) stockpile hundreds of millions of doses of a vaccine that has been shown for a century and a half to cause more problems than it solves. Although devious individuals (such as Bruce Ivins, if we believe the stories told) and nations (the Russians, among others) are willing to use disease agents as weapons, have they been successful in developing those bioweapons? If weaponized smallpox could kill only 3 of 10 people who were infected in Aralsk, Kazakhstan, in 1971 (Tucker & Zilinskas, 2002, p. 1), and if weaponized anthrax could infect only 22 persons and kill 5 when perhaps hundreds were exposed in 2001 ("Anthrax Attacks 2001," n.d. ●), we may wonder if the devious minds have not decided on another tack by now—perhaps to get the West to waste a lot of money on countermeasures to ineffective bioweapons. In the next chapter, we deal with attempts to control microbes and their sometimes inscrutable masters with the rule of law.

STUDY AND DISCUSSION QUESTIONS

1. Why are vaccines "hot" in the marketplace? What are some of the factors helping to keep them that way? Have you noticed any ads lately from the CDC?

2. What was Kevin de Cock's complaint about Bazin's story on Edward Jenner and the "eradication" of smallpox? Why, if smallpox has been eradicated, is the United States stockpiling smallpox vaccine?

3. Who was Bruce Ivins, and why is he an important part of the vaccine story in the new millennium?

4. How could vaccinia cause disease in an unvaccinated child in 2007?

5. Why would General Burgasov publicly come clean in 2001 about the weaponized smallpox accident in 1971?

6. Given the great importance of the claims made for vaccines, why is it so hard to come by systematic studies conducted by the CDC comparing vaccinated against unvaccinated populations?

7. In the cases examined in this chapter, where large relatively unvaccinated groups have been available for study (e.g., more than 200,000 cases in Leicester, England), what were the results and how do you account for them?

8. Given what we learned in earlier chapters about toxins, disease agents, and interactions, which arguments can you think of that would support or refute claims in favor of giving multiple vaccines simultaneously?

9. Considering the data from the twentieth century, during which 11 new vaccines in addition to the smallpox vaccine were introduced, what evidence is there that those vaccines reduced the incidence of death by infectious diseases?

10. What other factors besides the vaccines were at play in reducing deaths on the one hand and in causing disease on the other hand?

chapter eight

Thimerosal, Vaccines, and the Law

OBJECTIVES

In this chapter, we

1. Discuss current cases under review in the Vaccine Injury Court.

2. Analyze the law pertaining to vaccine injuries and neurodevelopmental disorders.

3. Discuss the rules of evidence in experimental science, logic, and mathematics as contrasted with those laid down by the U.S. Supreme Court.

4. Consider what is at stake from the government's side versus the privacy and social responsibility of individual citizens with respect to vaccines.

5. Discuss the difference between understanding the way things actually work (factual representations) versus the preponderance of opinion in science, politics, and law.

6. Analyze the "Aha!" experience in ordinary perception, in the scientific rejection of false theories, and in the precipitation of paradigm shifts in the sciences.

In this chapter, we begin with an analysis of the Hannah Poling case, and then proceed to consider how the individual's right to maintain the privacy and integrity of his or her own bodily tissues compares with the rights granted to government under the Constitution to provide for the common defense of the nation. To what extent, for instance, does the government have the right to insist on the vaccination of an individual on the theory that it is protecting the greater community from disease or even from attack, say, by bioweapons? We also consider the U.S. Supreme Court ruling in *Daubert v. Merrell Dow Pharmaceuticals* (509 U.S. 579, 1993) on what counts as "good" versus "junk" science under the law. In addition, we examine how scientific advances and paradigm shifts occur outside of the courts (Kuhn, 1962). We will see that a shift in what is regarded as good science, or rather in the general consensus among scientists, typically begins with innovative theories and ideas that eventually gain acceptance after a significant, and sometimes, prolonged period of resistance.

On February 29, 2008, Steven Novella summed up the issue in the cases included under the umbrella of the *Omnibus Autism Proceeding* still pending in Vaccine Injury court: Was the autism epidemic caused by vaccines? Did vaccines, in particular, play a significant role in the causation of autism in those cases? Novella said that the hypotheses under consideration by the Court are "that the MMR vaccine, or thimerosal in some vaccines (but not MMR), or the combination of both, is a cause of autism." ◐ According to Edlich, Son, et al. (2007), there were at least 5030 thimerosal-related lawsuits awaiting action in the Vaccine Injury Court in July 2006.

At the time of this writing in May 2009, the vast majority of the now more than 5300 cases (Fox, 2009) are still awaiting a decision or concession by the court. Setting aside cases that have been conceded (e.g., that of Hannah Poling and about a dozen others), four critical cases have been decided by the court. In the official test cases of Michelle Cedillo, Colten Snyder, and William Yates Hazlehurst, whose families argued that MMR plus thimerosal-containing vaccines had caused their autism, Special Masters Patricia Campbell-Smith, Denise Vowell, and George L. Hastings, Jr. each ruled against the families involved (Fox, 2009; Gupta, 2009; Office of Special Masters, 2009). The ruling in each of these three test cases declared unequivocally that MMR together with thimerosal-containing shots cannot cause autism and could not have done so in these cases. However, the following week the family of Bailey Banks, a 10-year-old boy on the autism spectrum, was awarded $810,000 by the same court. The damages awarded in this fourth case officially fall outside the purview of the *Omnibus Autism Proceeding*, but nevertheless present a strong contradiction to the three official test cases that had been decided only a week earlier.

The ruling in the case of Bailey Banks had been handed down by Special Master Richard B. Abell on July 20, 2007 (Office of Special Masters, 2007), but damages were not awarded until almost two years later on February 20, 2009 (Phillips, 2009). The court had ruled that MMR alone had caused autism in Bailey Banks (R. F. Kennedy, Jr., & Kirby, 2009). More specifically, Bailey's subsequent descent into autism was judged to be "both caused-in-fact and proximately caused by his vaccination" (Office of Special Masters, 2007 ◐). It is noteworthy that the case of Bailey Banks, like many of the other 1322 cases decided in favor of families claiming vaccine injuries (see Edlich, Son, et al., 2007) involved one or more seizures followed by brain damage placing him and others solidly on the autism spectrum. However, the Banks case was deliberately handled outside the scope of the *Omnibus Autism Proceeding* as reported to Robert F. Kennedy, Jr., by Bailey's attorney. The lead attorney for the Banks family, Mark McClaren, said: "[W]e thought we'd have a better chance . . . away from the spotlights and the precedent setting pressures that attend these *OAP* [*Omnibus Autism Proceeding*] test cases—and it worked."

Another attorney involved in vaccine injury petitions, Bob Krakow, told Kennedy, "There's a growing conviction that if you have a[n] autistic client who has also been diagnosed with encephalopathy/encephalitis or seizure disorder, you are better off not mentioning the word 'autism' if you want to win the case" (R. F. Kennedy, Jr., & Kirby, 2009 ◐). The other cases involving damages awarded at taxpayer expense typically, according to interviews reported by David Kirby (2009; also R. F. Kennedy, Jr., & Kirby, 2009), involved the very sort of regression following vaccinations that occurred in the case of Bailey Banks. He had his first seizure just 16 days after the MMR vaccination. His case, like that of Hannah Poling, involved a typical, sudden descent into autism after vaccination. The contradiction presented by the Banks ruling is this: If MMR by itself, according to the Vaccine Injury Court, can cause brain damage and autism, how was it possible for the same court to rule in three test cases under the scope of the *Omnibus Autism Proceeding* that both MMR and thimerosal-containing shots together were powerless to cause autism?

THE CASE OF HANNAH POLING REVISITED

The first case of autism introduced in Chapter 1 was that of a beautiful little red-headed girl who was developing normally up to her 18-month vaccinations. After receiving the recommended shots at 19 months, Hannah began showing classic signs of autism—namely, loss of language and of social contact, accompanied by self-stimulatory behaviors (commonly called "stimming"), fixation on spinning objects, and so on. Interestingly, CDC spokespersons have taken two distinct positions on the Hannah Poling case.

Hannah's Diagnosis After Multiple Vaccinations

On November 9, 2007, the Division of Vaccine Injury Compensation (DVIC) of the Department of Health and Human Services conceded that Hannah Poling's case merited compensation:

> . . . the facts of this case meet the statutory criteria for demonstrating that the vaccinations Hannah received on July 19, 2000, significantly aggravated an underlying mitochondrial disorder, which predisposed her to deficits in cellular energy metabolism, and manifested as a regressive encephalopathy with features of autism spectrum disorder. . . . Hannah's complex partial seizure disorder, nearly six years after her July 19, 2000 vaccinations, was not related to her vaccinations. (Office of Special Masters, 2008a, p. 3 ●)

However, on February 21, 2008, DVIC reversed itself on the seizure disorder and conceded that it, too, was caused by vaccines, although its onset was detected six years after the vaccinations occurred. The official wording recommended "compensation for Hannah's seizure disorder as sequela of her vaccine-injury" (Office of Special Masters, 2008a, p. 4).

Hannah's case is of interest because it was, allegedly, the first of the 5030 claims filed by July 2006 that was conceded by the court. Of course, all of the other cases also complained of a causal relationship between vaccines and the neurodevelopmental disorders known loosely under the umbrella of "autism." Dr. Julie Gerberding, director of the CDC, said on March 7, 2008, in an interview with Dr. Sanjay Gupta:

> We've got to set aside this very isolated, unusual situation, that the court apparently made the decision that it was fair to say that the vaccines may have been one of the precipitants of symptoms in this child with the genetic disorder but that has nothing to say about the thousands and thousands and thousands of children that need immunization day after day after day. (CNN, 2008. As of January 31, 2009, the video record of this conversation was no longer available at CNN; however, it is quoted in part by Kirby, 2008; and the segment in question can be found at Adventures in Autism, n.d. ●)

Given what we know (see Chapters 4–6) about the impact of vaccine components and their interactions, especially the extreme effects of ethyl mercury on mitochondria in general, Hannah Poling's case cannot be exceptional in the way claimed by Dr. Gerberding.

The statement that Hannah's case was "isolated, unusual" and so forth was made on March 7, 2008. However, 22 days later, on March 29, in another interview with Gupta about the Hannah Poling case, Gerberding said, "I don't have all the facts because I still haven't been able to review the case files myself" (*House Call with Dr. Sanjay Gupta*, 2008 ●). Although Gerberding claimed that Hannah's case is exceptional and unusual, another influential vaccine defender, Dr. Paul Offit, has argued that Hannah's case is not unexpected. He says that it is statistically inevitable that some children will descend into autism immediately or soon after receiving vaccines. Offit gives the generalized CDC position on the question: Do vaccines cause autism? He says:

> Vaccines don't cause autism. I mean about 20% of children with autism will regress between often the first and second birthday. So statistically it has to happen where some children will get a vaccine who have been fine. They get the vaccine. Then they're not fine anymore. (CNN, 2009 ●; also found in *House Call with Dr. Sanjay Gupta*, 2008)

In view of what we know about toxins, disease agents, and their interactions from Chapters 4–7, Offit's statistical argument is a little like saying that because a certain percentage of injuries to military personnel engaged in training exercises—say, 20% just for the sake of argument—are expected to be caused by random events, that none of those injuries can be attributed to training exercises.

Training Exercises and Injuries

Vaccinations are analogous to military training exercises. Vaccines are supposed to strengthen the immune system and make it more resistant to attack by certain disease agents. Vaccination with multiple disease agents is a little like a training exercise with multiple sorts of live ammunition, including degraded bioweapons and chemical weapons being fired at or near the trainees. The injuries suffered by military trainees would be analogous to the neurodevelopmental disorders, anaphylactic shock, SIDS, and "regressive" autism experienced by recipients of vaccines. Offit's statistical argument that vaccines don't cause any injuries of this sort—that is, the kind of injuries that occur during or after vaccines are administered—is like claiming that military training exercises do not cause injuries, disease, or death in personnel exposed to munitions, bioweapons, and hazardous chemicals.

One factor that was supposed to make the case of Hannah Poling exceptional was the mitochondrial dysfunction discovered well after she was diagnosed with autism. In fact, the diagnosis pertaining to mitochondrial dysfunction was confirmed by Dr. John Shoffner in February 2004, after four years and five months of multiple intermittent laboratory tests. All of this testing took place subsequent to Hannah's inoculation with multiple vaccines, which preceded her descent into severe autism. According to the CDC, mitochondrial dysfunction is a rare and exceptional genetic disorder that is not caused by vaccines.

Mitochondrial Involvement

Although the CDC has maintained that the mitochondrial dysfunction in Hannah Poling's case was exceptional, it is well known that the ethyl mercury in thimerosal universally attacks the mitochondria, but especially in nerve cells because of the affinity that mercury has for the sulfur-laden proteins that are abundant in nerve tissues. Therefore, we should expect to find mitochondrial dysfunction in a large percentage of, if not in all, cases of "regressive" autism. So, what does the research evidence show?

As early as 2003, Filipek et al. suspected a close association between mitochondrial dysfunction and autism. In fact, these researchers suggested that the "candidate gene loci for autism within the critical region may affect pathways influencing mitochondrial function" (p. 801). In 2004, based on a single case study, T. Clark-Taylor and B. E. Clark-Taylor also proposed mitochondrial dysfunction as a possible "cause of autism" (p. 970). G. Oliveira et al. (2005) found that 7.2% of the 120 cases of typical autism they examined had evidence of mitochondrial dysfunction. Correia et al. (2006) commented that mitochondrial dysfunction is "one of the most common medical conditions associated with autism" (p. 1137). In a later follow-up study with a much larger population, G. Oliveira et al. (2007) found that 20% of children diagnosed with autism in Portugal and the Azores Islands had measurable mitochondrial dysfunction.

Is it only coincidence that well over 20% of all autism cases are of the "regressive" kind? Increasingly, in part because of mitochondrial involvements in autism, the entire spectrum of such disorders is being viewed as a metabolic disease (Manzi, Loizzo, Giana, & Curatolo, 2008; Zecavati & Spence, 2009).

Respiratory Chain Disorders

Because the normal functioning of the mitochondria is essential to the biochemical conversion of fatty acids and sugars into energy that can be used by the body's cells, mitochondrial dysfunction is at the base of a large class of conditions that are loosely called **respiratory chain** (**RC**) disorders. Skladal, Halliday, and Thorburn (2003) estimate that there are hundreds of genetic varieties of RC disorders. According to these authors' research, however, those disorders are relatively rare—affecting about one person in 7634. If this is true, and if it is also true that as many as 20% of the persons diagnosed with autism have such a disorder, it follows that mitochondrial dysfunction is excessively common in persons with ASDs, at least as compared to the general population.

More recently, Haas et al. (2007) estimated that, on average, only one child in 5000 will be diagnosed with mitochondrial dysfunction. Using the latter estimate for mitochondrial disorders and the standard CDC estimate of 1 case per 150 of the whole population for diagnosis of autism (still the CDC estimate current at the time of this writing), if the two conditions—autism and mitochondrial dysfunction—were completely unrelated, the chance of a child being diagnosed with both disorders should be 1/150 times 1/5000, or approximately 1/750,000. Instead, the probability of being diagnosed with both disorders is estimated at 1/5. This makes the coincidence of both disorders 30 times more likely than merely being diagnosed with autism alone (1/150 divided by 1/5) and 1000 times more likely than being diagnosed with mitochondrial dysfunction without autism (1/5000 divided by 1/5). The odds against finding the unlikely coincidence of both autism and mitochondrial dysfunction in any one child with "regressive" autism, as we find it in the case of Hannah Poling, ought to be 750,000 to 1—but it is not. In fact, the odds appear to be less than 5 to 1. If this is so, the argument made by Gerberding and Offit (both CDC representatives) that Hannah's case is exceptional would fail by a margin of 150,000 to 1 (that is 750,000/5 = 150,000).

Hannah's case is not exceptional in the way that Gerberding has argued and it cannot be attributed to a mere statistical coincidence of unrelated factors, as suggested by Offit. Vaccines are implicated. Could it be that this is why the Vaccine Injury Court conceded the case?

Mitochondrial Dysfunction and Mercury Toxicity

Like mercury poisoning (discussed in Chapter 4), mitochondrial dysfunction, as explained by Rotig and Munnich (2003), can affect all the organs of the body. Although RC disorders involving the mitochondria are generally classified as cell disorders (i.e., **cytopathies**), it is interesting that they especially involve the brain, gut, and interactions between them and the muscles. The RC disorders share neurological and neurodevelopmental symptoms both with autism spectrum disorders and with mercury toxicity. Like mercury poisoning, mitochondrial dysfunction (as documented by G. Oliveira, Ataide, et al., 2007; G. Oliveira, Diogo, et al., 2005; Pereira & C. R. Oliveira, 2000; Rotig & Munnich, 2003; and Tsao & Mendell, 2007) can lead to seizures, gastrointestinal "pseudo-blockage" (a condition resembling constipation), chronic vomiting, and glomerular kidney disease. All these disease symptoms are also known to occur in autism.

As discussed in Chapter 4, because of its genotoxicity mercury can disrupt both intercellular and intracellular communications at the level of DNA, RNA, and proteins. As Cannino, Di Liegro, and Rinaldi (2007) have shown, the normal functioning of the mitochondria in cell respiration depends on interactions between all such elements, nuclear DNA, RNA, as well as mitochondrial DNA, RNA, and proteins. For this reason, the toxicity of ethyl mercury in particular plays havoc with the mitochondrial systems. Also, because ethyl mercury has a great affinity for sulfur-containing proteins, which are especially common in the brain and nervous system, the combined effects of mercury on the mitochondria and nerve cells in particular are especially conducive to development of RC disorders. Pereira and C. R. Oliveira (2000) argue that any sort of depletion of glutathione, the body's main detoxifier, will tend to produce additional oxidative stress, tending to cause mitochondrial dysfunction. Case studies by Tsao and Mendell (2007) confirm these expectations as do many studies with toxic buildup attributable to certain drugs in the treatment of AIDS (Kline et al., 2009).

The mitochondrial dysfunction that is common in the "regressive" type of autism can certainly be caused by ethyl mercury and it can be made worse through interactions with other toxins, foreign proteins, and disease agents in vaccines. There is no reason to doubt that mitochondrial dysfunction is common in autism.

An Unexceptional Onset of Regressive Autism

According to the published record from the U.S. Court of Federal Claims (the Vaccine Injury Court), Office of Special Masters, the diagnosis of autism for Hannah Poling occurred on February 8, 2001. At that time, pediatric neurologist Dr. Andrew Zimmerman evaluated Hannah at the Kennedy Krieger Children's Hospital Neurology Clinic (also known as the Krieger Institute). Quoting from the court record:

> He noted a disruption in CHILD's [Hannah's] sleep patterns, persistent screaming and arching, the development of pica [a fearful emotional reaction] to foreign objects, and loose stools. . . . Dr. Zimmerman observed that CHILD [Hannah] watched the fluorescent lights repeatedly during the examination and would not make eye contact. . . . He diagnosed CHILD with "regressive encephalopathy with features consistent with an autistic spectrum disorder, following normal development." (Submitted by the Special Masters, Keisler et al., 2008 ◕)

Zimmerman also noted that Hannah's "encephalopathy" had "progressed to persistent loss of previously acquired language, eye contact, and relatedness" (Keisler et al., 2008). These symptoms, of course, have been the main defining traits of autism since Kanner's original cases in 1943.

Not an Exceptional Fall

Contrary to Gerberding's claim that Hannah Poling's case is exceptional, the *DSM* from 1987 forward says that approximately 20% of the cases of "autistic disorder" involve normal development up to about 18 months followed by a "regression." The term "regression" is somewhat misleading, however: It implies either that the child is regressing to an earlier stage of development or that the child is returning to the disorder. In fact, neither is correct.

The regression in what is called "regressive autism" is not like walking back down a stair case to a previous position, but rather is more comparable to falling from a height because of an injury. The descent in the regressive cases is often like that of a flying bird that has been shot on the wing. The fall does not consist of a return to a prior disordered state or a previously achieved normal stage of development, as is suggested by the term "regression." Typically the child who descends into autism never exhibited the symptoms of autism before—that is, never had seizures, panic/pain tantrums, stereotypical hand-flapping, social unresponsiveness, screaming bouts that last for hours, and other symptoms prior to the fall. Thus the term "regression" is misleading: It is not a return to anything, but rather a new occurrence comparable to falling into a dark pit from which it may appear impossible to escape.

Johnson and Myers (2007) estimate that children diagnosed with autism who exhibit the rapid descent pattern after a year or more of normal development account for as many as 30% of all diagnoses. Hughes (2008) puts the estimate at one in three. Both estimates are considerably higher than the "1 in 5" estimate found in the *DSM-III-R* (1987). In view of the fact that the so-called regression may occur in almost unnoticed downward steps, rather than taking the form of an obvious sudden slide, the actual percentage of instances of normal development followed by descent into autism is probably higher than any of the previous estimates suggest. Also, research reported by the DAN! organization suggests that the percentage of diagnoses in recent birth cohorts arriving at schools over the last few years is closer to 80% (see Pangborn, 2005, p. 149). The implication that vaccines were involved was hinted at in Kanner's third case, who seemed to lose ground gradually, over a period of two years. According to his mother, after his "smallpox vaccination at 12 months," the child began to go "backward mentally" for the next 24 months into severe autism (Kanner, 1943, p. 225).

Hannah Poling's Case as Typical

Hannah's case of autism, in addition to demonstrating a typical "regression" after vaccination, was typical in other respects as well. Hannah was born in December 1998. During the first 19 months of her life, her verbal, social, and motor development were unexceptional; indeed, she was quite normal. According to the court record, at approximately 10 months of age, on October 5, 1999, Hannah "was mimicking sounds, crawling, and sitting" and by her "12-month pediatric examination . . . she was using the words 'Mom' and 'Dad'" and was "pulling herself up, and cruising" (Keisler et al., 2008). Then, on July 19, 2000, Hannah received five distinct vaccinations on the same day: DTAP, Hib, MMR, Varivax, and IPV.

Without knowing the specific manufacturer of each vaccine, it is impossible to determine just which toxins in addition to the disease agents were present in each of these five shots. However, according to the most authoritative and up-to-date information from the CDC (2008b), at a minimum, on a single "well-baby visit" to the pediatrician, Hannah likely received 9 disease agents and about 15 additional toxins including thimerosal. She received shots containing thimerosal about 5 months after the July 1999 public commitment "to remove thimerosal as soon as possible" (see American Academy of Pediatrics & Public Health Service, 1999 and the quote in Chapter 3 on p. 98). According to comments from her mother in interviews after the fact, the parents were shocked to learn that the neurotoxin thimerosal was in the mix of agents to which Hannah was exposed.

The disease agents Hannah received included at least one each for the following: diphtheria, tetanus, pertussis, bacterial meningitis, measles, mumps, rubella, live chickenpox virus (varicella), and inactivated polio virus. She also received various toxins in addition to the ethyl mercury in thimerosal. The additional toxins included aluminum in one or more forms, bovine extract (proteins from cow's blood or other tissues), formaldehyde or formalin, potassium sulfate, ammonium sulfate, chick embryo **fibroblasts** (cells that form the connective tissues of the chicken's body), human **serum albumin** (the yellowish white fluid in tissues and blood that accounts for approximately 55% of the body's weight), gelatin, glutamate (an amino acid), neomycin (an antibiotic), sorbitol (a sugar alcohol), sucrose, amino acid (unspecified), and phosphate buffers (used to maintain the acid–base balance of vaccines in solution).

On the day of her vaccinations, Hannah "spoke well" and was "alert and active" (retrieved from the court record submitted by Keisler et al., 2008). After her vaccinations on July 19, 2000, however, Hannah regressed within a few days into classic and severe infantile autism. In addition to loss of her verbal gains, she became unresponsive to social contact. Also, along with fevers, over the next

10 days, she began to exhibit "intermittent, high-pitched screaming" during which she "began to arch her back when she cried" (Keisler et al., 2008). Four and a half months later, in November 2000, Hannah's condition had not improved. Throughout that time she exhibited other symptoms typical of autism in 70% to 80% of the cases: She had chronic diarrhea, vomiting, and rashes. Also, just one month later, in December 2000, her doctor entered a notation concerning "speech delay" (Keisler et al., 2008). Later on, as noted by her mother (a registered nurse) and her father (a neurologist), Hannah would also show the classic symptoms self-stimming, fixation on spinning objects, and hypersensitivity.

DETERMINING FACTS IN PERCEPTION, SCIENCE, AND THE LAW

Did vaccines and their components—thimerosal and other toxins—or some combination of them cause Hannah Poling's autism and mitochondrial dysfunction? What about the 5000-plus other cases pending decisions in the U.S. Court of Federal Claims? And how many other children have been injured or killed by vaccines—tens or hundreds of thousands? How are the facts to be determined? Is it possible for us to say just which facts are relevant to these critical questions?

In this section, we consider how facts are normally determined in perception, in empirical sciences, and in the shaping of public policies, especially the law. We show that there is a logicomathematical basis for the expectation that ordinary true reports concerning factual occurrences must tend in the long run to prevail over wishful thinking, errors, and even well-funded public propaganda. The logicomathematical argument showing the superiority of ordinary true representations over all manner of fictional ones is simple, comprehensive, and consistent within itself, and is grounded in a series of logicomathematical proofs that stand more firmly than the Rock of Gibraltar against all opposition. We will summarize and illustrate that theory here, in addition to referring the interested reader to publications where it is presented in much greater detail. The main point of this section is to show that there is an irrefutable basis to suppose that any ordinary true report of accessible facts must be simpler, more comprehensive, and more consistent than any fictional representation that aims to account for the same facts. The upshot is that true accounts are better and will prevail.

Schopenhauer's Hopeful Cynicism

The following quotation—though overstated—sums up a well-known problem in scientific change. It is attributed to a man known as the "philosopher of pessimism," Arthur Schopenhauer [1788–1860]:

> All truth passes through three stages. First, it is ridiculed. Second, it is violently opposed. Third, it is accepted as being self-evident. (Schopenhauer, ca. 1860)

This statement is false of ordinary perceptions because they are generally regarded as true and are self-evident right from the start. The difficulty with perceptions, however, is that they are sometimes not true. Thus Schopenhauer's case is overstated. As soon as a perceptual judgment is made, it is generally regarded as valid, and, in the vast majority of cases, perceptions really are valid. In fact, it takes a lot of intellectual work and abstract thinking to realize that perceptions alone can never be fully trustworthy, but the necessary conclusion that *perceptions are never fully to be trusted* is a difficult, abstract, and certainly not a self-evident truth.

The truth that perceptual judgments have to be tested so that we can be sure they are not illusions or errors is not regarded as "self-evident" and it never will be. But it is still true, nevertheless.

So why quote the philosopher of pessimism on the subject of scientific advances? The reason to keep Schopenhauer's argument in mind is that it comes fairly close to summarizing the actual stages of doubt concerning a reasonable theory. After it is proposed, it is typically followed by investigation that may involve conflict of emotions if not fisticuffs, then, by newly won understanding that is often emotionally, intellectually, and in every way liberating.

The old cynic Arthur Schopenhauer summed up a reasonable basis for genuine hope. It is reasonable to suppose that we can discover, factually determine, and communicate to the world the basis of the autism epidemic. To the naysayers, this hope may sound like a "pie in the sky" fantasy or a pipe dream of some sort, but Schopenhauer was right in predicting the all too common irrational and pessimistic response to out-of-the-box rational thought. He was also correct in supposing that the common irrational response to valid new ideas can be overcome by persistent, diligent, and honest communication.

Attaining Perceptual Recognition

Schopenhauer's cynicism, however, was partly justified. When it comes to gaining acceptance, valid ideas in science—as Kuhn (1962) argued and documented in his work about scientific revolutions—are commonly resisted by reigning majorities. This is plainly the case when it comes to the widespread and continuing use of mercury in dental amalgam and in vaccines that are being exported throughout the world. Such practices continue to be widely supported by the CDC, the WHO, and other organizations and persons with vested interests.

The key proponents of the continued use of mercury in vaccines and in dentistry have enormous and very real legal and financial liabilities for the harm their products are causing. Perhaps this is why the American Dental Association and the FDA continue to hold on to the patently false idea that the mercury in dental amalgam is safe—though the same organizations admit that the same mercury is unsafe when it is removed from your mouth, flushed down a drain, swallowed by a tuna fish, or held in your hand. Similarly, the CDC, the WHO, and their collaborators continue to say that the mercury in vaccines is safe in spite of the fact that biochemistry and toxicology show that claim to be unquestionably false (even ridiculous). These actions show, as Thomas Kuhn demonstrated and as Schopenhauer complained, that scientific advances tend to be resisted.

The Moment of Truth

The process of advancing from a paradigm grounded in errors of judgment to a paradigm based on a more complete, consistent, and simpler theory depends on reaching what might be described as a moment of truth. In perception, it is referred to as the "Aha!" experience. The key moment was described by C. S. Peirce (1897) as that point in ongoing experience where suddenly we know a great deal more than we needed to know to reach a correct perceptual judgment about some formerly doubtful issue.

For instance, suppose we see someone walking toward us, say, in a dimly lit corridor, or just in an unfamiliar setting. At first, we think that the movement and silhouette look vaguely familiar. Then, suddenly, we know for a certainty who the person is. What follows may be a virtual flood of additional, but now superfluous evidence that our hunch was correct. However, after the "Aha!" experience, there is no longer any doubt. As soon as we have enough information to make the correct perceptual judgment, we have a great deal more than was necessary to justify it. We think something like, "Aha! Now I have it!" and then everything suddenly falls into place and any remaining doubt vanishes.

The Perceptual "Aha!"

A beautiful illustration of the perceptual "Aha!" experience is the reunion between the male African lion named Christian with his former owners, Anthony Bourke (also known as "Ace Berg") and John Rendall, just nine months after the young lion was returned to the wild. There were actually two reunions and the first one is so remarkable that you have to see it (perceptually) to believe it.

It illustrates well how preconceived ideas can be overwhelmed by factual evidence and by the unity of a coherent story.

In 1969, Bourke and Rendall (1971, 2009) bought the lion they named Christian. In effect, they rescued him, when he was a cub, from a Harrods exhibit in London. However, by the time Christian was 12 months old, he had grown from a 35-pound kitten, when he first went to live in his new apartment home, to a 185-pound male lion. About that time, Bourke and Rendall learned from Bill Travers and Virginia McKenna, a husband and wife team of actors who had appeared in the film *Born Free* about an orphaned lion cub, that the naturalist George Adamson had successfully rehabilitated the domesticated lions of that film to the wild in Kenya (Hill, Adamson, & Cole, 1966). Because of that conversation, Bourke and Rendall first corresponded with Adamson and then traveled to Nairobi to release Christian at a camp near the Tana River in Kora National Park. The vast wilderness dedicated to the park lies about 220 miles northeast of Nairobi on the western side of Kenya, just north of where the equator splits the hemispheres. Beforehand, Adamson stressed to Bourke and Rendall that their chances of seeing Christian again after his release in Africa would depend primarily on Christian's survival in competition with the wild male lions and other hazards of Kenya and secondarily on the extent to which his rehabilitation to the wild was successful. The greater the success, the less their chances of ever seeing him again after his release.

During the time the lion remained with Adamson over the next two years, Bourke and Rendall would stay in touch with Adamson and would visit the lion twice: They would see Christian again just about nine months after he began to acclimate to wild Africa, and then once more, for the very last time, a year after that. At the first reunion, the lion had grown to 300 pounds, and by the time of their second and last visit, Christian had fully acclimated to the wild and had become the largest male lion in the region with a full dark main and weighing in at about 500 pounds (Bourke & Rendall, 1971, 2009, p. 206; Adamson, 1971).

At the first reunion, according to one account (Moore, 2007), when they arrived at the remote desolate park, along with a film crew doing a documentary about the return of the lion to the wild, Adamson told them that he had not seen Christian and the female lions that had become his pride for several days. However, Adamson reported that Christian and his pride had come back to Kora the night before. According to Moore (2007), Adamson had told them, "Christian arrived last night. . . . He's outside the camp on his favorite rock. He's waiting for you" . After waiting several hours for the cool of the day when the lions would be up and moving, Bourke, Rendall, Adamson, and the film crew went out to see if they could find the right lion. As Bourke told the story in a letter to his parents, on that visit, when he and Rendall saw Christian at some distance, at first there was hesitation both by the lion and the men, and then there was recognition (Celizic, 2009).

Bourke and Rendall had found and recognized the very same male lion (Snopes.com, 2008) as they had left behind some nine months earlier. As the video of the event clearly shows, the lion also recognized them by their looks, sounds, smells, and their behaviors. Perhaps the lion knew by "a sixth sense" that his former masters were coming to Africa to see him one last time, as Adamson had suggested on an earlier occasion (Bourke & Rendall, 1971, 2009, p. 169). Whatever doubt had existed before the moment of certainty that Bourke and Rendall had found the right lion was removed as the male lion confirmed to them his identity by rearing up and hugging, nuzzling, and nearly knocking them over, first one then the other, with unrestrained affection for several minutes. The three men and the male lion then walked back to the camp at Kora, where Christian spent the rest of that day and all the following night romping and visiting intermittently with his friends.

In the morning, all of them exhausted, Christian returned to his lionesses and swatted them when they seemed to complain of his man-ish smells. Bourke and Rendall would see Christian one more time about a year later and that encounter too, with a much larger, more mature, and more dangerous full-grown African lion would be captured on film (Celizic, 2009 ●). Later, Adamson would write in his autobiography about his home in Kenya:

> Promises of solitude, of wild animals in a profusion to delight the heart of Noah, and of the spice of danger, were always honored. Today, of these three you are only likely to encounter the danger. (Snopes.com, 2008)

In 1989, George Adamson was murdered by bandits near Kora National Park. He is gone, but the story of Christian the lion will be told for generations to come. It is surely one of the most remarkable illustrations ever of the amazing process of perceptual recognition. It shows in flesh and blood, across cultures, continents, species, and genders, what is meant by the tipping point where that vague and uncertain line is crossed that separates a mere hunch from virtually certain perception that is suddenly followed by reasonably certain knowledge.

On the other side of that vague line, we meet a flood of information and a kind of abstract knowledge that overwhelms and washes away any reasonable former doubt. From the other side of that line, the virtual certainty of the recognition that has been achieved defies the vanishing remains of the former skepticism.

Consensus Building in Science, Law, and Politics

The tipping point of perceptual recognition is a microcosm of consensus building in mass communication. The same basic processes that are at work in tipping a perceptual judgment in favor of a particular conclusion—and against countless other possibilities that are ruled out (e.g., the male lion approaching Bourke and Rendall that day could have been an unfriendly wild lion and not their old pal Christian)—occur on a grand scale in science, law, and politics. Rational judgment in the sciences moves from imagining a hypothetical possibility or, usually, several hypotheses, to suspicion that some of those conjectures can reasonably be ruled out, while one or more others cannot. As the understanding of theories and of empirical evidences builds, the progress sometimes reaches the tipping point where all the evidence points toward one theory (or possibly several theories) and weighs decisively against others that are conclusively ruled out.

In the sciences, as in perception, the careful examination of empirical evidence and of theoretical arguments for and against alternative hypotheses often leads to a settled conclusion that some of the alternatives can certainly be ruled out, whereas others cannot reasonably be doubted. For example, Bourke and Rendall could no longer doubt the almost unbelievable conclusion that the lion hugging and nuzzling them really was their old pal Christian and not some other wild African lion. They thought it might be Christian when they first saw him at a distance, but at the start that was only a possible theory. The animal could have been some other lion. The differentiation of the alternatives in science, much as in perception, is accomplished by an interplay between abstract theory and empirical observation.

The work in the sciences has little to do with voting or consensus, except that scientists are obliged to communicate their findings in such a way as to make them comprehensible to others. This requirement is implicit in the whole process of scientific investigation, where it is essential that findings can be tested both theoretically and empirically. As a result, consensus in the sciences is virtually assured over the long haul. Nevertheless, as Schopenhauer complained, the consensus may sometimes be slow in coming and there can be a great deal of resistance to findings that require changes in widely accepted practices that are doing harm.

The Resistance Phase

The fate of ideas in the arenas where policies are shaped and where laws are made is fraught with struggle, uncertainty, and conflicting motives and interests. If the CDC and the FDA had been left on their own, presumably the hypothesis that vaccines were doing harm would not have been formed by them, much less publicly expressed. After all, why would proponents of vaccines be inclined to suppose that they had done any harm to any particular individual, much less to tens of millions of children who received vaccines containing the neurotoxin thimerosal? However, as the number of injuries—especially neurodevelopmental "regressions"—being produced in the early 1980s reached a critical tipping point, the public outcry became sufficient to push the U.S. Congress to pass the Vaccine Injury Act of 1986.

Perhaps Congress may have been moved to act more by a desire to protect pharmaceutical companies from civil lawsuits than to protect members of the public from injuries by vaccines. Whatever the underlying motive for the Vaccine Injury Act, the change brought about by this legislation was significant in terms of policy and law. It was also a step by the U.S. government acknowledging that vaccines were doing harm. What was unknown at that time was just how much harm was being done and on how vast a scale.

The Growing Public Awareness

The passage of the Vaccine Injury Act of 1986 set the stage for the discoveries that are now being made known to the general public. In 1986, there was little public awareness of the role played by ethyl mercury in the DTP, HepB, and Hib vaccines, and neither was there any public knowledge of the potential for interaction between MMR and DTP, not to mention the other vaccines.

These interactions would eventually be revealed, in part because of the policy change achieved in the passage of the 1986 Vaccine Injury Act. At the time of the enactment of that law, the public was largely unaware of the role being played by the tons of dental amalgam being used all over the world, including in pregnant women. There was little or no general awareness of the harm being done by ethyl mercury in contact lens solutions, spermicides, Rh-negative gamma globulin, and other sources.

Likewise, there was no general awareness of the interactions between the toxins, disease agents, and animal proteins in vaccines in 1986. Clinical trials of vaccines and medicines (not to mention studies of toxins in general), however, overwhelmingly showed that combining medications, vaccines, and toxins invariably increases the likelihood of injuries. The concept of free radicals and the role of oxidative stress could be found in the scientific literature, along with the growing literature on toxicology, but public awareness had not yet reached the critical point concerning such theories. Similarly, the implications of relevant theories and research for the growing epidemic of neurological disorders were barely beginning to come up on anyone's radar; hardly anyone had put two and two together yet.

The research showing the remarkable correlation between poliomyelitis and the use of pesticides, especially DDT, was virtually unknown to practitioners and the general public. But along with the exponential growth in the diagnosis of neurodevelopmental disorders, especially autism spectrum disorders, there was a growing understanding of the importance of toxicity and oxidative stress inside human bodies, and the amazing contributions made by vaccines, medicines, and medical procedures in producing it.

Admittedly, the law is a sluggish beast. In particular, changes in federal law often require enormous public pressure. However, as the lapse of time between the discovery and public availability of necessary and relevant information shrinks, the time necessary to achieve huge changes in public policy and the law can be in theory, and is evidently being, reduced. The Internet and its search engines have radically reduced the time lapse between the discovery of new information and its dissemination. Although propaganda can also be disseminated more rapidly, it can be exposed for what it is more easily than ever before.

COMMUNICATION AS THE KEY TO ADVANCES

The growth of worldwide access to the Internet, which includes increasingly universal access by the general public to information sources that were previously unavailable or difficult to access, has greatly speeded up the time from theoretical and empirical advances to changes in public policy. Valid information can be presented more vividly and more swiftly than ever before, and propaganda can be refuted more rapidly and more convincingly than at any prior period of history.

The Public Impact of Valid Information

As valid information about relevant facts is made increasingly accessible to the public, the pent-up demand for needed policy adjustments grows more and more rapidly toward the critical mass required for a course correction. Even an act of Congress can—in theory, at least—be produced more rapidly today than ever before.

As examples, we can compare the time required for passage of the Vaccine Injury Act of 1986 with the time it took to enact the Partial Birth Abortion Act of 2003. It took a little more than a century of mandatory vaccinations to lead to a sufficient growth in civil actions to precipitate the Vaccine Injury Act of 1986. Nearly universal administration of vaccinia (the so-called smallpox vaccine) and the addition of 10 more vaccines into the mandatory vaccination schedule took place over approximately a century before the Vaccine Injury Act of 1986. However, it took just three decades—from 1973 (with the *Roe v. Wade* decision) until 2003—for the American public to bring sufficient pressure on the Congress to pass the Partial Birth Abortion Act. Videos of unborn babies in the womb (see links and videos in the DVDs that accompany our 2006 *Milestones* book), together with public knowledge of the horrifying procedures actually employed by doctors in performing partial birth abortions, helped to cause radical changes in public opinion and policy.

We can hope that it will take less than another decade for reasonable independent researchers and citizens across the United States and around the world to begin to take a much more critical look at the contents of vaccines and at the inconsistent doctrines of the FDA and CDC about them. Most thinking individuals who would formerly have unquestioningly delivered up their infants for vaccinations at birth and at intermittent intervals thereafter are stunned to learn that the FDA and CDC, along with practicing pediatricians injecting the children, all hold to the doctrine that "one size fits all." The CDC schedule for vaccines (see Figure 8-1) also shows that pediatricians and parents who comply with the mandated program are very busy injecting toxins and disease agents of many different sorts into children.

It does not take a medical degree or a PhD to be astonished at the supposition that a premature baby weighing 3 pounds, a newborn weighing 5 pounds, and a full-term child weighing 12 to 13 pounds should all receive the same dose of disease agents, toxins, and vaccine contaminants. Similarly, it seems unbelievable that the watchdog agencies—the FDA and CDC, not to mention the professional medical associations and the vast majority of individual pediatricians—would routinely recommend the same dose in a prepackaged vaccine for a newborn baby as for a child of six months, or for a six-month-old as contrasted with a two-year-old or, in some cases, with an adult. The toxicology on dose-response ratios (e.g., see Hunt & Rai, 2008, and their references) renders all such practices absurdities on their face. The "Catch Up Immunization Schedule" (CDC, 2008a) crams even more doses of one-size-fits-all toxins and disease agents into children in an even shorter and more compressed time frame.

The idea espoused by the vaccine manufacturers, the CDC, and the AAP that "one size fits all" when it comes to vaccines for infants and children at all ages and all maturity levels is ludicrous. When well-meaning, compliant parents who are vaccinating their children in good faith discover

Recommended Immunization Schedule for Persons Aged 0–6 Years—United States • 2008

For those who fall behind or start late, see the catch-up schedule

Vaccine ▼ Age ▶	Birth	1 month	2 months	4 months	6 months	12 months	15 months	18 months	19–23 months	2–3 years	4–6 years
Hepatitis B[1]	HepB	HepB		*see footnote* 1		HepB					
Rotavirus[2]			Rota	Rota	Rota						
Diphtheria, Tetanus, Pertussis[3]			DTaP	DTaP	DTaP	*see footnote* 3	DTaP				DTaP
***Haemophilus influenzae* type b**[4]			Hib	Hib	Hib[4]	Hib					
Pneumococcal[5]			PCV	PCV	PCV	PCV				PPV	
Inactivated Poliovirus			IPV	IPV		IPV					IPV
Influenza[6]								Influenza (Yearly)			
Measles, Mumps, Rubella[7]						MMR					MMR
Varicella[8]						Varicella					Varicella
Hepatitis A[9]							HepA (2 doses)			HepA Series	
Meningococcal[10]										MCV4	

Range of recommended ages

Certain high-risk groups

This schedule indicates the recommended ages for routine administration of currently licensed childhood vaccines, as of December 1, 2007, for children aged 0 through 6 years. Additional information is available at **www.cdc.gov/vaccines/recs/schedules**. Any dose not administered at the recommended age should be administered at any subsequent visit, when indicated and feasible. Additional vaccines may be licensed and recommended during the year. Licensed combination vaccines may be used whenever any components of the combination are indicated and other components of the vaccine are not contraindicated and if approved by the Food and Drug Administration for that dose of the series. Providers should consult the respective Advisory Commitee on Immunization Practices statement for detailed recommendations, including for **high-risk conditions: http://www.cdc.gov/vaccines/pubs/ACIP-list htm.** Clinically significant adverse events that follow immunization should be reported to the Vaccine Adverse Event Reporting System (VAERS). Guidance about how to obtain and complete a VAERS form is available at **www.vaers.hhs.gov** or by telephone, **800-822-7967**.

Figure 8-1 Recommended CDC schedule (CDC, 2008b) for at least 36 vaccinations from birth to the age of six years. Children in the high-risk groups could receive 39 different shots.

Source: Reproduced from National Center for Immunization and Respiratory Diseases, *Recommended Immunization Schedule for Persons Aged 0–6 Years*, CDC (2008). [http://www.cdc.gov/vaccines/recs/schedules/].

that no allowances are made for smaller and less mature infants at birth, or for children of different weights, levels of maturity, and health conditions later in the schedule, they are shocked.

Shock and Grief Followed by Anger

Jenny McCarthy (2007a) described her own feelings and those of mothers everywhere during her September 18, 2007, appearance on Oprah Winfrey's television show: "We vaccinated our baby and *something* happened. *Something* happened. Why won't anyone believe us!" The audience began a slow rumble of applause as the tears began to come to the eyes of many moms.

McCarthy continued to talk about the CDC vaccine policy of "one size fits all" and described the reaction she saw around her and that she felt and imagined from parents across the nation who were watching the interview:

> I felt them jumping up and down on their couches, I felt them glued to their TV screens crying and raising up their arms, I felt them calling their own moms on the phone scream-ing, "Are you hearing this?! She said it!" (McCarthy, 2008, p. 9 ●)

When the general public discovered, through legal actions initiated by individual citizens on the basis of the Freedom of Information Act of 1966–2001, that the CDC experts at the Simpsonwood Conference were hard-pressed to think of any research showing that body mass and maturity are certain to be huge factors in the ability of a child to cope with multiple disease agents, toxins, and their interactions in vaccines, public confidence in the government watchdogs (the CDC and FDA, in particular) was reasonably shaken. As we saw in Chapters 3–7, there can be no reasonable doubt that body mass and maturity dramatically affect an individual's ability to cope with the challenges presented by vaccines or any other sources of toxins to be placed inside the human body.

True Reports Versus Invented Fiction

There is no reason for honorable scientific researchers—persons of integrity seeking to understand diseases and disorders—to fear the potential flood of propaganda that can be generated by vested interests on the part of the CDC, FDA, the pharmaceutical companies, and the mainstream medical profession. On the contrary, the propagandists and vested-interest groups have every logical reason to tremble in fear at the prospect of valid information getting out to the public. It is already hap-pening and it is certain to continue. At this juncture, it is important to consider the logicomathemati-cal proofs underlying the assertion that true reports are certain in the long-run to prevail over fictions.

Logicomathematical reasoning shows why simple, ordinary true reports (such as the story of Anthony Bourke, John Rendall, and Christian the lion, for instance) absolutely have the upper hand over invented fictions. It is important to realize that the proofs only require that the "true" reports be so in the most mundane and ordinary sense of "truth." They do not have to be "perfect" in the sense of reporting all details, or exact in the sense of "perfect measurement," or in any absolute sense of "perfection." They only have to be true relative to what they purport to say. Of course, clever writers may come up with fictions, and, of course, errors may be contained in "scientific" studies. Similarly, deliberate lies may be invented to deceive the public by propagandists or by indi-viduals and agencies just trying to protect their vested interests from legal or financial liabilities. Nevertheless, the logicomathematical proofs show why ordinary true representations of facts are, all else being equal, absolutely better than false ones trying to explain away, hide, or distort the same facts.

Even some skeptics will admit that public access to scientifically valid information and true representations is growing—that knowledge is actually increasing faster than ever before in history—

but they are apt to point out that the potential for disinformation, false defenses of false beliefs, and for outright lies and propaganda is also increasing. Thus they will want to know why it is so—if, indeed, it is so—that widely held false ideas cannot stand up against true representations of valid empirical evidence that is widely accessible.

Logic: True Reports Must Prevail

True representations of the facts of ordinary experience, if all else is held equal, are certain to be simpler, more comprehensive, and more consistent than false representations purporting to explain the same facts. The first proponents of logicomathematical proofs along this line were C. S. Peirce (1897) and A. Tarski (1949, 1956). The mathematician Gottlob Frege [1848–1925] may have been the first to suggest in print that ordinary true representations form the basis for all possible meaningful representations, but it was Peirce and Tarski who provided the first actual logicomathematical proofs of this grand proposition.

However, their proofs are not apt to be consumed with much comprehension by the general public. Simpler and more complete proofs, however, have been developed and have been shown to account for a vast research literature in mass communication, advertising, and discourse processing (J. W. Oller & Giardetti, 1999). The same general proofs and the principles derived from them account for findings in the assessment of language abilities and human intelligence (see J. W. Oller, 1993; J. W. Oller, L. Chen, S. D. Oller, & Pan, 2005). They also show how measurement in the sciences absolutely depends on true reports of the distinctly narrative kind (J. W. Oller & L. Chen, 2007). Following the tradition of C. S. Peirce in particular, a series of logicomathematical proofs has been produced, critiqued, and published in a variety of peer-reviewed contexts, ranging from the Internet and scholarly books to technical journals; all of these proofs have reached the conclusion that true representations of ordinary facts are necessarily *simpler, more comprehensive*, and *more consistent* than false ones. The logicomathematical proofs in question are completely general (i.e., they apply to all possible instances of meaningful representations without any exceptions). Without going into any technical detail, we can illustrate the upshot of them all with the still-fresh example of Christian the lion.

The Proofs Exemplified

If it is true that the lion approaching Ace Bourke and John Rendall in the video ("Christian the Lion," 2009 ●) is their former pal, Christian, this representation of the facts at hand (the representation that *the lion approaching really is Christian*) is *simpler* than any other competing fictional theory. It is simpler to suppose that the lion really is Christian than that it is a different African lion, an elephant, a tiger, an illusion, a dream, a shadow, a trick of a clever videographer, a digitally manufactured lie, or anything else.

Also, the true representation that the lion in question really is Christian, given that it is true, is *comprehensive*. It connects the current experience of a viewer of the video, for instance, with the particular lion in question and with the whole history of that lion, with the two men in question, with their girlfriends back in London, with the life and death of the naturalist named George Adamson, with the actors who recommended him to Bourke and Rendall, and so on—right out to the limits of the material history of the world. Any false or fictional representation pertaining to the same facts would necessarily break down with respect to some of the facts in evidence, or else it would not be fictional. Also, fictional representations, propaganda, and the like can be accounted for by true representations, while the reverse is not so. Fictions cannot fully account for true representations of anything whatsoever—not even the least significant of mundane facts.

Similarly, the representation of the lion in question as Christian is *more consistent* with the known facts than any false or fictional representation of the same facts can possibly be because any false or merely fictional representation will fail to be consistent with some of the determinable facts. If a fictional (false) representation turned out *not* to be false (or fictional), it would, logically speaking, have to agree with the details of the true reports and video of Christian and of the two men, Bourke and Rendall. In that case, the fiction would turn out to agree completely with an ordinary true representation and would not be a fiction! Therefore, it follows that any false or fictional representation pertaining to the facts at hand absolutely must be inconsistent with some of the facts in evidence precisely to the extent of its falseness or fictionality.

As a result, it follows by absolutely strict logic (irrespective of the truth or falsehood of any example we might choose to illustrate that logic) that an ordinary true representation of any facts in question must be more consistent with all of the facts at issue than any false or fictional representation can possibly be with respect to the same facts. The next step is merely to show that the argument generalizes to all possible representations of all possible facts irrespective of their complexity.

False Theories and Propaganda Will Fall

With the foregoing points in mind, it follows that successful communication concerning valid representations of publicly accessible facts can defeat well-supported false ideas and even huge propaganda machines. It does not follow that the contest will be without risk or cost, but we can illustrate the certainty that ordinary truth will prevail by using a metaphor from Archimedes. Archimedes said he could move the world with a lever if only he had a place to stand. Here is where the metaphor breaks down: He didn't have a place to stand. But so long as ordinary facts of experience have any warrior moms and dads left to represent them, ordinary true representations do have a place to stand. Also, the lever with which Archimedes said he could move the world is pitifully weak by comparison to the power of a fully abstract but true representation of ordinary facts.

According to the fully abstract logicomathematical proofs summarized here, any ordinary true representation of facts already has a place to stand in the facts that it represents, and it can absolutely defeat any propaganda about those same facts, if that ordinary, mundane truth is merely made known. Therefore, by the strictest of proofs of the logicomathematical kind, it follows that all that is needed to defeat propaganda about ordinary facts is a valid representation that is made publicly accessible. This is what this book is for, and that is why its authors determined to take no royalties for it (we have committed the royalties to the medical treatment of autism spectrum disorders). Our singular purpose is to get the information before the public.

The Shrinking Half-Life of Errors and Propaganda

As the accessibility of valid information and data sources becomes increasingly rapid, detailed, and global, commonly held false ideas, including all kinds of propaganda and any mere consensus of opinions based on false information, can be expected to have an increasingly shorter half-life. Theoretically, that half-life approaches and reaches its complete vanishing point at the moment when valid information becomes instantly accessible. We cannot quite achieve instantaneous communication even through the Internet, but we can achieve more rapid dissemination of information than ever before.

As false claims are held up to scrutiny and are compared in the light of overwhelming logical and empirical evidence, simpler, more comprehensive, and more consistent perspectives are certain to be proposed. The latter theories, provided they are correct and comprehensible, are assured of being more likely to be understood and accepted by the general public because they will be simpler and more sensible. The likelihood that truer explanations will produce a general rejection of falsehoods and propaganda that purport to explain the same facts follows from the greater simplicity, comprehensiveness, and consistency of the truer explanations.

A War of Ideas

When false claims are tested logically and experimentally and are shown to be false, those opposing the correction of their own errors are apt to take all kinds of defensive postures. A failing paradigm may be defended by public denials, by flooding the market with propaganda insisting that the false paradigm is still true. Herculean efforts may be made to shore up the collapsing system of ideas. Even so, there comes a point in ordinary perception and in mass communication where false perceptions are shown up for what they are. As more individuals say something like, "Aha! Now I see the error," public momentum grows like water rising until it begins to breach the propaganda levee.

At first there may be merely a vague hunch that commonly accepted practices are doing harm. The water begins to trickle over the propaganda dam. Meanwhile, the power brokers with vested interests may try to shore up the propaganda levees to prevent the evidence refuting their position from becoming known, or, if the evidence is already known, they may seek to prevent its being accepted as relevant to the particular cases at hand. For example, look at how the CDC scrambled its resources to promote its vigorous denial that Hannah Poling's case is typical. Nevertheless, the evidence continued to accumulate in favor of the view that Hannah's case is not exceptional.

Thus, as independent researchers and highly motivated members of the public begin to take increasing interest in what is causing them pain, the tipping point where the public consensus begins to change in favor of the more consistent, comprehensive, and simpler explanation of the facts is virtually certain to be reached. When that happens, the essential representations of relevant facts begin to flow over the top of the propaganda dam and to erode it until it can no longer withstand the pressure. Then in a rush, the prevailing paradigm will fall, the propaganda dam will collapse more certainly than the Berlin Wall, and needed change will come.

Changing a Scientific Paradigm

The problem in the sciences is much the same as it is in ordinary perception. The change point in perception occurs when a settled judgment is reached that effectively rules out all other possible competing alternatives. Bourke and Rendall might think at first that they are looking at a wild male African lion about the expected size of Christian. Then, as the lion approaches, they think it might be him. When the lion runs up and starts embracing them, they know for sure it is Christian, and all the competing possibilities are dismissed.

The process of judgment in the theoretical and empirical sciences—as argued most comprehensively in the vast writings of C. S. Peirce, and as we have likewise argued in our own writings—is similar. In the case of the epidemic of neurodevelopmental disorders, at first the unfamiliar landscape of the upsurge in disorders seems vaguely strange, then alarming; finally, we see it as a genuine problem that must have discoverable causes. By careful investigation, we have already discovered the critical causes that are pushing many children beyond the tipping point.

THIMEROSAL, VACCINES, AND THE AUTISM EPIDEMIC

On July 3, 2002, the Office of Special Masters in the U.S. Court of Federal Claims (Vaccine Injury Court) issued Autism General Order #1. That special order (Office of Special Masters, 2002) explains how the vaccine injury autism/thimerosal cases are now being handled and why they are being dealt with differently from any prior cases heard by the Court.

The Force of Epidemic Numbers

By the date the order was issued, the Court said there were already 400 cases on file to be heard and that the Office of Special Masters was expecting thousands more cases to be filed. By July 2006, according to Edlich, Son, et al. (2007), 5030 cases had been filed. Part of the reason for the flood of cases was a decision made with reference to many cases pending in civil courts. The case of *Owens v. American Home Products Corp.*, 2002 WL 992094 (S.D. Tex. May 7, 2002), determined that the many civil suits against vaccine manufacturers that were pending in civil courts would have to be brought to the U.S. Court of Federal Claims. That landmark decision resulted in thousands of cases in the civil courts across the United States being transferred to the U.S. Court of Federal Claims and the Office of Special Masters in particular.

Now, the question facing the Office of Special Masters is whether vaccines—the MMR and the thimerosal-containing vaccines—separately or in combination have caused the neurodevelopmental disorders associated with the autism spectrum. Because ASDs form the core of the many cases already under consideration, the proceeding would subsequently be referred to as the *Omnibus Autism Proceeding* (Office of Special Masters, 2002, p. 4).

First General Causation; Then Specific Claims

Here is how the Office of Special Masters has decided to handle the many claims still pending. On the basis of an advisory panel formed by the lawyers representing the many petitioners (who would be the plaintiffs in a civil court—that is, the parties claiming they were injured) asked for additional time to prepare a case showing causation. They have also said that they need time for **legal discovery**, the process in which vaccine manufacturers, the CDC, the FDA, and other entities are ordered to hand over documents, research reports, and raw data relevant to the general causation issues.

The petitioners asked the Office of Special Masters for a two-stage process. The first stage would consist of a general hearing about causation in which the relevant documents, studies, and raw data would be made accessible to interested parties. That compilation would be referred to as the "Autism Master File" and would be open to "inspection by any interested persons" (Office of Special Masters, 2002, p. 3). The data compiled and presented during this hearing would constitute an evidentiary record with respect to the general causation issues and would be made available to the several thousand claimants and their legal representatives. The second stage of the process would then involve arguing and deciding the individual cases.

Evidently, the petitioners on behalf of the families are counting on the strength of numbers. If they combine their resources in building the case for causation, the individual lawyers and teams now representing more than 5300 different families (Fox, 2009) will be able to benefit from the collective momentum. Meanwhile, tens of thousands of other families who now believe their children with autism were also injured by vaccines are watching these proceedings with great interest. Outside the group of pending cases, it is estimated that there are perhaps 10 to 50 times as many families who would have filed in the Vaccine Injury Court but were prevented from doing so by the stringent three-year statute of limitations (SOL), as discussed in Chapter 3. Because it commonly takes more than three years to get a diagnosis of autism, the three-year SOL has left many would-be petitioners on the outside, yet monitoring the proceedings very closely. In addition to that group, there are hundreds of thousands of families who have been caught up in the autism epidemic, and there are hundreds of millions who have been and are being exposed to the disease agents, toxins, and interactions that are associated with the vaccines under examination.

The *Omnibus Autism Proceeding* affects more families than all prior vaccine injury claims that have ever been heard and decided by the U.S. Court of Federal Claims. According to the published report by Edlich, Son, et al. (2007), a total of 4259 claims of vaccine injuries were filed between 1989 and 2004. Of those claims, 1189 were judged to be compensable under the Vaccine Injury Compensation Program and 3070 were dismissed. Figure 8-2 shows that the peak activity for the Court occurred from 1990 through 2000, during which time 4190 cases were decided. From 2001 to 2004, only 48 cases were heard. What was happening during that time, apparently, was that after Wakefield et al. (1998) published evidence that the MMR vaccine was involved in the gut disease

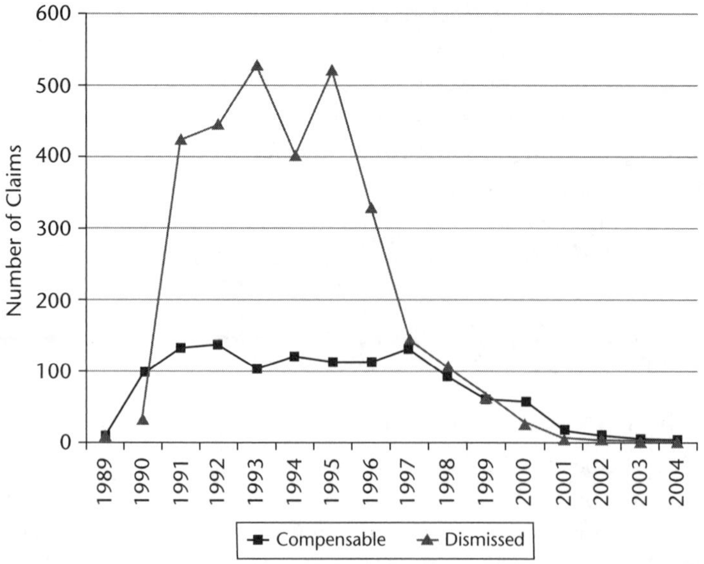

Figure 8-2 Number of compensable and dismissed cases (total = 4259) filed in the U.S. Court of Federal Claims between 1989 and 2004 for vaccine injuries not specifying either thimerosal or autism.
Source: Data from R. Edlich, et al., *Journal of Emergency Medicine, 33* (2007), 199–211.

of persons with autism, parents began increasingly to suspect that vaccines were causing autism. Then, when Bernard et al. proposed the mercury poisoning theory of autism in 2001—singling out especially the ethyl mercury in thimerosal, which was a major toxin in DTP, DTaP, HepB, and Hib shots—the focus of vaccine injury contests shifted to neurodevelopmental disorders, with autism at their center.

According to the Office of Special Masters handling the *Omnibus Autism Proceeding*, 400 cases concerning vaccines and autism were filed by July 3, 2002. It follows that if 5030 thimerosal/autism claims were filed by July 2006, 4630 of those cases must have been filed in a period of just four years. At the time of the publication of the Edlich, Son, et al. report in January 2007, no autism case had yet been decided. The case of Hannah Poling would not be conceded until March 7, 2007. That concession would be exceptional in singling out just one case out of the thousands already in the docket, but it would not be exceptional (as we have already shown) with respect to symptoms, diagnosis, or mitochondrial dysfunction. Clearly, the pressure on the government is growing to a crescendo.

Filing a Claim

Filing a claim proceeds through several steps that are summed up by Edlich, Son, et al. (2007). Initially, some individual (usually a parent, relative, or primary caregiver) files a petition claiming that injury or death was caused to a particular person (usually a child) from a vaccine. The petition requests compensation from the U.S. Court of Federal Claims and also goes to the Secretary of Health and Human Services (HHS; formerly known as the U.S. Department of Public Health Services). The HHS is the parent agency to the CDC and FDA, among a host of other government agencies. If the claim were heard in a civil court, the Secretary of HHS would be named as the defendant. However, the U.S. Court of Federal Claims is unique in the U.S. court system in offering, in theory at least, a "no-fault" system of adjudication.

In actuality, that is hardly the case. The HHS is very much on trial, as are the CDC, the FDA, the manufacturers of vaccines, the physicians who administer them, and the professional organizations that support their use and make all kinds of representations concerning the safety of vaccines and their components. Thimerosal, the ethyl mercury component found in many vaccines, is a primary focal point in view of the vast amount of research showing its generalized toxicity to nerves, to genes, to mitochondria, and to bodily cells, tissues, and organs in general (see Chapters 3–7). The idea that the still pending 5300 cases do not involve any fault or culpability on the part of the manufacturers and the promoters of vaccines is wishful thinking to say the least.

The next step in filing a claim involves the services of a physician at the Division of Vaccine Injury Compensation with HHS, who evaluates the petition. The question at this point is whether the claim meets the criteria for compensation. That physician then makes a recommendation through the Department of Justice to the Court. Although that recommendation is not binding, it is presented by a lawyer from the Department of Justice before a Special Master (SM), an attorney appointed by the judges of the U.S. Federal Court of Claims from the Office of Special Masters. The SM then acts as judge and jury on the claim and makes a decision about whether to compensate the claimant under the Vaccine Injury Compensation Program. Claimants who are not satisfied with the SM's decision may appeal first to a judge of the U.S. Court of Federal Claims, then to the Federal Circuit Court of Appeals, and finally to the U.S. Supreme Court. A key restriction on vaccine injury claims before the U.S. Court of Federal Claims is that the petition is automatically denied if an action is pending in civil court concerning the same alleged injury or if an award has already been made by a civil court.

No matter what the outcome in any given claim, the Vaccine Injury Act provides payment of reasonable attorneys' fees and costs. If the petition is filed by counsel, the filing attorney must be a member of the U.S. Court of Federal Claims Bar.

Physician Responsibility and Compliance

Under U.S. law, especially the Vaccine Injury Act of 1986 and its concomitant Vaccine Injury Compensation Program initiated on October 1, 1988, physicians are required to inform patients of the possibility that the vaccines to be administered may cause injury or death. The best study to date of the compliance of physicians with that law was done by T. C. Davis et al. (2004), who investigated compliance in the performance of routine vaccinations in response to a national survey of public health clinics (PHCs) that reported near-perfect compliance with the law. Davis and colleagues followed up this report by undertaking a more intensive look at 246 vaccine visits at two PHCs in Kansas and Louisiana. They found that the CDC-required "Vaccine Information Statement" warning patients of potential vaccine injuries was not provided to patients in 11% of the office visits. In addition, public health nurses failed to discuss vaccine side effects in 9% of the cases. The vaccine schedule mandated by the CDC was, however, discussed with 93% of the patients.

The most disappointing finding was that contraindications—instances where patients should have been warned about conditions that would prevent a vaccine from being used—were noted and screened in only 71% of the visits observed. Thus 29% of the children who should not have received a given vaccine owing to the risk of a possible adverse reaction got the injection anyway. It is commendable that 71% of the persons bringing children in for a vaccination were warned of conditions that should have prevented the child's being vaccinated, but what about the other 29%?

The most telling statistic was that although time for the whole visit averaged 20 minutes, time devoted to warnings about possible side effects, risks, and contraindications averaged less than 16 seconds. The latter time was also inflated by the fact that the researchers included the time it took for the staff to schedule the next visit to the clinic. No time—not for a single patient—was allocated for providing information about the Vaccine Injury Compensation Program (VICP).

Davis and colleagues noted that there is "room for improvement" in the "discussion of benefits, serious risks, and the VICP" (p. 228). Evidently, the PHCs studied had made little to no effort to inform patients of their rights under the Vaccine Injury Act of 1986 and devoted precious little time to discussing potential adverse reactions. Even in the 71% of cases where some discussion along those lines took place, it seems that the vast majority of the parents were persuaded to incur the risk of going ahead with the vaccination anyway, and none of them were told about their rights under the VICP.

THE LAW, SCIENCE, AND THE CITIZEN

In the ongoing court processes examining the *Omnibus Autism Proceeding* that began in 2007, many questions are at stake concerning the law, including what counts as scientific evidence in the cases and what the rights of individual citizens are under the law. The debates and legal battles currently under way in the courtroom, in the research arenas, and in the private sector reach out to touch all the citizens of the United States and the world. In the United States, the mandatory CDC vaccine schedule and the recommended shots that are not mandated directly affect virtually all of the country's citizens. Similarly, because the CDC influences the WHO, its policies affect not only residents of the United States but individuals in the rest of the world.

Looming in the background is the threat of bioweapons and the purported role of vaccines to defeat them or to minimize the damage they might do (see Chapter 7). In such a context, at such a time, comes the most pervasive epidemic of neurodevelopmental disorders in the history of our country and the world—the ubiquitous autism epidemic. The CDC and AAP can deny that this epidemic is real, but for reasons we have considered in detail in Chapter 2, those denials must be rejected. Exponential growth in incidence of the sort we are witnessing and documenting does not arise merely by chance. It is caused by something, and the implications of that causation affect us all—citizens of the United States and the peoples of the world alike.

In this section, we consider three aspects of law bearing heavily on legal determination of the causation of the autism epidemic. First, we consider the current rules for admitting scientific evidence about causation in courts of law as determined by the U.S. Supreme Court in *Daubert v. Merrell Dow Pharmaceuticals*, 509 U.S. 579 (1993). Second, we consider how the autism epidemic is leading toward changes in law with respect to the governance of insurance companies. Third, keeping in mind the evidence that vaccines are causally involved in producing the autism epidemic, we reflect on the freedom of individual citizens to decide what goes into their own or their children's bodies versus the arguments for mandatory vaccination under certain extreme conditions.

Daubert v. Merrell Dow Pharmaceuticals

In the ongoing litigation known as the *Omnibus Autism Proceeding*, there is a precedent referred to as *Daubert v. Merrell Dow Pharmaceuticals*, 509 U.S. 579 (1993 ◐), that is playing an important role.

In the *Daubert* case, two children and their parents claimed that an antinausea medication, Bendectin (manufactured and marketed by Merrell Dow Pharmaceuticals), which was taken prenatally by the mothers of both children, had caused serious birth defects in both of them. The children were Jason Daubert and Eric Schuller. In 1974, Jason Daubert was born missing three fingers on his right hand and a lower bone in his right arm. During her pregnancy with Jason, Mrs. Daubert had taken Bendectin. Schuller claimed similar injuries. Tests in lab animals showed that the drug could cause birth defects in rodents. However, a lower court had thrown out the evidence from rodent studies on the basis that such evidence was not generally accepted by the scientific community as valid. The case was then appealed and eventually was heard by the U.S. Supreme Court in 1993.

The majority opinion in the U.S. Supreme Court, written by Justice Harry Blackmun, noted that one of the issues was to prevent "junk" science from being presented in courts under the guise of "expert" testimony:

We conclude by briefly addressing what appear to be two underlying concerns of the parties and amici [their friends and supporters] in this case. Respondent expresses apprehension that abandonment of "general acceptance" as the exclusive requirement for admission will result in a "free-for-all" in which befuddled juries are confounded by absurd and irrational pseudoscientific assertions. ◐

The other issue was the fear that allowing judges too much latitude in ruling out some expert testimony would prevent genuine debate in areas where the truth about causal relationships, for instance, might not yet be generally known, much less widely accepted by stodgy scientific communities that may resist new findings not because they are wrong, but because they are merely unexpected. The majority held in Part III that there was a concern that

> . . . a screening role for the judge that allows for the exclusion of "invalid" evidence will sanction a stifling and repressive scientific orthodoxy, and will be inimical to the search for truth.

The majority of justices suggested different roles for law and science. According to them, the purpose of the courts operating under the law is "the particularized resolution of legal disputes," while the grand purpose of science is something more like "the exhaustive search for cosmic understanding" (at the end of Part III).

Reversing and Remanding

In the end, the question boiled down to whether the lower court judges had the right to throw out anything not "generally accepted" as "good" science by the relevant scientific community and then to render what is called a "summary judgment"—that is, a ruling in which the judge decides the case single-handedly. The U.S. Supreme Court ruled against that idea. The Court was unanimous in rejecting the idea that scientific evidence or expert testimony had to be "generally accepted" by the relevant scientific community to be admitted into evidence but expanded on that idea in Part IV of the ruling (to which Chief Justice William Rehnquist and Justice John Paul Stevens dissented):

> "General acceptance" is not a necessary precondition to the admissibility of scientific evidence under the Federal Rules of Evidence, but the Rules of Evidence, especially Rule 702, do assign to the trial judge the task of ensuring that an expert's testimony both rests on a reliable foundation and is relevant to the task at hand. Pertinent evidence based on scientifically valid principles will satisfy those demands.

As a result, the U.S. Supreme Court overturned both of the lower court rulings. The Ninth Circuit Court had granted a summary judgment in favor of the pharmaceutical industry on the grounds that the "general acceptance" criterion had not been met. Later, the U.S. Court of Appeals for the Ninth Circuit had upheld that decision. Both of the lower courts had disallowed expert testimony that the U.S. Supreme Court indicated must be heard. The highest court of the land, then, sent the case back for another round of hearings "consistent with this opinion"—that is, the published ruling in *Daubert* in 1993. The Supreme Court sent the case clear back to the Ninth Circuit Court. The lower court, presumably after allowing testimony that was disallowed earlier, still ruled in favor of the pharmaceutical company, just as it had in the prior instance. This result, of course, was applauded by the pharmaceutical industry as a victory, but it seems to have been the intention of the U.S. Supreme Court ruling in *Daubert* to provide greater latitude for introducing controversial scientific evidence in the courts. The question that remains is whether the Court achieved that goal.

Re-interpreting the Power of Judges to Admit Scientific Testimony

What the *Daubert* case did was to re-interpret the power of judges to assess what is or is not admissible expert testimony in court and what may be regarded as a valid scientific basis for that testimony. In a very important sense, the U.S. Supreme Court narrowed the power of the judges to throw out testimony and decide cases on a summary basis.

Prior to the *Daubert* case, in any U.S. court of law, the vague criterion for expert testimony was that it had to conform to whatever was "generally accepted" by the relevant scientific community. This rule was established by precedent in 1923 in *Frye v. United States*, 54 App. D. C. 46, 47, 293 F. 1013, 1014. In that case, the Court of Appeals of the District of Columbia threw out a "systolic blood pressure" test applied to show that the defendant, Frye, was lying concerning an alleged offense. The court ruled that the test had "not yet gained such standing and recognition among physiological and psychological authorities as would justify the courts in admitting expert testimony deduced from the discovery, development, and experiments thus far made" (Kadane, 2008, p. 51).

Under the *Frye* rule, a judge could decide that evidence was inadmissible only because it did not seem to be generally accepted in the scientific community. As a consequence, any controversial scientific finding could be thrown out of court by any judge on a whim. In its *Daubert* decision, the U.S. Supreme Court disallowed any such ruling. After *Frye,* when the Federal Rules of Evidence were enacted on January 2, 1975, and later amended (U.S. Government Printing Office, 2006 ◉), they provided a more explicit system for determining which expert testimony would be admissible in court. The 1975 rules contained just one section, Article VII, rules 701–706, pertaining to "Opinions and Expert Testimony" (pp. 13–15). However, in *Daubert* (Kadane, 2008, pp. 56–58), the Federal Rules of Evidence were re-interpreted.

Are Judges Competent to Assess Scientific Validity of Testimony?

A point that was contested in the dissenting opinion to *Daubert* written by Chief Justice Rehnquist and Justice Stevens was whether judges in courts throughout the land are competent to assess what is good or bad science:

> The Court speaks of its confidence that federal judges can make a "preliminary assessment of whether the reasoning or methodology underlying the testimony is scientifically valid, and of whether that reasoning or methodology properly can be applied to the facts in issue."

The dissenting Justices, with Chief Justice Rehnquist acting as spokesperson, reached the following conclusion:

> I [do not doubt that Rule 702 confides to the judge some gatekeeping responsibility] in deciding questions of the admissibility of proffered expert testimony. But I do not think it imposes on them either the obligation or the authority to become amateur scientists in order to perform that role. . . . (509 U.S. 579, 1 ◉)

The upshot of the case was to define more particularly the power of judges to decide which evidence is admissible in court. Succinctly put, the evidence presented by an expert only has to be relevant and reliable, not necessarily generally accepted by the larger scientific community. But how will ordinary judges make these decisions? They are usually trained in the law and are qualified to make judgments of ordinary facts. In contrast, the requirements of science are somewhat more abstract, general, and technical. A case in point concerns the use of the term **reliability**: It is often used in one way quite generally in the law and in another way, with a substantially different meaning, in the sciences. This difference in usage was pointed out in footnote 9 of *Daubert*. The majority opinion in *Daubert* explained that "our reference here is to evidentiary reliability, that is, trustworthiness." Contrasting with this usage, in the sciences, as the Court noted in footnote 9, "scientists typically distinguish between validity (does the principle support what it purports to show?) and reliability (does application of the principle produce consistent results?)."

Some have supposed that *Daubert* works to the advantage of defendants in cases of toxic injuries, but, as Yogi Berra has often been quoted as saying, "It ain't over till it's over." As yet, not all the facts are in on the long-range effects of *Daubert,* including how it will play out in the *Omnibus Autism Proceeding.*

What Counts as Reliable? Or, Reliability?

The U.S. Supreme Court established in *Daubert* that "reliable" evidence (trustworthy evidence) should have already been subjected to scientific tests that would refute it if it were false, should have been published in peer-reviewed journals or other peer-reviewed venues, and should have some established measure of its likelihood of being wrong. The earlier criterion of being "generally accepted" as a correct theory or standard knowledge by a relevant community of scientists was considered too demanding.

Obviously, the ultimate *Daubert* outcome, which went in favor of Merrell Dow Pharmaceuticals, was applauded by pharmaceutical companies. The long-term implications of the new criteria for allowing or disallowing "expert testimony" remain uncertain, however. If the new interpretations are strictly applied by the judges, the *Daubert* decision has made the task of plaintiffs in instances of toxic injury next to impossible. For that reason it is unsurprising that the *Daubert* precedent has been happily introduced in the *Omnibus Autism Proceeding* of 2007 by advocates for the drug industry. Those advocates include not only the companies' own employees and lawyers, but also at least some civil servants at the FDA, CDC, and Department of Health and Human Services. *Daubert* was not a particularly good result for people with any disabilities that may have been caused by prescribed drugs, medical procedures, or vaccines. Nevertheless, *Daubert* did establish as a matter of principle that "general acceptance" is not necessary for expert testimony to be admitted. It remains to be seen how the new and expanded power given to judges will be applied.

Insurance Coverage and the Autism Epidemic

One of the arguments that has been promoted by the CDC, the American Academy of Pediatrics, and the pharmaceutical companies and their amici (to use the legal term) is the strained notion that folks may have tended to prefer a diagnosis of autism to obtain federal funds (Fombonne, 2008) or to get insurance advantages. Neither of these claims is reasonable given that, in the vast majority of cases, until very recently, there have been no benefits provided to parents of children with autism. As J. Mitchell (2008) noted, in most instances, insurance companies have not even covered autism or pervasive developmental disorders at all. The argument has been that "treatments were either considered experimental or educational rather than medical." 🔊

In fact, according to an article published on September 2, 2008, in the *ASHA Leader,* by that time only eight states had laws requiring insurance coverage for the treatment of autism (Deppe, 2008). What is more, those laws had only recently been enacted and were passed over serious opposition. Among the states mentioned by Deppe with laws requiring some kind of insurance coverage for autism were Arizona, Connecticut, Florida, Hawaii, Louisiana, Missouri, and New Hampshire. South Carolina would be added to the list as of July 1, 2008, over a governor's veto (National Public Radio, 2007 🔊), and Pennsylvania as of September 12, 2008. However, not all commentators are in favor of the promised results of legislative acts requiring insurance companies to pay for the treatment of autism. What kind of treatment will be provided and how will the determination of which services to provide be made?

In many instances, as was the case in South Carolina until the new law went into effect in July 2008, if a child was ever diagnosed with autism (ASD or PDD), the insurance company would immediately cut off any funding of further medical treatment contending that the problem was "strictly an educational issue and that it was not a medical problem" (National Public Radio, 2007). This is exactly what happened to a child of Lisa Rollins and the parents of other children with autism in South Carolina prior to the passage of the new law. She and two other parents wrote the bill to mandate coverage by insurance companies for autism in South Carolina. The bill that she and colleagues pushed through the state legislature, however, covers only about 25% of the cases in the state. The law in South Carolina encountered vigorous opposition and required sufficient votes to push it through over the veto of South Carolina governor Mark Sanford. According to the Autism Speaks Web site (n.d.), at the time of this writing, there are now 10 states where insurance is provided for the treatment of autism spectrum disorders—Arizona, Florida, Illinois, Indiana, Louisiana, Montana, New Mexico, Pennsylvania, South Carolina, and Texas 🔊. In fact, it is because of the general practice of insurance companies to exclude the diagnosis and treatment of autism (ASD or PDD) from coverage that President Barack Obama has proposed the Federal Autism Insurance Reform Bill (n.d.). There would be no need for the discussion that is still going on at the federal level if it were not for the fact that insurance companies have routinely refused to cover the diagnosis and treatment of ASDs on the theory that they are genetic in nature and, therefore, are preexisting and medically untreatable conditions. Even now, it would seem that in 41 states, insurance companies do not have to cover autism under existing laws. Among the states that do have laws requiring insurance companies to cover autism is Louisiana.

Because the Louisiana Insurance/Health House Bill 958 is a relatively strong example and because it was signed into law relatively recently by Governor Bobby Jindal (July 16, 2008), it can serve as an example of the first step in requiring insurance companies to recognize the ASDs as medically and otherwise treatable. When Governor Jindal officially signed into law HB 516/SB 241 (formerly known as HB 958), Louisiana became one of 10 states, to date, that "have ended insurance discrimination against children with autism." The law requires insurers to cover up to $36,000 per year for applied behavior analysis (ABA) and other necessary treatments until a child reaches age 17. Governor Jindal formally signed the bill at a ceremony at the Greater Baton Rouge Families Helping Families office. An employee, Toni Peters, was instrumental in bringing the idea for the legislation to the attention of Representative Franklin J. Foil of Baton Rouge, the bill's sponsor.

Louisiana HB 516/SB 241 requires group health insurance plans and group benefits programs to provide coverage for diagnosis and treatment. The maximum benefit is $36,000 per year, with a lifetime cap of $144,000. Coverage begins after January 1, 2009, and extends to diagnosis, behavioral therapy, pharmaceutical intervention, psychiatric, psychological, and therapeutic care. The Louisiana law has been pointed to as a model for other states.

Immunity Under the Law

Finally, keeping in mind the evidence in previous chapters that vaccines are causally involved in producing the autism epidemic, we cannot close this chapter without dealing with the broader issue of laws pertaining to the use of vaccines. In 2003, Stuart Lieberman asked some penetrating questions about the association between the Homeland Security Act of 2002 and something he called "vaccine immunity." He was not speaking of any immunity produced in any individual by any vaccine, but rather of an immunity provided to vaccine manufacturers under the new law. Lieberman was formerly a New Jersey Deputy Attorney General assigned to the State Department of Environmental Protection from 1986 to 1990. In 2003, he was a shareholder associated with the environmental law firm of Lieberman & Blecher, P.C., in Princeton, New Jersey. Trusting that the pharmaceutical manufacturers would stop making thimerosal-containing vaccines, he wrote in 2003:

> While vaccines containing thimerosal are no longer made, it is reported that certain clinics in this country are still using stockpiled vaccines dating back to the time which they were made. ☁

The stockpiles have been verified, but the CDC, WHO, and vaccine manufacturers worldwide have indicated their clear intention to continue supplying thimerosal-containing vaccines to the less developed nations throughout the world. Lieberman's statement was correct only in supposing that stockpiled vaccines containing thimerosal were still being used in the United States. This point was also made by Dr. Jon Poling on March 6, 2008, in his interview with Dr. Sanjay Gupta (CNN, 2008). Given this fact, we will not be able to see the full effects of thimerosal's removal from vaccines in the United States, or the damage done prior to its removal, perhaps until the year 2009 or 2010, when the last of the cohorts of U.S. children who received thimerosal-containing vaccines finally arrive in schools where records are being kept and reported under current federal legislation. Even then, any effects of the removal of thimerosal will be clouded by the fact that many additional vaccines have been proposed and some have already been added to the schedule since the phase-out of thimerosal-containing vaccines began in the United States.

In the meantime, however, overwhelming evidence exists showing that a great deal of harm has already been done. Thimerosal is not the only culprit in the vaccines, but it is one of the most harmful ingredients known to be interacting with other toxins and disease agents.

Lieberman continued:

> At the end of the day, one must question why the Federal Government would pass a Homeland Security Bill seemingly hav[ing] nothing to do with vaccines [a]nd in the recesses of this Bill would be protection for American drug manufacturers.

He went on to say very politely:

> Children who have been affected by the use of this product may have been poisoned by mercury, and may have to struggle with ill effects for the rest of their lives. ☁

With the evidence now in hand, we can say that anyone receiving thimerosal in any vaccine was poisoned. When Morris Kharasch patented thimerosal in 1932 and 1935 on behalf of Eli Lilly, he already had data showing its extreme neurotoxic impact on human beings. In the end, it is necessary to ask, as Lieberman did, "What will Congress do for the victims?"

SUMMING UP AND LOOKING AHEAD

In this chapter, we considered the nature of the more than 5300 cases that are currently under review in the *Omnibus Autism Proceeding*. Hannah Poling's case cannot be regarded as isolated or extraordinary. In particular, the mitochondrial dysfunction discovered in her case is far less exceptional than claimed by the CDC's director Dr. Julie Gerberding. The attribution of Hannah's autism disorder to preexisting genetic traits also seems unlikely in view of the research showing that mitochondrial dysfunction can certainly be caused by thimerosal. Her so-called regressive type of autism is also unexceptional. If parents had known in 1943 what is now known about the interactive effects of disease agents and toxins in vaccines, it might have turned out that the descent from a perfectly normal sequence of developmental milestones into autism has always been characteristic of the majority of cases, just as it is now.

Logicomathematical reasoning supports the rational expectation that ordinary truth, as noted by the majority of the U.S. Supreme Court Justices in the *Daubert* case, will prevail over fictional fantasies, errors, and junk science. Although as Kuhn (1962) showed, science often advances by leaps that are preceded by novel findings that are at first rejected and only later regarded as obviously true (as the cynic Schopenhauer observed), if an idea or hypothesis is correct, experimental facts and observations substantiating it will become known. General truths do not exist in completely unembodied forms. Rather, as our own logicomathematical arguments along with those of Peirce, Tarski, and others have demonstrated, they are discoverable only through particular facts. As a result, true representations of ordinary factual observations—the kind that science depends on—are certain to be more consistent, more comprehensive, and simpler than false, fictional, erroneous, or deliberately deceptive ones. The story and video evidence of Christian the lion both illustrate and exemplify these logicomathematical conclusions.

The best and most recent research on communication between pediatricians and patients on "well-baby" visits (i.e., vaccination visits) shows that the pediatricians and nurses, in the majority of cases, are more diligent in giving the shots than in telling patients about the dangers of vaccines—much less of their rights under VICP. This chapter also explored how the *Daubert* ruling re-interpreted the Federal Rules of Evidence, reviewed the changing insurance laws covering ASDs, and considered the strange immunization of vaccine manufacturers from liability for thimerosal-related vaccine injuries that was included and then removed from the Homeland Security Act.

STUDY AND DISCUSSION QUESTIONS

1. Weighing the evidence, do you think Hannah Poling's case is exceptional? Which factors persuade you in making this decision?

2. When speaking of the descent into autism from a formerly normal course of development, why should we call it a "regression"? Why not call it a "fall"?

3. What are some of the superfluous facts that are noticed after we already have enough information to make a correct perceptual judgment in a particular case—for example, in applying the term "autism" to Hannah Poling or in recognizing an old friend in an unexpected context?

4. What is wrong with the one-size-fits-all approach to vaccines?

5. How does communication in science, law, and medicine work in favor of advances toward a truer (more reliable and valid) understanding of facts and against propaganda and fictions? Consider the Internet as a tool in the ongoing warfare of ideas.

6. How does the power of unity work in favor of the *Omnibus Autism Proceeding* cases?

7. What did T. C. Davis and colleagues learn about the compliance of medical service providers with respect to vaccinations? How are the providers doing with reference to contraindications and informing patients of risks and remedies?

8. Why is the *Daubert* case considered an important precedent by both sides in the *Omnibus Autism Proceeding* cases?

9. Should judges at any level be called on to determine what is or is not junk science? Reliable evidence? Admissible expert testimony concerning scientific matters? Why or why not?

10. Which factors will make it difficult to measure the effects of removing thimerosal from vaccines manufactured in the United States? Also, why will this determination, if any, have to be made sometime after 2009, according to Dr. Jon Poling?

chapter nine

Germs, Genes, and Viruses

OBJECTIVES

In this chapter, we

1. Discuss the contrast between theories of discrete germs, genes, and viruses with theories of integrated systems.

2. Compare the role of sanitation as contrasted with trying to kill infections already under way.

3. Discuss the communication systems underlying genetically regulated metabolism, growth, development, immunity, and detoxification.

4. Revisit the theory of the "toxic tipping point" and reconsider the plausibility of the idea that a mix of toxins, disease agents, and genetic factors is causing the autism epidemic.

5. Show why a systems approach grounded in communication and complex language-like systems is required to amplify the discrete germ theory.

6. Discuss the fact that wellness depends on a balance between all of the bodily systems interacting with each other and with the environment.

The germ theory of disease has a peculiar place in the history of science and especially in medicine. Some have argued (e.g., Abedon, 1998) that its introduction was the single greatest advance in the history of medicine and perhaps in the history of science. Although the widespread acceptance of the germ theory did not occur until Louis Pasteur's experiments between 1859 and 1864 became well known, the idea was proposed somewhat earlier by others, especially a Hungarian obstetrician, Ignaz Semmelweis [1818–1865]. By 1847, in the Vienna General Hospital in Austria, Semmelweis had reduced the high incidence of death caused by infections that occurred during childbirth to less than 2%. It is noteworthy that this accomplishment took place without the benefit of antibiotics, and well before the marketing of any vaccines. Semmelweis's method consisted of nothing more than simple handwashing and cleaning of instruments and bedclothes at the hospital (see "Ignaz Semmelweis," 2009).

In this chapter, we consider the essential history leading up to the widespread acceptance of the germ theory. From there, we look forward to the current autism epidemic. As we have discovered through evidence discussed in earlier chapters, it now appears that the autism epidemic is caused by multiple factors, including exposure to disease agents (germs and viruses of various sorts) and toxins, all of which interact with genetic factors.

As important as the germ theory of diseases was and is today, it is now clear that its widespread acceptance was an important historical factor in helping to set the stage for the rise of the pharmaceutical and medical industries and professions. In considering what has been learned from the germ theory of disease, we also see the crucial roles played by sanitation measures, antiseptics, natural and synthetic antibiotics, and, finally, vaccines and the widespread experiments with them that have been going on for a century and a half with animals and humans. Taking a holistic, systems-oriented view of health, we revisit the theory of the toxic tipping point as the basis for the autism epidemic. First, however, we discuss the discrete germ theory in some detail.

DISCRETE GERMS AND VIRUSES AS DISEASE AGENTS

It was Louis Pasteur who conclusively refuted the prevailing view that microbes could just form themselves spontaneously from inorganic matter. Prior to Pasteur's demonstrations, and before the **germ theory of disease** was taken seriously, the even more radical idea that insects, crustaceans, frogs, and rodents (mice in particular) could arise spontaneously from rotting plants or even soiled clothing had been widely propagated. For citations of specific arguments that had been widely accepted up to his time, see the lecture "On Spontaneous Generation" by Pasteur (delivered in French in 1864; English translation by Latour & Levine, 1993). The acceptance of the germ theory not only ended the popular but false claims for the spontaneous generation of life, but also opened the way for new understanding of diseases and their causation.

Experimental Demonstrations

In 1859, Pasteur performed his award-winning demonstration that microorganisms do not arise by spontaneous generation. The key questions that he put to a series of experimental tests were these:

> Could not matter, perhaps, organize itself? Or posed differently, could not creatures enter the world without parents, without forebears? This is the question I seek to resolve. (Pasteur, 1864, p. 1)

After a series of brilliant, yet relatively simple experiments begun in 1859, Pasteur would give a lecture in 1864 at the Sorbonne in Paris summarizing those experiments that, as he described them, had already dealt the "mortal blow" to the "doctrine of spontaneous generation" (p. 17). Pasteur showed that even the tiniest of microbes do not arise by chance; in other words, even microbes have biological parentage. As demonstrated by Pasteur, they, like other organisms, come from similar organisms. At the same time, microbes can commonly be found on dust particles in unpurified air and water. Pasteur used this evidence to argue for the germ theory of disease. He illustrated and described the germ theory in this way:

> Which of you has failed to amuse himself by following with his eyes the capricious move-ment of those countless tiny bodies, so small in volume, so light in weight, that the air bears them as easily as smoke? The air in this room is replete with dust motes, with those tiny

nothings which ought not always to be despised, for they sometimes carry sickness or death, in the form of typhus, cholera, yellow fever, and many other kinds of flux. (p. 12)

Pasteur then demonstrated the dust in the air by turning out all the lights in the room except for a bright one, in the cone of which he showed particles of dust floating in the air. He pointed out that they were all, however, falling:

> At this very moment, dust falls on the objects before me: on these books, this paper, this table, and on the mercury in this vat. (p. 13)

As it would turn out, Pasteur would convince all the world of his theory of germs, and yet, in the process of doing so, he would inadvertently poison himself and his entire audience. The amount of the mercury vapors to which Pasteur, his assistant, and his audience were exposed is difficult to estimate, but the exposure, given the description of the amounts of mercury required for his demonstrations, must have been substantial. In any case, a little more than four years after his lecture in April 1864, at the relatively young age of 45, Pasteur would suffer a paralyzing stroke on October 19, 1868 (see Pasteur, n.d.).

Why the Vat of Liquid Mercury?

Pasteur's purpose in using the vat of liquid mercury during his demonstration was to illustrate how a certain series of experiments by Pouchet and Houzeau (1858) had accidentally been contaminated by dust particles containing spores of mold and other microbes. Pasteur quoted from the original authors:

> A liter-flask is filled with boiling water and, having been hermetically sealed with greatest care, it is inverted over a vat of mercury; once the water has completely cooled, the flask is uncorked below the metal's surface, and a half-liter of pure oxygen is introduced. (As quoted by Pasteur, 1864, p. 10.)

The purpose of all the care—and of the vat of mercury, in particular—was to prevent the introduction of any seeds, spores, or preexisting microbes into the flask.

Next, just as Pouchet described it in his experiments, Pasteur demonstrated to his audience how it was possible to immerse under the surface of the mercury a vial containing 10 grams of hay. After it had been hermetically sealed in the glass vial, the hay had been purified by cooking it at 100 degrees centigrade in an oven for 30 minutes (to kill any possibly remaining microbes). Beneath the surface of the mercury, the vial containing the hay would be inserted into the inverted flask containing the purified water, which would be sealed and returned to the surface. Pouchet and his assistant showed that approximately eight days later, even after this severe sterilization, the liquid would contain a visible culture of mold. Pouchet concluded that the source of this mold was spontaneous generation—that is, the mold came from nothing.

Any thought that the air in Pouchet's sealed flask might have been contaminated was removed, according to Pouchet, by the fact that he extracted the oxygen from "a chemical compound" (water) so that it could not have contained any microbes. The possibility that the water might have contained microbes was supposedly ruled out by the fact that it was boiling hot when placed in the vial. Finally, there remained, in his thinking, only the hay as the possible source of any parent microbes, seeds, or spores to give rise to the subsequent mold.

Concerning that possibility, Pouchet went to extremes. He showed that he could get the same results—the mold would arise within eight days inside the sealed container—even if he cooked the hay for 30 minutes at 200 or 300 degrees centigrade. In fact, he claimed that the same mold appeared inside the sealed flask if the hay was cooked to the point of carbonization. In other words, the experiment came out the same if the 10 grams of hay was burned down to a black cinder.

Pasteur's Solution in the Mercury Problem

Pasteur was more skeptical: Could microbes have contaminated the sealed flask in Pouchet's experiments? Recalling the dust particles in the air, Pasteur reasoned that dust would accumulate on the surface of the vat of liquid mercury. This fact he had demonstrated with the cone of light showing the dust motes landing on the surface of the mercury, but now he added more dust just for good measure for the sake of his lecture demonstration. Then he inserted a glass stirring stick into the liquid, showing that it would carry the dust under the surface of the mercury. The conclusive demonstration was described by Pasteur in this way:

> Here, gentlemen, we have a much deeper vat, in which this same experiment may be performed to more startling effect. It consists in an iron tube one meter in depth, topped by a shallow basin. The entire surface of the mercury has been covered with dust. As I insert the glass rod, bit by bit, the mercury's surface clears, recovering its former metallic aspect. All of the dust is now contained within the metal fluid, in the lower part of the vase. As the rod is withdrawn, the surface once again becomes covered with dust. (Pasteur, 1864, p. 13)

Because the glass repelled the mercury but carried the dust on its surface down into the heavy liquid, Pasteur had demonstrated how the dust could reach the mouth of the sealed flask beneath the mercury. As a result, he showed how the hermetically sealed vial of 10 grams of cooked hay that had been introduced into each of Pouchet's experiments was also contaminated before the flask was resealed and brought to the surface of the mercury.

Pouchet had himself inadvertently and unknowingly introduced the spores of the mold that would consistently appear inside the hermetically sealed vials in his experiments within about eight days. With the help of a microscope, a projector, and an assistant, Pasteur was able to show to his audience the mold spores found in the sealed vials from a replication of Pouchet's experiments. The audience could see and compare the mold spores from the sealed vials with identical spores found on particles of dust captured by filtering the air in the same room where the demonstration was taking place.

However, the several experiments that would clinch the case against spontaneous generation were still to come. Pasteur anticipated the next part of his presentation by saying, "Gentlemen, I hasten to provide you with experiments so gripping that you cannot fail to remember them, even if you forget the others" (pp. 15–16).

The Mortal Blow to the Theory of Spontaneous Generation

Having already shown his audience that particles of dust fall slowly through the air by the force of gravity, Pasteur next described how he could take a hermetically sealed beaker (i.e., a tube that was made air-tight in one way or another, such as the one shown in Figure 9-1, which was sealed by closing the end of the glass tube) and, by breaking off the sealed end of the S-shaped glass tube, he could expose the purified material inside the container to air through the now-open glass tube. Because of the bend in the tube shown in Figure 9-1, air can enter the tube from the outside and can come in contact with the purified materials in the liquid inside. However, dust particles cannot enter the flask where the liquid is because, being subject to gravity, the dust particles settle to the bottom of the bent tube without ever coming in contact with the liquid inside the container.

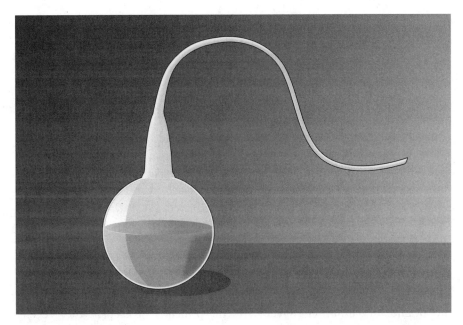

Figure 9-1 Pasteur's beaker, open to air, but not to dust particles in the air or the microbes associated with them.
Source: Adapted from an illustration by Yassine Mrabet.

If the glass tube were heated and bent so that it exposed the liquid to falling dust particles, on the other hand, the purified liquid would be contaminated by microbes. Pasteur's prediction was that purified liquid exposed to ordinary dust particles would soon culture microbes, just as happened in Pouchet's experiments. The same purified liquid exposed to air through a bent tube such as the one shown in Figure 9-1, however, he predicted would develop no such contamination. In fact, in flasks of purified materials exposed to air but not to dust particles, with a flask of the shape seen in Figure 9-1, Pasteur found no contamination no matter how long he waited for it:

> . . . the liquid in this second flask will remain completely unaltered, not just for two days, or three, or four, or even a month, a year, three years, or four! For the experiment just described has already been under way that long. (p. 16)

By contrast, identical beakers with straight tubes that allowed dust particles from the air to fall into the liquid developed flourishing microbial cultures within a few days. Pasteur found that by sealing, sterilizing, and preventing contamination, so that contact with the dust particles in the air could not take place, he could prevent the later appearance of microorganisms in any medium. Much earlier, Francesco Redi [1626–1697] had demonstrated that maggots do not appear in meat that has not been touched by flies. From Redi's experiments, it was understood that flies must lay their eggs for maggots to form. Nearly two centuries later, in 1864, Pasteur's experiments showed that even much tinier microbes depended on parentage of some sort. Pasteur's experiments catapulted him and the discrete germ theory to prominence.

When Pasteur showed his audience the seed spores of mold he announced, "These, gentlemen, are the germs of microscopic beings." He went on to say:

> The doctrine of spontaneous generation will never recover from the mortal blow inflicted by this experiment. (p. 12)

Pasteur's work did not end there, however. He went on to demonstrate that microbes do not occupy every bubble of air on the earth, as some had supposed. He did so by exposing 20 purified samples of a suitable culture medium to distinct layers of air and then resealing the flasks. Pasteur performed the experiment in the rarified air of the glacier at the top of Montblanc, then repeated it twice more as he came down the mountain. His results showed that some of the resealed flasks remained uncontaminated, indicating that the air in more remote regions and higher altitude was purer. Pasteur also experimented with sealed urine, blood, and animal tissues. Because he could not heat the latter elements without damaging or permanently altering their chemistry, he merely avoided contamination by contact with the air. He had begun experiments with biological fluids, urine, and blood in 1863, and he observed in his lecture in 1864 that

> the blood and urine remain just as they were when extracted from living animals. And so, once again, I conclude that the spontaneous generation of microscopic beings is a mere chimera. (p. 21)

The Long-Term Impact of the Germ Theory

Many consequences flowed from Pasteur's findings. Foremost among them was his having demonstrated the importance of sanitation—specifically, the principle of **asepsis**, the prevention of contamination by disease agents. Pasteur's findings showed plainly that by preventing exposure to disease-producing microbes, infections could be prevented. This idea had already been advocated, somewhat ahead of its time, by Semmelweis (Nuland, 2003).[1] It was Semmelweis who would be acknowledged—albeit after his death—by Dr. Joseph Lister, the surgeon who would actually receive the lion's share of public credit for advocating the use of **antiseptics** in 1865. The record shows that Lister credited Semmelweis as the person who first insisted on using antiseptic procedures in hospitals. In fact, he did so well before Pasteur's famous experiments gave a firmer basis and explanation for the germ theory of disease.

In 1847, 12 years before Pasteur's first experiments in 1859 gained him notoriety, Semmelweis advocated antiseptic procedures as the means to prevent infections. Before he began teaching medicine at Vienna General Hospital in 1847, Semmelweis noted between 1841 and 1847 that a remarkably high percentage of the women giving birth, almost 19% on the average (see Figure 9-2), developed **puerperal (childbirth) fever**. Semmelweis inferred that the high incidence of infections was caused by contamination carried by doctors who often went directly from the autopsy of a patient who had died of puerperal fever to deliver a baby. His faith in this idea was strengthened when his friend, Dr. Jakob Kolletschka, was accidentally cut with a scalpel used in an autopsy of a woman who had been infected and who had died of puerperal fever; Kolletschka himself also became infected and died. Semmelweis concluded that the contamination from the handling of cadavers by young interns was infecting healthy women during childbirth.

He supposed that infection was being transmitted through the soiled hands of the doctors. When he started teaching at the medical school in May 1847, he insisted that the interns at the hospital must wash their hands between the dissection area, where they handled cadavers at autopsy, before going to the live birthing rooms. For this purpose, Semmelweis used a cleanser (disinfectant) consisting of chlorinated lime solution. Subsequently, the number of women becoming infected with and dying of puerperal fever (see Figure 9-2) dropped markedly until Semmelweis was dismissed in 1849.

---

[1] We are indebted to our friend and colleague, Dr. David Kennedy, DDS, and former president of the International Academy of Oral Medicine and Toxicology, for first directing us to consider the importance of the historical findings and work of Dr. Semmelweis.

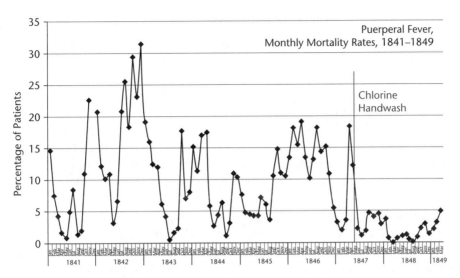

Figure 9-2 Statistics on puerperal fever from Vienna hospital 1841–1849 where Dr. Semmelweis taught medicine from 1847 until 1849 (and instituted the practice of hand washing).
Source: Data from Ignaz Philipp Semmelweis, 1862, *Offener Brief an sämtliche Professoren der Geburtshilfe* [*Open letter to all professors of obstetrics*]. Ofen (Budapest), Hungary: Royal Hungarian University of Buchdruckerei.

It seemed strange to historian J. H. Lienhard (1988–1997) that Semmelweis did not publish his findings. But, as Lienhard later learned, Semmelweis's supervisor felt criticized by Semmelweis's insistence on the new sanitation measures. He blocked Semmelweis from promotion, encouraged dissent by the Viennese doctors at the hospital who already thought the Hungarian strange, and arranged for his dismissal from the hospital in 1849. It appears from the records of Vienna General Hospital that the lowest rates of mortality by puerperal fever occurred when Semmelweis was insisting on handwashing and other cleanliness measures.

After leaving Vienna, Semmelweis moved back to Hungary, where he practiced obstetrics under much more primitive conditions in Budapest. Nevertheless, by practicing better hygiene, he reduced the rate of death in his new facility to about 1% (Nuland, 2003). We might have hoped that everyone working in hospitals would gladly embrace Semmelweis's findings concerning sanitation—but that is not what happened. For the next 12 years, Semmelweis collected additional data on his hygienic procedures. In 1861, he finally did publish his results recommending hygienic procedures and documenting their success with statistical data. The reception for Semmelweis's work by mainstream doctors, however, was not positive, and Semmelweis became angry and discouraged. He further alienated himself from the medical community by writing letters (e.g., the famous "Open letter . . ." of 1862) accusing his contemporaries of murdering their patients.

In 1865, Semmelweis was committed to an insane asylum and died within two weeks. According to Lienhard, Semmelweis cut his hand and died of infection, but the Semmelweis Society International (2009) suggests he was "severely beaten by guards." 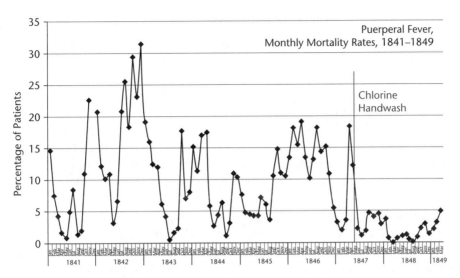. In the years after his death, owing to the importance of antisepsis and hygienic (asepsis) procedures, Semmelweis's work would save millions of lives. In the year following the death of Semmelweis, Dr. Joseph Lister [1827–1912] introduced the practice of washing surgical instruments with carbolic acid (Nuland, 1988). According to Lienhard, when recognized for his own work with antiseptic procedures, Lister protested, "Without Semmelweis, my achievements would be nothing."

COMBATING INFECTIONS AND DISEASE CONDITIONS ALREADY UNDER WAY

Trying to destroy an infectious agent that has already entered the body is like the military trying to deal with an invading army that is already inside the territory to be defended. The problem with "surgical strikes" against such invaders is the high likelihood of "collateral damage." When attacking an invader, innocent bystanders—not to mention property and real estate—tend to be damaged or destroyed. Sometimes the damage to friends may be greater than the damage to enemies. For this reason, dealing with an infection or disease condition that is already under way is generally less desirable than dealing with it before the invasion by disease agents, toxins, injuries, or any other disease condition can get started. It follows that sanitation (asepsis)—a means of dealing with the potential problem before it becomes a real one—is preferred over dealing with an infection that is already under way.

It is always better to prevent a disease or injury before it happens than to try to halt the disease or repair the damage from the injury after the fact. With toxins and disease agents, avoidance of exposure, asepsis, is generally preferred over antisepsis or antibiotic interventions. But how do we respond to diseases that have already gotten under way? How do we deal with toxins after we have already been exposed? In such undesirable cases, we generally aim first for survival and second to minimize future damage or repair any damage that may have already occurred.

Setting the Limits

In emergency situations, it may become necessary to differentiate conditions judged to be inevitably fatal from ones that can be treated successfully. The process of making such judgments is universally known by the French term **triage** (from the French verb *trier,* meaning "to sort" or "to sift"), though there are many variations in practice. In cases of extreme injuries or epidemic infectious diseases, persons affected may be sorted into categories. Color coding may sometimes be used, where a black armband or tape means "unlikely to survive under the constraints at hand"; red means "needs immediate medical care to survive"; yellow means "needs hospitalization but is not in imminent danger" (care can be delayed for a few minutes or longer); green means "in need of treatment but able to survive for hours or days without treatment"; and white means "has only minor injuries or disease conditions that do not require professional medical attention."

In dealing with the autism epidemic, the degree of severity of symptoms, in nontechnical terms, can be said to fall generally into the green or white category. Self-injurious behaviors such as head-banging, extreme gut pain, seizures, and combinations of these would, however, cross into the yellow category and move into the red zone. Moreover, in view of the research findings related to the pervasiveness of digestive problems, seizures, gut disease, toxicity, oxidative stress, compromised immune defenses, neurological abnormalities, and mitochondrial dysfunctions (to mention the more prominent of the chronic conditions associated with autism), it is reasonable to infer that the life expectancy of persons with any form of autism probably will not be in the normal range of 70-plus years, as has commonly been supposed (e.g., at the Autism Summit Conference in the lecture by Shestack, 2003).

On the contrary, as more data are collected on the large number of persons who have been diagnosed with autism over the last three to four decades, all research evidence and sound theoretical reasoning suggest that the diagnosis of autism must be tantamount to a significantly shortened life expectancy. In fact, research in Denmark with 341 individuals diagnosed with an ASD between 1960 and 1993 has already confirmed this prediction. The Danish data sample, at an average age of 43 years, showed a death rate twice that of the national average (Mouridsen, Hansen, Rich, & Isager, 2008). Approximately 31% of the deaths recorded in the Danish sample studied were attributed to epileptic-type seizures.

With the foregoing information in mind, we feel an increased sense of urgency about discovering the causes of the known chronic disease conditions associated with autism. Discovering the causes is essential so that effective treatment can be applied to alleviate those symptoms, to halt and possibly repair the damage, and to prevent additional problems wherever possible. Without question, when the additional risks that accompany chronic disease conditions are taken into consideration, as they must be for persons on the autism spectrum, minimizing exposure to toxins and disease agents should be a very high priority. Also, because the risks are much higher for persons already affected by chronic stress and disease conditions, it is, we argue, necessary to rethink the application of the standard discrete germ theory of disease.

As we understand more about genetic and epigenetic interactions throughout the body, it is becoming increasingly clear that the threshold of the tipping point for someone on the autism spectrum is certain to be much lower than for a person who is not coping with those chronic disease conditions. Exposures to disease agents and toxins that would fall well beneath the injury threshold for most persons may prove extremely dangerous, or even life-threatening, to persons on the autism spectrum. For this reason, we must think very carefully through the theories of preventive medicine, gathered loosely under the term **prophylaxis**, when those theories are applied to persons affected by the current epidemic of neurological disorders. In addition to avoiding unnecessary exposures to toxins and disease agents (e.g., as found in vaccines), it is necessary to consider what to do about the ongoing effects of toxins and disease agents that are already contributing to the symptoms of autism in most, if not in all, of the affected individuals.

As Pasteur demonstrated (see Abedon, 1998), the simplest, and perhaps the most effective, form of prophylaxis against infectious diseases is to avoid the germs or disease agents in advance—the method known as asepsis. If those microorganisms cannot be avoided, then perhaps we can kill them before they infect us. This latter method is the basis of sterilization, which works by heating or using a killing antiseptic such as Clorox or rubbing alcohol. Asepsis was the method demonstrated by Pasteur in his famous experiment where he simply prevented the entry of dust particles into an open flask by bending the tube. His experiments showed, in principle and in fact, that if there is no contamination by germs (the aseptic approach), there can be no infection by them.

In cases where an infection by a disease agent or contamination by a toxin has already occurred in a living organism, procedures can be followed after the fact to minimize or prevent damage to the body. If the disease agent progresses slowly, as is the case with an infection by the rabies virus (see Figure 9-3), treatment by a vaccine may be possible. Pasteur himself was involved in the development of the first supposedly successful rabies vaccine. Because the rabies virus takes time to damage the central nervous system, Pasteur inferred that it would be possible to introduce an attenuated form of the disease to produce immunity before the virile form could reach the central nervous system. It was generally agreed that he succeeded. In cases where too much time had elapsed from the exposure to the treatment, it was later found that the individual affected could be given immunoglobulin from a person (or animal) that had survived the disease. In the latter instance, the theory is that the defenses built up by the organism that has survived a previous exposure will assist a different organism in surviving an infection by the same disease agent.

Reexamining the Theory of Vaccines

As suggested by Stan Kurtz, and as borne out by empirical research, active disease agents are generally ranked near the top of the body's innate "Most Wanted" list for a counterattack. That is to say, the body's defense systems seem to devote major resources to capturing, disabling, interrogating, and eventually destroying active disease agents that penetrate its natural defenses (also see Jepson & Johnson, 2007). When the body is functioning up to par, it normally mobilizes considerable

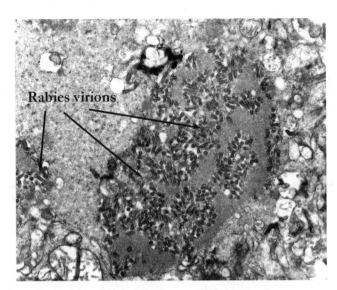

Figure 9-3 The rabies virus magnified by a factor of about 2 million times its actual size. An electron micrograph photo by Magnus Manske, April 6, 2008.
Source: Courtesy of F. A. Murphy/CDC.

immune defense resources against potential disease agents. Often the area under attack will become inflamed, feverish, and sensitive to the touch.

Toxic injuries, by contrast, seem to be assigned a lower priority. These injuries may sometimes be subtle and without overt signs that they are even taking place. The person affected may be **asymptomatic** or, at least, the symptoms may go unnoticed even by trained observers. There may be undefined symptoms or issues that are noticed only after the fact. Special tests or measurement procedures may be necessary to detect toxicity even when it is present.

Active disease agents—that is, invading microbes or viruses—are typically assigned relatively higher priority for active countermeasures, as indicated by inflammation of the lymph nodes, fever, swelling, mucus or pus accumulation, and so on. Whereas toxins are routinely handled at a lower level in the defense hierarchy, the body mobilizes highly sophisticated communication and defense systems to deal with what it perceives as active disease agents. Nevertheless, it is important to bear in mind that the immune and detoxification systems normally work hand in hand; as discussed in earlier chapters, disease agents commonly produce toxins of their own, and both disease agents and their toxins can interact with other disease agents and with toxins from other sources.

The discrete germ theory was not only very useful to the eventual development of the theories underlying vaccines and immunity, but also important in the development of essentially all of the known forms of prophylaxis. At about the time Jenner proposed using cowpox to strengthen the body's defenses against smallpox, the stage had already been set for the future development of other forms of prophylaxis. For instance, it did not take long to develop the idea that existing resources in an immune organism might be provided to an immune-deficient one to protect the latter organism against a particular disease agent. If the infectious agent was already present in an unprotected organism, perhaps the defenses developed by an organism with strong immunity against that particular agent could help.

The prophylactic theory of vaccines was exemplified from the beginning in the classic case of cowpox virus used by Jenner to try to prevent smallpox infections. The secondary development was to attempt to harness existing defenses of an already immune organism A to protect a different organism B—say, against an invading disease agent already in B's body. An excellent example of how this chain of events would unfold can be found in the history of the treatment of rabies. Because the disease progressed slowly from an infected area, typically where a person had been bitten by a rabid animal, up through the nerves of the infected person until the brain became inflamed, it was possible (in theory at least) to give the body advance warning of the coming onslaught of the rabies virus. What Pasteur did in the first "successful" treatment was to inject a weakened form of the disease agent into the infected person repeatedly over several months to stimulate the body's defenses. Later, this procedure would be supplemented by also giving the infected person the immunoglobulin of an organism known (or believed) to be immune to the infectious agent. However, there was a difference in the aims and urgency levels of Jenner and Pasteur in developing vaccines. Jenner wanted to make individuals immune to smallpox prior to exposure to it, whereas Pasteur was aiming to prevent death from rabies after the person to be treated had already been gravely, usually fatally (prior to Pasteur's vaccine), exposed to rabies infection by being bitten by a rabid animal.

Attacking the Disease Agents

The germ theory of disease also led to a series of other developments. As microbes became increasingly familiar to researchers and practitioners, the understanding of the role played by microbes in producing various diseases came under more intense scrutiny. In addition to advancing the theory of vaccines, researchers discovered penicillin, the first of the miracle **antibiotics**, and a little later a whole new type of disease agents known as viruses.

The first virus discovered was the tobacco mosaic virus, which was shown to produce disease in tobacco plants in 1892 but was not fully understood to be a virus until the mid-1930s. This virus was not isolated and cultured until 1936, and it was not found to be an RNA-type virus until 1937 ("Tobacco Mosaic Virus," 2006–2008).

The discrete germ theory also led, if not to the discovery of penicillin, at least to the elaboration of some of its functions from about 1870 forward (Wainwright & Swan, 1986). Large quantities of penicillin were produced and widely used as an antibiotic from the 1940s. In this case, researchers found that a toxin produced by a certain mold was deadly to some disease-producing microbes but harmless to most hosts, including most human beings. This interesting finding soon led to many others of its kind. Along with the antibiotics that could kill or render a bacterial agent harmless, antifungal and antiviral agents were discovered. With this approach, the key in combating disease agents already present in the body was to find ways to enable the body's natural defense systems to make these invaders harmless or to kill and remove their remains without leaving a lethal toxic mess of dead and damaged tissues behind in doing so.

Over time, the germ theory of disease led directly to our current understanding of bacteria, fungi, and viruses. It also provided the primary basis for the present pharmaceutical industries dealing in vaccines, antibiotics, antiseptics, antifungals, and antiviral medications. A great deal has been learned about the interactions of disease agents, toxins, and the body's own systems of immune defenses and detoxification. If there is any single conclusion that all of the research points to, and that the vast majority of researchers concur on, it is that the body's systems are extremely interactive and dynamic. For things to work normally within the complex biochemistry and metabolic activities of our bodies, the various systems need to maintain the balance that we think of as health or well-being.

It is now evident that in attempting to minimize the detrimental impact of disease agents (especially bacteria and viruses), the interaction and balance of the bodily systems necessary to health and well-being have been somewhat neglected. The discrete theory of germs has led to a dominant paradigm in medicine that has, to an important degree, failed to take adequate account of the complex systematic interactions that are essential to health and well-being. The biological, medicinal, and pharmaceutical means used to attack and destroy particular "germs"—regarded almost universally until recently as small harmful beings worthy only of destruction—have failed to take account of the interactions of biological systems. In fact, when we consider the larger picture and understand a bit more about the interactions, we discover that not all germs are bad, and that wholesale destruction of them without sufficient regard for their functions was not the good idea that it seemed to be during the heyday of the proliferation of vaccines (e.g., see the CDC's celebration in 2006 of the polio vaccines), antibiotics, antifungal, and antiviral medications, not to mention the widespread use of pesticides, food preservatives, and toxic industrial wastes that harm the entire biological spectrum (Bock & Stauth, 2007; Jepson & Johnson, 2007).

Disrupting the Microbial World

Future generations may look back to the present and think that people at the beginning of the third millennium were short-sighted in exploiting so many ways to poison specific bugs and germs while failing to notice the extent to which they were throwing whole ecosystems out of balance. It is already evident that this imbalance is happening not only at the macro level outside our bodies—largely as a function of the widespread use of pesticides and industrial pollutants—but also at the micro level inside our bodies' organs and cells.

At the micro level, ecosystems are being disrupted by toxins and disease agents in food preservatives and common household cleansers, by pollutants entering the food chain, and by medical procedures (e.g., dental amalgam) and vaccinations being the ubiquitous examples at hand. The shocking part of this picture—though it is hardly unpredictable—is that in attempting to kill off bugs and germs, we have also been poisoning ourselves along with plants, animals, and microorganisms that are, as the research is showing more and more plainly, vital to our own health and well-being, as is certain to become clearer over the long-term.

In fact, it is useful to notice the changing outlook concerning "germs" and "bugs." What is becoming increasingly evident is that most of the germs in our bodies are not only *not* harmful, but are actually *useful* to our own health and well-being. The same may well turn out to be true of insects and other organisms in the larger environment. We know that the good germs inside our bodies, when we are healthy, vastly outnumber the living cells of our own tissues. It is estimated that about 100 trillion bacteria inhabit our intestines and that when the gut is healthy, the helpful bacteria outnumber the harmful ones about 8 to 1 (Bourlioux, Koletzko, Guarner, & Braesco, 2003). The good microbes in our bodies also outnumber all the cells of our bodies by about 10 to 1.

Not all germs are harmful, and some of those that are harmful are highly useful if either kept outside the body or contained in the controlled environment of the gut. The first and most obvious barrier to infectious agents that might invade the body is the skin. It is generally not a good thing when something gets under our skin. Usually we do not want parasites, toxins, or potential disease agents to penetrate our bodies even at the level of the skin, much less to go deeper than that. Some toxins and disease agents can be harmful if they merely touch the skin, and we certainly do not want harmful toxins or disease agents in our mouths or in any of the other openings of the skin. Setting aside the interactions with the outside world that are involved in breathing, drinking liquids, consuming foods, sharing food or liquids, kissing, or having sexual intercourse—all of which involve the potential risk of introducing toxins and/or of transmitting disease agents—the importance of the skin as a barrier is easily demonstrated. For instance, when the barrier itself is broken, as it is with burns, puncture wounds, surgeries, and vaccinations, risks of infection are greatly increased and must be diligently guarded against. As Jepson and Johnson (2007, p. 48) note, the greatest threat to persons surviving burns is not the loss of tissue but the increased potential for invasion by undesirable microbes.

The second line of defense against invasion by microbes is found in the fluids contained within the gastrointestinal tract and in the multilayered mucosal lining of the airways, mouth, gut, and its communicating organ systems, including especially the liver, pancreas, kidneys, and urinary tract, as well as the entire rest of the body, which is connected to the gut through the bloodstream and the lymph. One organ system that is dramatically affected by what happens in the gut (though not commonly thought to be closely associated with the gut) is the brain. This fact is dramatically and conclusively demonstrated in many different ways—for example, by consuming a half a pot of coffee or a couple of shots of tequila.

In the case of the epidemic of neurological disorders, researchers have shown that problems occurring in the gut can markedly affect the states of the brain and, therefore, the whole body. At least since the 2005 publication of the research results reported by Vargas, Nascimbene, Krishnan, Zimmerman, and Pardo, it has been known that inflammation of the brain is common to individuals on the autism spectrum. To see why gut problems can affect the diverse systems of the body, and especially the brain, it is necessary to look beyond the discrete theory of germs. We must take account of the fact that the body's systems normally work in harmony and balance with each other and that to do so they must rely on effective and highly complex systems of communication.

As a result, the discrete theory of germs requires a major overhaul and amplification. It is incomplete because it cannot account for the fact that some germs, such as **Escherichia coli**, for instance, are bad in the bloodstream but (usually) good in the gut. Even *E. coli* O157, which can be deadly to humans, does no harm in the gut of a cow. The point is that germs interact with and communicate with their hosts in complex ways. For this reason, just killing them off—by spreading poisons helter-skelter all over huge crops to kill bugs—may not always be the best approach. The discrete theory of germs also cannot account for the fact that the 100 trillion microbes that inhabit the human gut are evidently not only in intimate communication with each other, but also with us. When the balance is within the normal range, in fact, the microbes in our gut form an important part of our immune protection against disease.

The End of the Discrete Germ Theory

Interestingly, as soon as we get past the skin, the outer barrier to most potential invading microbes, the center of our bodily defenses against potential invaders resides mainly in the gut. When we begin to penetrate the mysteries of this part of our bodies, we discover that it consists of a series of more or less hollow chambers—the mouth, esophagus, and stomach—connecting with the small intestine and colon from the mouth to the anus. The gut can be thought of as a complex connected tube of varying dimensions with multiple gates between its segments. Within that tube, along with potentially harmful microorganisms, there are normally found a great many "good bacteria" that populate our intestines. Technically speaking, as gastroenterologists are quick to point out, the material contained within the gut is not yet fully inside the body. To put it more accurately, if the gut is healthy, the material contained in it is in a controlled environment where potentially harmful agents can usually be kept from getting into the tissues outside the gut where they can do harm. For example, to return to *Escherichia coli* (shown in Figure 9-4) it is useful to stress that the most common strains are not only harmless but actually aid digestion in the intestines and form a large part of expelled fecal matter when the digestive tract is functioning normally (see "*Escherichia coli*," 2009).

In the case of *E. coli* O157 that produces the Shiga toxin (CDC, 2008e), what makes it harmful to humans is that the toxin breaks down the barrier in the human intestines so that the bacterium can escape into the bloodstream and organs where infections can be fatal. Figure 9-5 is an illustration of the propulsion system used by *E. coli*. Willard DiLuzio (2009) of Harvard University has produced a video of *E. coli* swimming in a micro-channel that is only 10 microns wide 💿. That video shows dramatically just how efficient the propulsion system diagrammed in Figure 9-5 actually

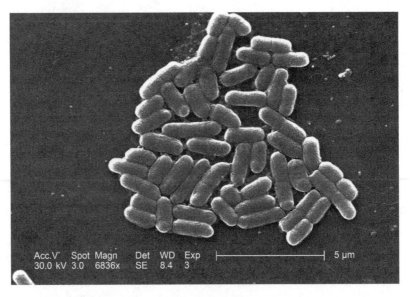

Figure 9-4 A micrograph of *Escherichia Coli* (*E. Coli*) bacteria.
Source: Courtesy of Janice Haney Carr and the National Escherichia, Shigella, Vibrio Reference Unit/CDC.

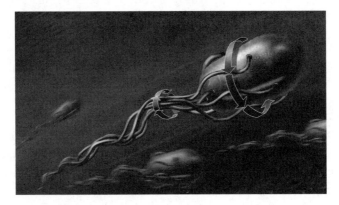

Figure 9-5 An artist's illustration of the *E. Coli* propulsion system.
Source: Courtesy of Nicolle Rager Fuller, National Science Foundation.

is. Presumably, even the **Shiga toxin**–producing *E. coli* O157 strain also serves some purpose in the gut of cattle. However, in compromised immune systems of human beings where the normal protections are dysfunctional, an *E. coli* infection can be fatal.

The vast majority of the bacteria and other microbes in the intestines form a critical component of the human digestive system and a useful, if not essential, component of the multilayered immune systems. Vighi, Marcucci, Sensi, Di Cara, and Frati (2008, p. 3) point out that "almost 70% of the entire immune system" is contained within the gut (also see H. Miller, Zhang, KuoLee, Patel, & W. Chen, 2007). No doubt this is one of the reasons why the National Institutes of Health has committed $115 million to study the microbes of the body and especially the gut (see "Human Microbiome Project," 2009 🌐). This five-year project is an extension of the well-known Human Genome Project (see Figure 9-6 and "Human Genome Project," 2008) and is expected to show that the genetic basis for the health of the 100 trillion biological microbes in the gut may exceed the length of the human genome by about 100 times.

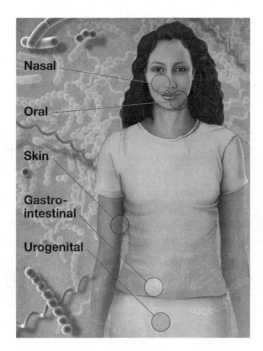

Nasal

Oral

Skin

Gastro-intestinal

Urogenital

Figure 9-6 The Human Microbiome Project will seek to determine the DNA sequences of microbes in the nose, mouth, skin, gut, and urogenital systems of the body.
Source: Courtesy of NIH [http://nihroadmap.nih.gov].

Into the Genetics of the Microbes

As the research shows, when everything is going swimmingly in a healthy gut, the good germs work in tandem with our own multilayered immune systems. In fact, some microbiologists argue that the good germs form an integral part of the immune system in a healthy body. The microbes to be targeted in the Human Microbiome Project include those that inhabit the areas highlighted in Figure 9-6. In addition to the skin (the body's largest organ and its primary defense against invading microbes and toxins), the project will target the genomes of the microbes in the nose, mouth, intestines, and the urinary–genital tract. All of these areas are known to be populated by microbes, although it is believed that many more in each of those areas have yet to be detected and investigated.

The majority of the microbes in the gastrointestinal tract are bacteria. Many of them (perhaps 70% or more) are benign to us and seem to constitute an integral system within the immune hierarchy. In ways that are not yet well understood, those friendly bacteria not only act in ways useful to us, but also help to prevent overpopulation of the gut by undesirable bacteria and by yeasts, fungi, and parasites (Bock & Stauth, 2007). They may also be critical in maintaining a tightly guarded boundary within the gut, thereby keeping invaders and toxins out of the bloodstream—that is, they may help to prevent the condition known as a leaky gut (Theoharides, 1990; Theoharides & Doyle, 2008; Theoharides, Doyle, Francis, Conti, & Kalogeromitros, 2008).

The Largest, Most Densely Packed Microbial Ecosystem on the Planet

Is it surprising to discover that a healthy gut contains the largest recorded (scientifically known) microbial ecosystem? It also has a higher bacterial cell density than any other known microbial system (Whitman, Coleman, & Wiebe, 1998). It appears that the entire ecosystem may itself constitute a significant component of the body's immune system—perhaps serving as the lowest layer

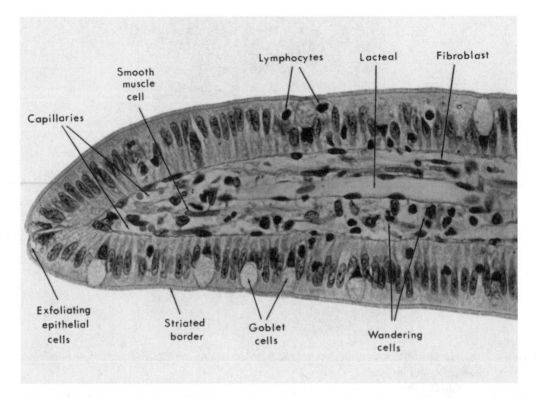

Figure 9-7 Layers of tissues in the wall of the intestine of a cat showing (at the top) that the convoluted inner surface area of the innermost lining, the intestinal glands, contain on their surface the densely packed microfold or M-cells (see Figure 9-8), the so-called "sentinels" of the gut.
Source: © Dr. Donald Fawcett/Visuals Unlimited.

of the multilayered hierarchy. The gut itself is the largest mucosal membrane surface in the human body. According to various sources (e.g., J. P. T. Ward, R. Clarke, R. W. Clarke, & Linden, 2005, p. 79, and references there), if the many intricate folds within the lining of the adult human's small intestines could be spread out in a single sheet, they would cover an area about as large as a full tennis court.

What makes the surface area of the inner lining of the gut so much larger than it would be if it were simply a smooth tube are the densely packed convoluted intestinal glands that protrude from the inner wall of the intestine into the long cavity formed by the folded tube that constitutes the gut. Figure 9-7 shows what this lining looks like in the gut of a cat, which shares some of the features of interest with the gut of a human being.

Within the lining, inside the small intestine (as can be seen at the top of Figure 9-7), the inner surface area—the **epithelium**—of the intestine has many densely packed, protruding intestinal glands. These glands, which are called **villi**, appear as a thick coating of relatively tiny protrusions shaped more like a finger or tongue than a hair. In humans, the surface exposed to the inside of the gut (the darker edge on the inside of the U-shaped segment of Figure 9-8) is covered by tiny hair-like protrusions called microvilli that form what, because of their somewhat shaggy look, is aptly called the "brush border" of the gut.

As seen in Figure 9-8, the surface cells of the human intestine consist of a densely packed layer of **microfold cells** (**M-cells**). They are called "microfold" cells on account of the form of the folds of the intestinal lining. The M-cells have also been called **membranous cells** (H. Miller et al., 2007)

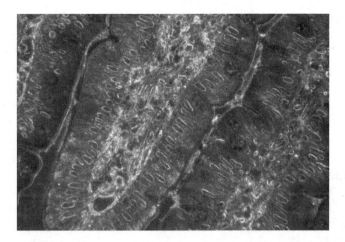

Figure 9-8   Densely packed M-cells in a gland from the human small intestine.
Source: © Dr. Cecil H. Fox/Photo Researchers, Inc.

because of their evident capacity to identify potential disease agents and toxins and actually hand them over to the immune system.

In certain specialized areas of the gut, called **Peyer's patches**, the microfold cells are closely associated with lymph glands (see H. Miller et al., 2007). Because the healthy M-cells are normally tightly packed together (as shown in Figure 9-8), some have supposed that damage to the gut produces what is commonly known as **leaky gut syndrome** in autism (Bock & Stauth, 2007, pp.178ff). In addition to the M-cells' normal physical closeness, which ensures that no material can leak past them into the tissues and bloodstream of the organism, the M-cells are dynamic participants in the immune system in living persons.

H. Miller et al. (2007) point out that an M-cell can literally reach out and grab a bacterium or large particle out of the intestinal fluid. The cell then engulfs the foreign material, a process referred to as **phagocytosis**. At this point, the bacterium may be either destroyed or handed over to a more specialized immune cell for a process of interrogation, dismantling, and analysis. Thus the M-cells "play a sentinel role for the intestinal immune system" (H. Miller et al., 2007, p. 1477): They deliver potential disease agents from the "lumen" (i.e., the hollow part of the gut) right through the "brush border" at the innermost surface of the gut to the immune cells of the lymph.

Communication Systems' Regulation of Immunity and Detoxification

A healthy person's immune system works something like an efficient police system supported by a strong border patrol, backed up by a national guard that can be called out in national emergencies and by a powerful array of elite military forces. The body also has the capacity to manufacture dynamic intelligent weapons systems to attack particular enemies. Within a healthy body, a vast military and industrial capability exists that can be mobilized to deal with almost any sort of invading forces. The immune system also has available expert teams of commandos that can search out and capture or kill small pockets of invaders. Likewise, it has sophisticated intelligence-gathering capabilities, including systems of confinement and interrogation used to gain information about potential invaders and to benefit from the information obtained from them.

The interrogations can be followed by commando sorties and surgical strikes at a great distance from where the body was first attacked. The troops sent out on search-and-destroy missions (e.g., ones focused on specific invaders) go through quick and efficient recruitment and training programs designed to help them deal with specific threats and to do so with sufficient resources. To extend the analogy, there appears to be the capability to communicate specialized training broadly to essentially every level of the defense hierarchy—from the domestic police, to the border guards, to the national guard, to all branches of the military.

The first step is to identify potential threats before they penetrate the mucosal lining of the gut, nasal passages, lungs, or the urinary–genital tract. The next step after a potential threat has been identified is to capture or control the potentially threatening agent, which is referred to by the broad term *antigen*. In extreme instances, the antigen is captured by immobilizing and encapsulating it; in some cases, it is then immediately destroyed and its remains—some of which may be toxic—are disposed of. The toxins are also dealt with, and repairs may be ordered for any damage that may have been done in the process.

In addition to its killing and cleanup capabilities, the immune system can deliver an antigen to another component of the immune system for interrogation before its destruction. The newly discovered information about the antigen in question may then be evaluated and transmitted. The process of communicating the intelligence gathered from the capture and interrogation process is amazingly like the sort of thing that might be expected from a highly intelligent police and military hierarchy.

WHY A SYSTEMS VIEW IS REQUIRED

In light of the scientific evidence and rational theory, it is clear that the discrete germ theory is inadequate. It cannot account for the known interactions of bodily systems, and neither can it account for disruption of communication systems by toxins, or the effects of antibiotics that—in the case of *E. coli* O157, for instance—increase (rather than decrease) the risk of death from an infection. Using generalized antibiotics is a little like carpet bombing the ecosystem in the gut: It is almost impossible to get the antibiotic agents to focus exclusively on specific targets. For this reason, antibiotics tend to disrupt the normal balance of the gut in ways that open it up to infections by parasites, yeast (fungi), and undesirable bacteria.

Also, the discrete germ theory is deficient in not being equipped to account for interactions—for example, the fact that combinations of antigens, toxins, and ongoing imbalances and allergies greatly increase the risk of doing harm with vaccines. Although the body's multilayered systems that protect against invading microbes and that normally rid the body of toxins are robust and effective when functioning properly, research shows that the body's systems can be pushed beyond reasonable limits. There is a tipping point beyond which disease conditions are certain to occur. The universal evidence of this fact is mortality. Nevertheless, apart from the fact that long-term exposure to physical and chemical injuries is guaranteed to bring an individual to the tipping point that ends in death, much can be done to prevent exposures and to both extend the life and improve the health of an individual.

Conditions Found in Autism Disrupt Many Systems

In the case of chronic neurological conditions such as autism, which is accompanied by gut disease in 70% to 80% of cases (D'Souza, Fombonne, & Ward, 2006; Jepson & Johnson, 2007; Valicenti-McDermott et al., 2006), as well as by full-blown epileptic seizures in about 40% of cases and by epileptiform seizures in an additional 20% of cases (Oslejskova et al., 2008a, 2008b), the evidence that an interactive systems view is necessary is compelling. Figure 9-9 shows the dramatic abnormality of microbes in the feces of children with autism as contrasted with normal controls. The data, which were gathered by Cosford (2008; also see T. A. Evans et al., 2008), show plainly that children with autism have a substantially smaller percentage of *E. coli* in their bowel but have a much higher proportion of *Enterococcus* and *Streptococcus* bacteria in their intestines than normal children (i.e., children not diagnosed with autism). All such bacteria are interactive and are known to affect

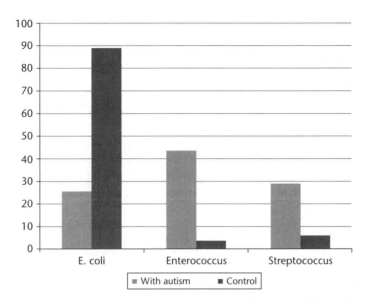

Figure 9-9 Distinct and abnormal distribution of microbes in the feces of children with autism (N = 88, 27 from New South Wales; 45 from Queensland; and 16 from Victoria) as contrasted with normal controls (n = 117) in a compilation of three studies of children in Australia by Dr. Robyn Cosford and colleagues from data presented at DAN!

Source: Compilation of three studies of children in Australia by Dr. Robyn Cosford and colleagues from data presented at DAN! 2008 in San Diego, California.

the overall balance of the ecosystem in the gut. On account of the fact that the *Streptococcus* bacteria are known to produce the toxins involved in such imbalances, it seems highly likely that they are up to mischief in many cases of autism.

PANDAS

A review of the class of disease conditions known as **pediatric autoimmune neuropsychiatric disorders associated with *Streptococcus* (PANDAS)** is particularly appropriate to show the critical need for a more holistic view of disorders in general and especially autism spectrum disorders. PANDAS is hypothesized to be caused by a latent streptococcal infection, which appears to be associated with, and possibly to cause, tics, **Tourette syndrome** (a violent cyclic subtype of **obsessive–compulsive disorder**), and ADHD (Leslie et al., 2008). The PANDAS-type condition is sometimes **comorbid** with a diagnosis of autism. This class of disorders was first hypothesized to exist by Swedo et al. (1997); although it remains a disputed classification (Singer, Gause, Morris, & Lopez, 2008), substantial positive evidence seems to be emerging in its favor (Cardona, Ventriglia, Cipolla, Romano, Creti, & Orefici, 2007; Kurlan, Johnson, & Kaplan, 2008; Segarra & Murphy, 2008).

The original theory behind PANDAS is that an initial streptococcal infection triggers an episodic (cyclical) self-immune response in certain genetically susceptible individuals. The result is cyclic outbursts that are caused by toxic build-up generated by self-immune attacks owing to a lingering streptococcal presence, followed by an explosive release, another build-up, and so on, in one cycle after another.

Simple, Single-Minded Theories: One and All Are Incomplete

Because many cases of autism are of the so-called regressive kind—20% to 50% according to Hrdlicka (2008) or more than 80% according to Pangborn (2005, p. 149)—it is perfectly reasonable to look for environmental conditions and factors that can and do produce such crashes. Food allergies, immune imbalances, and intestinal infections by parasites, bacteria, and fungi can all produce neuroinflammatory conditions. The sort of imbalance demonstrated in Figure 9-9, along with disease conditions previously noted, can also increase toxicity and oxidative stress.

It makes little sense, therefore, to suppose that chronic intermittent conditions (e.g., recurrent vomiting, cyclic self-injurious episodes of violence) are caused by a single gene or by one type of parasite, germ, fungus, or virus acting by itself and independently of other factors and systems. Indeed, Dr. Jon Pangborn (2005) asserts that "a single faulty gene that by itself accounts for all the increased incidence of autism is an impossibility in my opinion" (p. 154).

We would argue strongly on a strict logical basis that any single causative agent for autism or other epidemic chronic disease conditions is an absolute impossibility on account of the imbalances in multiple systems known to be involved in their manifestations. In the face of evidences already in hand (especially the kind depicted in Figure 9-9), the idea that autism is, or ever has been, a strictly genetically based complex of behavioral and psychological disorders is more than just implausible—it is a theory that must be incomplete.

Moreover, when removal of disease-producing conditions can produce dramatic improvements of the sort seen, for instance, in the case of Ethan Kurtz, the notion that any combination of behavioral interventions (e.g., speech therapy, applied behavior analysis, occupational therapy, or physical therapy) could have caused the observed transformation is untenable. The changes observed have to be attributed to overall balance in multiple biological systems that affect the internal metabolism, health, and neurological well-being of the individual.

With all such evidence in mind, searching for a single autism gene, or a complete genetic explanation of the diverse group of disorders under consideration, seems to hold very little promise. Neither does it make any sense to suppose that the changing prevalence of the chronic disease conditions observed in persons on the autism spectrum is uncaused.

The Always-There-But-Unnoticed Theory

Similarly, the notion that such conditions along with the noteworthy, blatant, accompanying behavioral and neurological symptoms could have existed at about the same prevalence without being noticed at least for decades, and perhaps even for centuries, is hard to believe. No one has made this clearer than Dr. Jay Gordon at the UCLA Medical Center. To hold that hundreds of thousands of neurologically impaired individuals with autism were always out there, but unnoticed, requires the supposition that parents, teachers, doctors, and so on have just gotten many times better than they used to be at noticing (and diagnosing) extremely debilitating communication and behavioral disorders. Gordon says, "I know that I am not 400% to 800% smarter than I was years ago" (McCarthy, 2008, p. xvii).

The Tipping Point

So where should we look? What are we left with? There appears to be no alternative to embracing the theory, as suggested by Dr. Bryan Jepson and others, that there is a natural "tipping point" beyond which we will notice events such as loss of verbal skills, social withdrawal, seizures, full-blown epilepsy, gut disease, neurological inflammation, and even death. Gordon agrees with Jepson and hundreds of DAN! doctors in saying that "we have to look much harder at what happens when we inject toxic material into babies, toddlers, and children" (J. N. Gordon, 2008, p. xvii).

Putting the case very simply, in view of all the evidence cited in this book, can any rational person doubt that a sufficient dose of toxins and disease agents, combined with genetic susceptibilities, appears to be causing the rising incidence of pervasive developmental disorders and a host of related disease conditions such as allergies, asthma, PANDAS, childhood multiple sclerosis, type 1 diabetes, rheumatoid arthritis, and, in later life, Parkinson's disease, Alzheimer's disease, and a host of other disabilities?

The gross load of factors necessary to push any individual beyond the tipping point no doubt differs across individuals and genetic types. Also, surely there are many different mixes of toxins, disease agents, and injuries sufficient to reach the critical level in some subset of any large group of individuals. For these reasons, the notion that one dose size or a single schedule of antigens, toxins, and repeated challenges is equally safe for all individuals is ill founded. Yet the one-size-fits-all and the same-schedule-fits-all philosophy remain standard doctrines for vaccinations promoted by the CDC. More unconscionable still are the ideas that neurotoxic metals such as mercury and aluminum are safe in vaccines, and that mercury is safe to use in dental restorations. Irrespective of a person's genetic make-up, there is, logically speaking, still a burden of toxins, disease agents, and injuries sufficient to kill any individual. If this were not so, some genetic types would be immortal. But they are not, so there is a tipping point beyond which a sufficient challenge will make any healthy person very sick and/or dead.

Health and Wellness

Just as the notion that a child of age six or seven years can say what ordinary truth is troubles many professional philosophers, who gave up long ago on the possibility of ever understanding a difficult concept like truth (e.g., Anderson, 1996), similarly, the idea that the health and wellness of their own children can be defined by parents without any medical training seems to trouble mainstream medical professionals. For instance, Paul Offit (2008) argues that parents who say their children got sick because of vaccines are just mistaken (see also CNN, 2008). Researchers who see a connection between autism and vaccines, or between autism and the mercury in dental amalgam, he says, are "false prophets" (Offit, 2008).

When asked what is causing the upsurge in the diagnosis of autism, Offit insists that the trend is a mystery, but one that is surely not linked to vaccines. He boldly asserts that children can theoretically cope with "about 10,000 vaccines at any one time" (Offit et al., 2002, p. 126). Meanwhile, he profits from the RotaTeq vaccine manufactured by Merck and continues his work in the $1.5 million Merck-funded chair he holds at Children's Hospital in Philadelphia. At the same time, many parents keep telling their doctors that their child was well up to the time of a series of vaccines but was never well after that.

Meanwhile, mainstream practitioners in dentistry, pediatrics, and other fields continue to hold that the toxins and disease agents they are putting inside human bodies, sometimes very tiny ones, have nothing to do with the explosion of neurological conditions and chronic diseases observed over the last three decades or so. Although the mainstream practitioners claim to have no idea what could be causing all those problems, they keep reassuring themselves and their patients—against all contrary logic and empirical evidence—that the problems cannot possibly be related to vaccines or their components, dental amalgam, the interaction of drugs and antibiotics with vaccines, or other medical practices. To many professional mainstreamers, both wellness and the causes of autism are undefinable abstractions. As Pangborn and S. M. Baker (2005, 2007) note, the prevailing view is that parents just should drop the whole idea of finding the causes of autism because the mainstreamers are convinced in their own minds that it just can't be done.

Standing Logic Right Side Up

There seems to be an inherent contradiction in the claim by Offit and like-minded vaccinologists who advocate the idea that a newborn can tolerate as many as 10,000 disease agents mingled with toxins at a single dose while, at the same time, contending that the same marvelous immune system that can handle 10,000 disease agents at a time needs special training from CDC-sponsored vaccines so that it can learn how to combat a select few—say, 11 to 200—of the multiple billions of disease agents that the natural immune system is equipped to deal with (Fanning, Connor, & Wu, 1996). To train the system for those special disease agents, the CDC proposes injecting a child with a potpourri of chemicals 36 times, according to the current CDC vaccine schedule. If the child can handle 10,000 disease agents at a time, what is the benefit in exposing that same child to one or even a hundred injected toxins and disease agents in any given vaccine? Also, why should the military training of the immune system begin before it reaches maturity?

There is something wrong with this picture. If the immune system can adequately handle 10,000 challenges from disease agents simultaneously, why not leave it alone and let it do its work of maintaining health and wellness? Of course, as the research shows, Offit's arguments are not correct. The truth is that even a half-dozen vaccines and toxins are enough to push many children into disease and disorder. Some of those children will die from even less exposure to toxins, foreign animal proteins, and disease agents.

Besides, there is another alternative: nurturing and strengthening the existing systems of the body through a healthy diet, good hygiene, plenty of rest, and good exercise. Meantime, we could just avoid, as much as possible, unnecessary exposures to toxins, foreign animal proteins, and disease agents. We could just say "No, thanks" to the vaccines. What would be wrong with an experiment like that? It worked in Leicester, England. It seems to be working well in the Amish communities in the United States (see Pangborn, 2007, p. 35). Who is to say that it wouldn't work everywhere? The defenses of the natural immune system seem to have worked for all the years of recorded history, and logically speaking they must have been working for whatever period preceded that. If the immune system can deal with 10 billion or more disease agents (according to Fanning, Connor, & Wu, 1996), why not give it a shot without the interference from poorly researched vaccines that are being rushed onto the market at an accelerating rate?

Recall the figure from Dr. Walter Orenstein's presentation (Figure 4-2) where he struggled to understand why parents seemed increasingly to be questioning vaccines. We know why: As the number of vaccines mandated by the CDC has grown, it has been matched by growth in the number of children being diagnosed with autism. Also, as Bock and Stauth (2007; see also S. M. Baker, 2005a, 2005b) have documented, autism is not the only growing epidemic where vaccines and their components are known to be playing a causative role.

At the Edge of a Shift

In this chapter, we have come to the brink of a necessary paradigm shift that is now taking place in medicine and in the related sciences. Empirical research findings and sound theoretical reasoning show that it is necessary to expand discrete theories of particular germs (genes, parasites, or viruses) as the single-minded causal agents for any chronic disease condition in favor of a perspective that accounts for the exquisitely complex communication systems of the body and their known interactions. Those systems range from genetics through every aspect of the body's epigenetic systems for metabolism, immunity, and detoxification, right on up to the highest levels of the neurological systems enabling human language, cognition, emotion, and social behavior. Also, as we are learning, in a large part from the studies focused on the autism epidemic, the systems of communication at the deeper levels of genetics and metabolism seem to be interacting with what is going on at much higher levels of communication with the internal ecosystem of the gut as well as the external environment where volitional actions pertaining to diet and social connections come into play.

Over time, changes in sanitation, hygiene, waste disposal, sewage management, and access to relatively uncontaminated food and water undoubtedly have had a much greater impact on the reduction of death by infectious diseases than the vastly more expensive vaccine industries have had. Contrary to the view espoused by the CDC and its pharmaceutical partners, vaccines—except for their cost and worldwide use with hundreds of millions of persons—have played a comparatively minor role in disease control. In fact, the research we have reviewed and critically examined here indicates that vaccines have played a major role in causing the modern epidemics of autism, self-immune diseases, and a host of related neurological disorders and diseases. Attacking suspected disease agents one at a time with, say, 11 to 100 vaccines, such as the smallpox virus, the polio virus, and so on, while disrupting entire healthy immune systems that are well equipped all by themselves to deal with billions of distinct disease agents, makes about as much sense as risking all the police forces and all the military capabilities of all the civilized world (i.e., all the body's natural defense systems) to try to kill at most a few dozen individual terrorists (i.e., the germs and viruses targeted by vaccines).

Even the miracle antibiotics must be reexamined in light of a better informed view of the body's internal communication systems. In general, it is probably not as good an idea as it once seemed to be to many pediatricians to use multiple antibiotics indiscriminately in the treatment of common illnesses. Current research on the ecosystems of the gut suggests that helping the body to kill off a minor bacterial infection by conducting a general antibiotic war on all the body's microbes is apt to be more harmful in many instances (though perhaps not in all) than supposed by many practicing pediatricians. Continuing with the military analogy, killing off most of the body's microbes through a generalized antibiotic regimen in an attempt to help the body rid itself of a particular bacterium is analogous to destroying approximately 70% of the world's police and military personnel while aiming to rid the world of a few terrorist cells.

It is plain from the research evidence that repeated use of antibiotics kills off nearly all of the 100 trillion mostly beneficial microbes in a person's intestines. As a result, the immune system may be thrown out of balance for weeks, months, or even permanently. In some types of bacterial infections (e.g., *E. coli* O157), the use of a generalized antibiotic is a bad idea. By incidentally killing off the helpful microbes of the intestines with friendly fire from the antibiotic, a well-meaning doctor can disrupt the balance of the body's immune systems and increase the likelihood of the patient's death by about 333.33% (Boedeker & Serna, 2008).

Can there be any doubt that holistic communication-based theories are required to upgrade the outdated discrete germ theory of disease? Study of the autism epidemic has revealed that normal development, immunity, and detoxification are all intensely dependent on biological systems of communication. Although these processes are normally robust and resilient in the face of natural challenges, the evidence shows that they can be seriously disrupted by repeated and persistent attacks engineered—sometimes unintentionally—by well-meaning dentists, doctors, and pharmaceutical advocates. There is, logically speaking, no reasonable doubt that every healthy person has a necessary "tipping point" beyond which a given quantity of toxins, disease agents, and foreign proteins will harm that individual irrespective of his or her particular genetic make-up. At the same time, there is also little doubt that genetic susceptibilities amount to a lowered tipping point for some individuals. Also, when stress factors (such as viral, bacterial, or parasite infection) are combined with increasing toxicity (e.g., from pesticides, preservatives, industrial wastes), and with explosive growth in burdens presented by medically implanted or injected toxins, disease agents, and foreign proteins, we have a sure-fire recipe for the autism epidemic and all of its epidemic "kissing cousins."

SUMMING UP AND LOOKING AHEAD

There is a paradigm shift under way in the health sciences that is being brought about in part by the autism epidemic. The discrete germ theory, as important as it has been in pointing the way toward better hygiene and sanitation, was incomplete from the beginning and encouraged other discrete theories of causation—namely, those promoting the idea that single genes, viruses, and the like should be searched out and treated individually in order to defeat specific diseases, disorders, and syndromes. Those theories may be good up to the tipping point where things go drastically wrong, but they are necessarily incomplete from the start. It is necessary to amplify them.

In this chapter, we examined evidence that massive repeated antibiotic assaults on the ecosystems of the gut have a debilitating impact on the body's natural immune systems. We showed that a richer, more integrative, communication-based, systems approach is required to fully understand the body's functioning. Evidence was provided from the autism epidemic showing that ecosystems in the gut are definitely out of balance, thereby permitting the emergence of opportunistic infections by *Enterococcus* and *Streptococcus* bacteria, not to mention worms, fungi, and many other bacteria. In the next chapter we discuss the paradigm shift that is under way.

STUDY AND DISCUSSION QUESTIONS

1. Which specific advances in medicine can be attributed to the germ theory of disease?

2. After reading about Pasteur's experiments and the results obtained by Semmelweis, are there any particular practices in the way that you handle food and drink or any personal hygiene practices that you might want to change?

3. Were you surprised by the reactions of the supervisor and contemporary physicians to the results obtained by Semmelweis? How different are those reactions from ones going on today in connection with the autism epidemic—for instance, the reactions to the research findings of Andrew Wakefield? The reactions to the work by Stan Kurtz? The reactions to Jenny McCarthy's claims?

4. What are some of the reasons why we might expect the ecosystem in the gut of children with autism to be substantially out of balance? Refer to Cosford's results.

5. What are some of the advantages afforded to medicine and science by the germ theory? How does the germ theory contrast with systems theory?

6. In view of the cyclic (episodic) nature of self-injurious behavior, or of violent and destructive outbursts, in some individuals with ASDs, what are some of the trial remedies that parents might want to discuss with their doctors?

7. Why does Dr. Jon Pangborn flatly reject the idea of a single gene causing autism?

8. Suppose you were asked to give a definition—a practical everyday description—of "health." What would you list as its main characteristics?

9. Based on the information in this chapter and preceding ones, why should we expect treatment with an antibiotic that attacks the ecosystem in the gut to increase the likelihood of death from approximately 15% to approximately 50% after an infection with *E. coli* O157?

10. What reasons can you think of to prevent modern medicine from taking a more holistic view of health than can be provided by the discrete germ, gene, or virus theory of disease? Assuming that we are on the brink of a paradigm shift toward a more comprehensive, consistent, and simpler view of what health is, do you have any thoughts on the future of vaccine policies?

chapter ten

The Paradigm Shift Under Way

OBJECTIVES

In this chapter, we

1. Discuss the military analogy for the immune systems.

2. Consider some of the dangers involved in the immune systems doing their work.

3. Show that communication is critical to the balance and smooth functioning of immunity.

4. Discuss the levels and interactions of the immune systems and their fail-safe procedures.

5. Consider some of the balances that must be maintained for the immune systems to function normally, avoiding allergies and self-immune attacks.

6. Consider why accurate diagnosis and monitoring over time are crucial in trying to understand autism and its treatments.

7. Discuss toxicity and interactions of toxins with disease agents that must be taken into account in a more holistic theory.

In this chapter, we examine the military analogy for the immune systems of the body in depth. We see why that analogy is the only one taken seriously in the research literature. The body has enemies, but it is innately well equipped to deal with them. By examining some of those enemies—including parasites, bacteria, viruses, and combinations of them, and the toxins they produce—we see why it is essential in dealing with the chronic conditions that epitomize the autism epidemic to take the immune systems into consideration.

Communication breakdowns caused by disease agents, toxins, and their interactions can cause sufficient imbalances that lead to the immune systems attacking the very body they are designed to protect. Specifically, mistaken immune responses caused by breakdowns in communication within the body can lead to allergies and/or self-immune diseases. In allergic reactions, the body, in effect, mistakes relatively harmless **allergens** for disease agents and attacks them, sometimes injuring itself in the process. In active immune diseases, the body becomes confused in its communications and directly attacks its own living cells, tissues, and organs.

As doctors, researchers, clinicians, and patient/clients come to better understand the intricate communication systems found within the body, their new knowledge is inspiring a paradigm shift in health care. We are rapidly moving away from the discrete germ and gene theories of past decades into an era where attention focuses mainly on the communication systems inside and outside of the body that enable the dynamic balance that we can reasonably call health or well-being.

THE MILITARY ANALOGY FOR THE IMMUNE SYSTEMS

The only drawback to the military analogy for the human immune system, perhaps, is that no military in the world is as efficient as a healthy immune system in maintaining communications across so many distinct systems. However, the military analogy is especially appropriate to the description of the networks of connections of the immune systems to other bodily systems. All of these systems are critically dependent on interconnected communication networks. In defense systems, even simple police patrols are especially dependent on good lines of communication. When it comes to complex and costly military campaigns, getting advance information about potential enemies, identifying targets, deciding when and where to engage, and determining how to limit damage control on the battlefield are even more important than in routine police actions. The immune systems engage in advance intelligence-gathering; maintain communications with attack units at a considerable distance from the site of any infection; and take prisoners and interrogate them—right down to their design systems as expressed in DNA, RNA, and proteins. In addition, command and control units maintain communication with other units performing commando raids on distant and diffuse targets.

Collateral Damage, Friendly Fire, and Military Take-Overs

Within the body's immune systems, all the former kinds of activities can be found when those systems are functioning properly. In contrast, extreme disease conditions may occur in which such systems fall out of balance or go completely awry when the military itself goes haywire. To the extent that communication networks break down, there is no way to keep any military system functioning well. Collateral damage (accidental damage to the body's own tissues) and friendly fire (in which the immune system kills the body's own healthy cells) are much more likely to occur when lines of communication within the immune system are disrupted or broken. It is possible, in fact, for the whole process of immunity to go wrong such that a self-destructive shooting match is undertaken. In such cases, the body may attack harmless entities that have been mistaken for deadly invaders, as happens in allergic reactions, or it may begin to attack its own cells, tissues, and organs, as occurs in self-immune disorders and diseases.

Allergies are popularly regarded as harmless, but they are a warning that things are not as they should be with the body's immune system. Allergies are undoubtedly involved as predecessors to many chronic diseases and can themselves be fatal even in what is called "hay fever," not to mention asthma, eczema, hives, full-blown epileptic seizures, and anaphylactic shock (Bock & Stauth, 2007; Richet, 1913). Allergies can also progress to conditions where the immune system begins to attack the body it is supposed to protect, as in the case of so-called **autoimmune disorders**—literally, "self-immune" disorders, such as rheumatoid arthritis, multiple sclerosis, lupus, and type 1 diabetes (see "Helper T-cells," n.d.; also T Helper cell, 2009 ☻). In addition, the brain inflammation associated with autism and the neuroinflammation associated with multiple sclerosis and neuroAIDS, along with many other diseases and disorders, involve self-immunity.

A Coup or Civil War

The military analogy is appropriate right up to the extreme case where the military goes berserk and takes over the whole country. In such instances, the economy—that is, the overall health and well-being of the person—usually slides to the level of a country engaged in one or more civil wars, where the enemies are factions within its own population. Life-threatening allergies and serious self-immunities fit this scenario.

To truly appreciate the crucial importance of the balance that is ordinarily maintained by a healthy immune system (actually a deeply layered system of interacting systems), it is essential to get a general idea of how it all works in a healthy body. It is also useful to see some of the ways that things can go radically wrong whenever we inadvertently throw one or more components of the multilayered system out of balance. In doing so, we will see further evidence that the discrete germ theory is seriously incomplete. Simply put, the discrete theory of germs cannot account for the dynamics of the many components of the immune system, nor can it account for the necessary communication networks that enable a healthy immune system to function well.

Among the most persuasive demonstrations that a healthy immune system can be disrupted by generalized attacks aimed at specific germs is what happens in a healthy gut when it is exposed to an antibiotic such as penicillin. The destruction of the good germs in the gut leaves it more vulnerable—rather than less so—to attacks by many germs other than the ones that may have been targeted. When penicillin has been administered in an effort to minimize the impact of an *E. coli* O157 infection, for instance, the fatality rate increases from approximately 15% to 50% of the persons infected (Boedeker & Serna, 2008). The difference appears to be attributable to the effect of killing off the good bacteria of the gut with the antibiotic. To understand how such harmful effects—potentially deadly ones—can and do occur in autism and related chronic disorders and diseases, it is necessary to take account of the multilayered interactions of the immune systems.

Layers and Interactions

Generally, it is supposed that the immune system can be divided into two distinct levels, each of which contains multiple subsystems and layers within those subsystems. However, if there is anything clear about the nature of the immune system, it is that this system is exquisitely complex from top to bottom. For this reason, there is probably no other area of human physiology where the discrete germ theory is more apt to mislead researchers and theoreticians. The idea that the components of the immune system are developed or that they act independently is probably mistaken in almost all of the cases where it has been proposed. The known functions of the immune system defy any rigid piecemeal explanation. The many layers of the immune system in a healthy body work together with such efficiency that it is necessary to suppose that they are interrelated to such a degree that just about any single component presupposes the existence of the rest.

At what is supposed (by many) to be the most basic level of the immune defense systems, there is what is somewhat misleadingly called the **innate immune system**. This part of the whole complex is called "innate" to distinguish it from the vast diversity of immune systems that appear to be "acquired" or "learned." It is a little misleading, however, to suppose that the rest of the immune system is not also provided for in the innate part. That idea appears to be incorrect. Nevertheless, what is called the "innate" system consists of a well-armed and well-distributed police force backed up by something like an Army Corps of Engineers with some really sophisticated demolition capabilities. At a higher level, but in close contact with the basic "innate" system, is a complex of related systems that are popularly (and roughly) referred to as the **adaptive immune capabilities** (see the discussion by Jepson & Johnson, 2007, p. 50). In between these two layers we find a distinct demolition capability known as the **complement cascade**. Whenever large numbers of enemy combatants or debris from battle needs to be disposed of, the complement cascade, which consists of an enormously complex system of proteins, working something like an organized tornado kicks in, mulches, vacuums up, and disposes of whole armies of attackers and the toxic wastes they leave behind.

As in mortal combat, the units and individual cells involved in any given conflict within the body must act somewhat independently, but the efficiency of the whole complex of immune systems depends greatly on communication between its components. In fact, it is probably easy to underestimate the importance of such communications and difficult to overestimate just how critical they are. From the very beginning at the deepest and earliest levels of innate immune responses, communication is the key. With adaptive responses, communication is crucial.

Communication at the Base of the "Innate" Immune System

The main police force in the "innate" immune system consists of the very numerous and powerful white blood cells known as **neutrophils**. These cells are usually found in the bloodstream, though they can migrate out from there to attack invaders in other bodily tissues. The neutrophils constitute approximately 70% of the total number of white blood cells (S. Cohen & Burns, 2002, p. 465). Secondary to the neutrophils in the innate immune system are the *macrophages,* which have some of the same powers to attack and destroy perceived foreign microbes; they can also perform cleanup functions. Both macrophages and neutrophils are able to communicate with other parts of the whole immune system. For instance, the macrophages seem to be able to activate the complement cascade to demolish and remove difficult enemies and large amounts of debris.

In Figure 10-1, a pair of white blood cells (neutrophils, with darkly stained nuclei) are surrounded by many more red blood cells. Such neutrophils serve more or less as cops—"constables on patrol." Like armed police officers who have the authority to use lethal force, they are always on the lookout for foreign cells, microbes, parasites, or anything else that cannot identify itself as native to the host organism. Neutrophils are also available to respond to any distress call from anywhere in the neighborhood. In performing their first-response functions to injuries or infections, neutrophils have the capacity to exit the bloodstream and travel to a point of infection or injury. They do so in

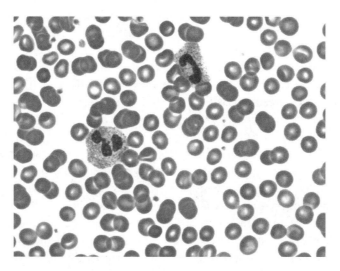

Figure 10-1   A smear of blood showing a couple of neutrophils surrounded by normal red blood cells. *Source:* Courtesy of Wadsworth Center, New York State Department of Health.

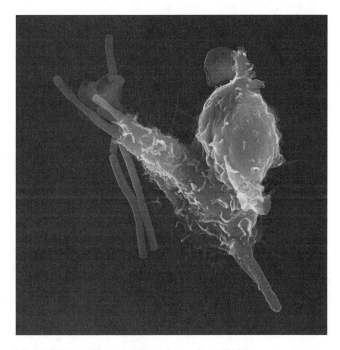

Figure 10-2   A neutrophil (right) engulfs an anthrax bacterium (left).
Source: Reproduced from A. Mayer-Scholl, R. Hurwitz, V. Brinkmann, M. Schmid, P. Jungblut et al. (2005). Human neutrophils kill *Bacillus anthracis. PLoS Pathogens, 1*(3), e23. [doi:10.1371/journal.ppat.0010023].

response to chemical signals received from body cells in distress. For example, they migrate quickly to a site of a physical injury, such as a bruise or a cut, or to the site of an infection. The communication process by which the white blood cells navigate to the site of an injury or infection is termed **chemotaxis**.

Halt—Who Goes There!

As they move around communicating with other cells, the first question neutrophils put to any suspicious cells within their vicinity is something like this: "Do you belong in this neighborhood? Let's see some identification." In the event that no identification is forthcoming, the neutrophil springs into action by arresting, interrogating, and dispatching the invader. Neutrophils have the capacity to attack and engulf from 1 to about 100 invaders while they are on patrol. Figure 10-2 shows a single neutrophil attacking an anthrax bacterium and engulfing it. Neutrophils can also hunt down particular suspects.

Figure 10-3 shows a still picture from a video on the DVD where a neutrophil is seen engulfing spores of a fungus known as ***Conidia***, one after another. Colonies of *Conidia* can infect the lungs and create problems in persons with compromised immune systems. As can be seen from the actions of neutrophils in the videos associated with Figure 10-3 and also especially in the one associated with Figure 10-4, neutrophils are capable of targeting one specific type of invader while ignoring others. In the video associated with Figure 10-4, a neutrophil can be seen attacking and disposing of several ***Candida*** spores while it ignores various *Conidia. Candida* and other parasitic fungal infections are common in autism. The targeted fungus in Figure 10-4 is the kind that overpopulated the gut of Ethan Kurtz after he received multiple rounds of antibiotics.

Neutrophils are relatively short-lived cells, usually completing their mission of capturing and destroying up to about 100 potential disease agents or foreign particles within a day or two

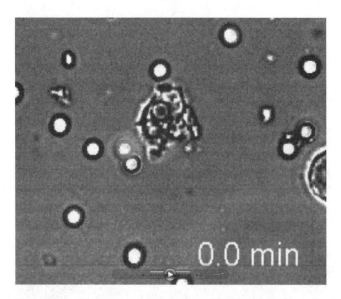

Figure 10-3 A neutrophil (entity at the right just below the midline) is seen here. In the moving video on the DVD, the neutrophil can be seen over a 2-hour time period with a frame shot every 30 seconds, capturing several *Conidia*.

Source: Reproduced from Behnsen, J., Narang, P., Hasenberg, M., Gunzer, F., Bilitewski, U., et al. (2007). Environmental dimensionality controls the interaction of phagocytes with the pathogenic fungi *Aspergillus fumigatus* and *Candida albicans*. *PLoS Pathogens*, 3(2), e13 [doi:10.1371/journal.ppat.0030013].

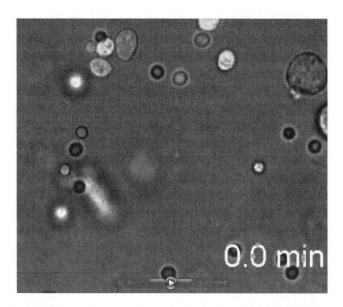

Figure 10-4 A neutrophil (entity in the upper left corner) engulfing *Candida* spores and passing up *Conidia* spores. In the moving video on the DVD, the neutrophil can be seen over a 2-hour time period with a frame shot every 30 seconds.

Source: Reproduced from Behnsen, J., Narang, P., Hasenberg, M., Gunzer, F., Bilitewski, U., et al. (2007). Environmental dimensionality controls the interaction of phagocytes with the pathogenic fungi *Aspergillus fumigatus* and *Candida albicans*. *PLoS Pathogens*, 3(2), e13 [doi:10.1371/journal.ppat.0030013].

before they systematically disperse their own parts at the end of their life cycle. While on patrol, the neutrophils are on the alert for chemical messages informing them of specific outbreaks of trouble in the neighborhood. After migrating to the point of an injury or infection, they also have the capacity to release chemical messages that call for reinforcements, consisting of additional neutrophils, and/or for the cleanup and repair crews (i.e., macrophages) that reinforce and back them up. In addition, they can initiate a higher-level immune response from the complement cascade, whereby the invading organisms—many of them more or less simultaneously—are systematically ripped open and dismantled by removing their proteins in a predetermined sequence.

The Adaptive Layers of the Immune System

Whereas the initial question put to potential invaders by the "innate" immune system merely focuses on whether they belong to this body, the follow-up questioning by the adaptive immune system is more detailed. The deeper problem for the immune system is to determine the identity and nature of the foreign invader, including whether the invader has any friends, how many of those compatriots there are, and where they may be lurking.

The adaptive immune system hierarchy includes numerous specialties and branches, each with its own complement of capabilities. For instance, the body has multiple ways to capture, interrogate, and use information from antigens (potential disease agents). The cells that have this capability are a diverse group, beginning, as we have already seen, with the macrophages. The function of identifying and then publishing the identity of malefactors (antigens) is performed by a diverse group of police and military-type cells known as **antigen-presenting cells** (**APCs**). The macrophages that can perform this function attack, ingest, disassemble, and then display the identity of the antigen on their surface—akin to an all-points police bulletin warning other cells and the police especially to be on the lookout for disease agents meeting the following description. The antigen presented on the surface of APCs is a symbolic descriptor of the suspected disease agent—something like a wanted poster with a photograph and a name of the wanted person.

In addition to the macrophages that can perform the function of APCs, other immune cells have appendages resembling the dendrites of a nerve cell. Because of that resemblance, they are called **dendritic cells** (Figure 10-5) though they are not nerve cells at all. They are special capture cells that function something like a net-throwing police wagon that can collect multiple live and intact specimens of the offending type of antigen. Whereas the antigen-presenting macrophages act a little like lethal cops—Dirty Harry characters that tend to kill potential suspects while interrogating them about their friends—the dendritic cells take live prisoners. They deliver these specimens to something like a specialized union of the Federal Bureau of Investigation and the Central Intelligence Agency, all rolled into one organization—an efficient one—for further questioning. To get to one of the local interrogation stations, which are found in the lymph or spleen, the loaded-up dendritic cells may travel either through the bloodstream or through the lymphatic ducts and fluids to get to a lymph node.

For example, in the video associated with Figure 10-5, a single dendritic cell can be seen dragging a conidium a distance of about 9 micrometers (roughly three times the width of the body of the dendritic cell itself). After antigens are taken prisoner by dendritic cells, they may be delivered directly to a lymph node for further interrogation. The lymph, in its turn, extracts information from the prisoners and determines how best to combat whatever threat seems to be posed by the invaders. In addition to issuing bulletins directly through APCs, including the dendritic cells themselves, the lymphatic system can deploy resources in the form of two major types of specially equipped military personnel. These two major types consist of additional lymphocytes, each with multiple subtypes and peculiar specializations.

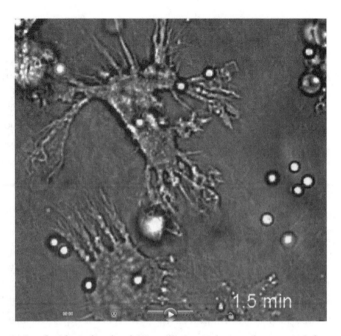

Figure 10-5 In the associated video, the dendritic cell situated near the upper left center of the picture can be seen dragging a conidium (at the right just below the midline) as if in a net.
Source: Reproduced from Behnsen, J., Narang, P., Hasenberg, M., Gunzer, F., Bilitewski, U., et al. (2007). Environmental dimensionality controls the interaction of phagocytes with the pathogenic fungi *Aspergillus fumigatus* and *Candida albicans. PLoS Pathogens,* 3(2), e13 [doi:10.1371/journal.ppat.0030013].

Communication and Cavalry

The so-called **T cells** form the communication and command components for the whole police/military hierarchy, the entire immune system. They also provide the basic hand-to-hand fighting units that go door to door in the street, with the capacity to enter the houses (i.e., the body's cells) and fight inside them. In contrast, the **B cells** are the body's mobile cavalry systems: They move fast and far on the body's major thoroughfares (the bloodstream and lymphatic ducts) and have the capability to manufacture a vast arsenal of effective weapons within highly mobile factories consisting of specially equipped B cells.

Both kinds of lymphocyte cells originate in the bone marrow. Later they are differentiated into multiple subtypes, but the T cells are especially well differentiated and provide the backbone of the command and control systems for the entire hierarchy. All of the T cells and B cells go through rigorous testing and training, comparable to special boot camps where failure is not a viable option. Some T cells are eventually selected for what might be termed Officer Training School; they become the ranking officers and communication specialists for the entire immune system.

The Killer T Cells

Some of the T lymphocytes, which are manufactured in the bone marrow, will become the fighting and killing type known, unsurprisingly, as **killer T cells** or "cytotoxic T cells." (These cells go by several other more or less synonymous designations.) After going through the do-or-die series of boot-camp training sessions within the **thymus**, the potential killer T cells are tested to make sure they are neither too strong and inclined to attack and kill healthy cells of the host (that would be us) nor too weak and unable to kill cells infected by foreign microbes.

The first level of authorization after reporting for duty is obtained by killer T cells by communicating first with APCs within the lymph. Usually a dendritic cell—but always an APC—presents the T cell with the antigen describing the invaders to be attacked. This step is analogous to providing a photograph and description of the targeted enemies.

The second level of authorization, which occurs after the killer T cell receives its antigen assignment, involves a thorough check of communication capabilities. Prior to the authorization to go "weapons hot" and apply lethal force to any cell marked by the antigen in question, there is evidently a check by a communications expert to make sure that all the channels are functioning properly so that the killer cell can distinguish friend from foe and can communicate with the rest of the immune system. That second authorization comes from another T cell that functions as a field agent, a kind of high-class technician, specializing in communications. At this level, the communications capabilities of the killer T cell are tested to make certain that it can send and receive signals properly. In particular, it needs to be able to differentiate friendly host cells (us again) from the enemy that it is equipped and designated to attack and kill. If the killer T cell passes this final test, it is authorized to go weapons hot and will not subsequently need any additional authorization to find and kill enemies of the known description. If it fails the communications test, it is promptly decommissioned and consigned to an inactive status.

After a killer T cell has been informed, equipped, and authorized to activate its weapons, it may also be authorized to reproduce itself by cloning and to go hunting for the particular species of invaders defined by the assigned antigen.

T-Helper Cells (Communication and Command)

The interconnections of the entire immune system are intricate and depend on well-developed systems of communication and command. The type of invader that the killer T cells are licensed to kill is the sort shown to them by some APC, usually a dendritic cell that has captured and presented the foreign cells to the lymph for further interrogation by intelligence analysts there. These guys are rough: Their system of interrogation consists of ripping the other guy apart, protein by protein. Later, a communications officer—a particular **T-helper cell**—will issue the weapons activation order to the newly trained and authorized killer T cell.

Obviously, the success of the killer T cell is critically dependent on prior intelligence gathered by other cells, usually dendritic cells that have presented prisoners to the lymph for interrogation. Information gained there concerning the nature of the antigens to be attacked is subsequently communicated to the killer T cells by "type 1" T-helper (**Th1**) cells. These particular command and communication specialists seem to play a critical role in activating and maintaining the balance of what is called the **cellular immune response** (i.e., the foot soldier response that involves going inside cells to kill enemy combatants), as contrasted with the **humoral immune response** (i.e., the highly mobile killing units and weapons manufacturing systems that operate outside cell walls moving rapidly in the bloodstream and lymph ducts). While the killer T cells work a lot like foot soldiers (with boots on the ground, as they say), the really sophisticated mobile military systems and the capacity to mass-produce specially designed capture systems known as *antibodies* are primary functions of the mobile cavalry of the humoral systems. The basic elements of the humoral systems consist of B cells. However, the command and control systems issuing orders to those B-cell units depends on T-helper cells.

The B Cells (Mobile Weapons and Factories)

In their book, Bock and Stauth (2007) refer to what they call "the wisdom of the body" (e.g., on p. 49 and in the surrounding text on pp. 46–50). These authors are not just referring to the general intelligence systems built into the immune capabilities of the body; they are also acknowledging the capacity of the humoral (fluid and mobile) immune system, and the body's B cells in particular. The B cells' capacity to form appropriate and specific antibodies is one of the most amazing manifestations of that wisdom. Within the B cells, antibodies are formed to combat specially targeted invaders.

As we have emphasized throughout this book, and in other publications on communication and communication disorders in general (see J. W. Oller et al., 2006, 2010), communication systems form the foundation of all the body's systems, from genetics to the unique linguistic intelligence systems found only in human beings (per Chomsky and colleagues). The multilayered and highly integrated systems of human immunity are no exception when it comes to depending on successful communications. They, too, depend on intricate systems of communication. When those systems of communication break down, as they often do in disorders such as autism, things can go badly wrong. The many ways that bodily systems are designed to achieve and maintain essential balances within the immune system are only just beginning to be understood. Also, some of the T-helper cells that were formerly thought to have only a precursor (command and control function) are now believed to be more actively involved in producing the inflammation that is associated with infections and allergies (Awasthi & Kuchroo, 2009).

Like the killer T cells, the mobile B cells originate in the bone marrow and go through similarly rigorous screening and training before they reach their mature stage. If the B cell fails any of the tests along the way, unlike a killer T cell that remains inactive (technically referred to as **anergic**), a B cell that fails is programmed to commit something like hara-kiri. They self-destruct through *apoptosis,* a generalized process that all bodily cells undergo at the end of their life cycle whereby they dismantle themselves. Like the rough interrogators, the B cells are what we might think of as extreme organ donors. They offer up all of their parts for reuse or disposal. Also like killer T cells, B cells are normally—but not always—dependent on authorization by a specialized communication officer, in this case, a type 2 T-helper (**Th2**) cell, to become activated and thus to enter the battle against a particular invader. Once they are activated, they have a unique capability to produce antibodies.

Like killer T cells, B cells have the capacity to reproduce themselves in large numbers by cloning. The replication process is authorized, it is believed, by a different type of T-helper cell called an **effector cell** that issues special orders for killer T cells and B cells to replicate. Presumably, effector cells are themselves authorized to issue such orders on the basis of information gathered elsewhere concerning the size and nature of the threat from a particular antigen that has been discovered in the body.

COMMUNICATION THROUGHOUT THE IMMUNE SYSTEMS

Although it is commonly supposed that the immune systems developed piecemeal and that distinct components operate independently to a high degree, there are, in fact, many indications that the systems are in communication with each other. The processes of manufacturing distinct types of cells in the bone marrow, their subsequent differentiation through a series of processes of development, and the intricate systems of communication, all the way from the bottom to the top of the immune hierarchy, indicate that communication is evidently occurring throughout the systems. Some of the means by which this communication occurs are understood. However, the systems of interaction are certain to be more complex and intricate than anything that is as yet fully understood.

Fail-Safe Checks for Authorization

The first level of authorization for a B cell to get into the fray is to be released into the bloodstream or lymph. When the B cells get this far, they have already shown that they are not sensitive to self-proteins displayed in the **major histocompatibility complex (MHC)**, the identifying, **glycoprotein** of the body's own cells. Any B cells that prove to be sensitive to the body's own glycoproteins either self-destruct by apoptosis or render themselves inactive (anergic) for the duration of their relatively short life, which usually lasts from a couple of days to about a week. The exceptions are **memory B**

cells, which survive for a much longer period (possibly the lifetime of the host) and are reactivated much more quickly if a second infection by the same antigen should occur later on.

Each day in a healthy body, millions of B cells are released into the bloodstream and lymph ducts and dispersed throughout the body on the lookout for antigens. Supposing that a B cell gets that far and then encounters what it identifies as a foreign antigen, it will normally take a sample of that antigen, internalize it, and then seek a briefing session with a communications officer that is able to confirm the foreign identity of the antigen in question. According to current understanding (Jepson & Johnson, 2007, pp. 53–54; also "Helper T-cell," 2009, and references there), the communication officer called for is a Th2 cell, which can display the antigen in question and confirm the foreign identity of that antigen to the B cell. Once the identity of the foreign antigen is confirmed by the Th2 cell, the B cell is authorized to get down to business. Usually the first order of business will be to clone itself into many **plasma B cells**—that is, B cells capable of producing many antibodies that can immobilize and defeat the identified antigen. However, several other types of B cells are also produced. The best known are the plasma cells that produce the greatest number of antibodies or **immunoglobulin** of type G (IgG). In addition, there are four other major types of antibodies, each of which has its own special functions.

Isotypes of Immunoglobulin

The five distinct known types of human immunoglobulin (referred to as **isotypes**) are labeled "Ig" for "immunoglobulin" (meaning "antibody"), followed by the letter A, D, E, G, or M (as shown in Figure 10-6). Each isotype consists of an arrangement of glycoprotein material that works mainly based on its stereoscopic shape and by the chemical attractions that enable it to capture up to 2, 4, or 10 antigens before it is filled up. In the greatly simplified diagram presented in Figure 10-6, the V-shaped ends of each stereotype (shape) show the number of places where antigens can be captured. In reality, of course, antibodies are vastly more complex than the diagram suggests, and each one is specially designed to deal with a particular antigen. Each distinct antibody is shaped to fit its particular antigen like a key fits a lock. With respect to our immune systems, the difference is that the keys and the locks are much more intricate and dynamic than the lock-and-key analogy or Figure 10-6 suggests. Antibodies have billions of distinct possible shapes, and each of the distinct

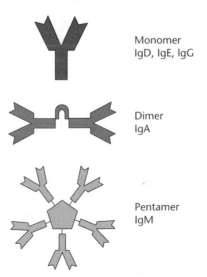

Monomer
IgD, IgE, IgG

Dimer
IgA

Pentamer
IgM

Figure 10-6   The three stereotypes (shapes, viewer's left) and the five isotypes of immunoglobulins (named, viewer's right) in a simplified diagram.
Source: Diagram created by Martin Brändli.

isotypes has a somewhat different set of functions. For any particular antibody, however, all of its adhesion areas (suggested by the V-shaped ends in Figure 10-6) are tuned to just one particular antigen. The body's B cells can produce an estimated 10 billion distinct antibodies (Fanning, Connor, & Wu, 1996).

In a healthy and mature person, the most common of the immunoglobulins is one of the smaller ones, which can cross the placental barrier from mother to child. In this way the child can receive from its mother an adult-level immunity to protect it during its time in the womb and for a few months after birth while the infant's own immune system is getting up to speed.

General Immunoglobulin

IgG is the most common and plentiful of all the body's immunoglobulins and is currently believed to be the *only one* that can cross the placental barrier and provide the mother's immunity to the developing unborn baby. That immunity is effective up to about the baby's sixth month of life after birth, by which time the baby's own immune system begins to function. To help remember what IgG does and the fact that it is the most widely distributed immunoglobulin of all, we can arbitrarily call it "general immunoglobulin."

After birth, until the child is five to six months of age, the human infant's immunity is almost exclusively dependent on this inheritance from its mother. In some cases, if the mother has an immune deficiency or is susceptible to self-immunity, as may be the case in autism and various related neurological conditions, the infant may also be vulnerable to self-immune diseases and disorders from early on. Abundant research shows that individuals on the autism spectrum tend to have a much higher than normal incidence of self-immunity (Cabanlit, Wills, Goines, Ashwood, & Van de Water, 2007; Van de Water, 2008; Wills, Cabanlit, Bennett, Ashwood, Amaral, & Van de Water, 2007).

There is also compelling research evidence showing that self-immunity in autism appears to be communicable from mother to child (Van de Water, 2008). In an interesting study with Rhesus monkeys, Van de Water and colleagues showed that infant Rhesus monkeys injected with the IgG of human mothers who had borne a child on the autism spectrum behaved very differently from monkeys injected with IgG from human mothers of children who did not have the autism diagnosis. The monkeys that received the injections from human mothers of children with autism subsequently (almost immediately) behaved as if they were severely autistic, avoiding social contact even with their own monkey mothers. The IgG injections seemed to render the normal monkeys unable to recognize—or take any interest in—their own mothers. The upshot of that research is that the sort of self-immunity common to many cases of autism appears to be something that can be passed from mother to child through IgG.

Different Functions for Distinct Isotypes

The stereoscopic structure—that is, the dynamic physical shape—of IgG (the general kind) makes it one of the three smaller isotypes, as can be seen in Figure 10-6. No doubt this is one of the reasons that the general kind of immunoglobulin can cross the placental barrier. IgG is the most plentiful system of antibodies, accounting for approximately 80% of the total number of antibodies in a mature healthy body at any given time. IgG can also cross from the bloodstream or lymph ducts into bodily tissues, and it tends to be concentrated in areas of inflammation where infections or injuries have occurred or are occurring. The IgG antibodies are basic fighting tools—something like armored vehicles and capture systems that are maneuverable in tight spaces (e.g., in bodily tissues between tightly packed cells). They are widely used throughout the body in fighting disease and infection.

Another of the smaller isotypes, **IgE**, is produced in much smaller quantities than IgG, but constitutes an elite fighting force that is widely distributed and rapidly deployed throughout the

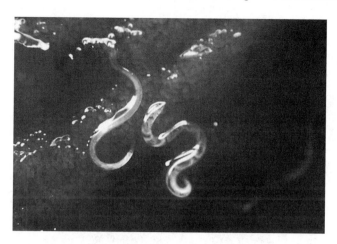

Figure 10-7 A common type of hookworm on the mucosal lining of the intestine where the peaks of microfold villi can be plainly seen.
Source: Courtesy of CDC.

body's systems. It may help to remember the function of IgE by associating it with the phrase "elite immunoglobulin." Although this type of immunoglobulin normally accounts for less than two-thousandths of a single percentage point of the body's total immune resources (Jepson & Johnson, 2007, p. 53), it may be overproduced in the case of extreme allergies and in anaphylactic shock (Gould et al., 2003; Gould & Sutton, 2008; Pier, Lyczak, & Wetzler, 2004). It is involved in the sorts of seizures commonly seen in autism.

The IgE isotype is also involved in the production of the **histamines**, which are critically associated with allergic reactions and inflammation. It is partly through the production of histamines that IgE helps to protect the body from attacks by parasites. The most common types of parasites found in humans, which are often passed to us from pets or from infected humans, are **helminths**, worms that live inside the bodily fluids and tissues of the host, but especially in the intestines. Examples of such parasites include the common hookworm (Figure 10-7) and the even more common pinworm (Figure 10-8). In addition to their frequent appearance in cases of gut disease (especially the sorts widely associated with the autism epidemic), these and other parasites are carriers of huge numbers of bacteria and viruses. They are often visitors to the human body, but not guests that we should welcome into our intestines. Parasites are undesirable elements commonly associated with gut disease and related problems.

Action at Distance

Because IgE can act at a distance from the site where a reactive agent is introduced, when things go wrong with IgE, a usually harmless protein (or a fragment of one) that happens to be mistaken for an antigen may cause a global reaction. For instance, in an allergic reaction to a toxin, protein, or vaccine, even an allergen derived from something that would normally be harmless (and hardly detectable) may cause hives on the surface of the skin, restricted breathing, asthma, or even fatal anaphylactic shock. As in a case well documented by Bock and Stauth (2007, p. 150), something in a vanishingly small quantity such as a whiff of the smell of peanuts can cause a severe and even fatal allergic reaction. It is clear that IgE is involved in such reactions and they are said to be **atopic** because they are far removed from the site where the allergen has been introduced. Because reactions can occur very soon after exposure to a tiny quantity of an allergen, disease agent, or toxin, the existence of IgE demonstrates the rich and almost instantaneous interconnectedness of the immune systems throughout the body.

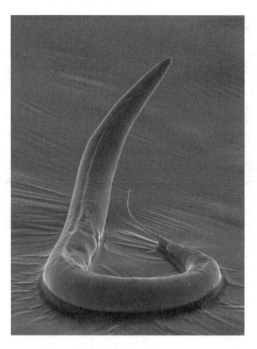

Figure 10-8 A pinworm of the sort commonly found in the intestines of human beings.
Source: Courtesy of Carolyn B. Marks and David H. Hall, Albert Einstein College of Medicine, Bronx, NY.

Another indication of that sort of interconnectedness is the fact that **IgD** appears to be involved in a peculiar way in the activation and authorization of B cells to begin mass-producing other B cells like themselves as clones, or to begin mass-producing one or another of the isotypes of antibodies. It seems reasonable to suppose that IgD is usually the means by which the final authorization to begin its warfare assignment is delivered to the B cell. There is also some evidence that IgD may be involved in the decommissioning of B cells, or their discharge at the end of the war. To help remember this particular type of function, it may be useful to associate IgD with the phrase "deployment and discharge immunoglobulin." When the IgD associated with a given B cell encounters the right antigen and captures—as confirmed by a different set of antigen receptors associated with a different isotype of antibodies, the type produced by **IgM**—the B cell is evidently authorized either to clone itself multiple times or to go into production of its particular type of immunoglobulin. Again there is evidence of fail-safe procedures.

Distinct Shapes: Monomer, Dimer, and Pentamer

As shown in Figure 10-6, the isotypes IgD, IgE, and IgG are all **monomers**; that is, they consist of a single structure with two ends, each of which can capture an antigen. The remaining isotypes of immunoglobulin, IgA and IgM, have distinct stereotypes. IgA is a **dimer**, a glycoprotein system consisting of two monomers joined in such a way that they can capture up to 4 antigens; IgM is a **pentamer** consisting of five monomers joined into a five-sided system that can capture up to 10 antigens.

IgA is normally found in the mucous linings of the body and in the lymph tissues. Next to IgG, it is the second most plentiful isotype in humans, normally accounting for approximately 15% of the body's total supply of antibodies. The IgA isotype helps to prevent the formation of colonies of associated antigens in the fluids and mucosal linings of the nose, mouth, lungs, gut, and urogenital tracts (Underdown & Schiff, 1986). A phrase that may help to fix its main function in memory is "anti-association immunoglobulin." Because bodily fluids provide convenient breeding grounds, preventing antigens from meeting up or hanging around in those fluids is a principal function of IgA.

IgM is the third most plentiful system of antibodies. It is produced by the body, along with IgD, ahead of IgG, and is involved in the activation of B cells. To help remember its functions. we can use the phrase "marshal management and manufacturing immunoglobulin." IgM is commonly found in the bloodstream and, like a marshal with lethal authority, has the special capacity to attack and dispatch pathogens that commonly circulate there. IgM accounts for about 10% of the body's total antibodies. Initially, before any B cell can be activated and put into active service either as a cloning factory to produce other B cells or as a mass producer of immunoglobulin, the B cell first produces IgM, which is expressed on its surface. It also produces IgD, which can aid in its activation and, it seems that it may, after the B cell has completed its work, participate in its decommissioning and discharge.

Meanwhile, with IgM on its surface, the B cell circulates in the blood or lymph looking for an antigen to latch onto. When it finds one and captures it, the B cell can be activated in one of two ways. First, a B cell can become an activated plasma cell and can initiate the production of a particular type of immunoglobulin by meeting up with a Th2 cell that confirms the antigen already captured by the B cell is, indeed, a foreign one and should be attacked. Second, activation can occur in a manner that resembles the B cell "hotwiring" itself. When it meets up with multiple antigens of the same type that do not have the right papers, the IgM can perform its "marshal managerial" function and activate itself immediately. It is believed that by grabbing onto more than one of the encountered foreign antigens of a given type, the B cell can achieve the same sort of activation of itself as would occur when it is briefed by a Th2 cell.

In any case, as soon as it is activated, the B cell can then begin to clone itself by producing multiple plasma B-cell factories tuned up to produce the required antibodies to attack the particular foreign antigen that has been discovered, or, alternatively, the B cell can begin itself to mass-produce antibodies.

Shuffling and Switching Systems

The B cells can achieve the production of a vast diversity of antibodies with relatively few genes because of ingenious built-in systems for shuffling components to get an enormous variety of distinct antibodies and, in some instances, for switching the manufacturing process from one isotype—say, an IgG (the general type of antibodies)—to another kind—say, an IgA (the anti-association kind) or an IgE (the elite attack forces that cause allergies when they are misdirected).

According to Borghesi and Milcarek (2006), the IgG isotype accounts for about 80% of the total number of antibodies in humans. In pregnant women, this type of immunoglobulin crosses the placental barrier to provide vicarious—often misleadingly referred to as "passive"—immunity to the developing unborn baby. Of course, there is nothing "passive" about immunity. It is less like a border fence than it is like a dynamic and fluid armed police force that is constantly engaging and dispatching potential threats. Likewise, antigens are not static. They can be expressed in many distinct varieties and consist of active bacteria, viruses, parasites, and chemically active toxins. They are moving targets.

The fact that the human immune system can produce billions of different antibodies, and many different varieties of the same antibody, undoubtedly makes it difficult for antigens to defend themselves against the body's dynamic police and military resources. Although an invariant portion of each antibody focuses on a particular antigen (i.e., a portion that fits the particular antigen in the way that a key fits a lock), other parts of the antibody are constantly changed to increase its versatility and effectiveness. The billions of different shapes of antibodies are necessary for the body's immune forces to have capturing and killing power over the great diversity of potential invaders.

The Theoretical Balance of Th1- and Th2-Helper Cells

In addition to producing the killer T cells that form the essential "boots on the ground" component of the body's military systems, a critical complementary role is played by T-helper cells. As noted previously, the better-known T-helper cells function as communication officers, intelligence couriers, and CIA-type analysts. Only in rare cases are T-helpers known to be armed with killing power (Awasthi & Kuchroo, 2009).

T-helper cells are differentiated into multiple types with different functions generally pertaining to communication. The better understood of the various T-helpers are Th1 and Th2. The Th1-helper cells are known to be involved in authorizing killer T cells to go after viruses and bacteria that are inside the cells of bodily tissues; whereas Th2-helper cells commonly play a role in activating lymphocyte B cells (macrophages) that circulate in the blood and lymph looking for particular antigens outside cell walls (Mosmann, Cherwinski, Bond, Giedlin, & Coffman, 1986). However, the research also shows that there are other types of T-helper cells and that some of them, notably Th17-helper cells, can also become participants in attacking invaders (Awasthi & Kuchroo, 2009).

As noted earlier, there is a basic division between the fighting cells that go after bad microbes inside cells and those that go after bad microbes and parasites in the blood and lymph fluids throughout the body. The killer T cells focus on the antigens inside cells, while the B cells (macrophages) focus on antigens in the bodily fluids—that is, the humoral systems. B cells, according to Mossmann et al. (1986), are authorized and commissioned by Th2-helper cells. According to the theory advocated by Mossmann et al., and as summed up by Jepson and Johnson (2007, pp. 53–55), an overproduction of Th2-helper cells (commissioning too many B cells) leads to allergies, whereas overstimulation of Th1-helper cells (sending out too many killer T cells) pushes the body toward self-immune disease.

All these authors, along with Bock and Stauth (2007), suggest that both types of imbalances are common among many individuals on the autism spectrum and help account for their frequently occurring (but often undiagnosed) allergic and autoimmune symptoms. However, as is generally acknowledged, the deeper control systems affecting allergies and self-immunity are without doubt more complex than the theory of the balance between Th1 and Th2 cells would suggest. For instance, research is bringing other control factors and systems to light. In addition to the involvement of Th17 helper cells in autoimmune disorders and inflammatory diseases (Awasthi, Murugaiyan, & Kuchroo, 2008; O'Garra, Stockinger, & Veldhoen, 2008; Veldhoen et al., 2008), the complicating presence of certain toxins seems to confuse Th17 cells in particular, leading to autoimmunity.

In addition to the various types of T-helper cells already discussed, the body produces **T-helper memory cells** that can last for years or a whole lifetime in the blood plasma and lymph. B cells also have the capacity to become memory cells. Such memory cells can remain in the blood and lymph for years, even a lifetime, always standing ready to reactivate in the event of a recurrent infection by a particular antigen. Besides this kind of T-helper cells, there is a class of **regulatory T-helper cells** (analogous in function to IgD) that help shut down an immune response after a disease threat has been sufficiently dealt with. These regulatory cells appear to do battle damage assessment after a conflict is under way; when they judge the damage to be sufficient to have destroyed the invading microbes, the regulatory cells may be authorized to issue ceasefire orders.

Along the way, there are various baffles and buffers set in place to help ensure that the immune systems stay balanced, remain effective, and do not run wild. It would seem that all of the T-helper cells serve regulatory—or at least communication—functions. Some of them authorize lethal weapons activation in lymphocyte cells (T-helper 1 in lymphocyte T cells and T-helper 2 in lymphocyte B cells). In addition to enabling lethal weapons activation in these distinct types of killer cells, they support proliferation of the cells themselves in the process referred to as "cell cloning." After receiving their marching orders, the active lethal cells are not only authorized to go into attack mode to search and destroy certain antigens, but also commonly (though not always) authorized to multiply their own numbers so as to meet the threat with sufficient force. In this way, T-helper cells are involved in threat assessment.

In view of the fact that such lethal activity—a form of microbial warfare—cannot be conducted without potential collateral tissue damage (especially in the case of the killer T cells that go after microbes within the cells of host tissues and organs), it follows that the T-helper cells must have the capability to assess their effectiveness against the enemy as well as friendly fire losses. All of these functions are performed by T-helper cells (possibly also by IgD). Battle damage assessments figure in the issuing of ceasefire orders—duties that appear to be handled by T-helper regulatory cells (perhaps in interaction with IgD).

In addition to all of the foregoing activity, another type of immune killer cell plays a role in the autoimmune system. These **natural killer (NK) cells** seem to possess advance authorization to kill any cell that has a missing or damaged set of identity papers. They are especially important in detecting and destroying tumorous tissue and cancer cells. When things are going well, the identity of cells in our bodies is defined mainly by the major histocompatibility complex (MHC), the complex system of glycoproteins that are expressed on the surface of each cell of the body. When that system is working properly it shows that the cell to which it is attached is a valid cell of that particular host organism rather than a cancerous creation or a tumor cell that should not be where it is found. NK cells can also kill a cell infected by a virus or a bacterium, or a cell damaged beyond recognition (e.g., by a toxin). In addition to "wearing their identities on their shirtsleeves," the body's cells display on their surfaces any antigens (additional glycoproteins) derived from infecting agents such as viruses or bacteria that may have invaded the cell. Oversimplifying the case, we could say that the MHC works like a passport or identity card, differentiating host cells from foreign invaders. It is actually a deeply layered system of identity markers that can be checked. The additional infection information serves as something like a detailed health certificate, the sort of thing required by the World Health Organization for reporting any infections. These "papers" concerning identity and health status of each cell of the body enable immune cells to determine whether to bypass a given cell or to destroy it. If an attack is called for, there is also the question of how best to carry it out.

NK cells have the highest-level authorization of any cells in the immune inventory. They have what might be described as the James Bond 007 rating. They are licensed to kill from the moment they are set apart and differentiated from the many other cells being produced in the bone marrow. Their license to kill, however, does not mean that they can kill indiscriminately. Like the other killer cells in the immune inventory (notably the killer T cells and the B cells), which must usually find the appropriate antigens before attacking and must avoid attacking cells that display appropriate identity and health information on their surfaces, the NK cells normally refrain from attacking cells displaying the right identity papers (the self-defining MHC). However, NK cells can move directly to attack mode if the papers are not in order or if strange antigens appear on the surface of any cell. Because of their capacity to read the MHC in some depth, NK cells are particularly well equipped to spot tumorous cells that do not belong in a given neighborhood. Also, because they are licensed to destroy any cell that cannot identify itself properly, or that is infected or damaged beyond recovery, they are critical for the body's ability to defend itself against disease and especially cancer cells.

WHY ACCURATE DIAGNOSIS IS CRUCIAL TO DISCOVERING CAUSATION

Just as the immune system depends on accurate identification and diagnosis of disease agents that may be attacking the body, at a higher level the health sciences and healing arts also depend on getting the diagnosis right. Likewise, it is important for healthcare providers to know when a condition is getting better or worse. Inaccurate information in terms of the initial diagnosis and failure to detect whether things are getting better or worse are both potentially harmful. The more serious the disorder or disease condition, the more critical a correct diagnosis and accurate monitoring of the progress of the condition and/or its treatments.

Not from Nothing

After the idea that disease agents could just pop into existence from nowhere and from nothing at all was shown to be false by Louis Pasteur, the germ theory of disease became the dominant idea in health care very quickly. An important part of that development was the building up of a theory about how to show that a particular germ was a cause of a particular disease. The series of steps is instructive with respect to the autism epidemic, and it involved an individual who helped shape the history of medicine and vaccines from near the beginning of the twentieth century.

In 1905, Dr. Robert Koch was awarded a Nobel Prize in Physiology or Medicine for his isolation of the bacterium involved in the causation of tuberculosis, **Tuberculosis bacillus**. Koch had earlier isolated the anthrax bacterium, **Bacillus anthracis**, and he or his students were credited with the discovery of many other causative disease agents, including the microbes causing diphtheria, typhoid, tetanus, bubonic plague, and dreaded venereal diseases including gonorrhea and syphilis (see R. Koch, 1905). He was even lionized in a Nazi propaganda film in 1939 as the hero in a drama about a tuberculosis epidemic titled in German, "Robert Koch, the Adversary of Death" [*Robert Koch, der Bekämpfer des Todes*]. As we saw in Chapter 9, Koch's discoveries were also important to the continuing advancement of the discrete germ theory.

Koch became known not only for his discoveries of disease agents for anthrax and tuberculosis, but also for his proposal of certain rigid criteria by which he believed the causation of a disease by a particular agent could be definitively established. He proposed four such criteria, which he termed "postulates" (as if they had something like the mathematical status of the postulates in Euclid's geometry). First, he supposed that the agent had to be demonstrable in all cases. Second, he argued that it should be possible to culture the agent and maintain it in a virile state. Third, Koch said it ought to be possible to show that the agent could still cause an infection leading to the disease in question after being cultured and recultured several times. Finally, he suggested that the chain of evidence concerning the causal agent ought to be traceable to an animal artificially infected with the agent, allowing it to be retrieved and recultured yet again. As it would turn out, the criteria for determining causation as proposed by Koch would later be relaxed following the discovery that latent infections could persist undetected for long periods of time with certain disease agents such as typhoid, and in many other diseases, especially ones involving viruses such as those associated later with polio and AIDS.

The most extreme relaxation of the criteria proposed by Koch would occur in the case of the polio virus and some other viruses discovered later on that were even more complex in their interactions with the systems of the body. In the case of the polio virus, causation would be inferred from the reduction in polio cases that was actually occurring well before the introduction of the polio vaccines (Salk and Sabin), as illustrated earlier in Figures 7-9 and 7-10. However, the decline in polio cases was generally credited to the vaccines, with this decline being seen as sufficient evidence to suppose that the virus in its various forms caused poliomyelitis.

An alternative causal explanation, first proposed and substantiated with animal models in the 1930s, involved toxic pesticides, including especially DDT (Figures 7-10). It was shown that such pesticides compromise the immune system and sufficiently damage the nervous system to produce the symptoms of poliomyelitis (Biskind, 1953; Rusiecki et al., 2008; West, 2003). Although the results of experiments with DDT were obtained mainly on the basis of animal models, the data also fit the case for humans. More recently, the research with mammalian animals and the central nervous system damage caused by pesticides has been shown to be generalizable to humans (Bornman, Pretorius, Marx, Smit, & van der Merwe, 2008; Fischer, Fredriksson, & Eriksson, 2008; Iwaniuk et al., 2008; Ton, Lin, & Willett, 2008). The theory that the polio virus was the primary cause of the disease, rather than a toxin such as DDT (per Biskind, 1953), was beneficial to the inventors of the polio vaccines; it also left the manufacturers of pesticides a way out of the obvious conclusion that DDT and related pesticides were involved in producing poliomyelitis. Nevertheless, the scientific evidence could not rule out the possibility that DDT, or some combination of toxins that were already known to compromise the neurological and immune systems in animal and human systems, were involved in causing outbreaks and epidemics of poliomyelitis.

Over time, Koch's original postulates would be relaxed significantly, though not entirely set aside, and the discrete germ theory would be retained on the basis of the less stringent criteria. In the meantime, research into toxins and their interactions with disease agents would continue producing evidence that the discrete germ theory at its best was still incomplete.

Toxins in the Mix

The theory that poliomyelitis was caused by the polio viruses in the Salk and Sabin vaccines also gained credibility in a sinister way. The weakened viruses found in both of these vaccines proved to be sufficiently virile in some individuals—especially in persons with compromised immune systems (see Mamishi et al., 2008, for discussion and a case study)—to produce full-blown symptoms of polio, including paralysis, limb atrophy, and the entire complex of symptoms. This finding, though contrary to the hopes of the creators of the vaccines, gave some credibility in an undesirable but empirical way to the theory that polio viruses were at least involved in the causation of some cases of poliomyelitis.

Nevertheless, the polio viruses by themselves could not account for the fact that 90% to 98% of the persons exposed to and infected by these viruses would never show symptoms of the disease. In fact, less than 1% of those infected would become symptomatic with poliomyelitis (Ryan & Ray, 2004). There had to be something more than just the polio viruses involved in their symptomatic forms. An agent that fails to cause symptoms of the disease in 90% to 95% of known infections would seem to be an agent that could not reasonably be regarded as the sole cause of the disease. The polio viruses did not, for instance, meet even the first of Koch's postulates for causation. Among other candidates for the causation of polio, as already mentioned, were environmental poisons such as the pesticide DDT and closely related toxins. In fact, the worst reported poliomyelitis epidemic in the history of the United States occurred in the summer of 1952 following the heaviest use of DDT in the country's history. In 1952, almost 58,000 cases of polio were reported, along with 3145 deaths and 21,269 persons left with mild to disabling paralysis (Zamula, 1991). The peak incidence, accounting in part at least for those infections, is plainly visible in Figure 7-10. The epidemic of polio after the summer of 1952 corresponds to the highest point in the graph in Figure 7-10.

That same graph also shows the peak in the use of DDT and related pesticides just prior to the polio epidemic, and it reveals that before the Salk vaccine was introduced in 1955, the incidence of polio was already falling. Was it merely a coincidence that the use of DDT was declining in a near lockstep pattern, just prior to the declining incidence of polio? In 1962, when the Sabin oral polio vaccine was introduced, the incidence of polio in the United States had already dropped almost to nothing, as had the production and use of DDT. In fact, incidence of polio in the United States had already reached an all-time low before the introduction of the Sabin oral vaccine in 1962. That also happened to be the year when Rachel Carson's award-winning book, *Silent Spring*, pointed out the long-term effects of DDT in poisoning not only insects, but also plants, birds, animals, and people. Her observations would come up short of connecting DDT with poliomyelitis, but the pesticide's neurotoxicity was made amply clear and its potential for long-range impact was brought to the attention of many.

At a press conference on August 29, 1962, following the publication of Carson's book, President John F. Kennedy was asked whether the Department of Agriculture or the Public Health Service was looking into the scientific evidence of the long-term effects of DDT and other pesticides. Kennedy said they were, and added, "I think particularly, of course, since Miss Carson's book." It would take 10 more years before DDT was officially banned from use in the United States in 1972. By then, the reduction in the number of cases of poliomyelitis, at least in the public mind, had long since been attributed to vaccines. It was virtually unknown by the general public that DDT, in combination with other pesticides, could cause the symptoms of poliomyelitis in animals and humans and that the widespread use of DDT in particular had fallen rapidly after the publication of Carson's book.

Toxic, Yes—But How Toxic?

Following Carson's exposé, the public discourse shifted from whether DDT and related pesticides were dangerous to just how dangerous they were and what sorts of problems they could cause. The nature of the complex interactions between disease agents—such as the polio-type RNA viruses—with pesticides came under increasing scrutiny and would demand a deeper and better account of the body's communication systems and the interactions of elements that had not been given sufficient consideration.

With respect to the autism spectrum, there is no longer any reasonable doubt that pesticides increase toxic burden and contribute to such developmental disorders. For instance, E. M. Roberts et al. (2008) found that expectant mothers exposed during the first two months of their pregnancy to organochlorine pesticides in farming areas of the central valley of California had an increased odds ratio by 610% of having a child who would later be diagnosed with autism. The controls in this study consisted of 6975 normal-weight babies who were born alive at full term. The offending pesticides included dicofol (a derivative of DDT) and endosulfan; both of these neurotoxic substances (Rosas & Eskenazi, 2008) were used widely in California agriculture during the period under investigation (Pesticide Action Network, 2006).

E. M. Roberts et al. (2008) were concerned with children born from 1996 to 1998, for whom they found that autism risk increased with increased dosage of one or both pesticides and decreased as the distance from the application of the pesticide(s) increased. The nearer and larger the exposure, the more likely a toxic injury would occur. According to their analyses, the period of greatest vulnerability for the unborn child to the particular organochlorine pesticides known as dicofol and endosulfan comes in the latter two months of the first trimester of prenatal development (roughly from day 26 to day 81). During this period, the unborn baby's brain and central nervous system are developing very rapidly. Although these authors call for "replication of these findings in other, larger populations" (p. 1488), the fact that there appears to be a causal relation is consistent with existing research showing that neurotoxins generally have a more potent impact when they are presented at an earlier—rather than a later—stage of development. It may well be that Roberts et al.'s procedure of eliminating low-birth-weight and premature babies from their data sample, and absolutely excluding stillbirths, prevented them from discovering the expected deleterious impact of the pesticides in question on unborn babies during the first month of prenatal development. It is virtually certain that the organochlorine pesticides have devastating effects on many vulnerable unborn babies during the first month of prenatal development as well.

There is little doubt that increasing the neurotoxic load of humans during the early stages of prenatal development increases the likelihood of a later diagnosis of autism. However, the CDC-sponsored research by Roberts et al., which looked for a dose-response relationship between pesticides and autism, is a little like looking for the spider that bit someone who died from multiple gunshot wounds. It is true that the pesticide involvements uncovered by Roberts et al. appeared to be causal factors in the later diagnosis of autism. This was so for a significant portion of the 465 children in their data sample who were born between 1996 and 1998 and who were later diagnosed with autism. However, it would be unwise to suppose that there were no other factors interacting with the organochlorines in causing the autism of those children. Among the other interactive factors that are known to be strongly correlated with the increasing numbers of children being diagnosed with autism are the disease agents, other toxins, and foreign proteins being introduced into the bodies of the same California children through vaccines.

With that caveat in mind, it makes sense to dig a little deeper into the Koch criteria for determining the causation of diseases as we continue to explore the research relevant to understanding the etiology of the autism epidemic. Again, the claims made for the efficacy of vaccines—and the polio vaccines in particular—must come under scrutiny. In 2006, David M. Oshinsky won the Pulitzer Prize for History for his book titled *Polio: An American Story* (2005; also see Oxford University Press, 2006). Among the surprises the book contained were some observations consistent with claims others have made concerning the polio research and the way in which the untested vaccines were widely used.

In an interview with Susan Dentzer on *PBS NewsHour with Jim Lehrer,* Oshinsky described the introduction of the polio vaccines in this way: "[W]hat they did when they thought they had a vaccine ready was to begin the largest public health experiment in American history. They lined up 2 million kids and basically gave them a vaccine that no one was certain was safe, that the government hadn't tested, that might not work. And what this really seemed to show was the enormous fear that people had of polio" (Oshinsky & Dentzer, 2005). In addition, Oshinsky pointed out that effective advertising with well-known public figures associated with the March of Dimes beginning with President Franklin D. Roosevelt, himself a victim of polio, and a long list of others including Elvis Presley, Jerry Lewis, and Richard M. Nixon, helped to raise money for research as well as to pay for worldwide polio vaccinations.

The final surprise is that David Oshinsky joins the mainstream in declaring the polio vaccines to have been almost, but not quite, fully successful. At the end of the interview, he urges everyone everywhere to vaccinate their children to help eradicate polio. He says, "Polio is a disease that can be wiped off the face of the earth, . . . break down the resistance to vaccination and you'll end polio forever." But Oshinsky missed a few points in the relevant research.

SV40 and HIV: Complex Interactions

Besides the evidence presented in this chapter (and in Chapter 7) showing the deep complexity of the causation of poliomyelitis and many other neurological diseases and disorders, another effect of the wide use of polio vaccines bears scrutiny. That effect is particularly relevant to our discussion of the ongoing autism epidemic, and it shows another reason why the discrete germ theory and other simplistic theories of the causation of diseases and disorders are mistaken in some cases, and incomplete in most, and probably, in all cases.

As noted earlier, in creating and mass-producing the Salk and Sabin polio vaccines, the researchers and government authorities who promoted them inadvertently introduced SV40 into the human population (CDC, 2007c; Simon, 2008; Sweet & Hilleman, 1960). Figure 10-9 depicts the **isocohedral structure** of this disease agent, which is estimated to be about five-billionths of a meter in diameter. The inadvertent spreading of this virus through the polio vaccines is instructive in relation to the autism epidemic.

In particular, the accidental spreading of SV40 through polio vaccines shows how medicine can get ahead of itself, so to speak, in trying to combat a supposed disease agent (or several of them)

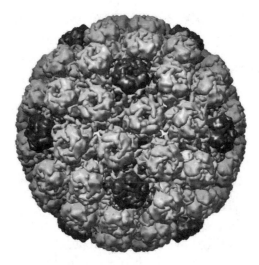

Figure 10-9 The simian virus 40.
Source: Courtesy of University of California San Francisco. Image produced with UCSF Chimera.

by inadvertently introducing one or many other agents that may prove in the long run to be even more threatening than the original agent that was targeted. We saw earlier, based on research with vaccinia—the cowpox virus that was supposedly used to "eradicate smallpox"—that the vaccine actually increased the likelihood of death from smallpox and from a host of other infectious diseases. Vaccines have never been the panacea that their proponents have often hoped for and imagined. On the contrary, in many instances, vaccine success stories have ridden on the coat-tails of reductions in infectious diseases attributable to advances in public sanitation (cleaner water and food and better waste disposal systems) and improved personal hygiene. As pointed out by Smallman-Raynor and Cliff (2004), worldwide epidemics have historically been associated with unsanitary living conditions, like those that still abound in crowded refugee camps in various parts of the world. Oddly, it is a virtual certainty that some vaccines and highly toxic medicines are helping to create worse problems than the ones they were designed to address if not to solve.

After gaining access to the human population through the polio vaccines, as conceded by the CDC (2007c; also see Sweet & Hilleman, 1960) and as is now common knowledge among researchers (Simon, 2008), SV40 has been linked to a huge variety of cancers and other disease conditions. Touching on just a few highlights of that research: M. White et al. (2005) found SV40 in human brain cancer cells; M. Carbone and Bedrossian (2006) reported findings linking SV40 to the asbestos type of lung cancer known as **mesothelioma**; Comar, D'Agaro, Luzzati, Martini, Tognon, and Campello (2007) found SV40 virus in the brain of an AIDS patient with dementia; and Shi et al. (2007) linked SV40 to the production of prostate cancer.

SV40 is believed to have been transmitted to 98 million people in the United States alone. It was probably transmitted to that many or more in the former Soviet bloc of nations, where if records were being kept from the 1950s up to the present, they have never been made public. However, it is certain that the same stocks used to produce the vaccines that infected the U.S. population with SV40 were also used widely in the Communist bloc and around the world.

After the first contaminations were discovered, some efforts were reportedly made to kill the SV40 virus in subsequent batches of the vaccines. Later research, however, has shown that not all the contaminated batches were destroyed or replaced as was commonly reported and supposed (Fiers et al., 1978). Batches of the vaccines manufactured long after the initial reporting of the SV40 contamination by Sweet and Hilleman in 1960 were shown still to contain SV40. Also, old batches thought to have been free of the virus were reexamined many years later and were found to contain it (Carlsen, 2001). The upshot of research concerning SV40 (14,076 hits were returned for peer-reviewed professional research papers from a search for SV40 or "simian virus 40" in "All Databases" at the Institute of Scientific Information's Web of Knowledge site on June 6, 2009) is that it has revealed interesting complexities in interactions across bodily systems.

In the light of the evidence uncovered concerning SV40, other polyoma viruses, and the more elusive **human immunodeficiency virus** (**HIV**), the single-germ/virus theories of disease causation, not to mention the overly simple single-gene theories, appear to have been generally incomplete, if not misleading. For instance, evidence has recently surfaced showing that the reported discovery of the AIDS virus by Robert Gallo and Luc Montagnier in 1983, believed until recently to be the primary cause of AIDS, was fraudulently reported in the journal *Science*. The person at fault was evidently Gallo; and, despite having been provided with ample evidence of the fraud, the journal has not retracted the earlier claims published there in 1984 (J. Cohen, 1993; S. Connor, 1993; Papadopulos-Eleopulos, Turner, & Papadimitriou, 1993).

Moreover, documentary evidence brought to light by an investigative journalist, J. Roberts, shows that Gallo amplified a report written by a colleague who had merely isolated a sufficient amount of what is now known as HIV, so that the possibility of an association with AIDS could be tested. Gallo modified the manuscript before it was published in *Science* and asserted that the AIDS virus had been found (as documented by J. Roberts, 2008). In making the modifications, Gallo crossed out explicit statements denying the claim that he would publish in four different articles in *Science* purporting to have discovered the AIDS virus (Gallo et al., 1984; Popovic, Sarngadharan, Read, & Gallo, 1984; Sarngadharan, Popovic, Bruch, Schupbach, & Gallo, 1984; Schupbach et al., 1984). Later, after Gallo was effectively found guilty of misconduct, he continued to maintain that he and his team had at least co-discovered the AIDS virus, along with Luc Montagnier at the Pasteur Institute in France.

The association of HIV with AIDS remains problematic. As is the case with the polio viruses, HIV comes in different forms and is never the sole cause of any of the disease conditions that constitute full-blown AIDS. We know that the diseases associated with AIDS involve factors other than HIV. In fact, research findings confirm this expectation and provide additional evidence of the incompleteness of discrete germ (and gene) theories and unexpected connections with neurological disorders and the autism epidemic.

Toxins and SV40 Interact with HIV

There is an extremely common neurological deterioration associated with full-blown AIDS that is widely attributed to HIV infection, but that is certain to involve toxins and other disease agents. Figure 10-10, from research by Dr. Clayton Wiley, a neuropathologist at the University of Pittsburgh, shows the inflamed brain tissue of a primate infected with simian immunodeficiency virus (SIV). In humans, a similar disease condition is referred to by a variety of names: **AIDS dementia complex** (**ADC**), **HIV dementia**, **HIV encephalopathy** (F. Gray et al., 2001), and neuroAIDS (Kopnisky, Bao, & Lin, 2008; Shaw et al., 1985; Soontornniyomkij & Wiley, 1998). In the first issue of the journal *NeuroAIDS* in May 1998, Soontornniyomkij and Wiley estimated that 25% of terminal AIDS patients develop neuroAIDS. More recently, the estimated percentage of HIV-infected persons with neurological disorders has been raised to between 40% and 70% (Boisse, Gill, & Power, 2008, p. 799).

The disruption of the central nervous system observed in both AIDS and autism is believed to be caused in part by toxins and in part by various disease agents. Both disorders also seem to involve disruption of the immune systems. In addition, just as studies of toxins show their impact generally to be more severe at early stages of development, so the neurological impact of HIV infection on

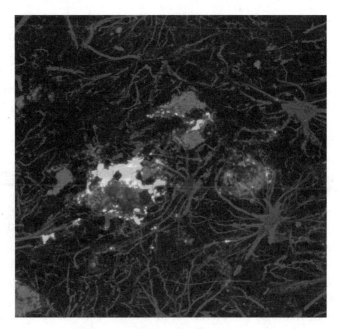

Figure 10-10 Reactive astrocytes (stained blue; darker gray in the black-and-white image) in the inflamed brain of a primate infected with *Simian* immunodeficiency virus (green; the lightest gray in the black-and-white image), and infected macrophages, averaging about 20 microns in diameter (red; e.g., the darker gray spherical form right of center in the black-and-white image).
Source: Courtesy of Clayton A. Wiley.

children appears to be greater than it is on adults. For instance, Mintz (1994) estimated that the incidence of HIV-associated neurological disorders was three to six times greater among HIV-infected children and adolescents than the incidence among HIV-positive adults. One fact accounting in part for the observed differences in the various age cohorts is that developing systems are more susceptible to injury by toxins and disease agents. In addition to being more severely affected than adults are by pesticides, food preservatives, industrial pollution, radiation, and so forth, younger cohorts of children are more apt to be exposed to the toxins and disease agents in vaccines and receive proportionately larger doses relative to their body size. In the case of AIDS, as with autism, the search for causes once again leads back to toxins, vaccines, and combined effects of multiple factors.

With respect to cases of AIDS dementia, it has been hypothesized by many different researchers that toxins and other disease agents are involved as causal elements. Comar et al. (2007), for instance, found both HIV and SV40 in an AIDS patient suffering from dementia and suggested that the SV40, introduced into humans through polio vaccinations, may be a causal factor in producing the dementia. There is also evidence of an interaction between the quantity of HIV and exposure to certain drugs. Carrico et al. (2008) studied 858 individuals who were on a program using prescribed drugs aiming to inhibit the action of HIV—namely, **antiretroviral therapy** (**ART**). Those individuals in their sample who reported regular use of stimulants—commonly including street drugs such as cocaine, methamphetamines (Liang et al., 2008), and especially **amyl nitrate** (a male performance enhancer in various forms referred to as "poppers")—had a 500% increase in their measured HIV load as compared to those individuals who denied regular stimulant use. Both physical and psychological interactions were observed among the stimulant users. On the psychological side, individuals who used stimulants were less likely to comply with the prescribed

ART regimen. However, even among those stimulant users who did stick to the regimen, a 50% increase in HIV load was noted.

Other sources of toxicity that are being examined along with opiates and drugs that are known to be factors in neuroAIDS (Hauser et al., 2009; Liang et al., 2008) and in the terminal diagnosis associated with the onset of ART are the prescription drugs that are most commonly used in the treatment of HIV infections. The prescription drug of choice for treatment of HIV infection is **zidovudine (ZDV)**, also known as **azidothymidine (AZT)**. This agent is believed to suppress the action of the retrovirus HIV, but is itself highly toxic. From early on, AZT was known not only to inhibit the action of HIV, but also to attack the bone marrow where the basic fighting cells of the human immune systems are manufactured. Based on 183 bone marrow examinations from 155 different AIDS patients who used AZT between the years 1984 and 1987, C. E. Harris, Biggs, Concannon, and Dodds (1990) concluded that one factor—in addition to the many different infections and other toxic exposures associated with AIDS, that was causing the many abnormalities they observed in more than two-thirds of the bone marrow specimens—was "therapy with marrow toxic drugs" (p. 146). Other disease agents that thrive in a body with a weakened immune system include tuberculosis (R. J. Patel, G. C. Patel, M. M. Patel, & N. J. Patel, 2008), hepatitis C (Cote et al., 2007), herpes infections (Knox & Carrigan, 1996), and numerous cancers.

After a few weeks of treatment, the drugs used to inhibit the HIV also destroy bone marrow, interfere with the mitochondria, and generally disrupt the immune systems while attempting to delay the impact of the HIV infection (McComsey et al., 2008). Caby and Catlama (2008, p. S45) note that "toxicity adverse events commonly observed with currently approved [drugs]" that aim to inhibit the multiplication of HIV include skin rash, kidney failure, and "neuropsychiatric disorder" (p. S45). A question that commonly arises is whether it is the HIV infection that is producing the observed causes of acute disease and death in most cases or whether it may be the prescribed medications. McComsey et al. argue that "mitochondrial toxicity . . . could be driven by ART and not by HIV itself" (2008, p. 715).

To complicate matters, as any toxicologist would predict and as relevant research consistently shows, adding street drugs into the mix increases the toxic load (Liang et al., 2008). Methamphetamines in particular seem to disable the inherent ability of the body's immune cells (especially the macrophages) to resist invasion by HIV. As a result, methamphetamines—and probably other stimulants, as noted in the research by Carrico et al. (2008)—speed up the disease course of infections that lead to full-blown, symptomatic AIDS.

Retroviruses: More Common Than Supposed

HIV is among those viruses that use an enzyme (a specialized protein system) to take RNA material and code it back into the DNA of the host. The process of genetic interpretation normally runs in the other direction: That is, the billions of words in the double-stranded DNA material of the host are normally interpreted into a vast array of single-stranded RNA molecules (Sanford, 2005). This process is referred to by geneticists as **transcription**, as if the body were taking dictation from the DNA concerning how to construct some protein or how to govern some aspect of its metabolism. However, some viruses, known as **retroviruses**, with the help of an enzyme known as **reverse transcriptase (RT)**—which was discovered in 1970 by independent researchers who shared the Nobel Prize in Physiology or Medicine in 1975 (Baltimore, 1970, 1975; Temin, 1975; Temin & Mizutani, 1970)—can make the process of transcription run backward.

In effect, the virus takes a bit of RNA coding and uploads it backward into the host's DNA with the assistance of reverse transcriptase. For this reason, viruses that use RT are called "retroviruses." When they were first discovered, they were thought to be rare. Now, however, it is known that possibly as much as 5% to 8% of the human genome—more than all the genetic material in the DNA that codes for functional proteins—is constructed with the assistance of the systems found in retroviruses (Bénit, Dessen, & Heidmann, 2001; Cho, Y. K. Lee, & Greenhalgh, 2008; R. Lower, J. Lower, & Kurth, 1996). In their report, Cho and colleagues (2008) review research showing that native retroviruses are richly incorporated into the human genome, these being called **endogenous retroviruses** (**ERVs**; as contrasted with retroviruses that come from outside the host organism, which are called **exogenous retroviruses**). Retroviruses also appear to be involved in cell communications at a distance within the body, thereby enhancing its response to stress factors including injuries, infections, and environmental changes.

SUMMING UP AND LOOKING AHEAD

A paradigm shift is now under way in our understanding of health and disease. Specifically, there is a movement away from the discrete germ, gene, and virus theories of disease and toward a more comprehensive understanding of the interactions and communications that are essential to health and well-being. Nowhere are these intense biochemical communications more evident than in the immune system. The immune system itself involves multiple interactive layers that must communicate with one another and with the rest of the body to function correctly. When defending against invaders such as parasites, bacteria, viruses, and combinations of them, effective communication among the body's own cells, tissues, and organs is essential. If nutrients are misidentified as invaders, allergies result. If the body's own cells, tissues, and organs are misidentified, self-immune diseases result. Everything depends on successful communication.

When research into cancers and AIDS revealed that SV40 and HIV were retroviruses capable of rewriting parts of the genetic text in the genome of an individual, it became apparent that the entire genetic system is more dynamic than realized previously. As a result of advances in theory and research, the interaction between genetics and disease has taken on a more dynamic aspect than ever before. Among the inferences to be drawn is the fact that getting the diagnosis right for both research and clinical purposes—particularly in dealing with the multiple dynamic systems involved in autism and neurological disorders—is more important than ever. In the next chapter, we introduce and review preliminary results with a scale of development based on critical milestones and we show how it can improve the benchmarks used in judging the efficacy of treatments of autism and in gauging the power of suspected or known causal factors in its etiology.

STUDY AND DISCUSSION QUESTIONS

1. How do allergies and autoimmune diseases demonstrate that discrete germ theories need amplification?

2. What empirical findings show that neutrophils can select and seek out a particular invader while ignoring others?

3. How do we know that dendritic cells can capture invaders and present them to the lymph for interrogation and dismantling?

4. How many distinct isotypes of immunoglobulin are there, and which ones can cross the placental barrier? How many functionally distinct immunoglobulin systems have been discovered, and why is there reason to believe that more exist?

5. Why are parasites, in addition to bacteria and viruses, of interest to parents, doctors, and researchers pursuing the root causes of autism? Why do hookworms and pinworms merit special concern?

6. What research findings suggest that a self-immune mother's immunoglobulin may play a role in the autism of her child? Also, what other evidence exists that self-immune diseases and allergies are more common in persons on the autism spectrum than among the population at large?

7. How do atopic reactions illustrate rapid and distant communications within the immune system?

8. In what ways are the problems of identification of diseases by the immune system itself comparable to the problems faced at a higher level by medical practitioners in trying to accurately diagnose and assess the effects of diseases such as autism?

9. How do diseases such as AIDS and cancers relate to neurological problems such as autism?

10. Why are retroviruses of special interest in the genetically linked diseases of the immune system and autism?

chapter eleven

Diagnosis and Treatment

OBJECTIVES

In this chapter, we

1. Consider how the diagnosis of autism and monitoring its course can be improved.

2. Provide a sound theoretical basis for a general scale of normal development.

3. Discuss why the highest and best semiotic representations used are diagnostic.

4. Demonstrate the practicality, validity, and reliability of the new diagnostic scale.

5. Consider why it is reasonable for parents of children with autism to seek answers about causation.

6. Show that effective treatment of autism requires putting ourselves in the position of the client/patient/student.

The diagnosis of disorders, diseases, complexes, and syndromes, and even the correct identification of symptoms of any of these, is crucial to the discovery of their causation and to successful treatment. In this chapter, we show why understanding causation is superior to merely treating symptoms. We do so by comparing treatments aimed at symptoms with treatments dealing with causes. In fact, to sort out the subtle epigenetic factors involved in the causation of the autism epidemic, the importance of accurate determination of levels of severity of any given symptom or combination of them can hardly be overestimated. Here we show how accurate knowledge of the steps involved in the development of normal systems of communication can provide a reliable and valid basis for differentiating levels of severity in autism and in pervasive developmental disorders in general.

The key to accurately assessing the overall impact of disease conditions on complex systems of representation, especially the human **semiotic systems**, is to look to the highest and best level achieved or maintained by an individual. As we will see in this chapter, there are multiple levels normally attained prior to the overt productive use of speech or manual signing, and multiple levels normally attained after that achievement. The highest and best level that is attained at any stage of development—or that is retained after the onset of a disease or disorder—forms the crucial watermark for diagnosis and intervention. In the short term, that watermark defines the starting point for effective behavioral and educational intervention. Looking to the long term, the highest level of representation attainable sets the rough limit on possible employment of the person affected. Clearly, theories of causation and approaches to treatment that enable the retention, restoration, and/or achievement of the highest possible levels of sensory, motor, and linguistic abilities are preferred. In assessing the effectiveness of any treatment, it is critical to be able to accurately measure the up or down movement in the highest and best level of representation that can be produced by the person receiving the treatment.

IMPROVING THE PROCESS OF DIAGNOSIS

In diagnosing a disorder as complex as any of those on the autism spectrum, any pervasive developmental disorder, or any disorders that are related to them, it is essential to consider all of the sign systems that are normally employed in cognitive, social, and emotional development. To say, for instance, that a child is delayed in speech development, or in social skills, or in any other aspect of social, behavioral, and semiotic development, we must know in advance and in some detail what sort of progression of milestones is normally expected. To say that some process of development is abnormal, aberrant, or disordered, it is crucial to have an idea beforehand of what normal, non-aberrant, orderly progress actually is like. When the main criteria for diagnosing an ASD have to do with "abnormal functioning" in "social interaction," "language as used in social communication," or "symbolic or imaginative play" as in the *DSM-IV* (APA, 1994, p. 71) and its successors, it is essential for the diagnostician to have some background and training in the normal milestones of social functioning, language development, and the abilities to represent things symbolically in imagination.

A Representational Problem Through and Through

Just as healthy, intact communication systems form the indispensable basis for the well-being of the genetic and epigenetic systems of the body and its defenses against disease and disorder, functional, intact communication systems also form the essential basis for the normal cognitive, social, and emotional growth and development of every human being. In studying the integrative processes of such development, we discover that systems of representation are critical to successful communications. The systems of representation range from genetics through the epigenetic systems and all the way up to the highest emotional and cognitive capacities that enable distinctly human social interactions. All of them depend on abstract representations that are manifested in some way through noticeable (physically manifested or perceivable) surface forms. These representations range from molecules to the words, phrases, and sentences of human language.

The developmental sequence from the bottom to the top is governed by representations. The meanings of the genetic material are at first manifested in the long molecules of DNA, later translated into RNA in various forms, then into proteins, and finally into the very organism itself that the DNA expresses in an extremely compact and abstract form. Exceedingly complex and detailed interactions across systems must proceed successfully over time if the organism is to be physically well formed. Assuming that all goes well from conception through embryonic development, the unborn child proceeds through an amazing series of rapid transformations, all of which utterly depend from start to finish on representational control systems. From conception forward, those representational systems involve interactions between the genetic and epigenetic systems of the developing unborn baby. The various transformations take place within a relatively controlled and protected biochemical and increasingly social environment. In a full-term baby, the senses are fully functional, integrated, and active well before birth. Even by the end of the first trimester, the developing unborn baby already has its distinct human limbs, fingers, and toes. It can take steps in the womb, jump around, turn a somersault, suck its thumb, rub its eyes, and scratch an itch.

The Unborn Baby Already Sensing, Moving, and Thinking

A few weeks later on, the fetus begins the processes of swallowing and, more importantly, breathing the amniotic fluid inside the placenta. This process, known as **fetal breathing**, begins about the time the unborn baby can smile. There is overwhelming evidence that this is a social smile in the womb, certainly not a response to gas pains (see J. W. Oller, 2006, 2010; also M. W. Sullivan & Lewis, 2003). The developing child can open its eyes, recognize the familiar voices of the mother and her frequent interlocutors, and distinguish the peculiar rhythms of its native language. It has already become highly responsive to bright sunlight as well as to the moods and emotions expressed in the mother's conversations and her physical interactions with others. The fetus is already sensitive to changes in lighting, sounds, tastes, and smells. For instance, unborn babies show significant increases in their rates of fetal breathing and swallowing if their mother consumes caffeine or has a cigarette (Huisman, Risseeuw, vanEyck, & Arabin, 1997).

Hepper, Dornan, and Little (2005; also Hepper, 2007) showed that unborn babies exposed to alcohol exhibit an abnormal increase in startle responses; Troese et al. (2008) showed that sleep abnormalities persist in babies exposed prenatally to alcohol use by mother. Babies exposed in this way, according to the research, are more apt to have neurodevelopmental delays or disorders and/ or to experience sudden infant death syndrome. It stands to reason from the study of such normal milestones of development, which can be impacted by even relatively mild toxins, that the more substantial interactions produced by vaccines, for instance, should be examined closely as prime causal factors in SIDS and neurodevelopmental disorders such as autism.

Layered and Ranked Representational (Semiotic) Systems

Before the normal child is born, all of the semiotic systems necessary for normal development are already in place. Contrary to the general notion that integration of the senses and complex motor expressions such as smiling must occur after birth, we now know from moving video of babies before birth, that the baby's senses are already fully functional and at work in the womb. Also contrary to the still popular view that a neonate's smile is caused by gas pains, we know from the technology developed by Dr. Stuart Campbell at London's Create Health Clinic that the unborn baby not only has integrated senses, but can produce unlearned facial gestures including the classic human smile well before birth (S. Campbell, 2004 ☺). His research, development, and clinical applications of four dimensional video technologies have opened new windows on prenatal development and his empirical work, along with theoretical advances in the general theory of sign systems (semiotics), have already demonstrated that the old "gas theory" of neonate smiling is an excellent modern example of a false idea that was widely accepted and propagated in the health sciences.

The current research on normal development shows that the baby in the womb is already processing information about voices, language, movements, and persons that the baby has come to know through the senses, especially sound and touch, before birth. If we look at what the normally developing baby can do in the womb, it is plainly false to suppose that social smiling is developed months after birth by imitation. If the unborn baby can produce a full-fledged social smile with upturned corners of the mouth and crinkled eyes well before birth, as we can see in the video from S. Campbell's work, the theory espoused by some—for example, by Feinberg (2007), the medical director of the Resnick Neuropsychiatric Hospital at UCLA—that babies smile "likely because they have gas" (p. xi) can be ruled out. To make valid judgments about developmental processes, we must have valid information about the normal sequence of the milestones and how they actually unfold.

There are three main systems of representation that must be distinguished, and, yet, that are intimately related from before birth. First there are the senses; second, there are sensations combined with intentional movements; and, finally, at the highest level, there are sensations together with significant intentional movements that form the basis for language and all of the higher cognitive, social, and behavioral functions dependent on the uniquely human language capacity.

From the Body and Senses Upward

As Aristotle pointed out long ago, without any of the senses (sight, hearing, touch, taste, and smell), no cognitive, social, or emotional development of any kind—and certainly no language development—could take place. In fact, a healthy, well-formed body is the normal (usual) basis for functional and intact senses. The senses, in their turn, are important to the development of coordinated movements within our bodily systems as we interact with other persons. Without sensible controlled movements, we could not acquire the normal abilities that are essential to the linguistic interactions that constitute the basis for families, communities, and the functional societies of the world. Without language, there could be no knowledge of history, law, science, mathematics, religion, art, music, choreography, or anything that is distinctively human.

For this reason, just as communication disorders have the potential to rob human beings of the capacity to interact with and relate to each other, in an analogous way toxins, disease agents, and their interactions can foul the inner workings of our biochemistry. Interestingly, all such disrupted conditions—from physical diseases to the most subtle of social, cognitive, and behavioral disorders—depend at their most basic level on things that go wrong in communication systems of one sort or another. With all that in mind, but setting aside the biochemical systems momentarily, we can divide and classify the traditional communication disorders (as we have shown elsewhere, with Badon, in our *Cases* book) into four major categories:

- Those that affect the form of the body—such as cleft lip, palate (**craniofacial disorders**), or spine (**spina bifida**)
- Those that adversely affect the senses—such as impairment or complete loss of sight, hearing, and so on
- Those that affect the capacity for intentional voluntary movement—for example, cerebral palsy, Parkinsonism, and epilepsy
- Those that affect the human language capacity and/or any of the related cognitive, social, and behavioral abilities that depend directly or indirectly on language (J. W. Oller et al., 2010)

Of course, many distinctions can be made within each of these major classifications of disorders, and there are many instances where more than one classification will fit a single individual. Disorders that occur together (i.e., that are comorbid) are especially common in autism and in all of the pervasive disorders that appear during development.

Pervasive Early Disorders

Because a disorder that occurs anywhere in the developmental sequence is apt to produce cascading effects, downstream consequences of any developmental disorder are not merely common, but are virtually inevitable. In the pervasive developmental disorders (i.e., the disorders associated with the autism spectrum), cascading effects and multiple simultaneous disorders—so-called *comorbid* conditions and diseases—must be anticipated and should be regarded, in most instances, as unsurprising.

Nevertheless, there is a great deal of controversy over categorical descriptions such as "Asperger syndrome" and "high-functioning autism" (HFA). Some have supposed, for instance, that it will be possible to draw a line between Asperger's disorder and HFA, that they are factually different conditions; others have supposed that the two cannot be distinguished at all. In fact, R. A. Ritvo and colleagues (R. A. Ritvo, E. R. Ritvo, Guthrie, & M. J. Ritvo, 2008; R. A. Ritvo, E. R. Ritvo, Guthrie, Yuwiler et al., 2008) could not distinguish these descriptors in their comparisons of groups of individuals who had previously been labeled with one or the other diagnosis. According to the criteria applied in the research by Ritvo and colleagues, the descriptors seem to fit the same cases equally well or badly. Although Nataf et al. (2006) found that "porphyrin levels [in urine samples] were unchanged in Asperger's disorder, distinguishing it from autistic disorder" (p. 99), these researchers did not focus attention specifically on HFA in the autism category. That is, they were really only able to distinguish Asperger's disorder from the broad spectrum of what is called "autistic disorder."

It remains unknown whether it will be possible to distinguish HFA from Asperger's disorder in the future, but there is no reason on the basis of present evidence to suppose that the distinction can be sharply made with any of the existing methods of diagnosis. It remains for researchers to find out to what extent (if at all) there are any behavioral, psychological, or biochemical differences yet to be identified across individuals and groups in the two categories. The fundamental question is whether the diagnoses of Asperger syndrome and HFA are the same or different.

In the meantime, more subtle measures of developmental processes may help to resolve that remaining question and others as well as the controversies underlying them. When it comes to development there are some major points that are not in doubt. For instance, there is nearly unanimous agreement among theoreticians who have concerned themselves with growth and development—especially in the unfolding of genetic systems and the development of the human language capacity—that the processes are constructive as well as layered and ranked. The idea that higher representational systems of language depend on lower-ranked representations involving movement and sensation can be traced back to Aristotle. Jean Jacques Rousseau (1712–1778) preceded Jean Piaget (1896–1980) by more than a century in proposing distinct stages of development. Later thinkers, however, would subscribe to the idea that we "learn to learn" by developing new systems of representation based on ones that preceded them.

The Theory of Abstraction in a Nutshell

Nowhere has the constructive process of sign building and the layeredness and ranking of the sign hierarchy been made so plain as in the recent development of the **theory of abstraction**. This theory (as we have noted and explained in detail in other publications) is grounded in irrefutable logic and supported by a great deal of empirical evidence. It can be summed up very succinctly. The analogy of a nut within its shell—take an ordinary acorn as an instance—is suggestive of the essence of the theory.

Suppose the nut falls to the ground, sprouts, takes root, and grows into an oak tree. As a nut, it was merely a bounded object. By falling to the earth and growing into a tree, it demonstrates the three main levels of the sign hierarchy:

- First, it shows the iconic level of bounded objects (**icons**) when it is merely an acorn.
- Second, it shows the indexical level consisting of meaningful movements (especially significant ones—**indexes**) of icons as it falls to the ground and sprouts.
- Third, it shows the symbolic level (of conventional genetic or linguistic **symbols**) by virtue of the fact that the icon (acorn) is linked through a series of indexes (movements of the acorn) with its conventional meaning as a symbol (which we see in the oak tree).

Through the process of abstraction, we can see that the acorn is connected through its history of movements with the oak tree. We can see, by virtue of the symbolic and historical (true) relationship between the acorn and the oak, that the icon (the acorn), through its actual relationship with the tree (an index connecting one with the other over time), constitutes an abstract symbol referring to the tree.

This is a surprisingly good metaphor for the whole theory of abstraction and for some of its most amazing logical consequences—ones that become obvious only as the process of mapping the icon through its indexical relations into its symbolic meaning dynamically unfolds over time. For instance, as the process develops over time it is easy to see that the tiny acorn must contain, in some way, a representation of the development of the oak tree including not only the tree itself but also all of its intricate living systems of communication and transportation as well as of the sort of environment that will be required to enable its development and to sustain it over time. Yet, it is certainly not obvious that all that could be contained within the tiny nutshell to start with. It can also be argued, on the basis of the theory of abstraction, that the meaning contained within the acorn anticipates the wind and weather; the microbes, insects, birds, squirrels, and other organisms that will interact with the tree over its expected lifetime; and the means by which the nut will produce other acorns like the one from which it came.

The acorn in our metaphor begins as an iconic representation that also points us to the beginning of the theory of abstraction. The noticing of distinct bounded objects (e.g., persons, things, spaces, and whatever parts they have or whatever they may contain) depends on the ability to discriminate boundaries, and to notice that the boundaries stay intact when an object or person moves—as when an acorn falls to the ground, or as we roll it around in our hand, or simply we move around the nut. Without taking account of the boundaries of things (e.g., the shell of the acorn), it would be impossible to develop any concepts of any objects whatever.

Next, moving upward in the sign hierarchy by the process of abstraction, we discover that meaningful intentional movements (e.g., meaningful gestures, or the articulate movements of speech and language) cannot be noticed at all without the objects that move in producing them. For instance, consider what would become of any movement of any person or thing if the bounded object itself had never existed, or if its boundaries were never known. Clearly, the movement also could not exist or be represented meaningfully.

It follows that meaningful movements depend on the prior discovery of objects that move. Logically climbing up to the next higher level of the sign hierarchy, it becomes obvious as we think through the process of abstraction that without objects that move intentionally and refer to other objects and their relations, no language system whatever would be possible. Thus the three main layers of the sign hierarchy—sensory representations, sensory–motor representations, and linguistic/symbolic representations—are established. Also, the fact that they are ranked is likewise established. Symbolic signs (especially linguistic ones) depend on and yet outrank sensory–motor signs, which likewise depend on but outrank sensory signs. Much more can be said along these lines from a theoretical and empirical point of view. The purpose here, however, is merely to sketch in the theory to provide the basis for a scale of development that can be used in diagnosing any given person's level of semiotic development, whether that person has a communication disorder or not.

The Basis for a Generalized Scale of Development

In view of the fact that development normally proceeds only in an outward and upward direction, and given that the theory of abstraction shows that higher systems of the sign hierarchy cannot be attained until the lower ones on which the higher ones absolutely depend are already in place, it follows that to diagnose the current level of development of any given individual, irrespective of any possible disease, disorder, or limiting condition, it is only logically necessary to find the highest and best level of representation and communication of which that individual is capable. That level, according to the theory of abstraction, provided only that it can be validly determined, will necessarily be diagnostic. It will show whether the person is developing normally or is significantly delayed. This outcome follows from logical and empirical evidence showing that normal semiotic development can progress at various rates, but must progress in a relatively rigid sequence. A person can always backslide to a lower level, or just reach back and use that level, but it is not possible without going through the normal sequence of acquisition to leap ahead from a very low level to a much higher one. This logical inference has been called the **reversion principle** (J. W. Oller & Rascón, 1999).

Each level of the sign hierarchy must be developed before the next level up, and there are many steps from the first level to the last. As a result, on the basis of the theory of abstraction, the level of attainment of any individual—and/or that individual's regression or progress over a period of time—can be determined with a high degree of validity by merely looking to the highest and best level of semiotic representation that is reliably manifested within a given time frame by that same individual. Determining that level, for any given time frame or across a given period of time during which, say, treatment has occurred, also forms the necessary basis for judging whether that treatment (or perhaps a combination of treatments) has resulted in a significant and measurable change. To attribute any gain over time to a treatment, however, it is necessary to subtract out any gain that would have been expected in the normal course of development without the treatment.

DETERMINING THE HIGHEST AND BEST LEVEL OF REPRESENTATION

For a normally developing fetus, neonate, toddler, or child at any age, the highest and best level of representation attainable is expected to advance over time. It is a moving target. According to the theory of abstraction, the moving level of the highest and best semiotic systems attained is expected to increase in richness, generality, and abstractness as the child progresses toward maturity.

Stages of Development

Perhaps the idea that psychologists and learning theorists are most apt to agree on is that physical, behavioral, cognitive, and social development are all fundamentally constructive. For this reason, the progress of the normally developing individual proceeds in steps. The normal progress itself can be thought of as something like a stairway going upward from the ground level. Although there may be disagreement and controversy about the steps to be taken, the levels to be attained, and how long it takes the individual to move between levels, there is fundamental and almost universal agreement that the process of growth and development is both constructive and somewhat layered.

Long ago, Jean Jacques Rousseau [1712–1778] wrote a generalized account of a partly fictional character named *Émile* of whom Rousseau was the teacher. In this book, which was really about education and teaching, he supposed that such a normal individual naturally progresses from a primitive pre-rational stage of development until approximately age 12, then begins to reason up to about age 16, after which, according to Rousseau, the individual is an adult. The twentieth-century psychologist Jean Piaget set quite different boundaries on the stages of development, but he, too, supposed that development proceeds upward through various levels. Piaget proposed four major stages. He supposed that the normal child first uses the five senses to discover the world during what he called the **sensorimotor stage** from birth to two years. Piaget did not place much emphasis during those first two years on the work being done by the child to acquire one or more particular languages.

Usually, by two years of age, the child has already reached the two-word stage of language development. Amplifying and correcting some of the inferences drawn by Piaget and others, T. G. R. Bower (1971, 1974) would later show that neonates already have fully integrated senses and are able to apply at birth fundamental logical principles and experimental procedures that Piaget attributed to a later period of development. The endpoint of Piaget's stages of learning was conceived in terms of what Piaget regarded as genuine logical reasoning. The highest level of such reasoning, according to Piaget, would be achieved by about the age of 12 years. Piaget's own daughters were the basis for most of his conclusions. According to his observations of them, by the time they were about 12 years old they were able to understand fully reversible abstract operations, such as adding 2 to 3 to get 5 and then taking 2 away from 5 to get back to 3.

Although a great deal of controversy persists about the order of stages and the means used to define them, the important thing to note here is that the idea that development progresses in stages, that it is constructive, has been widely accepted for a very long time. It is still perhaps the most fundamental point of agreement in developmental psychology and linguistics even today. It is almost unnecessary to mention that genetics and the study of embryology in particular also show that development is constructive, proceeding in stages.

The idea of constructive levels of development was amplified by Lev Vygotsky [1896–1934] a Russian genius who died of tuberculosis at the age of 38. In his most productive period (roughly from age 24 to 34), he produced a number of works that would shape the future of psychology and especially the study of learning disabilities and communication disorders—a field of study for which he proposed the term **defectology**. By this term, translated from an almost perfect Russian cognate (дефектология—[dIfik´talogjɛ] the reader can hear the Russian word on the DVD to appreciate just how close the cognate is 🔊), Vygotsky did not mean to disparage disorders, but rather to acknowledge their character. When persistent distortions, regressions, delays, plateaus, or other persistent deviations from the normal course of development occur, they are indicative of abnormalities.

Vygotsky's most important contributions, however, centered on his efforts to define the leading edge of normal growth and development. Concerning this idea—one deeply grounded in the constructive and layered nature of the processes of growth, development, and learning—there is also fundamental and widespread agreement. Vygotsky urged that special attention should be given to the level of development just beyond the one that the individual has already mastered. He called this next level upward the **zone of proximal development** (**ZPD**) (Vygotsky, 1962, 1978). If we think of the stairstep analogy, the ZPD would be the step on the stairway just above the one we already happen to be standing on.

The concept of the ZPD, if it could be determined for any given individual, would define the changing level of semiotic capacity over the course of time as the individual grows and develops normally. It is expected to be a growth curve resembling the curve shown in Figure 2-4 and 2-5, albeit with a very different basis. Logically, the moving point of the ZPD determines a line that fluctuates over time, normally rising. It also determines the benchmarks—or the growth curve—by which the efficacy of any treatment or intervention must ultimately be judged. If a "regression" is to be measured or if its reversal is to be documented, the changing level of Vygotsky's ZPD, to the extent that it can be determined, must show these changes.

Accurately determining the watermarks left by the upward movement of normal growth and development can also be critical to making valid inferences about the causation of upward movements, as well as of plateaus, regressions, and the sorts of crashes that we see in some instances of autism spectrum disorders. Logically, if a subtle causal effect of any causal impact (or treatment) is hypothesized, then a sufficiently sensitive measure of that impact will be essential to demonstrating the existence of the cause (or the effect of the treatment), if any genuine cause or effect does exist. To assess the distinct impact of any given factor or any combination of factors, or to tease apart contributions from distinct factors or interactive effects, accurate determination of the changing levels of abilities and skills before, during, and after a course of treatment(s) is logically indispensible. For all of the foregoing reasons, it is essential to look to the highest and best levels of cognitive, behavioral, and emotional capabilities. To do so, we need a concept such as the ZPD as proposed by Vygotsky.

Analogy: Severity of Disorder Is to Treatment as Highest and Best Is to Diagnosis

Just as the degree of severity of injuries, diseases, and disorders provides the basis for setting priorities in treating them, with the most threatening and urgent conditions usually receiving the highest priority, in assessing the efficacy of treatment outcomes in any given individual (or group) the highest and best capabilities that are enabled or restored by the treatment are diagnostic of the relative success or failure of the treatment itself. A treatment that produces no effect is of very little interest, if any. Conversely, a treatment that produces significant and substantial positive (or negative) effects may be of great interest. Usually, we think of the causes of diseases and disorders as producing negative effects, whereas effective treatments halt or, better yet, reverse those negative effects.

A treatment that produces no measurable change must be judged of no effect, while one that produces a substantial change—depending on whether the change is positive or negative—must generally be judged to be beneficial in the former case and harmful in the latter. Because treatments generally are costly in money, time, and effort, those that have no impact, or that have a negative impact, will generally be rejected in favor of treatments that produce significant and substantial measurable positive outcomes. For all of the foregoing reasons, in dealing with the causes of the present autism epidemic, and with proposed methods of prevention and treatment, it is essential to find the most practical, reliable, and valid methods that can be devised to diagnose, assess, and measure as accurately as possible the changing states of any given individual or group that may be affected by it.

In the following section, we present a generalized scale of development grounded thoroughly in the theory of abstraction along with preliminary pilot data showing that such a scale can be understood and applied in practice by persons with a modicum of training. It is hypothesized, and demonstrated in the pilot data reported later in this chapter, that persons with additional training can be expected to achieve even higher levels of accuracy. With such facts in mind, it is recommended (and we ourselves are engaged in research along this line) that such a scale be widely applied to treatment protocols for autism and related disorders.

A SCALE FOR DIAGNOSING THE SEVERITY OF COMMUNICATION DISORDERS

The following *Milestones Scale of Development* consists of 17 distinct levels of semiotic ability. It is derived from two earlier publications (J. W. Oller & Rascón, 1999; J. W. Oller et al., 2006) and from presentations by S. D. Oller and S. A. Oller (2008a, 2008b). Each level in the scale is defined with respect to the "highest and best" semiotic capability demonstrated by the individual in question. The Milestones Scale is based on normal development as understood in terms of the theory of abstraction. That theory is summarized briefly in this chapter but is discussed in detail in the publications just cited in this paragraph. The underlying premise for the scale in question is that abnormal semiotic development, and communication disorders in general, can be meaningfully defined and diagnosed only in relation to what is expected in normal development.

The Guiding Principle

In judging the manifest uses of meaningful sign systems—that is, what are called "nonverbal" or "preverbal" behaviors as well social and linguistic interactions—the question to keep in mind is this: *What is the highest and best level demonstrated by the individual in question when responding to the normal demands of day-to-day experience?* In making such a judgment, it is important to observe the individual in question for a sufficient amount of time and over a sufficient period of time to be relatively certain that the highest and best performance of which that person is capable (during that period of development) has been observed and accurately determined. Relatively small fluctuations in performance are normal and expected depending on such factors as alertness, intensity of interest, emotional state, and energy expended. Instead, what we are looking for is evidence of the highest level of development already attained in the performance of common (but demanding) behavioral, social, and cognitive tasks. We are interested in what the individual in question can do when fully alert, attentive, and motivated.

Each step up the Milestones Scale can be thought of as a "can do" ("has done" and "does do") behavior involved in representing things in relation to bodily persons, their meaningful movements, and the abstract signs (gestures, glances, facial expressions, and words) that form the main basis for social interactions. At each step on the scale, the sign systems involved increase in difficulty, complexity, and abstractness. As they do so, their power to represent the changing stream of experience also increases. As the developing sign user moves upward with each step, the sign systems that can be understood and produced at will progressively become more informative, more predictable, and more comprehensive. That is, as the sign systems that come into view become more complex, they also become more adequate to accurately and comprehensively represent what is going on in the stream of experience.

Piaget called this aspect of the constructive sign process **adequation**. Turning the same idea around the other way, we may suppose that failure to progress beyond a given level on the scale (i.e., a blocking or **plateau effect**) or falling back from a higher level to a substantially lower one (the sort of crash referred to as "regression" in much of the autism literature) are both indicative of the degree of severity of whatever communication disorder or disease condition has caused the halt in progress or the apparent loss of prior gains. In other words, every level of the scale defines a milestone that can be expected to be reached in a particular sequence and within a roughly defined time frame by someone progressing normally in ordinary, healthy growth and development. At the same time, every such milestone becomes diagnostic of the degree of severity of any delay, disorder, or disease condition that has interrupted progress at a particular level or that has set back prior gains of the affected individual (or group).

The scale to be presented has 16 levels pertaining to progress toward normal adult maturity. That level of maturity may be thought of as a seventeenth level that is just above the ceiling of the scale.

Level 0: Sensory Awareness of the Stream of Experience

Formerly, Level 0 on the Milestones Scale of normal development was believed to be attained by a normal infant some time between birth and two weeks of age. However, based on more up-to-date research and more informative technologies (especially ultrasound moving pictures of fetuses in real time), we now know that babies achieve this level by about the third or fourth week into the third trimester before their birth. This is the level of development where the senses are fully functional, well integrated, and already delivering valid sensory and motor information on multiple channels (visual, auditory, tactile, gustatory, and olfactory) about the baby's own body; the environment within the womb; the mother's bodily movements, rhythms, and emotional reactions; and so forth. The baby at this stage is also more or less aware of goings-on in the larger world outside the womb. Those external events are known to the developing unborn child through changes in lighting, sounds, movements that it can feel, as well as tastes and smells that it can sense from within the womb.

Because understanding of the behavior of babies in the womb is still in its infancy, so to speak, the extent to which the normally developing baby progresses beyond Level 0 while still in the womb remains to be further explored. However, with respect to autism and PDDs in general, a person who does not progress beyond this level or who falls back to this level is someone unable to process sensory information in such a way as to give evidence of perceiving, or taking account, of the bounded objects in his or her perceptual field. At this level, the individual with ASD seems not to be able to discriminate any boundaries and, we may suppose, fails even to differentiate the limits of his or her own body as distinct from everything else. A person plateaued or set back to this level of development will give evidence of not knowing at the most basic physical level the answer to the question, "What's me, and what's not me?" An example found on the DVD is the behavior characteristic of severe autism as displayed by Ethan Kurtz roughly from his second year to his fourth year, when he appeared to be unresponsive to other persons, toys, activities, and so forth 💿.

Behaviors to look for in defining Level 0 would include unresponsiveness to visual, auditory, or tactile stimuli. In extreme cases, what may appear as "stimming"—repetitive self-stimulating behaviors such as hand-flapping, rocking, spinning, or even self-injurious behaviors such as head-banging and other forms of self-mutilation—may be indicative of an inability, or a block of some sort, that prevents the individual from finding the physical boundaries of even that person's own body. It can be thought of as something like the situation of a person at sea, where things are constantly changing but not making any sense, and where there are no familiar boundaries or landmarks to be found. It has been suggested more than once by persons with high-functioning autism that the "stimming" behaviors that they tend to fall into unintentionally when stressed or distracted may provide something like a familiar place of retreat or a kind of "magic comfort zone" in which they commonly find themselves, without knowing how they got there. For instance, a highly verbal autistic individual, according to Cesaroni and Garber (1991, p. 309), observed "stereotyped movements aren't things I decide to do for a reason; they're things that happen by themselves when I'm not paying attention to my body" (also in Leary & Hill, 1996, p. 46).

Level 1: Discriminates Objects from the Background by Finding Boundaries

The normally developing individual can be expected to achieve Level 1 of development before birth. Formerly, J. W. Oller and Rascón (1999) supposed that the discrimination of bounded objects had to take place after birth, but it is now evident that the normally developing individual is able to discriminate the boundaries of his or her own body before birth by grasping a foot, scratching an itch, or sucking the thumb. However, there is no doubt that until about the fourth week after birth the normally developing infant continues to discriminate additional bounded objects, including persons—adding them to an expanding and increasingly familiar iconic repertoire of persons, objects, and scenes that the child discriminates.

To be assured that Level 1 development has been attained, there are several behaviors to look for, including mutual eye contact with someone else, shared interest in the mother's (or another adult's) cooing and gooing to the baby, and evidence of responsiveness to visual, auditory, and tactile stimuli. The normal baby will smile before it is born, and social smiling will also occur within the first few weeks after birth. When these things occur in response to close interactions with the mother or another caregiver, there is sufficient evidence that Level 1 has been achieved.

In abnormal or disordered cases, the key indicator that the individual has not achieved this level would be a blank stare as contrasted with mutual eye contact. However, in the event that the affected individual's attention can be drawn to a moving object, a person, or any bounded thing, we must suppose that Level 1 development, at a minimum, has been attained.

Level 2: Tracks a Slowly Moving Object

The capacity exhibited at this level involves the ability to track a moving object visually or otherwise. Again, we now have tentative evidence that Level 2 may be achieved even before birth. An instance of a behavior suggesting this level of development in the womb would be the act of an unborn baby striking and pushing away the barrel of a needle during **amniocentesis**—the procedure where a sample of amniotic fluid is drawn from the placenta to test for genetic abnormalities and/or infections (Chamberlain, 2007). A normally developing individual will continue to refine and speed up the capacity to perform these sorts of tasks. At birth, or very soon thereafter, the baby will be able to follow a slowly moving object within its visual field, performing what is known as **smooth pursuit**. Later, at a higher level of normal development, more complex pursuits will become possible, such that the individual's own eye and body movements can be coordinated with the changing movements of a fairly rapidly moving object.

However, at Level 2, the key behavioral demonstration is merely tracking the course of a slow-moving object. Additional behaviors showing that this level has been achieved include looking at an object while reaching and grasping. Also, avoidance behaviors, such as T. G. R. Bower and colleagues (Bower, 1974; Kaye & Bower, 1994; Walton & Bower, 1993) demonstrated in normal infants as young as two weeks, where the baby shows defensive posturing, wide eyes, open mouth, and hands up as a reaction to a moving object that seems to be on a collision course with the baby's face, provide ample evidence of the attainment of this level of representation.

By contrast, a person who shows no reaction to a hand or object moving in front of his or her own face, even if the object or hand appears to be on a collision course, must be diagnosed at a lower level than Level 2. (To determine which level, as always, it is essential to determine the highest and best level that the individual does demonstrate.)

Level 3: Recalls an Object No Longer Present in the Perceptual Field

Level 3 of semiotic development is demonstrated when the individual is able to think of an object that is no longer in the perceptual field. This ability might be called "perceptual memory." Although we cannot directly observe a behavior that unambiguously shows that this level of representation has been attained, we can infer that it must precede the capacity to dream. Supposing that **rapid eye movements** (**REM**) occur and can be observed while babies are sleeping in the womb, it should be possible to infer that dreaming occurs in babies before they are born. From studies with adults we know that such REM sleep is normally accompanied by dreaming in which the eye movements are associated with fictional, imaginary visual perceptions that occur in dreams. If such fictional experiences occur in the womb, this fact would seem to indicate that the unborn baby has already achieved the level of abstraction required, for instance, to think of its own body parts or of sensations of sound (as in hearing mother's voice) in the absence of the events that would normally produce such sensations.

Another way to diagnose the attainment of any given semiotic level of development is by inference. If any higher level than the one in question has been attained, clearly this one, for instance, Level 3 in this case, has also been achieved. When Level 3 is attained, we can infer that there is already in place an iconic vocabulary of things that can be thought of when they are not being perceived. In its absence—that is, in the case of a disorder where this level has either not been attained or has been lost—the individual will show no evidence of recalling, looking for, or otherwise showing a continued interest in an object that has disappeared or been removed from the perceptual field. By contrast, a person who has achieved this level will notice the change and show some interest in it (e.g., by fussing about it).

Level 4: Conducts a Search for an Object No Longer in the Perceptual Field

In a normally developing individual at Level 4, by about four to eight weeks after birth, the infant will be able to conduct a search for an object that falls on the floor from a highchair or that is removed, covered up, or otherwise occluded in the field of perception. Likewise, the individual may think of an object that has not been perceived for some time and initiate a search for it. The defining behavior is searching for a missing object, as demonstrated by the conclusion of the search when the object is found.

In the case of disorders (either failure to develop or loss of prior gains), a person below Level 4 may show annoyance at the removal or disappearance of an object, but without initiating any kind of search to retrieve it even if the object has just fallen a short distance, or has been occluded by another object, within the individual's perceptual field.

Level 5: Connects Distinct Appearances of a Moving Object in the Perceptual Field

Normally developing individuals seem to achieve Level 5 sometime between weeks 12 and 16 after their birth (at three to four months of age). When they arrive at Level 5, they are not only able to search for an object in its former location or in a location where the object may be expected to appear along a line of motion, but are also able to track the distinct movements of the same object to connect them with that self-same individual object.

Before they arrive at Level 5 of development, which usually happens near the end of month 4 after birth, normally developing infants have not yet discovered that a single object moving around is the same in all of its inertial states. For instance, in one of T. G. R. Bower's most famous experiments (Bower, 1971), he presented a baby with an interesting object, a small train car with flashing lights moving slowly to the baby's right along a track for a few seconds, then stopping for a few seconds, then moving slowly back to the baby's left, stopping again, and so forth. Bower correctly predicted that younger infants would expect to find the moving object in the position where it started out and returned on each of 10 cycles; when the car had ended up on cycle 11 by going farther to the baby's left, younger infants tended to look back to the position to the right where the car ended up on the 10 prior cycles.

What Bower did not expect to find, but did discover—contrary to essentially all of the popular theories of psychological development at that time—was that prior to about 12 weeks of age, the baby actually searched all of the former inertial states of the little car. That is, the child considered the train car going right, going left, back to standing in the middle of the field of view with its flashing lights, standing still at the left, standing still at the right, or standing off to the far left where it ended up on cycle 11. What the experiment showed, to the amazement of many theoreticians, was later explained by the theory of abstraction. The baby had to develop another whole system of coordinated indexical movements so that he or she could move smoothly with the object through each of its inertial states and discover that the object was the same one throughout the cycle.

At Level 5 of representation, which the normal baby seems to achieve (according to Bower's results) by about week 16, the developing individual is able to represent an object across its different inertial states. After this level of representation is achieved, when an object begins to move, the individual does not search the previous (stationary) location but continues to follow the object until interest is lost or the object quits moving.

Using Bower's experimental procedure or one like it, it is possible to test for the attainment of Level 5 by putting the child (or other individual) in a comfortable chair where a camera or observer can see that person's eye and head movements. Using a remote-controlled car or toy, we first move the toy back and forth in a relatively small area (6–10 inches) for five cycles, and then move the toy to a new location 24–36 inches away; if the child searches the previous locations for the toy, we conclude that the individual has not yet reached Level 5.

Level 6: Keeps an Object in Mind After It Has Left the Field of Perception

The normally developing individual seems to achieve Level 6 of development by about week 20. In saying this, we again draw on empirical research by T. G. R. Bower (Bower, 1974, 1984; Kaye & Bower, 1994; Walton & Bower, 1993) as informed by the theory of abstraction. At Level 6, the normally developing child correctly infers the continued existence of an object (or person) that not only moves around within the perceptual field periodically, but also may disappear entirely one or many times from the changing perceptual field. To represent the continued existence of such an object, the developing sign user must infer that the object that moves beyond the boundary/horizon of the perceptual field is still out there, even if it is beyond the limits of his or her perception. Once this achievement occurs, the child will no longer be greatly surprised if the object that formerly disappeared (e.g., the mother who left the room) should suddenly reappear.

The type of representational system possible at this level requires an abstraction beyond that of Level 5, where the object stayed within the perceptual field while moving around. In this case, the continued existence of the object that goes beyond the borders of the perceptual field and its mental association with prior experiences must be based on an inference that reaches beyond the borders of any particular perceptual field.

Behaviors that signal the achievement of Level 6 in the normally developing infant include evidence not only of awareness of routines that involve a familiar sequence of events (a person operating at Level 5 can do this), but also the ability of the individual at Level 6 to reach beyond the familiar sequence to its purpose in anticipation of an object that has not yet been introduced into the sequence (e.g., the baby who holds up the legs in anticipation of the clean diaper before it is even visible). In this case the child must anticipate the end result and purpose of the present sequence of events on the basis of prior sequences that must be recalled to know how the present sequence of events is going to end up—with a clean, dry diaper.

If a person with a communication disorder—say, an individual with ASD—insists on following a strict routine in a particular sequence, such as closing the door to the meeting room because it has been closed during previous meetings, or eating pizza at a particular place on a certain day of the week or after some other triggering event, then he or she must be operating at least at this level.

Level 7: Discriminates a Linguistic Surface Form Such as the Child's Own Name

At this level, which is reached by the normally developing individual at about the fifth month after birth, give or take a couple of weeks (Werker & Tees, 1999; Yoshida, Fennell, Swingley, & Werker, 2009), the child not only realizes that linguistic surface forms (spoken words or manual signs) are different from other skilled actions, but also discriminates at least one surface form from others (usually the child's own name) by showing special interest when it is produced. For instance, the child may orient his or her body toward whoever produces the familiar surface form and may demonstrate discrimination of that surface form by looking at and attending to the person who produced it as if to inquire what that person might have meant by doing so.

The form is often the name of the child, some other person, or a pet. In some cases, it may be another highly frequently encountered and salient word or phrase that interests the child. The discriminated surface form may be a word, phrase, or exclamation associated with some recurrent event such as calling the cat or dog, or saying "bye" to someone.

At first, the symbolic form is merely noticed as different from others. Its meaning is not yet understood. It is merely discriminated from other syllabic sequences (or manual signs) as one that occurs commonly and has a distinct shape, feel, rhythm, and sound to it. It is as if the child thinks something like, "Hmmm. I've encountered that sequence before. It must be important. I wonder what it's about." The child recognizes the sound sequence (or the manual sign) as unique, but does not produce or interpret it. An example of a similar action by an adult would be noticing someone using a particular sign in a manual signed language that the adult does not understand. Similarly, you might notice someone repeatedly saying some word in a foreign language that you recognize as being a repetition, yet you do not know what it means—just that it is a distinct form that is repeated often.

When an individual reaches this level, it may seem to people around the child that the orienting word is fully understood. It is possible that the surface form has already been connected with its meaning. However, before that can happen, logically speaking (according to the theory of abstraction) it is essential for the child to notice the surface form and discriminate it from others. Logically, that discrimination must occur before the child will be able to associate that newly discriminated surface form with its meaning (e.g., the child's name with himself or herself). Nevertheless, the key behavior to look for in diagnosing Level 7 is orientation toward a person saying a particular speech form or using a particular manual sign. It is also common that there will be a greater expression of interest in print and linguistic symbols (words or manual signs) relative to other auditory or visual stimuli. Intentional pointing with the index finger, possibly accompanied by nondistress vocalizations, may also commonly be observed at or just prior to the attainment of this stage of representation (Fogel & Hannan, 1985; Masataka, 1995).

In what is called "regressive autism," the orientation response to the child's own name or to familiar ways of calling that child's attention may be suddenly and completely lost. In severely delayed development, the child simply does not reach Level 7 at all.

Level 8: Repetitive Syllabic Babbling

The next expected advance in development, according to the theory of abstraction, is Level 8. It is defined by **canonical babbling** (D. K. Oller & Lynch, 1992), the kind of syllabic vocalization in which the infant repeats a given syllabic form, such as "ba-ba-ba" or "da-da-da," or any syllable. Normally developing children, according to the research evidence, usually achieve Level 8 sometime after month 5 and before month 10. Logically, it involves the process of gaining motor control over some of the surface forms of speech and is tuned from the beginning to the rhythms and sounds of the particular language to which the child has been exposed. The same sort of distinctly linguistic motor behavior can also be seen in **manual babble**—the kind that the baby does with the hands rather than the mouth and voice. This kind of babble occurs in normally developing infants who are deaf or in hearing infants whose parents or primary caregivers use a manual signed language.

For a person on the autism spectrum who has acquired fairly advanced language skills and then "regressed" back to Level 8, the defining symptom is the perseverative repetition of the surface form of some word, phrase, or bit of discourse that seems to have no discoverable connection to its context. This phenomenon, which is commonly associated with ASDs, is called *echolalia*. A person who does not progress beyond the level of canonical babble, or who falls back to that level, gives no solid evidence of understanding, or taking any account of, the meanings of the words or syllables that may be uttered.

Level 9: Receptive Vocabulary

In a normally developing child, Level 9 on the scale will usually be achieved sometime after the onset of canonical babbling. Commonly, it is achieved between months 6 and 8 after birth. We know that Level 9 has been achieved when the individual can demonstrate correct interpretation of a spoken, manually signed, or printed symbol. An easy-to-observe demonstration of the comprehension of a name, for instance, is the child's orienting himself or herself by looking at, sometimes moving the head and trunk in doing so, and thereby pointing out the person named. Alternatively, the child may indicate and demonstrate comprehension of a word or phrase by grasping and handing over the particular toy or whatever may be named, or by demonstrating the action referred to by someone else or even in a printed word phrase. An excellent example of Level 9 comprehension (prior to speech) is demonstrated by Aleka Titzer at 9 months after birth. She and all normal infants, as predicted by the theory of abstraction, are able to understand many spoken utterances and have the capacity to learn to read printed words and phrases with near perfect comprehension up to about six months before they will be able to produce the same words or phrases out loud themselves (see "Aleka Titzer Reading at Nine Months," 2009; also "Aleka and Friends Reading," 2009 ◉).

In addition to confirming a surprising prediction of the theory of abstraction, Dr. Robert C. Titzer has singlehandedly refuted essentially all of the prior theories of reading readiness (R. C. Titzer, 2009). He has also helped to sharply define Level 9 on the scale of development.

For a person with a developmental or other communication disorder, delay, or regressive condition, failure to demonstrate comprehension of or interest in responding to simple requests such as "Can you raise your hand?" or "Where is your nose?", or failure to orient toward the last known location of a mentioned object, would often be indicative that Level 9 has not been achieved or that a "regression" has taken the person back to a prior level of development. However, it is necessary always to keep in mind that a failure to demonstrate something in particular is never, by itself, a certain basis for determining anything in the sciences. Just as we cannot prove a null hypothesis, as discussed in Chapter 4, the fact that we do not observe evidence of comprehension does not necessarily mean that there is none.

Level 10: The First Word

When the normally developing child utters or signs the first meaningful word in a way that is recognizable and that can be repeated soon after by that child, parents and primary caregivers commonly (though not always) take notice. Because the very definition of the first meaningful word requires that it be produced and noticed by someone other than the developing child, logically it must be observed for it to occur at all.

According to the theory of abstraction, we can predict that this Level 10 on the scale of development cannot be attained before Levels 8 and 9, which cannot be achieved ahead of the ones below them, and so on all the way back to the beginning of the sequence. Level 10 has to come after Level 9 if the use of the first word is to be meaningful in the required way. Level 8 also has to occur before Level 10 if the motor control that is necessary to the production of the syllabic form is to occur. What distinguishes Level 10, however, from both Levels 8 and 9 is the fact that the production of the word at Level 10 is intentionally associated by the producer with a conventional meaning. That is, the word is used in a way that can be understood and verified as a valid application of the word by someone else. Prior to the attainment of Level 10, a child can demonstrate comprehension in all of the ways previously detailed in connection with Level 9, but the defining act at Level 10—the intentional production of the surface form of the word itself on an occasion where the purpose is to signify the conventional meaning of the word (e.g., to refer to a person named) is something new. Alternatively, the word may be used to signify an event, such as taking leave with the use of a word like "bye," or to signify something forbidden, as in an appropriate use of the word "no." To verify that Level 10 has been achieved, it is necessary for the symbol used—a word or a manual sign with the force of a word—to be recognizable (at least to the parents or caregivers), applied in an appropriate manner, and interpreted by the audience as the individual intends.

A person on the autism spectrum and/or with a communication delay or regression of some type that fails to reach Level 10 is typically described as "nonverbal." However, by distinguishing Levels 0–9, as derived from the theory of abstraction, the entire "nonverbal" class of developmental disorders can be sharply divided into nine explicitly distinct levels. The question for cases defined formerly as "nonverbal"—*a vague and inexplicit description at best*—is which of the preceding nine levels has the individual coming short of Level 10 already reached or to which level has that person fallen back.

Level 11: The Two-Word Stage

A normally developing child will usually achieve Level 11, which may loosely be described as the "two-word stage" of language development, by 18–24 months of age. The determination that Level 11 has been achieved depends on the person's use of more than one word in a meaningful sequence.

The defining trait of such a use is that the **syntactic arrangement** of the two words is such that the referential meaning and practical significance (the pragmatic mapping) of the whole sequence involves a distinctive contribution of each part of the sequence to the whole significance. A bona fide example of a two-word sequence manifesting this stage of development would be an utterance by a child of a phrase such as "Mimi house!" repeated several times, meaning I want to go to Mimi's (grandmother's) house, and not to my own house (which the child in question separately designates as "Mama house"). Or the child might say "Dada hat!" to refer to the father's baseball cap in contrast to "Pop hat!" meaning the grandfather's fedora. The distinctive character of genuine two-word utterances such as these, or manual signed sequences of a similar kind, is that the separate words are mapped onto distinct meanings that are syntactically joined to create a distinct pragmatic result that depends on both parts. That is, "Mimi" is clearly used to refer to the grandmother and "house" to the place where she lives, and the combined effect of the sequence is to direct the driver of the car to go to the particular house where the grandmother lives rather than the house where the speaker lives. Each element is pragmatically associated with its separate meaning, yet the meanings are brought together in a way that enables a more explicit reference and a useful, pragmatic differentiation of distinct referents and their conventional significance to both the producer and the consumer of the surface forms that are used.

Level 11 is not manifested in the holistic use of a phrase to refer to just one undifferentiated thing, event, or relation. The latter is what is meant by a single-word utterance or any utterance or sign sequence that has the significance of only a single word. For instance, suppose a child who wants to go outside produces a surface form such as "ohnfaway," which is a childish production of the phrase "Don't go far away!" as commonly told him by his mother before he is permitted to go out into the front yard; the word used by the child is called a **holophrasis.** It has the power and systematic complexity of only a single word (Level 10), because the individual parts of the holophrastic production are not differentiated. Similarly, a production such as "ohfirs" as a holistic construction of the phrase "Are you thirsty!" and meaning "I want a drink of water" is also an example of such a holophrastic production. Both of these cases would fall at Level 10, not Level 11, and for the same reason. To reach Level 11, the individual must show that the sequential syntactic combination of what appears to be more than one meaningful sign element involves the pragmatic intention to differentiate the conventional meanings of the component parts.

Level 12: Produces Predicates with at Least Two Distinct Referents

A normally developing individual at this stage, which is usually attained by about the age of three years, is able to produce sentences that contain two distinct referents that are brought together under the scope of a relation designated in a **predicate** that connects them in a meaningful way. For instance, a sequence such as "Gabby hug Brenden"—meaning that Gabby has hugged, is hugging, or is being directed to hug Brenden—is a predicate with two distinct referents. The referents are Brenden and Gabby, and the relation of Gabby hugging Brenden is signified in the predicate "hug" that joins the two referring terms "Gabby" and "Brenden." This level of development is relatively easy to diagnose because it is commonly demonstrated in simple **transitive sentences** of the subject–verb–object type.

An individual stranded at this stage will be able to handle most utterances of the subject–verb–object type, but not sentences with an indirect object. Productions at this stage may still have some telegraphic qualities. The limitation is the sort originally described in 1978 by Churchill. His test context consisted of three objects (block, ring, stick), three colors (red, yellow, blue), and three transitive actions (give, tap, slide). Churchill found that persons diagnosed with autism seemed to have an exceedingly difficult time in advancing to a higher level. DeLong (1991) interpreted Churchill's research as showing "a limited capacity for higher-order association," and went on to say that he believed it to be "cognitive: a limitation in the capacity to process multiple conjoined language elements" (p. 64). If any individual who has experienced a delay, disorder, or regression can handle predicates with up to two referents (or the equivalent), then Level 12 is indicated.

Level 13: Produces Predicates with Three Referents or Equivalent Complexity

For a normally developing child, usually sometime after age 3, sentence structures become enriched in several ways as the child moves up to Level 13. At this level, the predicates that the child can handle are expanded to account for at least one more referent under the scope of a single predicate. From two referents under a single predicate, the child moves up at Level 13 to predicates with three referents, or structures of equivalent complexity.

An example of this sort of expansion is seen in the production of predicates that require three referents—for example, "Brenden gives Gabby the crayon." A different manifestation of the achievement of this level is the consistent distinction between the shifting pragmatic values of pronouns such as "I," "you," and "it." When the child correctly and consistently produces sentences such as "I want you to hold me," where the distinct relations are correctly understood and indicated in the pronouns, in contrast with the earlier production of "I hold you!" where the clear intention was actually the reverse ("You hold me!"), Level 13 development has been achieved. That is, a structure equivalent in complexity to a predicate with three distinct referents in its scope has been produced.

Also, when Level 13 is achieved, the normally developing individual will be able to talk about how he or she feels about something or someone, but not necessarily understand talk about how someone else feels about the same thing, event, or person.

Persons on the autism spectrum who have failed to reach Level 13 on the Milestones Scale, or who have fallen back to a still earlier level, are often described in the literature as demonstrating *pronominal reversal,* where "I do it" is, for instance, a request for the person addressed to do something. To describe this problem as a "reversal" of pronouns is misleading, however, as we pointed out earlier in Chapter 2. It may seem to be a "reversal" of "you" to "I" from the viewpoint of a naive adult language user. In fact, careful analysis shows that the failure is something left undone rather than something done and then reversed to get the wrong result. The child who does what Kanner called "pronominal reversal" actually fails to change the pronoun from "I" (as in the mother saying, "I will do it") to "you" when the child making the request in fact wants the person addressed to perform whatever the task may be. It is actually a failure to make the expected reversal at the surface so as to get the required pronoun in the subject position. When the subject changes from the speaker ("I") to the person spoken to ("you"), the pronoun at the surface must also be changed.

Level 14: Produces Predicates with Four Distinct Referents or Equivalent Complexity

At this stage, which is commonly reached by about the age of 4 or 5 years, the normally developing individual can talk intelligibly about his or her feelings, but is not yet able to fully understand and produce talk of feelings about feelings. In other words, in a normally developing individual, at this stage we look for the person in question to be able to represent feelings in others, but not necessarily to be able to comment with full comprehension on feelings about feelings.

If a person is stranded at this level and does not advance higher, as Tantam (1988) observed, it may seem that the individual is an "assiduous pursuer of idiosyncratic interests" (p. 245), knowing about and yet not fully able to take account of the feelings of others. Such a person certainly has feelings, is able to talk about them, knows that others also have feelings and is able to talk about them, and yet is not fully able to understand or even to experience feelings about feelings.

We find Dr. Temple Grandin's discussion with Sacks (1993–1994) relevant here. She told Sacks, "When I look up at the stars at night, I know I should get a 'numinous' feeling, but I don't. I would like to get it. I can understand it intellectually. I think about the Big Bang, and the origin of the universe, and why we are here: Is it finite, or does it go on forever?" (p. 124). For Grandin, the meaning of a predicate referring to a feeling about a feeling—the "numinous" feeling about the intellectual questions she was able to refer to perfectly well—that higher feeling which would be the main referent of a higher predicate subordinating the referents of all the subordinate predicates, remained out of reach. In the same interview, Grandin said, "I do not fit in with the social life of my town or university. . . . My interests are factual and my recreational reading consists mostly of science and livestock publications. I have little interest in novels with complicated interpersonal relationships, because I am unable to remember the sequence of events" (p. 113)—and, we may add, presumably the complicated motivations of the characters involved in those events. To do so would require more complex predicates than a person stranded at Level 14 can manage.

An individual at this level on the autism spectrum, for example, may seem to manage complex syntax, morphology, and surface structures, yet nevertheless seem somewhat isolated emotionally and detached from full understanding of the feelings of other persons. A standard phrase for the isolation at issue is "lack of empathy."

Level 15: Produces Predicates with Five Distinct Referents or Equivalent Complexity

A person developing normally would usually reach Level 15 sometime after age 5 and before age 7. At this stage, we come to the lower edge of the normal limit on the number of referents that can be handled by average mature sign users—what George Miller (1956) described as the magic number seven plus or minus one or two. At this level, where predicates with five arguments, or ones of equivalent complexity, are within reach, the person is very near the full capacity of a normal mature adult.

If there is delay, plateauing, or a disorder diagnosed at this level, according to the theory of abstraction, it differs only in subtle respects from normal mature semiotic ability. Presumably, this is the upper edge of what is commonly diagnosed as Asperger syndrome (Wing, 1981a, 1981b). At this level, the individual may express humor and feelings about feelings, but not be able to complete activities of the sort "I know, that you know, what I'm thinking." That is, the individual can correctly identify feelings in others and can have feelings about their feelings (e.g., can say truthfully and with understanding, "I enjoy being happy"), but finds it difficult and tricky to try to adjust his or her expressions to account for the feelings and reactions of others.

Jerry Newport, for instance, a well-known celebrity and speaker diagnosed with Asperger syndrome, speaking in Monroe, Louisiana, at a meeting of the Autism Society of Louisiana in 2004, realized at one point in the question-and-answer session that he had used a tone of voice that was probably off-putting to his questioner. Newport said he had been told not to speak that way publicly by one of his therapists. He then gave essentially the same answer again, almost word for word, but in a more compatible tone of voice—something he had practiced with his therapist. He noted that he did so only because of special training and coaching he had received. Newport pointed out that this was not something he did naturally or that he understood as a matter of course (Leung, 2004).

Level 16: Mature Semiotic Ability

Persons progressing normally beyond about age 7 continue to enrich their vocabulary and specialized knowledge well into adulthood. However, the linguistic research shows that they do not advance a great deal more in their fundamental capacity to manage predicate structures of much greater complexity than those that were described in the now-famous paper by G. A. Miller (1956) about "the magical number seven." Although he himself has often hedged his remarks to exclude almost any simple understanding of his underlying point, as he did in that paper originally, his argument does seem to lead to a relatively simple logical conclusion about the number of referents that can easily be subordinated under the scope of a single predicate (even one that is complex). There seems to be a rough semiotic limit of seven to nine (or 10) referents that can be managed under the scope of a single predicate. Whether that limit is rigid, as it has seemed to be in many different sorts of psychological experiments, is an interesting question. Regardless of how that deeper theoretical question is resolved eventually, if ever, the fact is that once a person can handle predicates of about that level of complexity (7 to 10 referents or the equivalent), he or she certainly seems to be a member of the vast group called "normal language users." Within a wide range of limits, all of the people in that vast group appear to be able to participate in any social or cognitive activity that takes their interest.

Reviewing the Whole Scale

Altogether, there are theoretically 17 distinct levels on the proposed scale. They range from a low of 0 to a high of 16. The 0 on the Milestones Scale represents no ability whatever to divide up and make sense of the stream of experience; in contrast, the theoretical sixteenth position on the scale represents the range of abilities defined by any fully mature and competent person who is able to participate in essentially any normal social and cognitive interaction with mature individuals (or peers who have achieved linguistic maturity).

In the next section, we present some research evidence from a series of pilot studies showing that the Milestones Scale works well in practice when applied to autism spectrum disorders.

Assessing Practicality, Reliability, and Validity

In several pilot studies, audio/video clips of typical behaviors displayed by persons diagnosed with autism were rated. The problem set for judges in rating each sample of behavior was where to place that sample on the Milestones Scale. In other words, what is the highest and best semiotic ability of each individual as displayed in each of the 20 distinct video clips? Each group of raters was first given a training session of approximately 44 minutes by the second author prior to being asked to rate the 20 video clips. The video records exclusively pertained to persons who had already been diagnosed with autism or who would later (subsequent to the video in question) be judged to be on the autism spectrum.

The 20 clips, which ranged in length from a couple of seconds to 15 seconds in duration, were presented in no particular order. The entire sequence required slightly more than 12 minutes to present. Each clip was presented twice, with a brief interval between the first and second showing and a somewhat longer interval between the second showing and the next video clip in the sequence. The time between clips was sufficient to enable rater/judges to write down, on a form provided, the rating of the clip just viewed. The rater/judges were asked to assign a single rating—a number from 0 to 16—for each individual in the series. The individuals in the videos were not arranged in any particular order with respect to their degree of severity on the autism spectrum. The presumption understood from the training was that rater/judges should rate each performance as if it were the highest and best for the individual depicted in the clip.

The 20 clips were rated by 18 experienced speech-language pathologists (SLPs) at a hospital setting in Texas. The same clips were also rated by a group of 33 undergraduate students enrolled in an Introduction to Normal Speech and Language Development course at a mid-sized university in Louisiana. The undergraduate students had no clinical experience with autism. Of those students, 21 were undergraduates majoring in communication disorders, 9 in early childhood or special education, 2 in general studies (no declared major), and 1 in biology and communication disorders. In addition, there were 4 professional occupational therapists (OTs) and 4 physical therapists (PTs), and a small group of 3 professional researchers. The grand total was 62 raters. All of the professionals claimed at least some clinical experience in working with individuals diagnosed with autism. The average reported length of undifferentiated professional practice was 10.7 years for the SLPs,

Table 11-1 Reliability and Validity of the Milestones Scale of Development Applied to 20 Video Clips of Individuals Diagnosed with Autism

Group of Raters	Average *r* with Overall Mode Rating	Standard Deviation	Standard Error of Measurement	Number of Cases (*n*)
Undergraduates	0.802	0.164	0.029	33
Occupational/physical therapists	0.894	0.128	0.045	8
Speech-language pathologists	0.920	0.038	0.009	18
PhD specialists	0.954	0.051	0.026*	4
Top 40%	0.962	0.076	0.016	25
Top 20%	0.982	0.053	0.016	12
			Total *N*	63

*One of the raters in this group was a non-native speaker of English, and an outlier.

14.3 years for the OTs and PTs, and none for the undergraduate students. In general, SLPs have more training in dealing with the semiotic aspects of autism and substantially more experience in dealing with it.

Results of the Pilot Studies

In Table 11-1, in the first column of numbers we report the average agreement (expressed as a correlation, *r*) of the individual raters in each group with the most common ratings assigned to each of the 20 video clips—the overall mode rating. The second and third columns of numbers report the **standard deviation (SD)** of the correlation on each row and the **standard error of measurement (SEM)** of that correlation. The SD and SEM are both measures of the tendency of the correlations in question to differ across individuals in each group. The increasing agreement across groups, as they gain in experience and knowledge about autism, can be seen in the increasing correlations as we read down the rows, and also in the generally decreasing SDs and SEMs as we read down the rows. The agreement is least, though already substantial, between the relatively naive undergraduate students and it becomes increasingly more substantial for groups with more experience and knowledge, just as we would expect.

The average degree of agreement for naive undergraduates was .802, while for more experienced clinicians and researchers it ranged from .894 to .954. The last two rows in Table 11-1 show that if we select the top 40% of the 63 raters, their agreement averages .962; the top 20% achieved an agreement of .982. The fact that more experienced individuals agree more with one another shows both the validity and the reliability of the Milestones Scale. As persons gain more knowledge about normal speech and language development, about autism, and about disorders of communication in general, we must assume that their agreement increases because of their greater wealth of knowledge. Therefore, their tendency to agree with one another overall can be accounted for only by their understanding of the scale and its valid application to the problem of autism (in the case of the 20 clips presented). It follows from the strictest mathematical logic, and from classical test theory (H. H. Harman, 1976), that validity entails reliability. We cannot get strong indications of validity from measures that are not reliable. In fact, according to classical test theory (H. H. Harman, 1976; Nunnally, 1967), the reliability of a measure cannot be less than the square root of its validity. Therefore, the results in Table 11-1 can be read as showing both strong validity and reliability.

Agreement at the Foundation

The underlying premise for the Milestones Scale is justified by a general theory of signs as explained in other publications. The foundational idea is that agreement by competent judges on matters of abstract judgment, as established by C. S. Peirce (1897; see also J. W. Oller & L. Chen, 2007), is *the foundational basis for the determination of validity in representations of any kind.* The gist of this idea is illustrated by Jon Uebersax (1988, 1992; also see S. D. Oller, 2005). He used a seemingly trivial example concerning whether or not a certain joke is funny. Uebersax supposed that such a judgment is a direct and final measure of whether the joke is funny to the person, or persons, making the judgment. We agree. Similarly, moving to a nontrivial case, given the training provided to all the raters of the data referred to in Table 11-1, the agreement between them, on the whole, concerning the application of the scale to the 20 video clips in question would seem to be the best available criterion against which to judge the validity (and reliability) of the ratings by any individual or groups of judges.

For all of the foregoing reasons, the overall mode rating—the point on the Milestones Scale most commonly assigned to any given clip—was a reasonable criterion of validity for our pilot studies. Concurrence with that criterion, provided our underlying theory (according to the theoreticians and arguments already cited) is correct, constitutes a more or less direct measure of the validity (and reliability) of the ratings assigned by any individual rater, or by any group of raters. Judged by this criterion, the Milestones Scale has substantial validity (and reliability) as applied to the 20 audio/ video clips used in our pilot studies; this can be seen in several ways from Table 11-1.

As seen in the first column of Table 11-1, and as predicted earlier in this chapter and elsewhere (see J. W. Oller & Rascón, 1999), on the whole, more experience results in greater agreement in the ratings assigned on the scale. The fact that more experience accounts for greater agreement across rater groups suggests that as raters gain more experience in thinking about communication disorders in general, and about autism in particular, they are better able to make accurate judgments.

Also, as predicted and as can readily be seen from Figure 11-1, the agreement shown in the mean correlation of the individuals in the various groups with the overall mode rating increases with the experience of the groups doing the rating, exactly as predicted and as is required if the Milestones Scale is as valid as it appears to be. The increase in agreement between each successive level was tested by a standard *t*-test and found to be significant at the $p < .0001$ level in each case. Thus agreement, as predicted, does increase as more experienced raters do the assessments. This trend

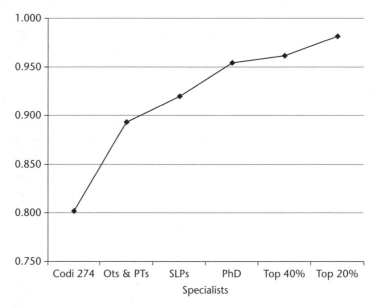

Figure 11-1 The validity (also reliability) of the Milestones Scale of Development applied to 20 audio/video clips of individuals with autism by groups of raters with increasing levels of experience (reading left to right).

holds true for groups ranging from undergraduates to clinicians outside of the speech-language area, to speech-language pathologists, and from there on to highly trained PhD-level researchers who are even more experienced in diagnosing symptoms of autism and levels of semiotic ability in general.

If the contrasts between the immediately adjacent levels in Figure 11-1 are significant, it follows that contrasts between nonadjacent levels must be significant as well as substantial. Therefore, we conclude on the basis of these pilot results that the Milestones Scale fulfills the requirements of practicality, reliability, and validity. It meets the criterion of practicality in view of the fact that high levels of validity and reliability were achieved within all of the rater groups with a bare minimum of training in the use of the scale for each group (no more than 44 minutes in each case). The practicality of the Milestones Scale, given the minimal amount of training, is demonstrated in the substantial degree of validity attained by all groups and by the substantial agreement overall across the various groups.

Discussion of the Preliminary Research

The evidence suggests that the Milestones Scale is practical, easily understood with a modicum of training, reliable, and valid as applied to the autism spectrum. As predicted, empirical evidence demonstrates that groups of judges become progressively more accurate and agree more with each other (and with other groups) as they gain more experience in understanding, diagnosing, and treating communication disorders. That said, it is important to note that even relatively naive judges, given a very brief period of training (44 minutes in the foregoing study), are able to achieve substantial agreement with each other and with more expert groups of judges in applying the scale.

Competent language users with a little training—even undergraduate university students—are evidently able to judge the highest and best level of any given individual's progress upward through the hierarchy of semiotic systems. This is not surprising because language users commonly make reliable and valid judgments about the intellectual and social abilities of their own children and of other interlocutors. Such judgments have been well documented with respect to naive (untrained) parents of young infants, mothers or primary caregivers, who can validly judge whether their baby has reached the stage of repetitive syllabic babbling, saying sequences such as "ba-ba-ba," "da-da-da," and so on. This is the stage technically known as canonical babbling (Ejiri, 1998; D. K. Oller, Eilers, & Basinger, 2001; D. K. Oller & Lynch, 1992).

Similarly, adults are quite good at making judgments about whether or not any given adult interlocutor understands and speaks their native language. If the interlocutor is judged to be a non-native speaker, even children and naive adults can usually make a reasonably accurate judgment about what the interlocutor will or will not be able to comprehend. Speakers of all languages, therefore, commonly adjust the level of complexity and the nature of their discourse to the level of their interlocutor(s) (see Wagner, 1996, and references; Duff, Wong, & Early, 2000). Evidence for such adjustments in adult–child interactions can be seen in the use of what is commonly called "baby talk" or **motherese** when addressing talk to a baby or small child (R. P. Cooper, Abraham, Berman, & Staska, 1997). A range of similar adjustments can be observed when cooperative adults address children of varying ages and abilities.

As the age and ability of the interlocutor advance, the level of discourse used by competent adults to address the person or persons in question also progresses upward. When we talk to a very young child, or to a person who does not know our language well, we are apt to speak more slowly, use fewer words, and employ simpler syntax (Yan, 2009). Also, we tend to rely on fewer and less complex inferences on the part of our less competent interlocutors than when we speak to native peers (i.e., adults who are able to manage our own highest and best use of our native language). There is no doubt that even relatively untrained but competent adults can learn to make valid judgments about the highest and best levels of semiotic functioning of almost anyone at any level.

The results of the pilot research with the Milestones Scale also show that with additional experience or training, significantly higher levels of reliability and validity can be expected. In fact, levels actually demonstrated approach perfect agreement between the individuals and groups with the highest levels of training and experience.

More importantly, with respect to the testing of theories about the causation of the autism epidemic and the assessment of the efficacy of different treatment protocols and methods of prevention, the Milestones Scale enables finer resolution concerning judgments about both so-called verbal and nonverbal communication abilities. Whereas the distinction between individuals who are "verbal" as contrasted with "nonverbal" has always been possible with the categories provided in the various editions of the *DSM* from 1980 forward and in the *ICD* series, the Milestones Scale enables us to reliably and validly distinguish nine different levels of "nonverbal" semiotic development. In addition, the scale provides for richer differentiation of distinct levels of "verbal" ability by distinguishing eight distinct levels of proficiency in that category as well. As a result, the Milestones Scale should enable more accurate judgments about the efficacy of treatments and thus more sensitive tests of theories about particular causal factors.

SETTING THE STAGE FOR TREATMENT

One of the main purposes of this book is to show that autism is preventable to a high degree and to demonstrate that when it does manifest the disorder can be treated. The preference is for prevention, of course, and even for individuals already on the autism spectrum, prevention of further injury is still a very high priority. The good news is that armed with better understanding of the immune system, toxins, and medical practices, we can unequivocally argue that ASDs can be successfully treated, even to the point of full recovery.

In the final chapter of this book, we deal with treatments that have some reasonable claim to bringing about improvement in individuals affected by autism. The still widespread myths associated with autism—that autism is an untreatable mystery, that it is a completely genetic problem, that there is no autism epidemic, that the causes of autism may never be understood, that there are no effective treatments, that autism is a diagnosis without hope, and so on—are mistaken. Such claims are theoretically illogical and empirically inconsistent with research findings. To parents, independent researchers, and all those clinicians and doctors seeking solutions to the autism epidemic, these autism-is-an-unsolvable-mystery myths are merely roadblocks that must be removed.

In 1964, Dr. Bernard Rimland succeeded in busting the myth that cold, unfeeling mothers cause autism. Thirty years later, he joined Dr. Jon Pangborn (a PhD researcher) and Dr. Sidney Baker (medical professor at Yale University) to establish the organization now known all over the world as Defeat Autism Now! (DAN!). Its purpose was "to provide parents and professionals with a timely consensus as to the safest and most effective treatment options for children with developmental problems in the autism spectrum" (see Pangborn & S. M. Baker, 2005, 2007; also see the Web sites established by DAN!, 2009, and its sister organization, also founded by Rimland, the Autism Research Institute, 2009).

The Road Not Chosen

In some instances, the myths associated with autism are superficial defenses of an absence of knowledge. The repetition of the mantras derived from the false stories about autism, however, are generally grounded in ignorance no matter how enthusiastically they may be embraced. The evidence suggests that, in many instances, mainstream professionals who have accepted the mythologies about autism have been misled by popular ideas that are simply false. In other instances, the same myths about autism are being knowingly promoted by propagandists for the vested interest groups. In light of the research contained in this book and in the many references cited herein, it is plain that the autism epidemic is among the most important medical problems of the modern world. It is, however, not untreatable.

Not long before his death in 2006, Dr. Bernard Rimland wrote of his quest in search of the causes of autism. After his son Mark, born in 1956, was diagnosed with severe autism, Rimland started down a road he would not have chosen for himself or for his child. The journey that he began and continued for the rest of his life was much like the one that every parent of a child with autism is drafted into. Rimland read everything he could possibly dig up, including translations of foreign works. He focused a lot of attention on the Kanner/Bettelheim myth that cold mothers cause autism. When Mark was young, the standard intervention was psychotherapy:

> [T]he mother was required to acknowledge her guilt, and disclose why she hated the child and wished it had never been born. The child, in so-called "play therapy," was provided with a paper or clay image of a woman (his mother) and was encouraged to tear it to bits, thus expressing his hostility toward his mother, whom the psychotherapists were positive had caused his autism. There were a few drugs that were also used with autistic children, but then, as now, the idea was not to treat the autism but to slow the children down enough to make life tolerable for those who must deal with them. (Rimland, 2005, p. 8)

The cold-hearted mother myth that Rimland demolished, according to Pangborn and S. M. Baker, was not just a mistaken view but was "wrong to the point of evil" (2005, p. 3).

It is noteworthy that Rimland's book *Infantile Autism* won the Century Award in 1964. In the three years following the publication of his book on autism, Rimland would found two other national autism organizations. However, it would require three decades of additional work before Rimland would be joined by Pangborn and Baker to undertake the task of creating and promoting a rational consensus of researchers, doctors, and clinicians concerning autism treatments that work. That is what the founders of DAN! set out to do.

The DAN! founders supposed that the parents are the best sources of information about how treatments work with the individuals affected by autism. Nevertheless, many mainstream profession-als continue to resist the notion that parents are able to evaluate treatments that help, or hurt, their children. Why wouldn't parents be able to do this? As a rule, they are with their children more frequently and for longer periods of time than anyone else is. As described earlier, even relatively naive raters with a 44-minute training session are able to judge the severity of autism in video clips of children with autism averaging less than 15 seconds in length. From this research we can conclude that even naive raters—who usually have far less experience with any given individual to be rated than the parents of that child—can rate the severity of the child's autism validly and reliably. In fact, 40% of the raters we studied achieved nearly perfect consensus with only 44 minutes of training in the use of the scale. The mode ratings not only differentiated severity levels reliably, but also did so in a way that was consistent with the theory of abstraction and with the published research on normal speech and language development. Follow-up work is planned to test the theory that parents of children with autism can also rate the severity of autism on the Milestones Scale with extremely high validity and reliability.

Listening to the Parents

After founding the Autism Society of America in 1965 (ASA, 2009) and going on to found the Autism Research Institute in 1967 (ARI, 2009) and DAN! in 1994 (DAN!, 2009), Rimland reported that he had found early on that "parents, especially the mothers of autistic children, were extremely effective at identifying treatments that were helpful to their autistic children. They were also very observant in detecting factors that caused their children to become worse" (2005, p. 10).

As early as 1967, Rimland had learned from questionnaires returned by parents of children with autism that many of them reported that their children became "markedly worse after the DTP shot." Although he did not know then about the mercury in that shot—as, in fact, almost no one outside of the manufacturers knew of the mercury at that time—in the 1967 survey sent out from ARI, Rimland included questions about dental mercury exposure of mothers while they were pregnant. The purpose of DAN!, taking its cue from the predecessor organizations ASA and ARI, rather than seeking to lay blame for harm done, much less to look for wrongdoing by vaccine manufacturers and the government, was to "identify treatments, safe treatments, for which there is credible evidence of efficacy . . . to find why they work, so their efficacy can be improved" (Rimland, 2005, p. 10).

Asking for Answers

The tide is turning slowly in favor of those who seek to defeat autism rather than merely to accept it as a life sentence, but the struggle is not over. Surprisingly, resistance to the idea that autism is treatable is coming from some professionals involved in diagnosis and intervention, and even a few parents of children with autism. We recently encountered opposition to the notion that autism is a treatable disease within a local chapter of the ASA, one of the three autism organizations founded by Rimland.

We proposed the idea of surveying the parents of children with autism in our region about demographic factors, the age of their child now and at diagnosis, their perceptions of possible triggering events, which treatments they had tried so far, and what, if anything, seemed to make their child better or worse. As Dr. S. M. Baker (2005a) points out, this information is essential and parents are the only reliable source of it. He calls this approach "patient-oriented integrative medicine" and describes it like this:

> The best time to discuss whether to use a (safe) supplement, drug, diet or other treatment is about three weeks after trying it. The first judgment based on symptoms is usually enough, but sometimes a change in a lab test will be needed as an extra measure of certainty or safety. . . . every treatment is really a diagnostic trial. (p. 43)

But, contrary to all logic and clinical experience, according to Baker, most people are willing to wait for the fog to lift all by itself on the basis of the "Don't look for answers" approach.

An articulate professional clinician provided us with an example. As a PhD-level clinician with multiple employees and new suite of offices substantially sustained by income from treating individuals with autism, this person objected to the idea of asking parents for any information about what they think is helping or hurting their children, what the triggers may have been before symptoms appeared or before the diagnosis was made, and so forth. This person argued that any questionnaire even touching on issues of causation or the efficacy of treatments was dangerous and unethical. According to this clinician, it would be unethical for anyone associated with ASA to ask such questions, because "We really can't claim to know anything about causes or treatments." This handsomely persuasive person with confidence and poise also asserted, "We could also be infringing on our charter, which is only for the purposes of education."

S. M. Baker (2005b, 2007) points out in the DAN! book on biomedical treatments of autism that Rimland more or less singlehandedly defeated the "It's your fault, mother" theory of the causation of autism. Nevertheless, as Baker sees it, we still have an uphill struggle ahead. From the beginning of the formation of the ASA, ARI, and DAN! organizations, the underlying premise was that parents are worth listening to and that we must identify causal factors if we are to find and verify safe and effective treatments.

As Baker points out, the difficult work—a task that Dr. Kenneth Bock describes as "working the clues" (Bock & Stauth, 2007, pp. 46ff)—is especially challenging in individual cases but has to be done there. All of the detective work centers on the problem of diagnosing and explaining symptoms in individuals. For this reason, Bock says, "A good diagnostician is a good detective" (p. 46). The whole of Baker's section on "Making a Plan" in the book about biomedical interventions could be construed as doing detective work (e.g., Baker, 2005b, refers to "the ongoing detective work" on p. 112) so as to identify specific details and understand causal relationships between known or likely causes, attempted treatments, and observed outcomes.

The difficulty of putting things right after the diagnosis of autism, as Dr. Boyd Haley has argued and as DAN! doctors universally agree (S. M. Baker, 2005a, p. 25), is a little like cleaning up a train wreck (see Haley, 2006). In getting the mess cleaned up and the train back together and moving again, many potential hazards must be dealt with. Many things can go wrong, in many different ways, in very different individuals. For that reason, finding the best next step for any individual requires careful planning, record keeping to sort out what is learned along the way, and thinking through the results obtained from prior steps and the likely outcome of the next step to be taken. All along the way, communication between the players—researchers, clinicians, parents, and patients—is the key to achieving successful outcomes.

The First, Second, and Third Rules of Treatment

The general rule in therapeutic interventions of all kinds is first to identify the most severe problem, which is sometimes a life-threatening one such as choking on solids or fluids during a seizure, and then to work downward to less threatening ones. That rule applies in dealing with every aspect of the autism epidemic and especially in dealing with individual cases. LaPointe and Katz (2002) put this first rule clearly in saying that, in setting priorities for therapy, we should seek "relief from the greatest evil." They illustrate this first rule with the following analogy: "When the lifeboat springs a leak, we do not worry about how soon it can be given a fresh coat of paint" (p. 500). Thus, if a person cannot breathe, and at the same time is bleeding from a finger, we would try to clear the airway before dealing with the cut.

Similarly, if an illness, toxin, injury, or some combination of factors has caused a bowel disease that intermittently produces seizures, injurious emotional outbursts, breakdown of the immune systems, and interference with emotional well-being, social connections, and cognition, doesn't it make sense to deal with the causes of the gut condition rather than merely concentrating on changing the resulting behavioral symptoms? After all, the first rule of treatment is to deal with the most serious need first. However, balancing this rule are two others that are equally important. With respect to the treatment of the autism epidemic and the individuals affected by it, attention has very reasonably been centered on the interaction of the gastrointestinal tract with the central nervous system (Bock & Stauth, 2007; Jepson & Johnson, 2007; Pangborn & S. M. Baker, 2005, 2007; Wakefield et al., 1997). As explained by Michael Gershon in his 1998 book *The Second Brain*, the interaction between the gut and the brain is so intense that the ecosystem contained in the gut can be regarded as a brain in its own right. We can think of it as a kind of "meta-brain"—a multitiered communication system of systems, acting like a virtual computer residing between the so-called hard-wired neurology of the brain and the physical pipes, valves, and processing chambers of the gut.

Once the priorities are determined on the basis of a ranking of needs from greatest to least, there is also the rule that we should minimize the risk of potential harm. The idea behind this rule is suggested by S. M. Baker: "Once the ballpark is found, you can back off and find the least inconvenient dietary change and the lowest doses of the least risk medication or supplements that maintain the desired effect" (2005b, p. 85). This can be done by always seeking the greatest positive effect with the least invasive and the safest treatment that is likely to produce the desired outcome.

Finally, there is the third rule: Treatment must address the whole person in the larger context of life. As Baker puts it, we need to look at things from "a functional as opposed to an anatomical, point of view" (2005b, p. 114). As far as we know, all of the DAN! doctors agree that it is necessary to treat the whole person. Bock argues that it is necessary to address "the human body as an integrated, interdependent, interrelated entity" (Bock & Stauth, 2007, p. 66), or to use what Baker refers to as "a systems approach" (2005a, p. 15).

Required: A Systems Approach

Obviously, such a systems approach ought to be universally accepted in mainstream medicine and clinical practices of all sorts. In writing this book, we aim to contribute to the needed sea change that is already taking place. If you have already gotten this far in pursuing the issues at stake, it is almost certain that you have already joined with us. If so, we welcome you to our worthy quest. If not, we invite you to reflect and consider joining with us in a common cause from which the whole world can benefit. We agree with S. M. Baker when he says, "I am sure that you realize that I have no axe to grind" (2005b, p. 78). We also declare the same sort of independence as do nearly all of the professionals who are now helping to change the mainstream paradigm of medicine and the health sciences from theories of discrete germs, genes, and isolated factors to more sensible integrative theories. As Pangborn argues, and as we have maintained in this book and elsewhere (see J. W. Oller et al., 2010), it is essential to consider "epigenetics"—that is, "how . . . diet, infection, toxicity . . . affect the activity and expression of genes" (Pangborn, 2005, p. 154).

This idea has also been suggested by mainstream geneticists studying autism. For instance, D. B. Campbell et al. (2006; also see R. R. Dietert & J. M. Dietert, 2008; Kinney, Munir, Crowley, & A. M. Miller, 2008) note that there must be "environmental factors" in addition to "vulnerability genes" that "precipitate the onset of autism" (p. 16838). There can be no doubt that epigenetic interactions between genes and environmental factors are involved in producing the autism epidemic. It is particularly relevant, as argued by Pangborn (2005, pp. 149–151, citing an article by Rimland, 2000) that the percentage of children with "regressive" autism with onset of symptoms after 18 months or later (Type II) outnumber children with autism who have metabolic problems associated with known genetic defects (Type I) by 9 to 1 or more. Pangborn, for instance, asserts categorically that late-onset (regressive) autism accounts for approximately 80% of the upsurge documented in Figure 1-1.

Addressing the Epidemic

For all of the foregoing reasons, we believe that the autism epidemic, perhaps more than any other single problem on the horizon in the health sciences, is forcing the needed paradigm shift toward a dynamic systems orientation. It is a certainty, we believe, that the mainstream health sciences must sooner or later come to embrace the obvious fact that autism is not alone in demonstrating that chronic illnesses are universally "multifactorial" (S. M. Baker, 2005a, p. 15). This finding is guaranteed and required by logicomathematical reasoning based in semiotic theory (J. W. Oller et al., 2010). The required paradigm shift, which we believe is already under way, is inevitably leading medicine toward a holistic, systems-based view of the rich and multilayered communication systems on which health, wellness, and the successful treatment of diseases and disorders in general necessarily depend. Discrete germ theories are fine up to a point. Nevertheless, when it comes to the interactions of germs (viruses), genes, and so forth within the ecosystems both within and outside living organisms—and especially human beings—discrete germ theories are necessarily incomplete and misleading if they are used as the sole basis for the treatment of multifactorial diseases and disorders.

To anyone who thinks about it, as researchers and theoreticians must, it is obvious that human beings are distinct individuals with somewhat different—yet always dynamic and changing—physical, behavioral, emotional, cognitive, and social needs. Therefore, it follows that successful treatments that deal with chronic disorders and the disease conditions that accompany them (certainly including persons on the autism spectrum) will usually be team efforts. These efforts will necessarily involve the individual with autism plus the primary caregiver(s), the whole family, and, to a greater extent than is commonly realized, the teachers, clinicians, doctors, extended family, and community at large with whom the affected individual interacts. S. M. Baker describes the teamwork that is needed as "an active collaboration" between the patient's family, the doctor(s), and the crucial data gained by researchers.

Active Collaboration: Three Positions of Discourse

A minimum of three components are essential to the active collaboration recommended by thoughtful doctors such as Dr. Sid Baker and his DAN! colleagues. Those three components can be thought of more or less as persons—namely, the patient, the clinician, and the researcher. In the sort of collaboration required, however, it is important to keep in mind from a more abstract point of view that each of the persons, or groups of persons, involved must occupy a logically necessary position of discourse. Also, though each position is best occupied by just one person at a time on any given occasion, there are many persons involved at any given moment at all of the positions. There are many different individuals who are patients, clinicians, and researchers. Also, we often exchange roles. To a greater extent than is commonly realized, the clinician can be both patient and researcher. The patient can be both clinician and researcher, and the researcher can be both patient and clinician.

Of course, there is a logical rank to the positions in terms of where we must start and where we must end up. First, there is the person who is experiencing the problem (the first person) together with his or her primary caregiver(s) who bring that person to the doctor or clinician; second, there is the doctor/clinician (the second person) who listens and interacts with the patient; and third, there is the researcher (the third person) who gathers information from all sources. The role of the researcher is to work with all the parties concerned to figure out what is going on—what are the causes of the problems and symptoms reported and how they are related to any treatments proposed and/or applied.

The Logical Ranking

As in normal communication, the three positions of discourse in this collaboration are shared by all the participants, though each position logically retains its distinctive underlying role. In other words, each role remains distinct even though it is shared by many persons. With respect to the first discourse position, clinician/doctors (and researchers, too) need to think as if they were patient/clients, or the parent of such a person. In the case of many—but certainly not all—DAN! doctors and researchers, the clinician or researcher *is* a parent of a person with autism. Even in those cases, however, clinician/researchers need to think of each patient, every person in a study, as if they themselves were the patient/client or the parent of the person being treated. The adoption of this perspective does not transform any of us into patient/client/participants, nor does it make us their parents, but in an abstract way we can still see persons as if we were those persons or their parents.

Even more so, it is important for the patient/client, and the parents of such persons, to think like clinician/doctors to understand why individuals with autism need the help of such professionals and to be willing and able to follow sometimes challenging treatment regimens. Patients and caregivers must themselves become clinicians so that they can understand and follow the regimens as successfully as possible. They need to become "medical detectives"; that is, the parents themselves have to become researchers. As Bock (Bock & Stauth, 2007, pp. 46ff) and S. M. Baker suggest, the parents must become detectives and what Baker calls "Dr. Moms" (2005b, p. 94). All of the parties concerned must think like researcher/theoreticians and, to a very great extent, must become active participants in the research and theory-building processes (as also argued by Jepson & Johnson, 2007).

Putting Ourselves in Their Shoes: Prerequisite to Communication

The necessity of taking into consideration the viewpoint of the other person is not extraordinary in human communication. It is normal. In fact, failure to take account of the viewpoints of other persons leads to breakdowns in what has been called "perspective taking" or "theory of mind" by Simon Baron-Cohen and others. These phrases loosely describe a huge complex of diverse behavioral, social, and linguistic symptoms associated not only with autism, but, indirectly at least, with a host of other disorders reaching out to dementias (including Alzheimer's disease and Parkinsonism, as well as delusional pathologies, e.g., see the comments from John Forbes Nash, 2002, 2009 on his amazing illness and research on **mythomania** 💿). The way that whole complex of symptoms is described with reference to autism demonstrates clearly that we normally understand the experience of other people by listening to them and by, in a very real sense, putting ourselves in their shoes. The emotive element that seems best to characterize, if not define, such perspective taking is referred to in the autism literature as **empathy.** Also, this aspect of communication is often supposed to be diminished or missing entirely in persons diagnosed with autism.

Recovery from autism is also often definitively associated with the demonstration of empathy. Consider the end of the video of Ethan Kurtz on the DVD, where he shows that he is able to take his father's reported point of view into consideration by offering him not one but two toys to play with. Ethan shows that he understands his father's reported feelings and intentions at a high level of abstraction and that he is able to help his father out by enabling the fulfillment of a perceived objective—access to the toy that Ethan is involved with. Ethan gives the toy up and offers another so Stan won't be sad.

The idea that "a friend is another self," as explained by Aristotle in his book *Nichomachean Ethics* (written about 350 B.C.), and the Golden Rule ("Treat others as we want to be treated"), as put in both the Old and New Testaments of the Bible, are not only foundational principles of ethics, but also describe the foundational basis of communication itself. When mainstream professionals fail to act on such true principles, we get results of the sort that Pangborn and S. M. Baker described as "wrong to the point of evil" (2005, p. 3). Conversely, when the foundational principles of communication are respected, taking account of the perspectives and needs of others, acting out of empathy and understanding is reasonable, ordinary, and it works. That is, collaborative genuine communication based on understanding is the most successful kind that can be attained.

Autism as Key Contributor to the Ongoing Paradigm Shift

As in the study of normal development, where communication disorders can often enable us to better understand systems and processes that normally go unnoticed and are taken for granted, the metabolic difficulties observed in individual cases of autism afford a living laboratory for the study of normal biochemistry. From the point of view of clinical work, as S. M. Baker points out, "The child is the best lab" (2005b, p. 128). The dynamic interactions between treatments and observed outcomes afford the best possible information concerning both the study of causal factors and their interactions and the effectiveness and means by which treatments work. In fact, the metabolic imbalances of individual children with autism can help us to better understand normal metabolic processes and interactions; if there were no disorders or disease conditions involved, such conditions might be exceedingly difficult or even impossible to detect.

For this reason—in addition to the fact that the autism epidemic is "one of the worst man-made public health disasters in history" (S. M. Baker, 2005b, p. 120)—the surge in autism incidence is a clarion call to all researchers and clinicians to find out more about how the body's biochemistry normally works. As the DAN! doctors stress, because of the nature of the autism epidemic (and related diseases and disorders), we cannot bide our time for several decades before getting serious about gathering information concerning the various treatments being used in individual cases. While many mainstream professionals appear content to wait for breakthroughs that may occur decades from now—the mythical anti-autism vaccine, or the miracle pill that drug companies may produce someday, the stem cell breakthrough that will change the genetic landscape, or some magic bullet that is yet to be invented—more and more children are being diagnosed with ASD. None of them, and none of us, can put our lives on hold, as is paradoxically recommended by the "Don't look for answers" brigade.

SUMMING UP AND LOOKING AHEAD

In this chapter, we have demonstrated a way to improve the diagnosis of developmental disorders by using a scale of the normal milestones achieved in ordinary growth and semiotic development. The scale begins with nonverbal abilities and works upward through nine levels of increasingly higher and distinct levels leading to the child's first word. It also differentiates eight additional levels within the scope of what is normally termed "verbal ability." One application of such a general scale of milestones is a more reliable and valid way of differentiating levels of severity in autism. The scale is bounded at the low end by cases where there is essentially no evidence of any representational ability and at the high end by normal adult-like linguistic maturity. The practicality, reliability, and validity of the Milestones Scale has been demonstrated both empirically and theoretically. Accurate diagnosis of autism followed by monitoring of progress is essential to assessing the efficacy of alternative methods of treatment and to judging the relative contributions made by known and suspected causal factors to ASD incidence. In the final chapter of this book, we compare the efficacy of the full range of treatments that have reasonable claim to being effective.

STUDY AND DISCUSSION QUESTIONS

1. Why is accurate diagnosis critical to the discovery of the causation of disorders, diseases, and chronic conditions such as those associated with the autism spectrum?

2. How can we know for certain that the sign systems to be developed by normal babies from conception forward must be layered and ranked in a hierarchy leading from the body, to the senses, to intentional movements, and finally to language and all that is associated with it? Is it possible for a child to speak English, say, before it is born? If not, why not? If so, how so?

3. What are some of the reasons that the baby's smile in the womb should (or should not) be taken as exemplary of the universal genuine social smile, one meaning contentment and security?

4. What is the reversion principle, and how does it work? Why is it easier to go down a level than up to a level not yet achieved in the normal course of development?

5. Why is it logically impossible for a person with no senses to acquire language?

6. Why is there, seemingly at least, universal agreement about the constructive nature of sign systems?

7. Why is the loss of any sign repertoire—for example, a vocabulary of icons, indexes, or symbols—an unexpected turn of events? Why is it universally regarded by parents, teachers, coaches, and other adults as symptomatic of a possibly serious illness or disorder?

8. What are some of the features of Asperger syndrome that you observe in the video clips of Jerry Newport and his wife Mary in the *60 Minutes* documentary about them?

9. Why is consensus among competent judges so crucial to the validity of judgments about the naturalness of human semiotic behaviors?

10. What are some of the myths about autism that you would like to help demolish? Is there one myth that you think is more important than the others?

chapter twelve

Comparing Treatments

Empirical research and sound theory show the gastrointestinal tract to be central to the chronic disease symptoms associated with autism. The tendency of mainstream pediatricians and clinicians, however, is to look to behavioral interventions that address symptoms rather than their causes. The treatments that have been attempted are too many to list exhaustively here, and new ones are constantly being proposed. However, we can sum them up, from bottom to top, from a semiotic perspective in terms of ones aiming to affect (1) the body; (2) the body and senses; (3) bodily movements, whether intentional or unintentional; and (4) intentional linguistic acts of cognition, self-expression, and socialization (see J. W. Oller et al., 2010, for elaboration of the disorders at each of these levels). Each of these levels of increasing complexity, comprehensiveness, and abstractness logically occupies a higher layer of the hierarchy of the communication systems that our health and well-being depend on.

Although parents and professionals may be inclined to think first of interventions aiming to advance, or restore, language and social skills, those are actually at the top of the semiotic hierarchy. Focusing therapies in this manner amounts to treating symptoms rather than causes. As logic shows, and as we will see in this chapter, the research is clear in demonstrating that it is far better to treat the causes of the behavioral symptoms rather than to treat the symptoms alone. This does not mean, of course, that we should neglect symptoms, but rather that there is little profit in pursuing behavioral therapies that do not address the deeper problems. Social experiences will not become meaningful to the person on the ASD spectrum, no matter how well thought out those therapies may be, if the gut and its related systems remain seriously out of balance.

FINDING TREATMENTS THAT WORK

The most effective dietary and biomedical treatments, according to a substantial, dynamic, and growing body of research, begin by (1) minimizing exposure to toxins and disease agents, (2) improving the diet, rest, and exercise of the affected individual, and (3) controlling and/or removing disease agents, toxins, and their interactions as soon and as fast as it can be safely done. Of course, treatment should be guided by the best available research and theory. It ought to proceed under the guidance of competent doctors and clinicians who are well informed and who are constantly updating and refreshing their knowledge of the relevant evidence and reasoning.

The Best Authority

Having said that, parents of children with autism should not underestimate the essential contribution that *only they themselves*—mostly in consultation with *other highly motivated parents of children with autism*—can make. The reason for this special parental authority is that only parents are more or less in constant contact with the person affected by the disorders and disease conditions. They know the relevant facts of the case better than anyone else. They may need some help from a good doctor/researcher/medical detective to help discover what they know, but they are the intimate observers of the relevant facts. Parents are the best authorities on what is going on in their child's illness. If the affected child is "nonverbal," the parents are the only advocates who are in a position to find out and speak up on behalf of what the child is going through.

Parents generally understand that they must shoulder the burden of responsibility of acting as advocates for their child. Also, as the research shows, and as clinicians and DAN! doctors point out, parents and researchers alike should keep in mind that the person showing the symptomatic disorder/disease condition(s) is by far the best laboratory—and the highest authority—for measuring and assessing the effectiveness of any proposed intervention for that particular individual. Parents need to become the primary researchers/clinicians/advocates for their affected children. This understanding does not let the rest of us—researchers, doctors, clinicians, teachers, and others—off the hook, but it does recognize the special authority and responsibility of the parents who are burdened with taking care of their children on a full-time basis.

The authors of this book speak as researchers. We are not medical doctors, and we are not giving any medical advice. However, we have decided to join with the doctors and others who have chosen to make common cause with the *Mother Warriors* whom Jenny McCarthy has written about (2008). Along with the DAN! doctors, we agree with McCarthy, Katie Wright, the Jepsons, the Poling family, and thousands more, that parents, patients, and clients are worth listening to. We are glad to add our voices as professional researchers to the growing number of parents—many of them doctors, clinicians, and researchers themselves—who are being inspired and informed by listening to and studying reports from families and individuals affected by the autism epidemic.

Dr. Kenneth Bock says, "I've often thought that there are two basic types of doctors: those who listen to their patients and those who don't." It is a common mistake of doctors to dismiss or underestimate the importance of what their patients are telling them. Also, as Jepson points out, "Surprisingly, most physicians do not regularly take the time to read the methodology of the studies and yet will often change how they practice based on faulty conclusions or incomplete evidence. Even worse, many physicians rely solely on the practice patterns of others and never read the literature themselves" (Jepson & Johnson, 2007, p. 6).

This being the case, we propose a three-way division, Eastwood style, into the good, the bad, and the really ugly:

1. The good clinicians listen to their patient/clients and their families, read the research, and work diligently to understand diseases and disorders in an effort to prevent, cure, or make things better.

2. The bad clinicians do not trust their patient/clients to know anything beyond whether their insurance is up-to-date (and even the bad clinicians and the really ugly ones will research this question!) while they repeat outdated and refuted textbook theories. They are apt to repeat absurdities to parents—the gas theory of infant smiling, the idea that you get more mercury from a single tuna sandwich than from wearing dental amalgam in your teeth, and so on. The bad clinicians rely on blind drug-pushing, where the next step is usually to increase the dose, or add another drug, even if the drugs already in play are killing the patient (see L. Smith & H. Smith, 2001–2010).

3. The really ugly clinicians feel entitled to fees and gifts from pharmaceutical companies and rely on research interpreted to them by well-paid sales representatives, who may not have gone to college but who are well dressed, well spoken, and smart enough to work for big drug companies (see Moynihan, 2008, and video clips there). The research shows that the big pharmaceutical manufacturers spend more than twice as much on advertising and marketing, often disguised as research and development, as they do on any actual research (Gagnon & Lexchin, 2008).

In fact, this last group is so important, so thoroughly entrenched, and so connected to the Washington, D.C., drug lobbyists that we need to give them some special attention.

Pushing Drugs

In peddling influence, the drug companies play hardball with legislators. They have two lobbyists for every person in the U.S. Congress. With practicing physicians, however, they play sweet talk, fine clothes, short skirts, free lunches, biased research papers in fancy briefcases, slick PowerPoint presentations with a blank slot for the doctor's name if he or she is willing to give the lecture to other doctors for a juicy consulting fee, and so on. According to Kimberly Elliot and Gwen Leslie Olsen, two former marketing strategists for pharmaceutical companies, things have gone from not good to really corrupt in pharmaceutical marketing over the last two decades during which Elliot and Olsen were in the business.

Elliot spent 18 years working for drug giants in the marketing company known as the Cutting Edge. It is not too hard to guess that this pharma marketing group targets physicians and surgeons (Cutting Edge Information, 2009). Elliot herself was the hospital marketing specialist for pharmaceutical giants such as Bayer, Bristol-Myers Squibb, Eli Lilly, GlaxoSmithKline, Johnson & Johnson,

Merck & Company, Procter & Gamble, Sanofi-Aventis, and Wyeth, among others. She tells her story in two short video clips accompanying the published interview with Ray Moynihan, guest editor of the *British Medical Journal* (Elliot, 2008 ●).

Similarly, Olsen, author of *Confessions of an Rx Drug Pusher* (2005), spent a decade and a half as a sales representative for such giants as Johnson & Johnson and Bristol-Myers Squibb (Olsen, 2007 ●). Her basic message is that pharmaceutical companies use some extremely sophisticated approaches not only in putting their best foot forward, but to the point of cleverly concealing negative evidence concerning the harmful effects of their products. Olsen shows that prescription drugs certainly can and do kill—just as Larry and Kelly Smith (2001–2010) discovered the hard way. She, too, has a sad but true story to tell that changed her life and her profession forever.

Extending and confirming what Moynihan, Elliot, Olsen, and the Smiths have said, a 2005 survey published in the *Journal of the American Medical Association* conducted at eight U.S. medical schools from California to New York found that, on the average, each student received at least one gift or attended one drug-company-sponsored activity each week while attending medical school (Sierles et al., 2005). Of those surveyed, 93% had been invited to a drug-company-sponsored lunch at least once by a practicing physician. While a substantial majority of the students surveyed, by a margin of about two to one, believed that they would be able to resist the influence peddling by pharmaceutical companies, they supposed that almost half their classmates could be bought. Paradoxically, more than 80% of the respondents supposed that they had a right to whatever gifts they might receive from generous pharmaceutical companies; of the 183 students who said even a gift of less than $50 value was too much to accept, just over 86% had already taken one gift worth that amount or more from Big Pharma. The authors of the report concluded that "student experiences and attitudes suggest that as a group they are at risk for unrecognized influence by marketing efforts" (p. 1034).

On the Brighter Side

Although treatments of autism with prescription drugs are exceedingly common, according to the research by the Autism Research Institute to be reviewed in this chapter, they are among the least likely candidates to make client/patients better. In fact, on the whole, pharmaceutical therapies are more likely than the other common treatment approaches included in the surveys to make patients worse. This does not mean prescription drugs should never be used, but it does suggest that all drugs should be used with caution and under the supervision of a competent medical doctor who has read and knows the relevant research. The only way to be certain that a physician meets those criteria is for parents to check up on their child's doctors.

In spite of the indispensable need for parents to check out the drugs, and the doctors, there is a hopeful side to the pharmaceutical industry's and professional organizations' promotion of prescription medicines for autism treatment. It comes from the profit motive. Most assuredly, drug companies want to make money. In the long run, the products that are apt to bring in the most profits in treating the chronic disease conditions associated with autism and other pandemic conditions are the products that really make people better. As we learn more about the causes of chronic neurological conditions, it will become increasingly more feasible for the drug companies to make products that effectively address those causes.

As a result, over time the pharmaceutical industry can be expected to shift from being contributors to some of the key problems—especially the ones brought on by medical toxins—to becoming contributors to their solution. Although nothing in industry happens instantaneously, the removal of offending toxins from medicines, blocking of their effects, and even their extraction from human bodies are all basic problems that the pharmaceutical companies can—and we believe will—help to solve.

Despite this cause of optimism, the current research findings show that we remain some distance from being able to recommend a particular protocol for treating even a subset of cases of individuals with autism for toxicity and/or oxidative stress. Nonetheless, we already know a great deal about the constellation of factors that is causing the current epidemic of chronic illnesses including autism. Armed with such information, a general plan for detecting the most important elements impacting any given case is within reach. The research shows that the ongoing epidemics of autism and related chronic illnesses are treatable.

A Double Dose of Reality

What does not exist and should not be expected, as the DAN! doctors are the first to point out, is any single "protocol" for treating autism. *There is no logical reason to expect that there ever will be a single-minded "magic bullet" protocol to fix everything that has already gone wrong in autism* (S. M. Baker, 2005b, pp. 67ff). Prevention is the only remedy that can achieve this goal. Of course, after things have gone wrong, it is too late for prevention.

Happily, the research base concerning the dynamic, thoughtful, and loving interventions that are being explored by parents interacting with other parents as well as with physicians, clinicians, and competent researchers gives the reasonable hope of full recovery for many cases. It shows that major improvements are probably possible in almost all cases with complete recovery as a reachable goal for many. There are already many well-documented cases where unique combinations of treatments have worked very well for certain individuals. Such dynamically tailored approaches have even resulted in full recoveries. In many other cases, ranging from severe autism to ADHD and a host of other chronic disease conditions, individualized plans and programs of treatment have led to substantial improvements in measurable symptoms.

As research evidence continues to accumulate, formerly disconnected theoretical streams and avenues of research are coming together. Biochemical processes that many different groups of specialists previously thought were unique to some particular chronic condition, disease, or disorder have—unsurprisingly—turned out to be very much the same across the whole range of human experience. Also, it is important to keep in mind, as Drs. S. M. Baker, Pangborn, Cave, and Wakefield, and about 1500 DAN! doctors are pointing out almost in a single thunderous voice, there is no "alternative" pretend kind of biochemistry; there is only the kind found in real, living human bodies. When toxins and disease agents are introduced into our medicines, domiciles, workplaces, and especially our crops, farms, animals, guts, bloodstreams, and brains by well-meaning persons, including doctors, dentists, legal drug peddlers, crop dusters, and petro-chemical industries, the actions and interactions of those agents affect real biochemistry.

Diets and food supplements, as well as exercise programs, oxygen enhancement programs, and the like, also affect real biochemistry. As Dr. Sid Baker emphasizes, "There is no alternative biochemistry." For that very reason, as Bock and Stauth (2007) have pointed out, and as the DAN! organization continues to show in case after case, when the biochemistry of the gut and the brain are set right, when toxins and disease agents are avoided (and or purged), and when the body is nourished with healthy foods, a whole raft of supposedly "incurable" chronic diseases disappear. In some cases, the chronic disorders and disease conditions in question are ones like AIDS that are supposed to require an almost lethal daily cocktail of medications for the rest of the patient's brief and increasingly miserable life.

When we address underlying causes, toxins, and disease agents, and their interactions with the body's systems, very sick people get better. Many of them get completely well—to look at these individuals, you would never know they had ever been chronically ill. Thus there is a general overall strategy for developing a suitable program of treatment. As we speak and write these words, it is being shaped by dynamic clinical experience and research. We offer this strategy here as an abstract—a summary—of what we believe can be learned from the currently available research about interventions that address the biochemical causes of the autism epidemic. We also believe that our analysis applies in a very general way to the ongoing successful treatment of a host of other chronic diseases, disorders, and conditions that have reached epidemic proportions in the last several decades.

THE HEALTH AND WELLNESS INTERVENTION CYCLE

Figure 12-1 distills some basic conclusions from research on the biochemistry of autism. The intention is to sum up a dynamic plan for developing individualized healing programs on a case-by-case basis. The figure itself is an abstract summary of a cycle of interventions that are being widely applied in treating autism. We believe that the proposed cycle is applicable to chronic disease and disorders in general.

In the following sections, we discuss that cycle beginning at the ground floor or Stage 0, the starting place that logically affords the least risk to the person being treated. From there, we progress through the remaining four stages of the healing cycle, each of which involves increasingly invasive and successively higher-risk procedures. At the end of the cycle, the last stage requires assessment of any progress made. If the desired recovery has not yet been achieved, the logical recommendation is to begin again at Stage 0 and to proceed through the alternatives again in the same recommended order. The idea is to examine and reexamine the alternatives at each stage and to continue the cycle either until recovery is achieved or until a limit of diminishing returns is reached.

Stage 0: Prevention

The health and wellness intervention cycle logically begins at Stage 0 with prevention. It is better, of course, not to be injured by toxins—pesticides, preservatives, dental amalgam, thimerosal, foreign proteins in vaccines, animal wastes in food or drink, industrial pollution, and so on. It is also better

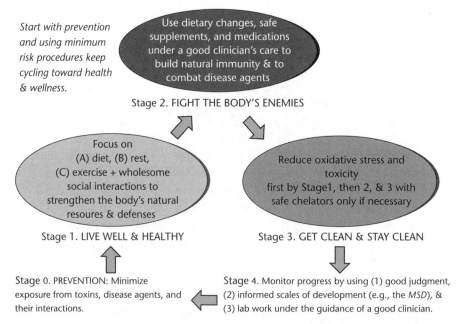

Figure 12-1 A summary of the health and wellness cycle distilled from research on the biochemistry and treatment of autism.

to keep ourselves from being exposed to disease agents—parasites, germs, viruses, and allergens, and their interactions.

We should diligently avoid being infected or injected, say, with a rusty nail, a dirty syringe, any unnecessary antibiotic, and any questionable vaccine. Also, because disease agents can produce toxins of their own and because they can interact, producing effects that are orders of magnitude more intense than they could produce if acting alone, we should be especially wary of multiple exposures. We should avoid piling drugs and disease agents on top of each other as a matter of general principle.

In the final analysis, the best way to prevent chronic diseases and disorders is, as Figure 12-1 suggests, to minimize exposure to toxins, disease agents, and their interactions. Although we cannot yet do much to change our genetic inheritance, we can limit our exposures to outside agents that might harm us by causing any genetic errors lurking in our genome to express themselves overtly. In dealing with autism in genetically susceptible individuals, the best way to cure the problem is to avoid the triggers that would set in motion the cascading series of biochemical events leading to the expression of autism as a chronic condition. If symptoms have already appeared, then steps to prevent the worsening of those symptoms and their underlying causes (Stage 0) are still the logical starting point.

In any case, the least invasive procedures are to be preferred in developing and initiating a treatment plan. In more severe cases, as the DAN! manual suggests (Pangborn & S. M. Baker, 2005, 2007), multiple treatments may be implemented more or less simultaneously. Nevertheless, the first and least invasive step is always to reduce exposure to toxins and disease agents, including pesticides, preservatives, food coloring, and vaccines. All of these substances are known to be particularly dangerous for individuals already on the autism spectrum or with a known related disorder or disease condition. Genetic susceptibilities can be anticipated in part by taking the family history into account and considering any incidence of immune diseases, scleroses, diabetes, Alzheimer's disease, Parkinson's disease, and the like in the child's family history. A child who is already sick should not voluntarily be loaded up with additional toxins and disease agents.

Also, what happened just prior to and during the mother's pregnancy may also be relevant. Exposures to disease agents and toxins during that pregnancy must be considered as risk factors for autoimmunity problems, metabolic imbalances, toxicity, and general oxidative stress. As a precautionary measure, couples planning a pregnancy should consider removal of any dental amalgam well in advance of the pregnancy. Also, they should sensibly avoid toxic substances, such as pesticides, flu shots, alcohol, cigarettes, and even caffeine immediately prior to and during the pregnancy and while breastfeeding or nurturing the baby after it is born.

To avoid or reduce the likelihood of toxic injury to a vulnerable child, parents can insist on dispensing with unnecessary vaccine exposures altogether, delaying others, and spacing out shots. If parents decide to go ahead with any given vaccine, it is only sensible, based on the research reviewed in this book, to check the known toxins and seek out the preparation that involves the least risk. Based on the research presented here and elsewhere, parents may want to refuse vaccines that deliver multiple disease agents simultaneously as well as vaccines that contain unnecessary toxins. Parents may also want to avoid unnecessary exposures to antibiotics, prescription drugs, and any procedures that do not have a very high likelihood of producing a positive and beneficial effect while having extremely low risk of injuring a person with their own child's unique history.

At Stage 0 of the health and wellness cycle, we think in terms of things that should be kept outside the body. If this approach is thought of as therapy, it is a negative, preventative, safe-side kind of therapy. At the next stage in the cycle, we consider the kinds of things we should actively seek to get into the body, moving from a negative kind of therapy to the least invasive kind of positive maintenance and repair.

Stage 1: Strengthening the Body's Natural Resources

The next stage up in the health and wellness intervention cycle, Stage 1 (shown in Figure 12-1 as the ellipse at the viewer's left), relies on the main positive pillars of health and wellness in the body itself—specifically, diet, rest, and exercise. There are several reasons why diet is mentioned so prominently among these three pillars of health. First, the gut and brain are connected. Second, we can usually control what we put in our mouths and swallow. Third, parents have greater control over what they offer their own child in the way of food and drink than over almost anything else in the child's environment. It cannot hurt, and may help a lot, just to do the simplest and safest things to improve digestion (use more organic vegetables) and to make every effort possible to improve rest and exercise.

Diet, Rest, and Exercise: Least Invasive, Most Effective

According to the most current information available at the time of this writing, the best approaches in combating autism (or other chronic conditions) involve dietary changes. To determine what will work best in any given case, as S. M. Baker has pointed out in the excellent materials prepared by himself, Pangborn, and others at the Autism Research Institute (also see Bock & Stauth, 2007; Jepson & Johnson, 2007), it is necessary to do some medical detective work in the research laboratory—that is, the lab consisting of the body of the person displaying the symptoms.

As we have seen, the gut and the brain are in intimate and constant communication. For this reason, diet will affect the ability to rest. In short, a healthy diet means better sleep. Rest is logically secondary to diet in priority, however, because the ability to rest well depends largely on metabolic balances that can be achieved and maintained only by consuming a healthy diet.

Next, still working at Stage 1 of the health and wellness intervention cycle, we come to exercise. It is no secret that everything in the body works better when the voluntary muscles are used vigorously and regularly, preferably on an everyday basis, as in walking, running, cycling, swimming, and the like. Calisthenics and weight lifting strengthen bones as well as the muscles. In general, engaging in vigorous daily exercise for 10 minutes to an hour, or longer, facilitates digestion, increases metabolic efficiency, and increases blood and lymph flow, thereby promoting healing and the elimination of wastes. A healthy, well-exercised body enables us to do everything better, faster, longer, and more completely. It provides for better digestion and rest, and it makes all our body's systems, especially breathing and circulation of the blood, more efficient and less strenuous. In addition, regular exercise reduces stress both physically and psychologically.

Treating the Senses

It has often been noted by Temple Grandin that deep firm touch is reassuring to persons with autism (see S. M. Edelson, M. G. Edelson, Kerr, & Grandin, 1999; Grandin, 1992). In fact, deep, firm massage stimulation is generally relaxing to everyone who experiences it.

In autism, one of the widely known characteristics is that the senses may either appear to be overly sensitive (**hyperactive**), such that the person experiences pain from ordinary sounds or textures, or unusually insensitive (**hypoactive**), such that the senses seem to be so deeply buried that self-stimulation to the point of injury appears to be the only way to awaken them. Generally speaking, the techniques discussed in the preceding paragraph and ones derived from them are loosely collected under the heading of "physical therapy."

In addition, a host of **sensory integration** therapies (Hess, Morrier, Heflin, & Ivey, 2008) have been employed to treat autism. These strategies involve everything from listening to classical music (Hall & Case-Smith, 2008 ◐) to active participation in activities such as riding or leading a horse (J. Brown, n.d.) or swimming with dolphins (NBC6.net, 2008; Servais, 2008 ◐).

Motor Therapies

A variety of relatively noninvasive (nonmedical) physical therapies can be seen as motor therapies. They range from massage to stretching to "passive" manipulative exercise where someone else—possibly a trained therapist, or perhaps a parent or grandparent—works the muscles of the patient/client's body. These interventions are probably helpful in stimulating the flow of blood and lymph, thereby reducing stress and tension, and there is evidence that they have many beneficial effects (Field, 1995; Silva, Ayres, & Schalock, 2008).

The use of animals in general, but dolphins in particular, connects therapies for autism with a fascinating research literature on the capacities of animals such as dolphins (Herman, Uyeyama, & Pack, 2008). Is it possible that dolphins are smart enough to know that a child or an injured person needs special care? Some individuals have made such an argument (e.g., Hyson, n.d. ◉). Others have tried to generalize this effect to many other species. Most types of animals, even a male lion like Christian, seem to have a kind of healing impact on human beings. Regardless whether we believe the ancient dolphin stories—which "although authenticated by undoubted evidence," still look very much like fables (as the Roman scholar, Pliny the Younger, said in his letter to Caninus, circa A.D. 100)—they can still move us to tears. We and our students were affected that way when we saw John Rendall and Ace Berg reunited with Christian. Something similar happens at a deep level when we see the interactions between children with autism and a horse or a dolphin. We find ourselves reacting like Ulysses when his dog Argos died:

> Soft pity touch'd the mighty master's soul;
> Adown his cheek the tear unbidden stole,
> Stole unperceived; he turn'd his head and dry'd
> The drop humane . . . (from *The Odyssey* by Homer, circa 1178 B.C., as translated by Alexander Pope)

Why do we react that way when we see a child with autism swimming with a dolphin or leading a horse that gently follows? It almost seems as though the animal can sense that the child is vulnerable and immature. In the case of some dolphins, they seem to go even further, realizing in some way that the child is injured (see the story by Hyson, n.d., about a dolphin named Dreamer).

All of the animal-assisted interventions targeting autism (and, in fact, any "activity-oriented" interventions) fit loosely into the category of occupational therapy. This sort of therapy aims to help the patient/client "participate in the activities of everyday life . . . by enabling people . . . or by modifying the environment to better support participation" (World Federation of Occupational Therapists, 2004). Adding a horse or a dolphin into the experience is one way an occupational therapist might modify the environment. As modest as it might sound, the goal of what is called occupational therapy is not the grand objective of enabling the client/patient to earn a living, as might be expected from the title, but merely to participate in one or more ordinary daily activities—occupations in the sense of passing the time or just doing something that has the potential to capture the client/patient's interest. Other environmental modifications to help a client/patient interact successfully with the world and with other persons might include such things as providing glasses or hearing aids. Because of the special difficulties of working with children affected by severe autism—and the common comorbidity of autism with other disorders—it is probably wise to appeal to specialists in vision and audiology to check for sensory deficits as well.

All of the foregoing sorts of therapy, but especially massage and physical manipulation, are believed to contribute to a sense of well-being and to healthy functioning of global bodily systems including the brain and gut, while laying the groundwork for development of social and linguistic skills (Field & Diego, 2008). Also, as we learn from the constructive theories of semiotic growth and development, improvements at the lowest levels have positive effects that can cascade upward, just as diseases, disorders, and deficits can have negative effects that work something like a series of falling dominoes. It follows that if things are going to go well at higher levels, the foundational systems need to be in place, functional, and whole.

Cognitive, Social, and Linguistic Therapies

Just above physical exercise, and often closely related to diet, rest, and exercise, are all of the healthy behavioral and social activities that we can undertake. These activities can be used in helping to maintain our own health and that of our children and our clients/patients/students. We can expect improvements in health as we increase the wholesome things we do not only in the way of diet, rest, and exercise, but also in terms of work, learning, and recreation. With respect to the treatment of autism (and other chronic disorders and neurological diseases), interventions from exercise upward, at Stage 1, are the main focal points of physical, occupational, and speech-language therapies.

Stage 2: Fighting Off the Body's Enemies

In some cases, it may be desirable and necessary, with the advice and guidance of one or more competent doctors or clinicians, to graduate to approaches that actively attack parasites, bacteria, and viruses, and/or to move up to procedures that rely on chemical agents to remove one or more specific toxins from the body. However, before undertaking any procedure that has a higher risk value than ones already tested in the laboratory of the patient's body, it is reasonable to first do everything else short of the riskier procedure to achieve the same objective with less risk if possible. In some cases (e.g., Stan Kurtz, Jenny McCarthy), parents have tested drugs, antibiotics, and injections on themselves before using them to treat their own child's autism. On the theory that the parent shares a lot of genetic material and the concomitant biochemical propensities with that child they have then screened out procedures to which they reacted or that seemed harmful in any way while keeping those that seemed to work effectively or that were, at the very least, harmless to the parent.

At a 2007 meeting in Long Island, New York, Stan Kurtz noted that after his son Ethan began to recover, while Stan was considering a chelation procedure for detoxification, Ethan started dumping mercury and other toxins on his own. However, before Ethan started to improve dramatically, there was evidence of disease in his gut that had to be dealt with. In Ethan's case, as in many others, it was necessary to take disease agents in the intestines into consideration. In many cases it is necessary to attack the disease agents that are attacking us. As explained on the video provided on the *Autism DVD*, the crucial treatments that turned things around for Ethan Kurtz were prescription drugs aimed at the fungus and yeast in his gut.

Stage 3: Removing Toxins

Perhaps the most controversial intervention used to treat autism has been the chelation of heavy metals and other toxins. The removal of toxins from inside the body potentially creates a situation in which molecules of poison released from one location are like loose cannons that may bounce around and do harm at many other sites. The chelation process must be done carefully and under competent medical supervision. However, as discussed later in this chapter, even nonprescription chelation has been found to be extremely effective in cases where it has been applied. Although this approach is not recommended until toxicity has been reasonably shown to be involved in producing symptoms, in the many cases where it has been safely used, it has been judged to be extremely effective.

Stage 4: Monitoring Progress

The least controversial, yet one of the least used approaches by many mainstream clinicians, is to carefully monitor progress. Without a good record of the therapies that have been applied and the results obtained while using those therapies, much of the process of intervention is reduced to guesswork while relying on imperfect memories. A written record of what was attempted and what happened just before, during, and after treatment is indispensable.

S. M. Baker (2005a) has some excellent recommendations about how to keep such a record. Noting that many doctors do not keep good records (p. 31), he recommends a simple chronology in a chart form, to be kept by the parent. He has also developed a 20-page questionnaire for keeping track of the details (S. M. Baker, n.d.), which is intended for use by parents in collaboration with their pediatricians. The questionnaire covers everything from the child's name, date of birth, and address; to the patient's blood type, known allergies, symptoms of disorder, and laboratory tests and their results; to caregivers, pets, therapies, nutrition, hospitalization, treatments, vaccination record, mother's pregnancy and delivery, mother's dental fillings, medications received during pregnancy, weight gain, antibiotics used, child's own milestones of development and dates when they were achieved, medications used, supplements, therapies, dietary restrictions and their impact, and so on, through the medical histories of parents, siblings, grandparents, and cousins.

One item to be included in the recommended records is a systematic, written narrative accompanying a summary timeline recording critical facts about diet, rest, exercise, supplements, and therapies (as also noted by McCarthy & Kartzinel, 2008, p. 27). In addition, we suggest that a periodic assessment of milestones achieved is essential. If an argument is to be made about causal relations, or about effective therapeutic interventions, it is important to be able to demonstrate and show a record of improvement in observable symptoms. The most important indicator by far, for reasons detailed in Chapter 11 in the discussion of the Milestones Scale of Development, is the highest and best representational performance of which the individual is capable at any given time during the course of the disorder and its treatment.

With all the foregoing in mind, parents generally need the help of one or more qualified clinicians (e.g., a DAN! doctor) who can guide the tailored development of a treatment program for their child based on a correct and current understanding of the relevant research. We are always looking for good doctors who listen. In the case of the often-nonverbal children affected by autism, the clinicians must also pay close attention to what the parents of those children are saying.

In his Carnegie Mellon lectures of November 17, 2005, Wakefield made this point emphatically:

> I cannot overemphasize the importance of the clinical history. The first lesson that I ever learned in medicine when I walked onto the ward is that the most important thing you will hear is the first thing the patient or the patient's parents tell you. Therein lies the clue to the origin of their disease. The day that you forget that, the day that in your arrogance you assume you know more than the patient, then that is the day that you walk off the ward and go into pathology [where biochemical assays are made in biopsies and autopsies rather than in working directly with live patients].

We could say that listening to patient/clients and, in the case of children with autism, to their parents, is the first rule of good treatment.

RESULTS OF THE ARI PARENT SURVEY

A case in point is the work conducted by the late Dr. Bernard Rimland and the Autism Research Institute (ARI). Rimland began his systematic research into the nature of autism with questions put to parents. In particular, he asked which treatments made their child better or worse, or had no effect. On the basis of the research that he started, a great deal of valuable information and research data have been compiled over a period of nearly 21 years coming from more than 26,000 returned questionnaires between 1967 and 2008. In this section, we review highlights of the results from that 21 years' worth of research grounded in the process of listening to parents of children diagnosed with autism.

In all, 47 prescription drugs have been studied, including antifungals, antidepressants, amphetamines, steroids, and antiseizure drugs. ARI researchers have also collected data on 28 nonprescription (over-the-counter) supplements, ranging from minerals such as calcium and zinc to vitamins A, B_6, B_{12}, and C, and chelators—plus **hyperbaric therapy**, which aims to increase blood flow and oxygen, thereby improving detoxification, metabolism, and so forth. Also, 10 special diets have been included in the ARI (2008) survey, which is titled "Parent Ratings of Behavioral Effects of Biomedical Interventions." The major lesson to be noted from the findings of the ARI research is that in the vast majority of cases, prescription drugs have been judged by parents to be less effective than nonprescription approaches in treating autism. The approaches judged to have the greatest impact have been dietary ones.

The Overall Comparisons

According to the latest chart published by ARI, on average the 47 prescription drugs covered in the parents' survey produced an improvement ratio (percentage of persons who were reported to get better divided by percentage of persons who were reported to get worse) of 1.2 to 1, while the nonprescription minerals, vitamins, hyperbaric therapy, and special diets produced an average improvement ratio of 7.7 to 1. The idea behind this kind of comparison is that it will especially help parents—as well as clinicians, researchers, and doctors—to judge the likelihood of achieving a beneficial effect from a treatment versus no effect or a negative one. This information can be especially useful when thinking about developing a plan of action to help an individual child.

When judging the overall effect of a particular biomedical intervention, it may also be important to take the middle ground into consideration. There are usually very few cases on the "got worse" side of the questionnaire, simply because parents and clinicians are quick to reject medicines and procedures that make things worse. As a result, there are likely to be only a relatively few cases where the intervention did make things worse. For this reason, where no change was reported by parents, we are simply taking account of more data.

Across all prescription drugs in the ARI data, this "middle ground" accounted for 42% of the cases; for the nonprescription approaches, it accounted for 45% of the cases. Thus, if we did not take the middle ground into consideration, we would be disregarding almost half the reports by parents. If our question is whether the supplement, dietary restriction, or other intervention seems to have a significant relation with symptoms of autism, we would not want to answer it while throwing out almost half of the relevant data. Given that, when we do take the middle ground into account, the nonprescription category in the ARI data has the advantage over the prescription approaches.

Table 12-1 gives the percentage of persons treated who got worse according to the person responding to the ARI questionnaire in the first column, the percentage unaffected in column 2, and

Table 12-1 Summary of Data from Parent Ratings of Behavioral Effects of Interventions from Autism Research Institute ($N = 26,000$)

Intervention Applied	Got Worse	No Effect	Got Better	Better/Worse	Chance of Getting Better
10 dietary interventions	3%	43%	54%	17.8 : 1	1.17
29 other biomedical approaches	7%	46%	46%	6.2 : 1	0.86
All 39 nondrug approaches	6%	45%	48%	7.7 : 1	0.93
47 different prescription drugs	26%	42%	32%	1.2 : 1	0.46

the percentage who got better in column 3. Column 4 reports the better-to-worse ratio, giving a best estimate of the odds against a negative result when using the intervention in question. Column 5 gives the odds ratio for those patients who got better against all patients who either appeared to be unaffected or who got worse with the intervention. The last column is an indication of the extent to which we can expect the given intervention, in similar cases, to produce an improvement. It is also the best indicator, from the ARI questionnaire data, of there being an actual causal relation between the intervention and the assessed outcome.

Overall, the ARI data clearly show that diet is the most important causal factor in the entire mix. If we are looking for a positive result, the chances are better by an odds ratio of 2.54 to 1 that dietary interventions, along the lines discussed in the DAN! book, will produce a better result, on average, than the use of prescription drugs. The odds ratio of seeing some improvement, rather than no result or a worsening of behavioral symptoms, is .93 for the nonprescription approaches versus .46 for the prescription drug options. That is, nonprescription biomedical approaches were 2.04 times more likely to produce a positive change in the person being treated.

Comparing Dietary Restrictions

Because dietary restrictions seem to be the most important factors in relation to the observed behavioral effects associated with autism, we consider the dietary changes next (Table 12-2). At any rate, they produced the greatest overall effects. S. M. Baker (2005b, pp. 52–53) has indicated that the **specific carbohydrate diet (SCD)** has turned up at the top of the list of dietary interventions. Although it was introduced relatively recently, and although only 278 parents have reported on it so far, this approach has taken the frontline position among the dietary interventions. When this diet is implemented, Bock recommends testing for specific food allergies or reactions and removing those particular items, often carbohydrates, from the diet. The procedure of working out the details for particular individuals on such a diet, or any other intervention, involves intense detective work with that particular person in view. We cannot overstress the fact that in finding out what works, the child is the best laboratory and informant. We must listen to the patient/client and pay close attention to changes over time: "Your child is the ultimate expert and the best laboratory" (S. M. Baker, 2005b, p. 137).

Recent data confirms Baker's prediction. The SCD diet is the most effective. The **gluten and casein-free diet** is next, then, the *Candida* **diet** tied with the **Feingold diet**. The *Candida* diet avoids refined and other sugars that encourage *Candida* overgrowth while Feingold aims to eliminate foods with preservatives and **salicylate**, which is found (Swain, Dutton, & Truswell, 1985) in medicines

Table 12-2 Comparing Dietary Restrictions in Parent Reports to the Autism Research Institute

Intervention Applied	Got Worse	No Effect	Got Better	Better/ Worse	Chance of Getting Better	Number of Cases
Specific carbohydrate diet	7%	24%	69%	10:1	2.23	278
Gluten-/casein-free diet	3%	31%	66%	19:1	1.94	2561
Candida diet	3%	41%	56%	19:1	1.27	941
Feingold diet	2%	42%	56%	25:1	1.27	899
Removed milk products/dairy	2%	46%	52%	32:1	1.08	6360
Rotation diet	2%	46%	51%	21:1	1.06	938
Removed chocolate	2%	47%	51%	28:1	1.04	2021
Removed wheat	2%	47%	51%	28:1	1.04	3774
Removed sugar	2%	48%	50%	25:1	1.00	4187
Removed eggs	2%	56%	41%	17:1	0.71	1386

such as aspirin and in foods such as licorice candy, honey, port wine, and tomato sauces. The next most effective approach in the list of diet interventions was removing milk and dairy products, followed by the **rotation diet**, then removing chocolate, wheat, sugar, and eggs, in that order.

The three principles behind a rotation diet are simple and foundational to healthy eating. The first principle is to avoid a monotonous repetitive consumption of too much of anything—which can generate abnormalities including food addictions (e.g., the autistic child's insistence on consuming only chicken nuggets and tater tots), toxic build-up, and allergies. The second principle is to dilute the impact of items to which a reaction may have occurred in the past (or one that could develop by overexposure) by reducing the intake at any given time (e.g., avoid allowing the child to eat a whole loaf of bread or an entire package of Oreos at one sitting). The third principle is foundational to allergy therapies in general. It involves, in theory at least, endeavoring to reduce the impact of known or suspected allergies by building tolerance through cyclic consumption of small quantities well mixed with foods and liquids which the child is known to tolerate well. Obviously, rotation dieting means something different in each individual case.

In fact, every one of the approaches discussed under the category of dietary interventions will vary across cases. It follows emphatically from that observation alone that we are not recommending any particular approach for any given individual. Rather, we are merely summing up the overall picture as seen by thousands of parents who have taken the trouble to respond to ARI surveys. The purpose of critical examination of that large data base is to reflect on what we know of causation from biochemical research in order to draw reasonable inferences about the efficacy of common approaches to treatments for autism as judged by many parents in consultation with many different doctors, clinicians, and so forth. For each individual case, parents should also study the data and then consult doctors and clinicians who know the research and who are able and willing to take account of the individual child's unique history. In our experience, DAN! and its affiliates are organizations that can help parents find competent doctors and clinicians who are informed as well as willing and able to help develop effective individual programs of treatment.

Nonprescription Interventions

The overall picture presented by the ARI data also includes information on the biomedical procedures that involve over-the-counter supplements. These items can be obtained without prescriptions for the most part, including injectable vitamins and chelators.

At the top of the list in terms of causal impact is the chelation alternative. This intervention has generally been undertaken only with a subgroup of very well-screened individuals for whom metal toxicity seems to be a factor that has not been resolved by prior interventions. Strictly speaking, it is not a dietary intervention at Stage 2 in our classification system (Figure 12-1), but rather a Stage 3 option, in which a specific chemical intervention is undertaken to get toxins out of the body. However, it is listed along with the nonprescription biomedical approaches because this strategy can be implemented using over-the-counter drugs. We must emphasize that we are not recommending chelation for any individual child: That decision must be made by parents, ideally in consultation with a competent DAN! doctor. Nevertheless, when undertaken in a thoughtful manner, according to the results reported by ARI, chelation has had a remarkable record of success in producing improvements in individuals with autism. It is substantially the best weapon in the entire arsenal.

Looking to the individual interventions in Table 12-3, as judged by the parents reporting on those specific treatments, the top performer overall as reported by 803 parents was detoxification (chelation), with 2.85 times as many parents reporting that their child got better (74%) as compared with those reporting either that the child got worse (3%) or experienced no change (23%) with this intervention. On the ARI Web site, ARI researchers note that DAN! doctors recommend chelation only in a minority of cases; where it is used, however, it appears to be effective in producing a

Table 12-3 Comparing Nonprescription Biomedical Approaches in Parent Reports to the Autism Research Institute

Intervention Applied	Got Worse	No Effect	Got Better	Better/ Worse	Chance of Getting Better	Number of Cases
Detoxification (chelation)	3%	23%	74%	24:1	2.85	803
Methyl vitamin B$_{12}$ (subcutaneous)	7%	26%	67%	9.5:1	2.03	170
Melatonin	8%	27%	65%	7.8:1	1.86	1105
Food allergy treatment	3%	33%	64%	24:1	1.78	952
Vitamin B$_{12}$ (oral)	7%	32%	61%	8.6:1	1.56	98
Hyperbaric oxygen therapy	5%	34%	60%	12:1	1.54	134
Digestive enzymes	3%	39%	58%	17:1	1.38	1502
Fatty acids	2%	41%	56%	24:1	1.30	1169
Methyl vitamin B$_{12}$ (nasal)	15%	29%	56%	3.9:1	1.27	48

Table 12-4 Comparing Prescription Drugs in Parent Reports to the Autism Research Institute

Intervention Applied	Got Worse	No Effect	Got Better	Better/Worse	Chance of Getting Better	Number of Cases
Antifungals: Diflucan	5%	38%	57%	11:1	1.33	653
Depakene: seizures	11%	33%	56%	4.8:1	1.27	705
Risperidal	20%	26%	54%	2.8:1	1.17	1038
Tegretol: seizures	13%	33%	54%	4:1	1.17	842
Valtex	6%	42%	52%	8.5:1	1.08	65
Antifungals: nystatin	5%	44%	50%	9.7:1	1.02	1388

positive result in a greater percentage of cases than any other intervention, including all 86 of the other drugs, diets, and treatments reported on.

Next in line among the treatments in the nonprescription category in terms of effectiveness was vitamin B$_{12}$ administered by injection, with an overall 2.03 advantage ratio; followed by melatonin (1.86); food allergy treatments (1.78); vitamin B$_{12}$ administered orally (1.56); hyperbaric oxygen (1.54); digestive enzymes (1.38); fatty acids (1.30); and vitamin B$_{12}$ administered in nasal spray (1.27).

Comparing Prescription Drugs

When it comes to prescription drugs (see Table 12-4), from the individual case perspective, the antifungals fluconazole (Diflucan) and nystatin had better-to-worse ratios of 11:1 and 9.7:1 with 653 and 1388 reports, respectively. Contrast this with the nonprescription category, where the *average* better-to-worse ratio among dietary treatments, all of which were substantial winners according to parental reports, was 17.8:1. The safest and best approach by that measure was removing milk and dairy products from the diet (32:1, with 6360 families reporting). However, if we take the middle ground into consideration in evaluating the drugs (i.e., reports where there was no change observed with the drug in question), the antifungal Diflucan was on top, with an advantage ratio of 1.33; the antiseizure medication valproic acid (Depakene) had a ratio of 1.27.

THE GASTROINTESTINAL TRACT AS A CENTRAL CONSIDERATION IN TREATMENT

One of the things that DAN! doctors agree on is that the gut is the place to begin treatment. Likewise, in their responses to the ARI questionnaires, parents are in agreement that treatments focusing on the gastrointestinal tract are doing more good, and are considerably less apt to make things worse, than any other form of intervention. We have already noted that behavioral interventions addressing symptoms rather than causes, however valuable they may be, are powerless to remove causes that originate in the gut. Among those known causal factors are oxidative stress, toxicity, out-of-balance metabolism, immune dysfunctions, and food allergies. Symptomatically, these conditions may be expressed as chronic acid reflux, recurrent vomiting, extremely putrid and sometimes bloody diarrhea and/or intermittent constipation, and full-blown seizures. There is commonly evidence of immune dysfunction, which is manifested by one illness after another and by a failure to thrive, listlessness, disinterest in social connections, and so on. As the father of a child with multiple disorders recently put it, "I've heard if your digestion is messed up, it can give you a real sorry attitude."

Chronic Enterocolitis

Although not always detected or recognized, it is now apparent that a substantial majority—if not all—of the individuals on the autism spectrum have a condition described by Dr. Andrew J. Wakefield as **chronic enterocolitis**. In his 1997 paper where this idea was first stated clearly, he wrote:

> We have identified a chronic **enterocolitis** in children that may be related to neuropsychiatric dysfunction. (p. 641)

In addition to overt symptoms of gut disease, by examining affected individuals endoscopically, Wakefield found evidence of general inflammation. This inflammation was particularly noticeable in the 13 to 23 feet of the small intestine, known as the **ileum**, found where the small intestine links through a valve system with the colon (the large intestine). As shown in Figure 12-2, the ileum is the last segment of the small intestine. At the initial segment of the gut where the stomach connects with the small intestine, we find the **duodenum**. It is followed by the middle section known as the **jejunum**, which in its turn is followed at the end segment of the small intestine by the ileum.

By flushing the gut and examining it with an endoscopic procedure, Wakefield found inflammation of the ileum manifested in enlarged, lumpy, lymph glands—a condition he described as

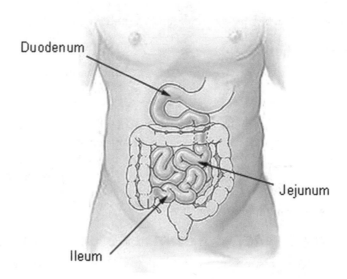

Figure 12-2 A schematic drawing of the intestines.

ileal–lymphoid–nodular hyperplasia. He also found that measles virus was associated with this condition.

When his article was first published, Wakefield's conclusions were shared by 12 co-authors in the highly respected *Lancet* journal of medicine. However, the co-authors soon exited from debate after the spotlight of the vaccine establishment was pointed in their direction. Wakefield was left standing alone under the intense critical and disapproving glare of an unfriendly group of mainstream critics who were willing to defend the vaccine industry against all evidence of harm done. Subsequently, however, independent researchers who examined the evidence (see Jepson & Johnson, 2007, and Bock & Stauth, 2007, for reviews) agreed that Wakefield was correct from the beginning. The abnormalities that he called **autistic enterocolitis** (Wakefield, 2007; Wakefield et al., 2000) are, indeed, associated with a large percentage of autism cases. Levy et al. (2007), by examining diaries kept by parents of children with autism, found that parents reported abnormal stool consistency in 54% of a cross-sectional sample of 62 cases.

Valicenti-McDermott, McVicar, Cohen, Wershil, and Shinnar (2008), in a similar sample of 100 families of children with a history of autoimmune disease, representing 35% of the total data sample, found that 78% of the autoimmune patients reported abnormal stools. It is unsurprising when the symptoms of gut problems in persons with autism come to the attention of doctors and clinicians treating gastrointestinal symptoms, such as constipation, diarrhea, acid reflux, and the like; such symptoms are commonly found to be associated with tissue damage ranging from the esophagus to the anus and with abnormal biochemistry in a majority of instances (Balzola et al., 2007; Horvath, Papadimitriou, Rabsztyn, Drachenberg, & Tildon, 1999; Wakefield, Stott, & Krigsman, 2008).

The Gut/Brain/Immune Systems Connections

The critical element that has puzzled many mainstream pediatricians and other clinicians is how the gut problems that are now well documented in a majority of persons with autism—and that were noticed but not given adequate consideration by Kanner (1943 and following)—could possibly cause the sorts of symptoms of neurological disorders that are the hallmarks of autism. Among the plausible suggestions about how such neuropsychiatric symptoms can be caused by abnormality, disease, or dysfunction in the gut has been proposed by Theoharides and colleagues (Theoharides, 1990; Theoharides & Doyle, 2008; Theoharides, Doyle, Francis, Conti, & Kalogeromitros, 2008). Allergies and autoimmune conditions commonly associated with autism are also implicated in the theory proposed.

Theoharides and colleagues focus specifically on a type of mucosal cell that resembles and functions somewhat like a white blood cell—the so-called **mastocyte** (or more simply **mast cell**). Mast cells appear to be centrally involved in the mucosal linings of the gut and are also involved in interaction with what is called the blood–brain barrier (BBB). They function much like white blood cells and the M-cells in the gut villi and microvilli (see Chapter 9), though they are different in structure and function from M-cells. Mastocytes appear to be crucially involved in immunity and the permeability of the gut. Figure 12-3, used by permission from Theoharides et al. (2008, p. 376), gives a capsulized account of the interaction between the brain and the gut. It also incorporates some of the known key factors and their known or suspected roles in the interaction. Briefly put, it is suspected that

> the mast cell could be activated by a variety of triggers in the intestines and the brain to release key molecules that could disrupt the gut–blood–brain barrier and lead to neurotoxic effects. (Theoharides et al., 2008, p. 375)

With that in mind,

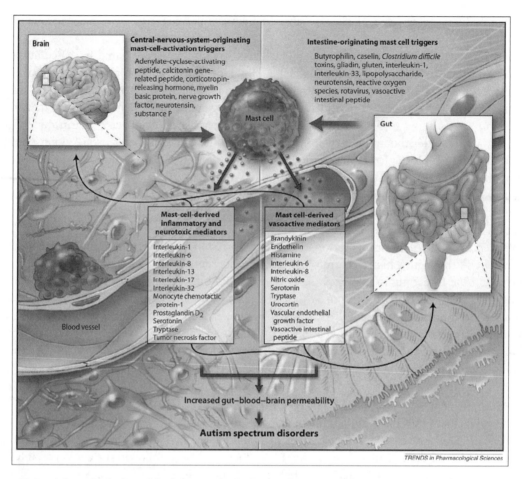

Figure 12-3 A hypothetical model of the gut–brain interaction according to Theoharides et al. *Source*: From "Novel therapeutic targets for autism," by T. C. Theoharides et al., 2008, *Trends in Pharmacological Science*, *29*(3), p. 376. Copyright 2008 by Elsevier. Reprinted with permission of the author and publisher. [http://www.sciencedirect.com/science/journal/01656147]

Dysfunctional or immature development of the gut–blood barrier or BBB would expose local mast cells to triggers derived from the gut and result in the release of mast-cell-derived vasoactive and inflammatory molecules that could increase intestinal permeability, in addition to disrupting the BBB. (p. 377)

Theoharides and colleagues have proposed a dietary supplement with natural ingredients (NeuroProtek) based on their research, which is scheduled soon to undergo clinical trials (personal communication by email from Dr. Theoharides, January 5, 2009). The idea underlying this intervention, as suggested in Figure 12-3, is that mast cells send messages affecting the BBB through **vasoactive mediators**, and at the same time send messages affecting the permeability of the gut in the form of **neurotoxic mediators**. If the mast cells are damaged by toxins, disease agents, or their interactions, it is plausible that the outcome is, on the one hand, increased permeability of the BBB, resulting in an undesirable cascade of inflammation and other symptoms of the neuropsychiatric sort, and, on the other hand, dysregulated permeability of the gut, resulting in the transport of undesirable toxins and disease agents from there into the bloodstream. Based on such gut–brain interactions, Theoharides and colleagues suppose that disruption of the functions of the mast cells in particular can result in autism spectrum disorders.

Although the theory that leaky gut syndrome causes autism has proved controversial, the existence of intense interactions between the brain and the gut is not at all doubtful. Wakefield's research showing inflammation and hyperplasia in the ileum of the small intestine (see Figure 12-2) has been intensely challenged, reexamined, and confirmed in multiple follow-up studies. Some authors have published null results to the contrary, though those reports are largely irrelevant and useless for the logical reasons already stated in this book (see especially Chapter 4). The fact is that positive associations between gut disease and autism have already been documented multiple times: There is no doubt that the gut and the brain are connected intimately.

Similarly, the fact that measles virus has been found in the guts of children with autism, coupled with the fact that subacute sclerosing panencephalitis (SSPE)—see the work of Brouns et al. (2001), Onal et al. (2006), and Akram et al. (2008)—occurs more commonly in persons who have been vaccinated against measles than in those who have not, all show again that the gut and the brain are interacting in complex ways. The incidence of SSPE is much higher in males than in females (by a ratio of 3.2 to 1), which raises suspicion that the link between that virus and SSPE may be similar to that seen in the measles virus infections associated with autism.

With all the foregoing in mind, wouldn't it make sense to deal with the root causes of the gut problems? It may not yet be possible to reverse intrinsic inherited genetic damage, but that fact certainly should not deter our pursuit of known causes of the most severe symptoms of autism. In the exemplary recovery of Ethan Kurtz, which was subsequently followed by the recovery of Jenny McCarthy's son Evan (McCarthy, 2007, 2008) and many other children, treatments focusing on the gut make excellent sense. Certainly, as S. M. Baker, Pangborn, Bock, Kartzinel, Cave, and others have argued, the gut is a reasonable starting point for dietary and biomedical interventions. Setting things back in balance in the gut seems to have been the crucial factor in substantial progress in many cases, and in the case of Ethan Kurtz, treating gut disease seems to have led to a full recovery.

Among the many cases that could be cited, one breakthrough case—that of Ethan Kurtz—is so well documented that it cannot be ignored. If it had not been so well documented by his father, Stan Kurtz (2005–2008a; also see Ethan Kurtz's recovery on the DVD 🌐), Ethan's recovery might be dismissed by the naysayers as either an incorrect diagnosis of a normal child, a "spontaneous" growth change, or an unexplained healing accident or fluke. Any such argument fails as soon as the documented facts of the case are examined closely. In addition to providing a reasonable basis for hope that autism is not a life sentence to a nonverbal, antisocial, listless. or even head-banging existence, the case of Ethan Kurtz is instructive in showing that interventions focusing on disease and imbalances in the gut can make a huge difference in treating autism.

PARENTS BECOMING MEDICAL DETECTIVES

Proactive parents such as Stan Kurtz, who are unwilling to accept the prognosis of a lifelong nonverbal disorder with social isolation and strange repetitive behaviors eventually leading to institutionalization, have turned to the research in an attempt to help their children. They have become doctor/clinician/researcher moms and dads, or what S. M. Baker and Bock call "medical detectives." In Stan Kurtz's case, his study led him to individuals such as Bernard Rimland, who helped him to think deeply and critically about some of the conclusions that others had already reached regarding autism.

Like many parents of children diagnosed with autism, Kurtz considered the least invasive procedures of intervention relying on dietary changes, food supplements, vitamins, and behavioral therapy early on. He systematically sought out physical, occupational, and speech-language therapy for Ethan. In the meantime, he also pursued every possible avenue of research information about the potential causes of his son's condition. He diligently tried the safe approaches that he thought would help, and he used no medications or treatments on his son that he had not first tried on himself.

Before Kurtz became convinced that the gut was central to the evolution of autism, like many other parents, he looked to the noninvasive therapies already mentioned in this book. However, it did not take Kurtz long to suspect the role of toxins, disease agents, and interactions between them.

The Miraculous Component

There was also a miraculous aspect to the undaunted persistence of Stan Kurtz. How and why did he keep on working toward what everyone around him kept saying was impossible? The question is not so much how he could resist the unfriendly critics—that's not so hard. The difficult part had to be the knowing looks of well-meaning parents and friends who thought Kurtz was, well, nuts. How could he ignore the folded arms of the seemingly well-informed physicians? They were doctors, weren't they? Why did they keep shaking their heads and raising their eyebrows? Even members of parent groups whom Kurtz might have expected to join in his quest rolled their eyes and shook their heads disapprovingly. Who did he think he was, anyway?

As the hours turned into days, months, and even years, Kurtz refused to give up. He persisted in seeking the recovery of his son against all the odds and the predictions of the naysayers who expected him to fail. His opponents, who had long since embraced the "hopeless" theories about autism, said: "It's all genetics; nothing can be done" or "We're sorry for you, Stan, but it's a sad, unresolvable, unfortunate situation. It's just a one of those things, a mystery with no solution, something you just have to accept." Other support groups cited funding fears in rejecting this line of research: "We can't afford to risk our charter status in the ABCXYZ organization by actually claiming that recovery from autism might really be possible. We're just an educational organization made up by parents and a few professionals. We don't do ground-breaking research and you shouldn't try it either. You could mislead or hurt someone! You're just a parent!"

But Kurtz wouldn't give up. He had that "extra ingredient" described so well in Bock and Stauth's book, *Healing the New Childhood Epidemics* (2007). That book focuses on dietary, clinical, and medical interventions that work in moving children with autism, and other chronic diseases and disorders, toward recovery. Over and above the "behavioral and educational interventions" that Bock (a medical doctor) recommends, he focuses his attention mainly on treatments based on investigative medical research and clinical experience, listening to and talking to parents and to his patients. Bock argues that in addition to therapies, medicines, supplements, or vitamins, children affected by the growing epidemics of autism and related disorders need one more thing:

> Their parents' love. Love, and all the attention, talking, teaching, helping, and work that comes with it—is the final element that brings these recovering children out of darkness, into light. (Bock & Stauth, 2007, p. 25)

When we view the video record of the recovery of Ethan Kurtz, it is clear that a miraculous element is involved in it—Stan Kurtz's love for his son. It is the unconditional and unstoppable love that never quits. The same ingredient brought hope into Jenny McCarthy's life when it seemed there was no hope for her son Evan. Love is that eternal virtue described by the Apostle Paul in his first letter to the Corinthians:

> Love is patient and kind. . . . is not selfish, and does not get upset with others. . . . does not count up wrongs that have been done. . . . is not happy with evil but is happy with the truth. . . . always trusts, always hopes, always remains strong. . . . and never ends. (Parsons Technology, 1998, *New Century Version of the Bible*, 1 Corinthians 13:4–8)

To discover that ZPD, and to define the series of steps involved in reaching it or surpassing it, requires knowledge of normal human development. To understand and to assist infants and children with severe communication disorders, as Howe observed, we require a detailed analysis of the dynamics of human communication.

"Typically developing" children, as is often noted by linguists, do not need any special tutoring beyond whatever they commonly receive from ordinary interactions with peers, siblings, and other interlocutors. In contrast, children with disorders may need more intensive assistance and may have to advance in even smaller increments than a child without a developmental disorder would require. Typically it takes a child about a year to 15 months to advance to the first word; for deaf–blind children such as Laura Bridgman and Helen Keller, it took eight to ten years to reach this milestone. Similarly, it may require many more exemplars in much smaller steps for a child affected by a developmental disability to acquire a gesture, sign, symbol, or naming relation. A child affected by neurotoxicity, for instance, will generally require more time and smaller-step sizes than a child who has not been injured by toxins.

The highest priority is to address the causes of the disorder; secondary to that, we must find the ZPD for the injured child and work within it to optimize advancement. The essential question is this: What can the child do when functioning at his or her highest level? The level just above that is the one we must aim for, and we must adjust our goals step by step as the child advances.

Applied Behavioral Analysis

One of the most widely used and most highly effective approaches to intervention—and an approach that zeros in on the ZPD—is **applied behavior analysis (ABA)** therapy. It aims to break down the processes of gesturing, vocalizing, signing, speaking, reading, and writing, and any other representational processes, into exceedingly small steps. The key is to move the child in very gentle steps from whatever the child is already able to do to a more advanced level that is within reach. ABA is grounded in the theory of behavior developed by B. F. Skinner (1957). His theory is sometimes loosely referred to as **behaviorism** because Skinner tried to explain away any need for reference to unobservable emotions and acts of thought. He emphasized observable behavior as contrasted with unobservable internal mental and emotional events.

B. F. Skinner

Skinner's theory is more accurately described as **operant conditioning**. Its underlying idea is that an actor/operator acts on the world and experiences the consequences of those actions. In Skinner's theory, an **operant** is a behavior that is, or is believed to be, subject to the consequences and conditions that follow from it. For instance, Skinner's best-known example of an operant **verbal behavior** was his claim that people learn to ask for water when they are thirsty on account of the fact that such a request often results in the consequence of getting a drink. The desirable result of the behavior—getting a drink of water after asking for water when thirsty—increases the likelihood of that behavior reoccurring in the future. A desirable consequence of an operant behavior, therefore, is said to serve as a **positive reinforcement** for that behavior; in other words, it makes the behavior more likely in the future. At the same time, Skinner's theory predicts that **negative reinforcement**, also known as **punishment**, will result in a reduction of the operant behavior. Research shows that punishment is less effective in controlling behaviors than positive reinforcement (see Holland & Skinner, 1961 ◉). The old adage that you can catch more flies with honey than with vinegar holds true in the research with operant conditioning.

Skinner's theory has been criticized as an oversimplification in the case of language, or what Skinner called "verbal" behaviors (see Chomsky, 1959; Morris, 1958). Nevertheless, it is generally agreed that Skinner's theory provides an excellent basis for many aspects of teaching, learning, and therapy for disorders. **Reinforcing stimuli** increase the likelihood of a given behavior (action), whereas **aversive stimuli** reduce its frequency or strength. Skinner observed that a rat that is fed a pellet of food each time it presses a bar will tend to continue the bar-pressing behavior. If no food is provided for bar-pressing for a sufficient number of instances, the bar-pressing will stop and the consequence for the behavior is **extinction**.

If every instance of a behavior is reinforced, the **schedule of reinforcement** is described as **continuous reinforcement**. If the reinforcement appears on every second, third, fourth, or *n*th occurrence of the behavior, the learner is said to be on a **fixed-ratio schedule of reinforcement**. If reinforcement appears unpredictably, the learner is on an **intermittent schedule of reinforcement**. Skinner discovered that behaviors on continuous schedules of reinforcement are easier to extinguish than ones on intermittent schedules. For example, if the computer starts every time we press the start button, we expect it to do so on the next occasion. If it does not start up as expected, we may give up trying after only one or two failures. But suppose we have an engine that is difficult to start and that requires multiple tries to fire. In that case, we will persist and try many times before we give up. Skinner's explanation for the difference in our persistence has to do with the differences in schedules of reinforcement. An intermittent schedule of reinforcement makes the behavior more difficult to extinguish.

Vincent Carbone

One of the therapists who has achieved significant advances with children who have various developmental disorders, including autism, is Dr. Vincent Carbone (2007). Not only is Carbone able to get individuals with severe disorders to advance in communication abilities, but he is also successful in training others in the ABA methods that he uses following Skinnerian principles.

The first step in ABA therapy is to observe and analyze what the child is doing in interactive contexts. Some of the observed behaviors may be desirable; others may be undesirable and counterproductive. For instance, the first objective may be merely to reduce certain disruptive behaviors and to encourage more cooperative ones. Screaming at a high pitch, for example, is not conducive to speech acquisition or to improved speech articulation. By contrast, looking at the parent/therapist to observe a modeled behavior is a step in the right direction. This behavior can help move the child toward functional speech and/or signing behaviors and better socialization skills.

Also, the analysis phase of the program must ask which events cause the child to do things that are undesirable, ineffective, and perhaps even disruptive from the point of view of interlocutors, as contrasted with actions of the child that are productive, acceptable, useful, and cooperative. In each case, what is the child under observation/treatment trying to achieve? What causes the child to express distress, glee, calmness, or agitation? Once this analysis has been done, it is possible to develop a program for the child in which desirable behaviors are shaped in the direction that the therapist/parent wants the child to go, and in a way that will enable the child to move in step-by-step fashion from less effective behaviors to more effective ones.

In his workshops on ABA, Carbone often shows video clips of real children as they progress from one therapy session to the next over a period of days, weeks, or longer. In one such clip, a child of five or six comes into the clinic with his mother. The little boy is agitated and pulls away. As the pair walks with the clinician from the waiting room to a play area, the little boy shrieks, pulls away from the clinician, and practically has to be dragged kicking and screaming from one room to the other. At this point, Carbone stops the video and asks his audience if they would like to see that little boy a few sessions later. During that later session, the same boy practically gallops, without the shrieking, down the same hall with the same clinician. What has happened in the interim?

Step by step, Carbone shows how during the first session, the clinician observes the boy as he calms down and begins to explore the toys on the perimeter of the room with his back to the clinician. In this way, the clinician discovers what interests the boy. As soon as she knows what the little child will regard as reinforcement, she puts him on a schedule to shape his behaviors so that the shrieking, kicking, and pulling-away behaviors are diminished to a vanishing point (i.e., to extinction), while eye contact and desirable vocalizations are shaped and enhanced in the direction of meaningful speech and effective communication. The key with this particular child, and a strategy that will work in much the same way with any similar child, is to provide the desired activity (reinforcement) shortly after the cessation of some undesirable behavior such as shrieking.

The Shaping Process

As Carbone describes operant conditioning, it is a process of shaping new behaviors little by little. Suppose the child shows interest in a particular toy. The clinician first observes this expression of interest. In the early going, it is essential to move away from the ineffective behaviors that prevent progress in communication. For instance, when the child is shrieking or pitching a tantrum, it is hardly possible to engage in productive communication or teaching. Thus the clinician must patiently extinguish the undesirable behaviors so as to shape and develop desirable ones. While the child is behaving in an undesirable way in Carbone's video (shrieking at the top of his lungs), the clinician gets between him and the toy, presenting her back to the child, and waits until there is a brief silence, about two seconds. Then she turns and produces the toy, and as Carbone says, "The circus begins."

The clinician smiles and talks to the child, facing the child, while the interesting toy dances between them. This "circus" continues until the shrieking or some other undesirable behavior recurs. Then the circus ends; the clinician turns her back and waits for the child to calm down again. After two seconds of silence, the circus returns, and so forth. Within a few short sessions, the child's behavior has been shaped to a degree that the shrieking is completely extinguished and the child is interacting with the clinician, vocalizing appropriately, and moving forward on the developmental scale toward speech and effective communication.

Carbone has video clips showing children who started as completely nonverbal and, after a few weeks or months of therapy, were able to begin talking or (in some cases) to use meaningful manual signs. The key is to find out what the child is interested in—that is, what is reinforcing to the child—and then use the "circus" to shape the desired behaviors bit by bit in the direction of effective socialization and communication. Examples can be given of moving from a completely nonverbal child in a first-grade class to a child who is effectively communicating with classmates through some verbalization and manual signing.

Appeals to All Available Modalities

One of the things that we particularly like about Carbone's adaptation and extension of Skinner's operant conditioning paradigm is that Carbone uses all of the modalities of sense, movement, and language, but adjusts his intervention to suit the particular strengths of the child in whatever modality seems to work best. He uses speech, manual signs, pictures, gestures, objects, food, tickling, hugging, bouncing on a trampoline, or whatever works to reinforce desirable socialization and to extinguish ineffective or disruptive behaviors. He finds and works within what Vygotsky called the ZPD.

One of Carbone's approaches involves the combination of manual signing, reinforcing action, and verbalization. For instance, the gesture for hugging with the arms crossed against the chest while rocking back and forth as if hugging a child can be combined with hugging the child so as to suggest the linking of the sign with the action. This is what we call a pragmatic mapping exemplar. The child sees the gesture and then experiences the meaning of it when his mother wraps him in her arms and hugs him. Carbone, however, takes matters a step further.

2. What can private citizens do to keep pharmaceutical companies and doctors honest?

3. Discuss your own thoughts about the evidence you can see in the videos on the *Autism DVD* dealing with the healing impact of animals on human beings.

4. We were surprised to see from the ARI data that dietary interventions came out ahead of prescription drugs in terms of effectiveness for the most part. Were you? Should anyone have been surprised by this outcome? Why or why not?

5. If we compare the remarkable success achieved by treating the causes of autism, as in the case of Ethan Kurtz, with the movement achieved by a behavioral intervention that enables a "nonverbal" individual to move up to saying a word such as "hug" for the first time (at age five), which is a larger advance? What sorts of advances might be expected for the child benefiting from behavioral therapy if the gut issues were addressed in an appropriate way?

6. What are some of the ways that the miraculous ingredient of love affects healing in your experience and in the data examined in this chapter? How do you think this factor influences human interactions in the doctor's office? What are some of its manifestations there?

7. Reflect on the ADA's positions on putting dental amalgam in and taking it out of human mouths. What does the research show us about removal of mercury-containing fillings?

8. Comment on the case of the dentist who removed the amalgam fillings from Michelle Kurtz's mouth. How reliable a witness do you suppose she is concerning the harm mercury did to herself and to her patients? Why might or might not the dentist misrepresent the situation given her terminal prognosis?

9. Why is the determination of the zone of proximal development crucial to the success of any behavioral intervention?

10. As we look to the future, what do you see as your own role in helping to halt the autism epidemic and to recover those affected by it?

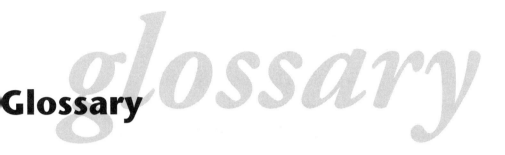

Glossary

acetylcholine: the main excitatory neurotransmitter of the autonomic nervous system and a key element in the control and regulation of voluntary movements.

acid reflux: the phenomenon commonly referred to as "heartburn," in which stomach juices rise into the throat; sometimes as a precursor to vomiting.

acrodynia: a form of mercury poisoning seen in early childhood, also known as "pink disease" because of the pinkish discoloration of extremities as well as the cheeks and nose.

actin: a globular protein forming the microfilaments of muscle tissue and involved in muscle contraction, cell movement, signaling, and the shape of cells.

adaptive immune capabilities: the complex of systems above the genetically supplied capacities of the body to defend itself, and also above the complement cascade.

ADC: abbreviation for *AIDS dementia complex.*

adequation: a term introduced by Jean Piaget, suggesting the process by which systems of thought, reasoning, and representation become increasingly well suited to their purposes.

adrenoleukodystrophy: a genetic disorder triggered by long-chain fatty acids that build up over time, preventing the normal functioning of *myelin.*

affective disorder: any one of many chronic conditions affecting the ability of a person to maintain emotional balance, to manage, and/or to experience and control emotions.

AIDS: the acronym and abbreviation for *acquired immune deficiency syndrome.*

AIDS dementia complex (ADC): the debilitating constellation of symptoms associated with AIDS, whereby the person affected experiences mental and psychological deterioration including loss of memory, inability to plan a sequence of actions, and ultimately inability to recognize others and self.

AIF: acronym for *apoptosis-inducing factor.*

alkyls: unstable compounds of hydrogen and carbon that are very reactive free radicals; they include methyl, ethyl, and pentyl types (among others) when joined, for instance, to mercury.

allergen: any substance, protein, or agent that produces an allergic reaction.

ALS: abbreviation for *amyotrophic lateral sclerosis.*

Alzheimer's disease: a condition first described by Alois Alzheimer (1906) that commonly affects older persons and has sometimes been referred to as "old-timer's disease"; it is known to be affected by toxins that damage cortical tissues.

amalgam: in dentistry, an unstable mixture of various metals consisting of about 50% elemental mercury, widely used in filling cavities in tooth and bone material.

AMD: abbreviation for *age-related macular degeneration.*

amniocentesis: insertion of a needle through the wall of the uterus to withdraw a sample of amniotic fluid to test for genetic defects and/or infections in a developing fetus.

amyl nitrate: a male sex performance enhancer found in street dugs known as "poppers."

amyotrophic lateral sclerosis (ALS): a progressive neurodegenerative disease of the nerves that control voluntary movements; also known as *Lou Gehrig's disease.*

anaphylactic encephalopathy: a brain-damaging and life-threatening form of allergic shock.

anaphylaxis: an extreme whole-body allergic reaction leading to life-threatening shock with sudden loss of blood pressure owed to cardiovascular failure.

anergic: unresponsiveness of the body's immune systems to an antigen or allergen.

antibiotic: any substance or compound that kills or inhibits the growth of microbial life-forms.

antibody: any of the gammaglobulin proteins found in the bodily fluids of vertebrates that can kill, capture, or neutralize bacteria and viruses that may attack the body.

antigen: any biological or other substance—but especially a microbe, virus, or protein—that can cause the immune system of a vertebrate to produce antibodies against it.

antigen-presenting cell (APC): a cell that displays a foreign antigen or some identifying component of such an antigen, together with its own *major histocompatibility complex*, on its surface. It acts much like a foreign visitor to another country who must present a passport to military or police authorities in international airports.

antioxidant: a biomolecule that reduces the rate of or prevents the oxidation of other molecules.

antiretroviral therapy (ART): any therapeutic intervention, usually with drugs, that aims to halt or reduce the impact of viruses that rewrite portions of an individual's DNA.

antiseptic: an antimicrobial substance applied to living tissues to reduce the possibility of and aiming to prevent infection.

antivenin: a biological product designed to prevent harm or raise tolerance for a poison from a snake, spider, or other organism; also known as *antivenom.*

APC: abbreviation for *antigen-presenting cell.*

aphasia: loss of ability to produce or comprehend speech, manual signs, or language.

apoptosis: the systematic disassembling of a cell; often referred to as "programmed cell death."

apoptosis-inducing factor: a protein in the outer membrane of the mitochondria that is involved in causing a damaged or diseased cell to disassemble itself (often referred to, somewhat misleadingly, as the "cell suicide" factor).

applied behavior analysis (ABA): a kind of therapeutic analysis and intervention aiming to change behaviors by discovering the reinforcing factors that shape them in the first place and gaining control over them by managing the controlling consequences.

argument: any entity or *logical object* that can be referred to or signified; a simple example is whatever is named in a naming operation, or whatever any other conventional *predicate* may be associated with.

ART: acronym for *antiretroviral therapy*.

ASDs: abbreviation for *autism spectrum disorders*; also known as *pervasive developmental disorders* (*PPDs*).

asepsis: a means for prevention of infection, or the condition characterized by the complete absence of any infecting organisms.

asymptomatic: without any noticeable signs or symptoms of disease or problematic conditions.

atherosclerosis: a chronic inflammatory response in the walls of arteries, commonly referred to as "hardening" or furring of the arteries. It is caused largely by an accumulation of white blood cells, fats, and proteins, which form plaques on the inside walls of the arteries.

atopic: characteristic or descriptive of an allergic reaction at a distance.

attention-deficit/hyperactivity disorder (ADHD): a poorly defined condition that is loosely described by what appears to be a shortened attention span and a tendency toward extreme, erratic, and relatively uncontrolled activity.

autism spectrum disorders (ASDs): a class of chronic conditions defined in terms of abnormal social interactions and communication, restricted interests, and stereotyped behaviors such as hand-flapping; also termed *pervasive developmental disorders*.

autistic enterocolitis: a condition associated with about 70% to 80% of persons diagnosed with autism, which involves inflammation of the colon and/or small intestine especially at the juncture known as the *ileum*.

autoimmune disease: any condition in which the body's defense systems begin to attack its own cells or over-react to perceived *antigens*, as in allergies.

autoimmune disorder: any chronic undesirable and abnormal state in which the body's defense systems begin to attack its own cells, organs, or products.

aversive stimuli: stimuli that engender a negative, possibly a mild, flight-or-fight response, or that merely repulse the organism or person affected.

avitaminosis: an abnormal metabolic condition caused by lack of access to or uptake of essential vitamins.

azidothymidine (AZT): one of the reverse transcriptase inhibitors; an antiretroviral drug used in the treatment of AIDS; also known as *zidovudine* (*ZDV*).

AZT: abbreviation for *azidothymidine*.

B cells: highly mobile cells of the immune system that move in the bloodstream and lymph ducts.

Bacillus anthracis: the bacterium that causes anthrax disease.

BBB: abbreviation for *blood–brain barrier*.

behaviorism: a philosophical outlook about human psychology that emphasizes observable actions that, according to the theory, come under the control of certain observable consequences.

benzene hexachloride (BHC): an organochlorine (marketed as Lindane) and *neurotoxin* used as an agricultural insecticide and a pharmaceutical pesticide. It has the undesirable effect of attacking the brain, liver, and kidneys. Although it has been banned for the most part as an agricultural product, it is still used in some medicines for treating infestations of lice and scabies.

beta amyloid: a peptide consisting of many amino acids that are the main constituents of the plaques found in the brains of patients with Alzheimer's disease.

beta-carotene: a form of vitamin A that is the main source of the orange color in carrots and sweet potatoes, and a potent *antioxidant*.

BHC: acronym for *benzene hexachloride*.

biopsy: examination of tissue or cells from a host to test for disease, especially cancers.

blood–brain barrier (BBB): a complex of membranous, metabolic, and cellular systems between the bloodstream and the brain that prevent passage of bacteria and some toxins, while permitting passage of other substances essential to the metabolic systems of the brain (e.g., oxygen).

bolus: from the Latin word for "ball"; any more or less coherent mass or quantity of a liquid or substance loosely contained within a bodily or other cavity (e.g., a syringe or blood vessel, to be injected or ingested in one gulp, swallow, or shot).

Candida: a fungus (yeast) capable of sexual reproduction that is known to cause oral and genital infections in humans; commonly *Candida albicans*.

***Candida* diet:** any procedure restricting the intake of refined and other sugars believed to contribute to the overgrowth of *Candida albicans*.

canonical babbling: the repetitive type of infant vocalizations—for instance, /bababa/, or /gagaga/—as produced by normal human babies by about their sixth post-birth month.

carcinogen: any chemical substance that causes cancers.

celiac disease: an autoimmune disease of the small intestine with symptoms consisting of chronic diarrhea, failure to thrive (in children), and fatigue.

cellular immune response: an immune response that involves going inside cells to kill enemy combatants, as contrasted with a *humoral immune response*, in which the combat or capture process occurs outside the boundaries of the body's cells.

cerebellar ataxia: neurological deficits in rhythms that are controlled in large measure by the cerebellum and that, depending on whether the damage is only to one side or to both, may disrupt the ability to produce a rapid sequence of syllables in speech, thus resembling *Broca's aphasia*.

chelation: any therapy using chemical substances, natural or pharmaceutical, to grab onto toxic chemicals and pull them from their molecular attachments in bodily proteins.

chelators: chemicals that serve as claws or grappling hooks that can latch onto toxins that are already attached to other molecules and break them loose.

chemical oxidation: the breakdown of a metal or other chemical through its combination (usually with oxygen) in a process by which it either gains electrons or, by borrowing from another chemical, increases its own oxidation number. An example is the rusting of iron. Chemical oxidation is the opposite of *chemical reduction*.

chemical reduction: a chemical reaction in which a metal or other chemical loses oxygen and gains hydrogen or, by sharing its electrons with another chemical, decreases in electrons (or, more accurately, decreases its oxidation number). Chemical reduction is the opposite of *chemical oxidation*.

chemotaxis: the means by which an immune cell navigates its way to the site of an injury, as if following a chemical trail.

childhood schizophrenia: the sort of hallucinatory loss of touch with reality that is believed to occur in childhood.

chronic enterocolitis: a persistent inflammation of the gut.

chronic vomiting: a persistent form of vomiting that is characteristic of autistic enterocolitis in many cases, sometimes involving repeated projectile vomiting of an extreme and persistent sort that requires intravenous fluid supply to prevent dehydration and death.

comorbid: said of any co-occurring undesirable or abnormal conditions or disorders.

complement cascade: a cell-killing attack complex that is part of the *innate immune system* but is activated by the *adaptive immune system*. It consists of proteins and protein fragments synthesized mainly in the liver and accounting for approximately 5% of the globulin in blood serum.

Conidia: a fungus that can infect the lungs of individuals with depressed immune systems— for example, persons undergoing chemotherapy, AIDS patients, bone marrow recipients, organ transplant patients, and others with debilitating chronic disease conditions.

conjugate vaccine: a vaccine in which an antigen is attached to a carrier protein, with the aim of giving the vaccine increased power to cause the immune system to generate antibodies to the antigen, which might otherwise go unnoticed or generate only a weak response by the immune system.

continuous reinforcement: a behavioral training schedule in which positive consequences are provided every time a certain behavior occurs.

craniofacial disorders: abnormalities, usually genetic and always developmental, that affect the bone structures and/or muscle systems of the face and head.

cyanosis: a blueness under the fingernails and in surfaces where capillaries come near enough to the surface to be noticed. It is caused by a lack of oxygen in the blood vessels that normally carry oxygen outward to the extremities from the heart and lungs.

cytopathy: any disease or disorder of the cells.

D-penicillamine: a product derived from penicillin, used as a chelating agent and in treating rheumatoid arthritis, as well as mercury and lead poisoning.

DDT: abbreviation for *dichloro-diphenyl-trichloroethane*.

defectology: Lev Vygotsky's term for the study of communication disorders as well as genetic and developmental diseases and abnormalities.

defendant: in a court of law, the person or party that is charged with wrongdoing.

delay technique: in *behaviorism* and *applied behavior analysis*, a technique advocated by Vincent Carbone in which a trainer/interlocutor/therapist withholds a reinforcement for a brief interval to allow the patient/client/learner an opportunity to take another step toward a desired behavior, such as saying a word or producing a manual sign, to get the desired consequence (*reinforcement*).

delayed echolalia: a repetition of all or part of a surface form of an utterance or linguistic behavior that occurs after a lapse of minutes, hours, or even longer.

delusions: representations that are imaginary, but are mistaken by the person producing the representations as valid perceptions or memories.

dementia: in general, any loss of mental ability, memory, or processing capacity, especially for linguistic and related systems of representation.

dementia infantilis: a disintegrative condition affecting essentially every aspect of a child's capacity to represent experience and to express such representations that is considered by some to be indistinguishable from a severe form of "regressive" autism; also known as *childhood disintegrative disorder (CDD)* and *Heller's syndrome*. Dementia infantilis is diagnosed by onset later than expected for "regressive" autism (after 3 years of age) and by delays or loss of language, social functions, and motor skills. Regression can occur from age 3 to 10. The actual diagnosis depends on "expert" opinion.

dendritic cells: immune cells that can capture and process antigen material functioning as *antigen presenting cells* and that can capture microbes and present them to lymphoid tissues. These cells are characterized by branched projections, called *dendrites*, from which they get their name.

dental amalgam: see *amalgam*.

diabetes: a syndrome of disordered metabolism yielding imbalanced (usually high) blood sugar levels owing to inadequate production and/or uptake of the hormone insulin, which is manufactured in the pancreas. The condition appears to be exacerbated—if not in some cases caused or precipitated—by toxins, disease agents, and their interactions.

dichloro-diphenyl-trichloroethane (DDT): an organochlorine insecticide, similar to the pesticides dicofol and methoxychlor. It is a colorless, crystalline solid with a weak, chemical odor that is marketed under many different brand names. DDT accumulates in body fat and human blood.

dimer: a chemical or biological entity, such as an antibody, consisting of two simpler subunits called *monomers* that are held together by molecular bonds.

dimercaprol: a chelating agent developed during World War II to help combat chemical warfare using arsenic derivatives. It is now used in treating poisoning by heavy metals such as arsenic, mercury, and lead.

dimercaptuosuccinic acid (DMSA): an FDA-approved sulfur compound that attracts and captures mercury molecules enabling the body to eliminate mercury mainly through the urine and feces.

disinfectant germicide: any substance intended to kill germs. *Thimerosal* is an example.

disintegrative psychosis: another name for *dementia infantilis*, which is also known as *childhood disintegrative disorder* and *Heller's syndrome*.

DMPS (2,3-dimercaptopropane-1-sulfonate): a chelator used to treat mercury poisoning. It is reported to cause a full-body rash as seen in cases of severe mercury poisoning.

Down syndrome: a genetic disorder named for John Langdon Down [1828–1896], who described it in 1866. This disorder is caused by an extra copy of chromosome 21. Affected persons are characterized by moderate to severe developmental disabilities, almond-shaped eyes, shorter limbs, poor muscle tone, and protruding tongue. Risks associated with Down syndrome include congenital heart defects, reflux disease, greater susceptibility to infections, and reduced life expectancy.

duodenum: the section of the small intestine that connects it to the stomach.

dyadic: having two parts, as in a typical two-person conversation, or a verb that takes two arguments as in "Bill kissed Mary," where "Bill" and "Mary" are arguments of the verb "kissed."

dysbiosis: a breakdown in the ecosystems of the gut.

E. coli: see *Escherichia coli*.

Ebolavirus: a virus believed to cause Ebola hemorrhagic fever that was named for the Ebola River of Zaire where it was first observed in 1976; characterized by long filaments; transmitted primarily through bodily fluids and/or through skin and mucous membrane contact; damages blood vessels and platelet cells so that about 90% of infected persons die of shock.

echolalia: a symptom of disorder that is often observed in autism; involves repeating, possibly after a considerable delay and without full comprehension, the surface forms of some utterance, discourse, or linguistic expression.

effector cell: a type of helper cell in the immune system that seems to authorize the replication processes, like an adjutant that issues an order for military manufacturing, cloning of fighters, and mobilization, that will be carried out by *killer T cells* and *B cells*.

electron: an atomic particle/wave that carries a negative charge and that is especially involved in the *oxidation* and *reduction* processes so important to the body's handling of *free radicals*.

elemental mercury: the kind of mercury that consists at room temperature of a heavy liquid metal. It readily vaporizes, especially when heated or disturbed, giving off extremely neurotoxic mercuric gas.

empathy: the kind of emotional comprehension and understanding that enables us to understand how someone else is feeling.

encephalopathic conditions: any disorder or disease involving the central nervous system and especially the brain.

endogenous retroviruses (ERVs): native retroviruses that are richly incorporated into the human genome. In contrast, invasive retroviruses come from outside the host organism.

enterocolitis: inflammation of the small intestine and colon.

epigenetic: a term applied to all of the systems above the genetic ones that can influence health and well-being. They include all the systems that influence metabolism, immunity, and detoxification as well as the neurological systems enabling human language, cognition, emotion, and social behavior.

epilepsy: a neurological disorder of unknown etiology characterized by repeated and chronic convulsive seizures.

epithelium: tissue composed of the cells that line the cavities and surfaces throughout the body both on the inside and the outside.

equine encephalomyelitis: commonly known as "sleeping sickness," a disease that most often affects horses (hence, "equine") but can also infect humans with a high fatality rate in young children; symptomatically somewhat similar to *West Nile virus*.

ERV: abbreviation for *endogenous retrovirus*.

erythrocytes: red blood cells.

***Escherichia coli* (*E. coli*):** a bacterium commonly found in the intestines, some strains of which are harmful—particularly the *serotype* that produces *Shiga toxin*.

ethyl mercury: an alkyl form of mercury found in the pharmaceutical product known as *Thimerosal*, *Thiomersal*, and *Merthiolate*, patented by M. S. Kharasch and marketed by Eli Lilly.

ethyl mercury *p*-toluene sulfonanilide: the killing ingredient in the fungicide used for seed-borne diseases of cereals; formerly marketed under the trade name *Granoson M* and produced by DuPont.

etiology: the causation and/or the study of the causation of a disease or disorder.

exogenous retroviruses: invasive retroviruses that come from outside the organism.

extinction: in *behaviorism* and *applied behavior analysis*, a training or shaping process that leads to the diminution of a particular behavior to the point that it finally disappears altogether from an individual learner/client's repertoire.

Feingold diet: a restrictive intake program developed by Ben F. Feingold that has been used in the treatment of various *autism spectrum disorders*, including those on the periphery such as *hyperactivity* and *ADHD*. This diet restricts artificial colors and flavors, aspartame, petroleum-based preservatives, and *salicylates*.

fetal breathing: a process by which an unborn baby in the womb actually breathes in the amniotic fluid. It is believed to be essential to normal pre-birth growth and development of the lungs and body.

fibroblasts: the stem cells that form connective tissues and make the collagen and fibrin that give the bodily tissues their shape and hold them together. Fibroblasts are important for healing of injuries and are the most common cells in the connective tissues.

first person: in grammar and in semiotic theory, the one who is doing the talking or producing the utterance, text, discourse, or signs.

fixed-ratio schedule of reinforcement: positive consequences for a particular behavior that are provided on every *n*th occurrence, where *n* may be any number greater than 1 but is usually smaller than 7.

forensic: a term applied to scientific investigations and research that are of interest to legal proceedings, as in the investigation of evidence pertaining to a crime.

free radicals: negatively charged atoms or molecules that are highly active from a chemical point of view; they are likely to participate in chemical reactions, often doing damage to bodily proteins and making them dysfunctional.

gastrointestinal: said of any bodily function having to do with the gut, especially the stomach, small intestine, and colon.

genetic theory of autism: the idea that autism is mainly caused by genes; more particularly by genetic errors.

genome: the entire inheritance of genetic material that is passed from one generation to the next in a given species; the organism's hereditary information encoded in DNA, or in the case of certain viruses, RNA.

genomics: the study of the nature and functions of the genome of one or many organisms; how the genetic material of the body works and functions, often focused on in a particular species of organism.

genotoxic effects: any that involve damage to genes or genetic material and that are caused by poisons.

genotoxins: poisons that damage the genes or the *genome*.

germ theory of disease: the idea that individual particular microbes—loosely called "germs" and including bacteria, fungi, and viruses, or their parts—cause diseases.

glomerular kidney disease: damage to the capillaries and the capsules that contain them as those tiny blood vessels flow through the walls of the kidneys and enable the filtration of poisons and waste matter, especially creatinine, from the blood in the production of urine.

glomeruli: the filters of the kidney; they consist of Bowman's capsule, which surrounds a cluster of tightly packed capillaries (tiny blood vessels), from which the capsule extracts creatinine and other wastes under pressure.

glutathione (GSH): an antioxidant containing glutamate as one of its main components that sequesters certain free radicals and enables their removal from the body.

glutathione peroxidase (GPx): a chemical form of the antioxidant *glutathione* that reduces the highly reactive hydrogen peroxide to water, thereby enabling the replenishment of the supply of *glutathione*.

gluten- and casein-free diet: a diet that restricts or completely eliminates foods or liquids containing the protein gluten, which is found in grains such as wheat, barley, and rye, along with the protein casein, which is found in milk and its by-products.

glycoproteins: proteins consisting mainly of certain sugars—some of which are rare and must be produced by the body—that are involved in cell communications, immunity, and metabolism.

GPx: abbreviation for *glutathione peroxidase*.

Granoson M: a fungicide containing ethyl mercury which was used to kill fungi infecting cereal grains; *ethyl mercury* p-*toluene sulfonanilide*.

GSH: abbreviation for *glutathione*.

hallucinations: representations that are marginally coherent, such as a vivid dream, and that are mistaken for actual perceptions.

Heller's syndrome: another name for *dementia infantilis*; also known as *childhood disintegrative disorder*.

helminths: worms that live inside the bodily fluids and tissues of the host, but especially in the intestines.

heme: the iron-containing part of hemoglobin that enables the blood to capture and transport oxygen molecules; also a critical component of *porphyrins*.

hemoglobin: the oxygen-transporting iron containing protein in red blood cells.

hemolyze: to burst open; as applied to red blood cells, to break open as in the release of hemoglobin from red blood cells into the surrounding fluid.

heritability: the tendency or even possibility for traits, including diseases and disorders, to be passed from one generation to the next.

heterolytic reactions: in chemistry, reactions that involve splitting of covalent bonds between different atoms or molecules; in biological ("organic") chemistry, reactions that involve energetic chemical reactions within or between cells, especially ones leading to *apoptosis* caused by inflammation or toxic injury. Heterolytic reactions form the basis for the development of modern theories of *oxidative stress*; Kharasch discovered that in these reactions two electrons from a broken covalent bond are assigned to the same fragmented chemical product, which makes it a *free radical*.

histamine: an organic compound of the amino acid histidine that acts as a neurotransmitter affecting arousal and attention, and as a pro-inflammatory signal involved in allergic reactions or response to tissue damage. Histamine acts as neurotransmitter by increasing the permeability of the capillaries to immune cells so that they can attack, capture, and transport invaders to the lymph nodes.

HIV: abbreviation for *human immunodeficiency virus.*

HIV dementia: any disease or disorder of the brain and central nervous system attributed to the *human immunodeficiency virus*; also known as *HIV encephalopathy.*

HIV encephalopathy: see *HIV dementia.*

HLA: abbreviation for *human leukocyte antigen.*

holophrasis: the use of a phrase, or of a sequence of distinct words or morphemes, to indicate the sort of meaning, reference, or significance that involves the simplest sort of pragmatic mapping relation—the sort of mapping best exemplified by the relationship between an object, person, or event and the name, verb, or signifying term that calls attention to it.

human immune (immunodeficiency) virus (HIV): the elusive and controversial virus that many believe is the main cause of AIDS.

human leukocyte antigen (HLA) system: a long, complex, multidimensional and dynamic specification of the *major histocompatibility complex* (*MHC*) that identifies cells belonging within the body itself to prevent attack by the body's own immune cells on the same body's own tissues; functions as a name or password identifying the cell to the body's defense systems.

humoral immune response: that portion of the bodily defense system that operates in fluids—particularly within the bloodstream and lymph system, and outside the boundaries of individual cells.

hyperactive: overexcited; more active than expected or judged to be normal.

hyperbaric therapy: an intervention using a special chamber where the atmospheric pressure is increased, somewhat as it is when descending under water, but where the person is able to breathe normally. As the atmospheric pressure is increased within the chamber, oxygen transport by the blood is enhanced, thereby supporting better uptake of oxygen by bodily organs including the brain, and especially the liver, kidneys, and transport systems involved in detoxification.

hypoactive: characterized by a state of arousal that is lower than expected, as if the person were drowsy or far less alert and less active than normally expected.

hypomanic: characterized by a persistently irritable mood accompanied by morose thoughts and actions that are consistent with a dangerously depressed state of mind that seems always almost on the verge of an explosive expression.

icons: signs that resemble their objects in some but not all respects; hence, incomplete signs that are analogs of what they represent. Sensory impressions are almost universally of this kind. Icons are distinct from *indexes* and *symbols*.

IgA: the "anti-association immunoglobulin," which tends to prevent invaders from congregating in the mucous linings of the body and in the lymph tissues. IgA is the second most common type of *immunoglobulin* in the human body, accounting for approximately 15% of the body's total supply of antibodies.

IgD: the "deployment and discharge immunoglobulin," which appears to be involved in the activation and authorization of B cells to begin mass production of other B cells like themselves as clones, or to begin mass production of one or another of the isotypes of antibodies. IgD also may be involved in the decommissioning of B cells, or their discharge at the end of the war.

IgE: the "elite immunoglobulin," consisting of a fighting force that can be widely and rapidly deployed throughout the body's systems. IgE normally accounts for less than about two-thousandths of a single percentage point of the body's total immune resources (Jepson & Johnson, 2007, p. 53), but may be overproduced in extreme allergies and anaphylactic shock (Gould et al., 2003; Pier, Lyczak, & Wetzler, 2004; Gould & Sutton, 2008). This type of immunoglobulin appears to be involved in the sorts of epilepti-form seizures commonly seen in autism and autism spectrum disorders.

IgG: the "general immunoglobulin"; the most plentiful of all the body's immunoglobulins and the only one believed to cross the placental barrier. IgG provides the mother's immunity to the developing unborn baby; this immunity is effective until approximately the baby's sixth month after birth.

IgM: the "marshal management and manufacturing immunoglobulin"; the third most plentiful of all immunoglobulins, which seems to be involved in authorizing B cells either to clone themselves or to begin production of a particular type of antibodies.

ileal–lymphoid–nodular hyperplasia: an inflammatory bowel disease characterized by swollen and inflamed lymph glands at the junction between the small intestine and colon—that is, in or around the *ileum*.

ileum: the junction between the small intestine and colon; the segment after the *jejunum* and at the opposite end from the *duodenum*.

immune system(s): the body's built-in defense systems. The plural form should be preferred on account of the fact that there are multiple layers of defenses—that is, systems within systems that communicate with one another in ways that are still being discovered.

immunoglobulin: any antibody, of which there are at least five distinct types, produced by the body's defense systems; a protein structure (better thought of as a dynamic system of moving parts) found in blood or other bodily fluids and deployed there and in bodily tissues to identify unfriendly foreign bacteria, fungi, and viruses.

immunologic glomerular disease: a disease in which the body's defense systems attack the capsules in the kidneys where bundles of tightly packed capillaries pass waste products from the blood into the urine.

indexes: signs that function as such by dynamically connecting one icon with another; to be understood they must always involve actions. Indexes are distinct from *icons* and *symbols*.

innate immune system: the first layer of a deeply layered and interconnected system of bodily defenses. It consists of first-line physical barriers to keep bacteria, fungi, viruses, and toxins from getting inside the body. The next level up provides an immediate police response that attacks and destroys foreign invaders without discrimination; if that layer fails to resolve the problem, the problem is referred to the higher layer known as the *adaptive immune system*.

inorganic mercury: a term loosely applied to *elemental mercury* prior to any uptake by an organism.

intermittent schedule of reinforcement: in *behaviorism* and *applied behavior analysis*, a plan for providing positive consequences for a given behavior on an unpredictable and irregular schedule.

intravenous immunoglobulin (IVIG): a blood product containing antibodies extracted from the plasma of other blood donors that is inserted directly into a person's veins. This therapy is usually applied only in cases of severe immune deficiency where the recipient's body is no longer producing antibodies in an attempt to confer what is misleadingly called "passive" immunity—misleading because immunity is like combat, it is always active and when an attack is under way it is extremely so. Also, foreign antibodies in blood plasma are a little like a foreign police force—not always welcomed by the locals.

iron ion: an atom of iron with a positive or negative charge depending on whether it has gained or lost an electron. Being a metal, iron readily gives up an electron (thus metals are generally good conductors of electricity). The most common form is positively charged because of having given up an electron, leaving it as a *free radical*. The sort of iron ion captured in the *porphyrin heme* is no longer a dangerous free radical because it is part of a stable framework where its missing electrons are supplied by stable covalent bonds with nitrogen atoms; the positively charged iron ion captured in the *heme* of *hemoglobin* is essential for normal respiratory functions of the body.

isocohedral structure: any approximately regular shape of two or three dimensions, the surface of which is covered, as if by tiling, with approximately equal and regularly distributed geometric shapes of the same dimensions and size that completely, or almost completely, cover the surface.

isomorphic: having the same structural or logical configuration; being exactly the same at some level of abstraction.

isotypes: objects of a physical or logical kind; in this book, antibodies that are the same with respect to their shape or structure, making them examples of the same "type" or of a common kind. An analogy would be coins or bank notes of a given denomination, say, quarters or dollar bills, produced by a standardized minting or printing process; each would constitute an exemplar of a given isotype.

jejunum: the middle section of the small intestine, following after the *duodenum* and preceding the *ileum*.

killer T cells: the type of T lymphocytes manufactured in the bone marrow that go on to become the fighting and killing type; also known as "cytologic T cells."

LD$_{50}$: the dose of a toxin that kills 50% of the test species.

leaky gut syndrome: the hypothesized disorder in which the densely packed *M-cells* lining the small intestine become damaged, thereby allowing toxins and disease agents or undigested matter to enter the bloodstream and other body tissues, where they can cause damage and infection.

learning disabled: a term applied to persons with communication disorders that are sufficiently severe so as to impede normal cognitive, emotional, and social growth and development.

legal discovery: the process by which teams of lawyers are permitted to examine the sources of information available to their opponents in a court of law.

logical object: as contrasted with a physical thing, an abstract representation to which reference is made—for instance, the thing, person, event, relation, or whatever that may be referred to by an abstract representation. It may actually be a physical object or event, but need not be real or even possible. For instance, the raft built by Tom Sawyer is strictly a fiction, and a square circle is impossible, yet both can be referred to as logical objects.

low birth weight: born with a subnormal body mass; a defining characteristic of fully developed neonates at risk, or of newborn babies who are born prematurely, who may have been injured or malnourished during development, or who may have undetected genetic problems. Low birth weight is a warning sign of possible risk for later health and development problems.

lupus erythmatosus: a chronic, inflammatory autoimmune disorder affecting connective tissue (bones and joints), kidneys, mucous membranes, and blood vessels.

lymphocytes: white blood cells.

M-cells: microfold cells. These cells are found in the epithelium of the small intestine; they can deliver an antigen from an *antigen-presenting cell* through the wall of the intestine to *lymphocytes* on the opposite side of the intestinal wall where the antigen can be transported to be further examined in the lymph.

macrophages: cells in the *innate immune system* that act like border police, capturing and destroying foreign invaders; they can also initiate a higher immune response from the *adaptive immune system*.

macular degeneration: loss of vision that typically occurs in genetically susceptible individuals with aging. It is characterized and caused by fatty acids and damaged protein deposits in the central area of the retina, the *fovea*.

magnetic resonance imaging (MRI): a radiological technique used to see the inside of the body. It employs a powerful system of magnetic fields in three dimensions to differentially align hydrogen atoms in water in the body, thereby picturing its internal configuration on the basis of distinct densities of atoms within the organs, tissues, and systems.

major histocompatibility complex (MHC): a genomic region in most vertebrates that contains the descriptors that identify the nature of the self in jawed vertebrates. It plays a crucial role in the immune system and avoidance of self-immunity. Proteins encoded by this complex appear on the surface of cells to inform T cells of the cell's identity and to indicate whether it has been infected by a pathogen, and if so, by which kind.

manual babble: the sort of verbal work/play that babies do with the surface forms of linguistic signs before they start producing meaningful applications of them; in this case, the kind of verbal work done by deaf infants.

mass spectroscopy: a labor-intensive means of investigating the composition of a molecule. First, a molecule—say, a piece of DNA—is bombarded with an electron beam to break apart the molecule; then, the fragments are accelerated through a magnetic field and sorted by mass-to-charge ratio; finally, they are reassembled to reconstruct the original molecule.

mast cell: a type of cell that originates in bone marrow and that is involved in immunity and defense systems; also referred to as a *mastocyte*. Mast cells reside in several types of tissues and contain granules loaded with *histamine* and the anticoagulant protein known as heparin. They are known to be involved in allergies and *anaphylaxis*.

mastocyte: see *mast cell*.

membranous cells (M-cells): see *microfold cells*.

memory B cells: after certain B cells are exposed to a given antigen and activated, they multiply and differentiate themselves into (1) antigen-presenting B cells that go out and consume offending foreign agents; (2) B cells that are in the business of manufacturing antibodies; and (3) regular B cells that serve as memory cells—like survivors whose main purpose is to store information about the enemy just in case he comes back again; these memory cells can last years, or even a whole lifetime.

meningococcal meningitis: the type of inflammation caused by *Neisseria meningitidis* (a meningo-coccus); a sometimes fatal infection of the *meninges*—the protective membranes that cover the brain and spinal cord.

merbromin: an organomercuric disodium salt compound; formerly marketed as *Mercurochrome*, *Merbromine*, and under several other names as a topical antiseptic. It is still readily available in many places around the world, but not in the United States because it contains mercury, a neurotoxin.

Mercurochrome: in its dry form, a green crystalline powder that turns a deep orange-red color in water; see *merbromin*.

mesothelioma: a form of cancer associated with exposure to asbestos and now known to involve SV40.

methyl mercury: the compound with the chemical formula CH_3Hg^+ (sometimes written $MeHg^+$); a positively charged ion (*free radical*) that has high affinity for sulfur-containing molecules found in nerve tissues. Methyl mercury migrates easily to other metal-binding sites in proteins; acute methyl mercury poisoning has occurred in the past (as in Minamata disease). This compound is not readily eliminated from organisms, so it is biomagnified. It has a half-life in human blood of approximately 50 days; when ingested, it is readily and completely absorbed by the gastrointestinal tract and is transported throughout the body and across the *blood–brain barrier* and in pregnant mothers to the unborn baby. Because of its strong binding to proteins, methyl mercury is readily eliminated from the body.

methylcobalimin: one of the essential vitamins; a form of vitamin B_{12} that is evidently deficient in persons on the autism spectrum and that is especially important to the health and functioning of the nervous system. Methylcobalimin is known to be depleted in anemias, inflammatory bowel disease, and measles infections.

methylmalonic acid: an indicator both of inflammatory bowel disease and of vitamin B_{12} deficiency.

MHC: abbreviation for *major histocompatibility complex*.

microfold cells (M-cells): the densely packed surface cells on the inside (*lumen*) of the human small intestine; also referred to as *membranous cells*.

microglia: a type of glial cell that serves as the first layer and the primary active defense in the brain, accounting for approximately one-fifth of all glial cells found there.

mitochondria: membrane-enclosed organelles often referred to as "cellular power plants"; they are also critical to communication between cells, tissue differentiation, *apoptosis*, and defense systems. Some cells have only a single mitochondrion, while others may have thousands. These organelles act like cities within a larger city, each with its own independent genome and its own distinct DNA.

monomer: any small molecule that can be bonded to others to form **polymers**, including *dimers* (consisting of two monomers) and *pentamers* (consisting of five monomers), as are found among the *isotypes* of immunoglobulin.

mortality: the inevitable fact that the cumulative errors and damage to the representational systems that maintain any organism ultimately overwhelm their capacity to repair themselves, resulting in aging and ultimately in death.

motherese: the special adjustments in linguistic forms that are common to speech, signs, and linguistic forms addressed to infants and children.

motor aphasia: a loss of speech- or sign-producing capacity that results in halting, dysfluent, or arrhythmic sequences of articulated movements.

multiple sclerosis: also known as *disseminated sclerosis* or *encephalomyelitis disseminata*; a disease in which the immune system attacks the brain and spinal cord, stripping nerve fibers of their myelin sheath. Symptoms include episodic loss of muscular control that waxes and wanes until the disease overwhelms the body with paralysis, ultimately ending in death by asphyxiation.

multivalent vaccine: a vaccine that contains more than one disease agent and/or toxoid derived from one or more disease agents.

mythomania: a delusional disorder also known as "pathological lying," where the person affected by it at the inception of the actual disorder, in theory at least, begins to believe his or her constructed falsehoods.

natural killer cells: cytotoxic *lymphocytes* that act like the police/border guards in the *innate immune system*; they enable destruction of diseased cells and/or of invading intruders. Natural killer cells can generally penetrate the wall of a cell under attack by shooting it with cytoplasmic granules of *perforin* and then presenting *granzymes* to the inside of the cell to induce *apoptosis* (the orderly form of disassembly) or *necrosis* (the disorderly form of disassembly).

necrosis: a less orderly form of destruction that leaves more of a mess behind, somewhat as if the cell had been exploded. It stands in contrast to *apoptosis*, in which the disassembled parts are carried off to be reused on other construction projects or are disposed of in an orderly manner.

negative reinforcement: in *behaviorism* and *applied behavior analysis*, the withholding of *reinforcement* (i.e., a positive or desirable consequence) or the provision of an actual punishment.

nerve growth factor (NGF): a protein that initiates the differentiation of particular nerve cells and enables them to survive.

neuroAIDS: the brain disorders, degenerative neurological conditions, and evidences of nervous system damage attributed to HIV.

neurofibrillary tangle: a confusion of tiny nerve fibrils seen in the autopsied brains of patients with Alzheimer's disease; a type of damage that has been demonstrated to be caused by the introduction of the neurotoxin mercury in the nerves of other organisms built of proteins similar to our own.

neurotoxic: a characteristic of poisons that affect the nerves or the nervous system.

neurotoxic mediators: factors that enhance or diminish the impact of poisons on the nerves or the nervous system.

neutrophil: the most common type of white blood cell in the bodily defense systems of humans. It is normally found in the bloodstream, but can migrate to sites of inflammation and accounts for the yellowish-white coloring of pus.

NGF: abbreviation for *nerve growth factor*.

no-fault: in law, the sort of compensation system in which injuries are treated as if there were no entity responsible for them; the sort of system followed in the Vaccine Injury Court, also known as the U.S. Court of Federal Claims.

nuclear DNA: the kind found in the nucleus of a cell as contrasted with mitochondrial DNA, which is found in organelles outside the nucleus.

obsessive–compulsive disorder (OCD): a disorder generally attributed to psychosis in which persistent impulses seem to force a person to do things in a particular way every time, even though there is no good reason to feel compelled to do so. If the rules are not rigidly followed, the person with this disorder may feel certain that something awful will happen or may be severely depressed and anxious in an extreme way.

occupational therapy: a behavioral intervention that aims to enable the performance of some mundane activity, such as tying a pair of shoelaces or regaining a skill that was lost after a brain injury.

operant: the sort of consequence that follows a given behavior and has the power to gain control over that behavior, according to the theory underlying *behaviorism* and *applied behavior analysis*. For instance, if ringing a bell produces food for a hungry lab rat, the rat is apt to ring the bell again to produce more food; the consequence of obtaining the food becomes an operant controlling the ringing of the bell.

operant conditioning: the process or result of using contingent consequences to shape, establish, or extinguish some behavior or set of behaviors.

orbital: the probability distribution of an electron in an atom or molecule; a somewhat indefinite layer or shell of space around the nucleus of an atom that is occupied, according to quantum theory, approximately 90% of the time by an electron that occupies that orbital. This depiction is an oversimplification because different electrons repel each other (they are all negatively charged).

organic chemistry: the study of chemicals that are used or produced inside living organisms.

oxidative number: the number of electrons that a given molecule or atom can either give up or receive so as to achieve a relatively stable and balanced state. A negative oxidative number is indicative of a capacity to reduce an oxidizer, while a positive number indicates the capacity to oxidize.

oxidative stress: a state of imbalance in the body's capacity to react to its normal reducing environment that is essential to metabolism and detoxification. The result is a build-up of peroxides and *free radicals* that damage the proteins, lipids, and DNA of the body's tissues.

oxidizer: any reactive chemical (but especially a metal) that is (or is susceptible to becoming) a negatively charged ion with one or more unattached electrons; any chemical that is capable of contributing to an increase in oxidation number when it reacts with another atom or molecule.

PANDAS: acronym for *pediatric autoimmune neuropsychiatric disorders associated with* Streptococcus.

paradigm shift: a change in theoretical and empirical approaches to a problematic study in the sciences; a term popularized in the sciences by Thomas Kuhn (1962) in his book about scientific revolutions.

Parkinson's disease: a disease characterized by tremors, muscular rigidity, and jerky movements. It involves, among other things, damage to the *substantia nigra* in the basal ganglia of the brain, evidently leading to or produced by inadequate production of the neurotransmitter *dopamine*. This disease was first described by Dr. James Parkinson in 1817.

pathognomonic: a defining character of a disease or undesirable condition.

PDDs: abbreviation for *pervasive developmental disorders*.

Pediarix: a brand name for a *multivalent vaccine* marketed by GlaxoSmithKline aiming to prevent diphtheria, tetanus, whooping cough, hepatitis B, and polio.

pediatric autoimmune neuropsychiatric disorders associated with *Streptococcus*: a complex of chronic conditions hypothesized to be caused by a latent streptococcal infection, which appears to be associated with, and possibly to cause, tics, *Tourette syndrome*, a violent cyclic subtype of *obsessive–compulsive disorder*, and *ADHD*.

pentamer: a chemical consisting of five simpler components referred to as *monomers*; therefore, a *polymer*.

peroxide: a typically unstable compound containing an oxygen–oxygen single bond. Peroxides tend to form part of highly reactive *free radicals*.

perspective taking: the process or result of seeing things the way someone else does by correctly imagining the other person's position and point of view.

pervasive developmental disorders (PDDs): any combination of a host of persistent undesirable bodily, sensory, sensory–motor, or sensory–motor–linguistic conditions that may begin in genetic damage prior to conception, or that may involve injuries or errors that arise in fetal growth or after birth.

petitioner: the entity, person, or parties bringing a request to a court of law or arbitrator seeking resolution of a problem or dispute; occupies the place of a *plaintiff* in the U.S. Court of Federal Claims.

Peyer's patches: specialized areas of the gut, especially the small intestine, where densely packed *M-cells* are closely associated with lymph glands and are known to be particularly active components of the immune systems that prevent microbial infections beginning in the gut.

phagocytosis: the engulfing of bacteria and solid particles of dead tissue, as well as small mineral particles, by a cell of the body, especially a white blood cell; the engulfed material is enclosed and possibly isolated still further within the walls of the engulfing cell in a special cavity referred to as a vacuole, somewhat as garbage might be encased in a sealable bag for later disposal.

pharmacokinetics: the dynamic tendencies of drugs or medicines to interact chemically.

phenol: a chemical also known as *hydroxybenzene* (partially oxidized *benzene*) and as carbolic acid. It can be distilled as a white crystalline solid and is said to have a kind of "hospital odor."

physical therapy: clinical treatment usually by a licensed practitioner focusing on musculoskeletal movement, range of motion, and ordinary skills such as walking, bending, and so forth.

plaintiff: the party or parties seeking redress in a court of law against a *defendant*.

plaque: an accumulation of protein debris that creates an obstructive covering of a tissue.

plasma B cells: specialized *B cells*, also called *plasmocytes*, that are differentiated into antibody producers.

plateau effect: a tendency in developmental processes to reach a growth level beyond which little or no additional progress is made.

pneumococcal viruses: viruses involved in many types of diseases, including pneumonia, but also commonly found in other disease conditions diagnosed as sinusitis, otitis media, meningitis, and so forth. These viruses are distinguished from bacteria such as *Streptococcus pneumoniae*.

polymer: a chemical consisting of any number of multiple smaller components referred to as *monomers*.

porphyrins: complex cyclic systems of molecules involved in metabolism, energy production, and waste elimination—for example, in the oxygenation of the blood and in the formation of urine. They are typically deeply colored in dark red (as in the porphyrin *heme* in *hemoglobin*) and purple—hence, their name, which comes from the Greek word for "purple."

porphyrinuria: the excretion of a greater quantity of *porphyrins* in the urine than is normally expected to be found there.

positive reinforcement: a consequence that follows a given action and increases the likelihood that that particular action will occur again; in *behaviorism* and *applied behavior analysis*, the process or result of providing a desirable consequence for a behavior whose probability of recurring is thereby increased.

pragmatic mapping: the process or result of associating a referring or signifying term with whatever it refers to or signifies; for example, the process of connecting an entity (or event) that is named with whatever name (or signifier) may be associated with it.

predicate: any abstract sign or symbol that is associated with a given *argument*; a simple example would be the name that is applied to an object.

prevalence: in the theory of diseases and their spread, the number of persons in a whole population who are believed to have the disease, disorder, or condition in question.

Prevnar: the brand name of a vaccine manufactured by Wyeth consisting of a *multivalent conjugate* vaccine with seven serotypes of *Pneumococcus* joined, conjugated, with diphtheria proteins.

pronominal reversal: a misleading designation for the failure of many children with autism, and perhaps the majority of normally developing toddlers, at some point to use "I" to refer to a person spoken to or about, and "you" to refer to self. Actually, there is no "reversal" from the child's perspective, so the term is misleading in this respect.

prophylaxis: the prevention of an infection, or any procedure that is intended to achieve that effect.

proton: a positively charged subatomic particle that makes up the nucleus of a hydrogen atom.

psychosis: theoretically, any abnormal condition of the mind, but generally limited to those conditions that involve what is loosely termed a "loss of contact with reality."

psychotic symptoms: any loss of the capacity to distinguish what is real from what it merely imagined, dreamed, or thought of; examples include hallucinations and delusions.

puerperal (childbirth) fever: any infection associated with the delivery of a baby. Such infections commonly led to death prior to the practices of cleaning hospitals and surgical instruments, scrubbing before surgeries, avoiding contamination of wounds by breathing on them (wearing of masks by doctors and nurses), and using antiseptics.

punishment: the withholding of *reinforcement* or the provision of a consequence to a given action that decreases the likelihood of that particular action's recurrence; in *behaviorism* and *applied behavior analysis*, the process or result of providing an undesirable consequence for a behavior whose probability of recurring is thereby decreased. Punishment is generally regarded as a less satisfactory means of *operant* control than positive reinforcement.

quantum physics: according to a theory first advocated by Max Planck, units of energy and momentum are bundled together in discrete numerical quantities, as if the matter/energy itself can come only in certain relative sizes or quantities, in spite of the fact that each bundle might contain many particles.

rapid eye movements (REM): with the eyes closed while sleeping, movements of the eyes beneath the eyelids as if the sleeper were visually perceiving a changing scene. Such movements are commonly associated with dreaming.

RC: abbreviation for *respiratory chain*.

redox: a shorthand form of *reduction–oxidation*; in these cycles in biochemistry, atoms are affected so that their oxidation number (oxidation state) is changed—usually this involves either the loss of electrons (oxidation) or the gain of electrons (reduction).

reducer: any biochemical protein system contributing to a decrease in oxidation number when it reacts with another atom or molecule.

referent: the *logical object* of a term or expression that refers to that object; for example, the person that is named by a certain name.

regulatory T-helper cells: T cells that are believed to control and especially to shut down an immune response.

reinforcing stimuli: in *behaviorism* and *applied behavior analysis*, any factors to which an organism responds that are judged to increase the rate of a particular response.

reliability: the degree to which a test, assessment, or measure produces similar results on different occasions.

REM: acronym for *rapid eye movement*.

replication: in the sciences, the demonstration of the *reliability* of an experimental procedure and/or result by obtaining it again following the same procedure.

resin composite: in dental restorations, an alternative to the use of the mercury-loaded amalgam.

respiratory chain (RC): the complex sequence of metabolic events by which energy in the body is made accessible through its association with oxygen; a process that critically involves the *mitochondria*.

respondent: the person in a *no-fault* court system who occupies the position of a *defendant* in a court of law.

retroviruses: viruses that have the capacity to reverse the normal flow of information from DNA to RNA, thereby rewriting the sequence in the DNA.

reverse transcriptase (RT): the key ingredient—an enzymatic catalyst—necessary to the process of reversing the normal flow of information from DNA to RNA.

reversion principle: the general rule that regression or descent to a much earlier level of development, or a lower level of representation (abstraction), is generally possible in sign systems, whereas advance to a much higher level than the one already attained at any given point in development requires growth and progress step by step.

rheumatoid arthritis: a debilitating and commonly fatal degenerative form of self-immunity disease in which the body attacks its own joints, producing painful swelling and inflammation, and ultimately ending in the destruction of tissues.

Rho(D)-immune globulin: an injectable plasma containing antibodies to Rhesus factor disease produced by Johnson & Johnson; formerly containing *Thimerosal* as a preservative, and associated with Creutzfeldt-Jakob disease attributable to the mercury in *Thimerosal*.

RotaTeq: the trade name of a rotavirus vaccine manufactured by Merck and developed in part by Dr. Paul Offit. This vaccine is designed to induce production of antibodies to four distinct serotypes of the seven known types of rotavirus, all of which types are associated with gastrointestinal problems characterized by vomiting and diarrhea.

rotation diet: a system of avoiding reactions and/or reducing food allergies by spacing out the periodic intake of foods to which a person may have a mild intolerance, and then cyclically reintroducing them no more frequently than about every four days; a phrase also applied to dieting for weight loss where the person intermittently takes a break from the diet and/or combines dieting with a cyclic exercise regimen.

RT: abbreviation for *reverse transcriptase*.

salicylates: natural hormones in licorice, honey, port wine, tomato sauce, and aspirin; the root is derived from the Latin word referring to the "willow" or "Salix" tree, from the bark of which *salicylic acid* (the key ingredient in aspirin) can be extracted.

salt: a stable inorganic chemical as contrasted with any *alkyl*.

savant traits: characteristics that seem to entail an unusual or extraordinary type or extent of learning or ability; for example, the ability to correctly identify very large prime numbers.

savantism: the result of possessing many *savant traits*.

SCD: abbreviation for *specific carbohydrate diet*.

schedule of reinforcement: in *behaviorism* and *applied behavior analysis*, any systematic plan for providing reinforcing stimuli as consequences to a particular behavior.

schizoid disorder (SD): a psychiatric diagnosis probably confusing Asperger syndrome or high-functioning autism with a *psychosis*. This condition is characterized by disinterest in social relationships, a solitary lifestyle, secretiveness, and emotional coldness.

schizophrenia: a psychiatric diagnosis associated with persistent hallucinations, delusions, or other symptoms of being disconnected from reality.

schizophrenia praecox: the sort of *schizophrenia* supposedly originating in childhood.

scleroses: a diverse class of diseases in which nerve tissues are affected by plaques that interfere with or destroy the myelin sheath.

SD: abbreviation for *schizoid disorder*; also for *standard deviation.*.

second person: the person addressed or spoken to by some other person (the *first person*).

secondary trauma: the sort of injury that follows bruising or bursting of cell walls and that is caused by the release of toxins or disease agents into surrounding tissues.

semiotic systems: the systems involved in representation at any level from genetics to language.

senile dementia: any loss or distortion of mental capacities attributed to aging.

sensorimotor stage: in the psychological theory of growth and development created by Jean Piaget, that phase of development during which the child's representations consist mainly of perceptions and movements.

sensory aphasia: a type of aphasia that hypothetically should involve a loss of speech production or, presumably, manual signing capacity, because of a loss of sensation (we do not think this is a valid conception); in other words this is probably a nonexistent type of aphasia.

sensory integration: the process by which a person learns to associate seeing with hearing, touch with sight, and so on.

serotype: the means by which, in part at least, a tissue identifies itself as belonging to a particular "person" identified as "self" to the immune system, and, in particular, to the white blood cells of the *human leukocyte antigen system*. Each individual can get two different antigen proteins for each genetic locus in the genome, one from each parent. During development, the immune systems note and remember that these proteins belong to the "self"; thus, when they appear on the surface of a cell, it recognizes them and does not attack the cells and tissues bearing that *serotype*.

serum albumin: the most common plasma protein in humans, which is essential for maintaining necessary fluid pressure in the blood and lymph.

Shiga toxin: the potentially deadly poison produced by *E. coli* O157.

SIDS: acronym for *sudden infant death syndrome*.

simian virus 40: the fortieth virus associated with monkeys; also with the manufacture of vaccines, especially, the polio vaccines. Known to be associated with many cancers and AIDS.

smooth pursuit: the tracking of a moving object by coordinated movements of the eyes. This term is also applied to any fixation by which the eyes stay focused on an object irrespective of the movements of the head, trunk, neck, or other movements of the body of the perceiver, almost as if the eyes were anchored to the object outside the body more securely than to the body itself.

spasticity: a continual contraction of a muscle or bundle of muscles, creating rigid tenseness.

Special Master: a lawyer appointed by a judge and authorized to act with final authority in certain matters under the jurisdiction of the court.

specific carbohydrate diet (SCD): a restricted intake of starches and sugars that is discovered by investigation and experimentation and that is tailored, in theory at least, to the needs of the individual undergoing the intervention.

spina bifida: a congenital condition, possibly genetic and/or owed to toxic injuries during fetal development, in which an infant is born with an exposed spinal column.

SSPE: abbreviation for *subacute sclerosing panencephalitis*.

standard deviation (SD): an algebraically standardized measure of variability in a distribution of scores, measures, or ratings that are at least differentiated by order or rank if not by standardized intervals. Technically, the standard deviation is the square root of the sum of deviations from the mean distributed over the number of degrees of freedom (usually the number of cases minus one) of the entire distribution.

standard error of measurement (SEM): an estimate of the variability of a mean, or score, from its true value. It is most commonly calculated algebraically as the *standard deviation* of the distribution of scores (measures or ratings) in question divided by the square root of the number of cases or observations.

***Staphylococcus aureus*:** a spherical bacterium whose name means "golden cluster seed" or "seed gold"; it appears in golden grape-like clusters in infections. This bacterium is found in pimples, impetigo, boils, and abscesses; it may also be found in pneumonia, meningitis, bone infections, and heart disease. *S. aureus* is the most common postsurgical infection.

statute of limitations: a rule restricting the amount of time under which damages or penalties may be sought by a petitioner/plaintiff against a respondent/defendant.

Stevens-Johnson syndrome (SJS): a disorder characterized by a skin rash similar to the sort observed with mercury poisoning and other extreme allergic reactions where the skin sloughs off.

subacute sclerosing panencephalitis (SSPE): a condition whose symptoms include cognitive decline, stereotyped tics sometimes accompanied by seizures, and deterioration of the central nervous system. SSPE is more common in males than females by about a 3-to-1 ratio. It resembles regressive autism initially but is usually fatal and diagnosed only by tissue sampling, usually after death.

sudden infant death syndrome (SIDS): "the sudden death of any infant or young child, which is unexpected by history, and in which a thorough postmortem examination fails to demonstrate an adequate cause of death" (Bergman et al., 1970, p. 18).

surface forms: the manifest forms of language that can be perceived by seeing, hearing, or touching (as in Braille reading and in Deaf-Blind manual signing).

symbols: signs that serve as such by conventional use; contrasted with *icons* and *indexes*.

syntactic arrangement: the differential sequence of two or more signs in a way that affects either their conventional meaning or use.

T cells: the white blood cells also known as *lymphocytes*.

T-helper cell: a type of regulatory cell involved in managing the responses of the immune systems.

T-helper memory cells: cells that persist indefinitely, storing and able to recall the specifics of an antigen long after it has ceased to be a current problem, just in case it comes up again.

teratogens: toxic substances that damage the germ cells sufficiently to cause extreme noticeable effects; these are the "monstrous" toxins causing major deformities.

Th1: type 1 *T-helper cell* believed to regulate the immune response to infections that attack the insides of cells.

Th2: type 2 *T-helper cell* believed to regulate the humoral immune response to infections that attack through the blood, lymph, and bodily tissues outside of individual cells.

theory of abstraction: an explanation of the manner, logical constraints, and relatively rigid sequence in which sign systems must be built during early development, language acquisition, and maturation.

theory of the broadened definition: the idea that the definition of autism has changed in such a way as to account for the growth in the number of cases being diagnosed over the last three decades.

theory of diagnostic substitution: a theory that attempts to account for the upsurge in diagnoses of autism by supposing that persons previously diagnosed as mentally retarded, learning disabled, or in some other category have been recently moved into the classification of autism.

theory of intellectual diversity: the notion that autism is just another mode of being, such as being Caucasian or being Asian; the idea that autism is not a true disorder or disease condition, but rather another way of representing the world and existing within it.

theory of mind: a phrase that has been associated with the notion that autism consists mainly of a loss of ability to take account of perspectives other than one's own; see *perspective taking.*

theory of public awareness: the explanation of the upsurge in the autism diagnoses as a consequence of greater knowledge by doctors, teachers, and especially parents, which, according to proponents of this idea, has led to more cases being noticed and thus diagnosed.

thiosalicylic acid: the non-mercury component in *Thimerosal.*

third person: a person (or the logical/grammatical position occupied by a person) spoken about rather than to; distinct from the speaker (*first person*) and from the listener (*second person*).

thrombocytopenia: an abnormally low platelet count in the blood.

thymus: a glandular organ located just behind the sternum and between the lungs where *T-lymphocyte* maturation occurs; it can be thought of as a training and screening station for immune cells.

tort liability: the kind of legal responsibility that adheres to a person or legal entity as a result of an injury done to someone else or to some other entity.

Tourette syndrome: a disorder usually diagnosed in childhood, which is characterized by symptoms of physical (motor) tics and at least one vocal (phonic) tic. It is named for Gilles de la Tourette [1859–1904], who first described the condition in nine patients.

toxicity: the result of poisoning.

toxicodynamics: see *toxicokinetics.*

toxicokinetics: the study of, or the results of such study of, the dynamic physical and chemical interactions of poisons, especially with biochemicals in a living organism; also known as *toxicodynamics.*

tracheotomy: a surgical procedure in which an incision is made in the throat to permit breathing when the nasal and oral passages are completely blocked.

transcription: the process of representing a sequence of actions, especially an articulate utterance of a sequence of syllables, or possibly a sequence of manual signs or gestures, in a written or printed form.

transitive sentences: sentences in which two or more *arguments* are associated under the scope of a single *predicate* in such a manner that one of the arguments serves the role of an agent that affects another of the arguments, which serves the role of a recipient or patient of the action of that agent. "Sam kissed Susan" is an example of such a sentence.

triage: the procedure of separating surviving injured persons in a mass-casualty incident into groups based on whether they can be saved by treatment.

Tuberculosis bacillus: the germ agent, a bacterium, judged to be the primary causal agent in tuberculosis.

tubulin: the protein critically involved in the formation of the protective sheath that insulates the tiniest nerve fibrils.

type 1 diabetes: an autoimmune disease involving destruction or malfunction of insulin-producing cells in the pancreas.

type 2 diabetes: often referred to as "adult-onset diabetes" and characterized by not requiring shots of insulin to survive; a condition linked to toxins and disease agents known to increase oxidative stress.

ulcerative colitis: an inflammation of the colon leading to the formation of open sores inside the lumen that are visible with an endoscopic procedure.

Vaccine Adverse Events Reporting System (VAERS): one of the systems set up under the scope of the federal Vaccine Injury Act of 1986 that was supposed to help monitor injuries caused to the public by vaccines.

VAERS: acronym for Vaccine Adverse Events Reporting System.

validity: the degree to which a test, assessment, or measurement varies proportionately as the object that it is supposed to test, asses, or measure varies.

variolation: the process leading to smallpox vaccination that involved rubbing the pus of an infected individual in a cut or abrasion deliberately produced in the skin of an uninfected person.

vasoactive mediators: drugs or biochemicals that affect the flexibility—especially the relative constriction or dilation—of the blood vessels.

verbal behavior: any use of language, but commonly restricted in speech-language pathology circles to spoken language; in *behaviorism* and *applied behavior analysis*, generally applied to productive use of language as in speaking or manual signing.

villi: tiny valleys between the hair-like protrusions that vastly increase the surface area of the inner lining of the small intestine.

vitamin A: a vitamin found in healthy retinas and essential in light perception; its deficiency can cause visual loss or blindness.

vitamin C: a well-known antioxidant; its inclusion in the diet prevents scurvy or Rickets disease.

vitamin E: an antioxidant that reduces tissue scarring in certain injuries.

weaponized variants: known disease agents that have been manipulated in a laboratory context so as to manufacture a more lethal or otherwise specially designed type or combination of agents.

well-baby visit: a visit to a physician whose sole purpose is to administer one or more vaccines.

ZDV: abbreviation for *zidovudine*.

zidovudine (ZDV): a reverse transcriptase inhibitor; an antiretroviral drug used in the treatment of AIDS; also known as *azidothymidine (AZT)*.

zone of proximal development (ZPD): on a scale of development, the next step upward that an individual is prepared to take with some assistance.

ZPD: abbreviation for *zone of proximal development*.

References

Abedon, S. T. (1998, March 23). Germ theory of disease. Retrieved June 10, 2009, from http://www.mansfield. ohio-state.edu/~sabedon/biol2007.htm

Adventures in Autism. (n.d.). Julie Gerberding admits on CNN that vaccines can trigger autism. Retrieved June 10, 2009, from http://adventuresinautism.blogspot.com/2008/03/julie-gerberding-admits-on-cnn-that.html

Agency for Toxic Substances and Disease Registry (ATSDR). (1989). *Toxicological profile for mercury*. Atlanta, GA: ATSDR/U.S. Public Health Service.

Akram, M., Naz, F., Malik, A., & Hamid, H. (2008). Clinical profile of subacute sclerosing panencephalitis. *Journal of the College of Physicians and Surgeons Pakistan, 1*(8), 485–488.

Al-Kassab, S., & Saigh, N. (1962). Mercury and calcium excretion in chronic poisoning with organic mercury compounds. *Journal of the Faculty of Medicine Baghdad, 4*, 118–123.

Alarcon, M. (2002). Evidence for a language quantitative trait locus on chromosome 7q in multiplex autism families. *American Journal of Human Genetics, 70*, 60.

Aleka Titzer Reading at Nine Months. (2009). Video demonstration on the *Autism DVD*.

Aleka and Friends Reading. (2009). Video demonstration on the DVD.

Alibek [alias Alibekov], K. (1998, May 20). Terrorist and intelligence operations: Potential impact on the U.S. economy. Retrieved June 10, 2009, from http://www.house.gov/jec/hearings/intell/alibek.htm

Allen, A. (2002, November 10). The not-so-crackpot autism theory. *New York Times Magazine*, retrieved June 10, 2009, from http://www.nytimes.com/2002/11/10/magazine/the-not-so-crackpot-autism-theory.html?sec= &spon=&pagewanted=1

Alzheimer's disease. (2009, February 5). Retrieved June 10, 2009, from http://en.wikipedia.org/wiki/ Alzheimer's_disease

American Academy of Pediatrics. (n.d.). Friends of Children Fund corporate members. Retrieved June 10, 2009, from http://www.aap.org/donate/FCFhonorroll.HTM

American Academy of Pediatrics & Public Health Service. (1999, July 9). Notice to readers: Thimerosal in vaccines: A joint statement of the American Academy of Pediatrics and the Public Health Service. *Morbidity and Mortality Weekly Report, 48*(26), 563–565. Retrieved June 10, 2009, from http://www.cdc.gov/mmwr/ preview/mmwrhtml/mm4826a3.htm

American Academy of Pediatrics & Public Health Service. (2008, March). Facts for parents about vaccine safety from the American Academy of Pediatrics. Retrieved June 10, 2009, from http://www.aap.org/advocacy/ releases/autismparentfacts.htm

American Dental Association (ADA). (1995–2009a). Amalgam. Retrieved June 10, 2009, from http://www. ada.org/prof/resources/topics/amalgam.asp

American Dental Association (ADA). (1995–2009b). Amalgam fillings. Retrieved June 10, 2009, from http:// www.ada.org/public/topics/fillings.asp

American Dental Association (ADA). (1995–2009c). Best management practices for amalgam waste. Retrieved June 10, 2009, from http://www.ada.org/prof/resources/topics/amalgam_bmp.asp

American Dental Association (ADA). (2005). Concise international chemical assessment document 50. Retrieved June 11, 2009, from http://www.ada.org/prof/resources/topics/amalgam.asp

American Health Assistance Foundation. (2000–2008). Plaques and tangles. Retrieved June 10, 2009, from http://www.ahaf.org/alzheimers/about/understanding/plaques-and-tangles.html

American Psychiatric Association (APA). (1952). *Diagnostic and statistical manual of mental disorders (DSM)*. Washington, DC: Author.

American Psychiatric Association (APA). (1968). *Diagnostic and statistical manual of mental disorders* (2nd ed., *DSM-II*). Washington, DC: Author.

American Psychiatric Association (APA). (1980). *Diagnostic and statistical manual of mental disorders* (3rd ed., *DSM-III*). Washington, DC: Author.

American Psychiatric Association (APA). (1987). *Diagnostic and statistical manual of mental disorders*. (3rd ed. rev., *DSM-III-R*). Washington, DC: Author.

American Psychiatric Association (APA). (1994). *Diagnostic and statistical manual of mental disorders* (4th ed., *DSM-IV*). Washington, DC: Author.

American Psychiatric Association (APA). (2000–2008). *Diagnostic and statistical manual of mental disorders* (4th ed. Text Revision, *DSM-IV-TR*). Washington, DC: Author.

Andrews, N., Miller, E., Grant, A., Stowe, J., Osborne, V., & Taylor, B. (2004). Thimerosal exposure in infants and developmental disorders: A retrospective cohort study in the United Kingdom does not support a causal association. *Pediatrics, 1*(3), 584–591.

Anthrax Attacks 2001. (n.d.). Retrieved June 10, 2009, from http://en.wikipedia.org/wiki/2001_anthrax_attacks.

Anundi, I., Hogberg, J., & Stead, A. H. (1979). Glutathione depletion in isolated hepatocytes: Its relation to lipid peroxidation and cellular damage. *Acta Pharmacologica et Toxicologica, 49*, 45–51.

Apoptosis. (2009, February 5). Retrieved June 10, 2009, from http://en.wikipedia.org/wiki/Apoptosis

Aposhian, H. V., Bruce, D. C., Alter, W., Dart, R. C., Hurlbut, K. M., & Aposhian, M. M. (1992). Urinary mercury after administration of 2,3-dimercaptopropane-1-sulfonic acid: Correlation with Dental Amalgam Score. *FASEB Journal, 6*(7), 2472–2476.

Aristotle. (ca. 350 BC). *Nichomachean ethics*. Retrieved June 10, 2009, from http://en.wikipedia.org/wiki/Nicomachean_Ethics

Ashcraft & Gerel, L. L. P. (n.d.). Autism caused by childhood vaccinations containing thimerosal or mercury. Retrieved June 10, 2009, from http://www.ashcraftandgerel.com/thimerosal.html

Asperger, H. (1944). Die "autistischen Psychopathen" im Kindesalter. *Archives für Psychiatrie und Nervenkrakheiten, 117*, 76–136.

Asperger H. (1961). Die psychopathologies des coeliakakranken kindes. *Annales de Pediatrie, 197*, 146–151.

Asperger, H. (1968). Zur Differentialdiagnos des kindlichn Autismus. *Acta Paedopsychiatrica, 35*, 136–145.

Asperger, H. (1979) Problems of infantile autism. *Communication, 13*, 45–52.

Attkisson, S. (2008, July 25). How Independent Are Vaccine Defenders? Sharyl Attkisson investigates vaccine advocates taking funding from the companies whose vaccines they endorse. Retrieved June 10, 2009, from http://www.cbsnews.com/stories/2008/07/25/cbsnews_investigates/main4296175.shtml

Autism Developmental Disabilities Monitoring Network. (2007). *Prevalence of the autism spectrum disorders (ASDs) in multiple areas of the United States, 2000 and 2002*. retrieved June 10, 2009, from http://www.cdc.gov/ncbddd/autism/documents/AutismCommunityReport.pdf

Autism Research Institute (ARI). (2008, February). Parent ratings of behavioral effects of biomedical interventions. Retrieved June 10, 2009, from http://www.autism.com/treatable/form34qr.htm

Autism Research Institute (ARI). (2009). Retrieved June 10, 2009, from http://www.autism.com/

Autism Society of America (ASA). Retrieved June 10, 2009, from http://www.autism-society.org/site/PageServer

Autism Speaks. (n.d.). Where in the U.S. is there an Autism Speaks insurance reform initiative? Retrieved June 10, 2009, from http://www.autismvotes.org/site/c.frKNI3PCImE/b.3909861/k.B9DF/State_Initiatives.htm

Awasthi, A., & Kuchroo, V. K. (2009). T(h)17 cells: from precursors to players in inflammation and infection. *International Immunology, 2*(5), 489–498.

Awasthi, A., Murugaiyan, G., & Kuchroo, V. K. (2008). Interplay between effector Th17 and regulatory T cells. *Journal of Clinical Immunology, 28*(6), 660–670.

Autism spectrum disorders (pervasive developmental disorders). (n.d.). Retrieved June 11, 2009, from http://www.nimh.nih.gov/health/publications/autism/complete-index.shtml

Axton, J. H. M. (1972). Six cases of poisoning after a parenteral organic mercurial compound (Merthiolate). *Postgraduate Medical Journal, 48,* 417–421.

Bacchelli, E., & Maestrini, E. (2006). Autism spectrum disorders: Molecular genetic advances. *American Journal of Medical Genetics Part Seminars in Medical Genetics, 142c*(1), 13–23.

Badon, L. C. (1993). *Comparison of word recognition and story-retelling under the conditions of contextualized versus decontextualized reading events in at-risk poor readers.* Unpublished doctoral dissertation. Louisiana State University, Baton Rouge, LA.

Baird, G., Robinson, R. O., Boyd, S., & Charman, T. (2006). Sleep electroencephalograms in young children with autism with and without regression. *Developmental Medicine and Child Neurology, 48*(7), 604–608.

Baker, J. P. (2008). Mercury, vaccines, and autism: One controversy, three strands. *American Journal of Public Health, 98*(2), 244–253.

Baker, J. P., & Katz, S. L. (2004). Childhood vaccine development: An overview. *Pediatric Research, 55*(2), 347–356.

Baker, S. M. (n.d.). Questionnaire for children with autism and related developmental and/or attention problems. Retrieved June 10, 2009, from http://www.autism.com/families/questionnaire.pdf

Baker, S. M. (2005a). Individuality. In J. Pangborn & S. M. Baker, *Autism: Effective biomedical treatments—Have we done everything we can for this child? Individuality in an epidemic* (pp. 69–148). San Diego, CA: Autism Research Institute.

Baker, S. M. (2005b). Making a plan. In J. Pangborn & S. M. Baker, *Autism: Effective biomedical treatments—Have we done everything we can for this child? Individuality in an epidemic* (pp. 16–68). San Diego, CA: Autism Research Institute.

Baker, S. M. (2007). Autism is an ecological problem and a gastrointestinal disease. In J. Pangborn, & S. M. Baker, *2007 Supplement to the 2005 Edition of Autism: Effective biomedical treatments—Have we done everything we can for this child? Individuality in an epidemic* (pp. 1–33). San Diego, CA: Autism Research Institute.

Bakir, F., Damluji, S. F., Amin-Zaki, L., Murtadha, M., Khalidi, A., Al-Rawi, N. Y. A., et al. (1973, July 20). Methylmercury poisoning in Iraq. *Science, New Series, 181*(4096), 230–241.

Bakulina, A. V. (1968). The effect of subacute Granosan poisoning on the progeny. *Soviet Medicine, 31,* 6063.

Ball, L. K., Ball, R., & Pratt, R. D. (2001). An assessment of thimerosal use in childhood vaccines. *Pediatrics, 107*(5), 1147–1154.

Baltimore, D. (1970). RNA-dependent DNA polymerase in virions of RNA tumour viruses. *Nature, 226,* 1209–1211.

Baltimore, D. (1975). The Nobel Prize in Physiology or Medicine 1975. Retrieved June 10, 2009, from http://nobelprize.org/nobel_prizes/medicine/laureates/1975/baltimore-autobio.html

Balzola, F., Clauser, D., Curri, F., Caldognetto, M., Repici, A., Barletti, C., et al. (2007). Autistic enterocolitis in childhood: The early evidence of the later Crohn's disease in autistic adulthood? *Gastroenterology, 1*(4), A660.

Banthia, J., & Dyson, T. (1999). Smallpox in nineteenth-century India. *Population and Development Review, 25*(4), 649–689.

Barclay, L. (2005). Autism: "Epidemic?" A newsmaker interview with Morton Ann Gernsbacher, PhD, and Craig J. Newschaffer, PhD. Retrieved June 10, 2009, from http://www.medscape.com/viewarticle/508429_print

Barkin, N. (2006, February 9). Autism at the movies again. Retrieved June 10, 2009, from http://autismdiva.blogspot.com/2006/02/autism-at-movies-again.html

Baron-Cohen, S. (1991). Do people with autism understand what causes emotion? *Child Development, 62,* 385–395.

Baron-Cohen, S., Leslie, A. M., & Frith, U. (1986). Mechanical, behavioural and intentional understanding of picture stories in autistic children. *British Journal of Developmental Psychology, 4,* 113–125.

Barr, L. (2004). EPA's draft use reduction program. Retrieved June 10, 2009, from http://www.epa.gov/region5/air/mercury/meetings/Nov04/barr.pdf

Bartleby.com. (2008, November 27). Figure 1062. An intestinal gland from the human intestine. Retrieved June 10, 2009, from http://www.bartleby.com/107/illus1062.html

Basel Action Network. (2004, March 17, 2004). Green groups call on European Commission to "Stop toxic trade in mercury." Retrieved June 10, 2009, from http://www.ban.org/ban_news/2004/040329_green_groups.html

Bauer, A. (2005). *A wild ride up the cupboards*. New York: Scribner.

Bazin, H. (2000). *The eradication of smallpox: Edward Jenner and the first and only eradication of a human infectious disease*. New York: Academic Press.

BBC News Channel. (n.d.). In pictures: Chad refugee camp. Retrieved June 10, 2009, from http://news.bbc.co.uk/1/shared/spl/hi/picture_gallery/04/africa_chad_refugee_camp/html/1.stm

BBC News Channel. (2006, February 9). Snow Cake opens Berlin festival. Retrieved June 10, 2009, from http://news.bbc.co.uk/1/hi/entertainment/4696262.stm

Becker, H. (Director), Pearson, R. D. (Novel), & Konner, L. (Screenplay). (1998). *Mercury Rising* [Motion picture]. United States: Imagine Entertainment.

Behnsen, J., Narang, P., Hasenberg, M., Gunzer, F., Bilitewski, U., et al. (2007). Environmental dimensionality controls the interaction of phagocytes with the pathogenic fungi *Aspergillus fumigatus* and *Candida albicans*. *PLoS Pathogens*, 3(2), e13 [doi:10.1371/journal.ppat.0030013].

Bellinger, D. C., Trachtenberg, F., Barregard, L., Tavares, M., Cernichiari, E., Daniel, D., & McKinlay, S. (2006). Neuropsychological and renal effects of dental amalgam in children: A randomized clinical trial. *Journal of the American Medical Association*, 295(15), 1775–1783.

Bénit, L., Dessen, P., & Heidmann, T. (2001). Identification, phylogeny, and evolution of retroviral elements based on their envelope genes. *Journal of Virology*, 75(23), 11709–11719.

Bergman, A. B., Beckwith, J. B., & Ray, C. G. (Eds.). (1970). *Sudden infant death syndrome Proceedings of the Second International Conference on Causes of Sudden Death in Infants*. Seattle: University of Washington Press.

Bernard, S. (2004). Association between thimerosal-containing vaccine and autism. *Journal of the American Medical Association, 291*, 180.

Bernard, S., Enayati, A., Redwood, L., Roger, H., & Binstock, T. (2001). Autism: A novel form of mercury poisoning. *Medical Hypotheses, 56*, 462–471.

Bernard, S., Enayati, A., Roger, H., Binstock, T., & Redwood, L. (2002). The role of mercury in the pathogenesis of autism. *Molecular Psychiatry*, 7(suppl 2), S42–S43.

Bernard, S., Redwood, L., & Blaxill, M. (2004). Thimerosal, mercury, and autism: Case study in the failure of the risk assessment paradigm. *Neurotoxicology, 2*(4), 710.

Bettelheim, B. (1950). *Love is not enough; the treatment of emotionally disturbed children*. Glencoe, IL: Free Press.

Bettelheim, B. (1967). *The empty fortress: Infantile autism and the birth of the self*. New York: Free Press.

Biggs, J. T. (1910). Diagram G. Illustrating smallpox in the first column of Table 42. Smallpox Leicester 1838–1910. Retrieved June 10, 2009, from http://www.whale.to/a/table_42.html

Biggs, J. T. (1912). The Leicester method. Retrieved June 10, 2009, from http://www.whale.to/a/biggsext.html

Bishop, D. V. M., Whitehouse, A. J. O., Watt, H. J., & Line, E. A. (2008). Autism and diagnostic substitution: Evidence from a study of adults with a history of developmental language disorder. *Developmental Medicine and Child Neurology*, 5(5), 341–345.

Biskind, M. S. (1949a). DDT poisoning and elusive virus X: A new cause for gastro-enteritis. *American Journal of Digestive Diseases*, 16(3), 79–84.

Biskind, M. S. (1949b, January). DDT poisoning and X disease in cattle. *Journal of the American Veterinary Medical Association, 114*, 20.

Biskind, M. S. (1949c, February). DDT Poisoning a serious public health hazard. *American Journal of Digestive Diseases, 16*, 73.

Biskind, M. S. (1949d). Endocrine disturbances in gastrointestinal conditions. *Review of Gastroenterology*, 16(3), 220–225.

Biskind, M. S. (1953). Public health aspects of the new insecticides. *American Journal of Digestive Diseases, 20*, 331–341.

Biskind, M. S., & Bieber, I. (1949, April). DDT poisoning: A new syndrome with neuropsychiatric manifestations. *American Journal of Psychotherapy*, 3(2), 261–270. Retrieved June 10, 2009, from http://www.whale.to/a/biskind11.html

Blair, A. M. J. N., Clark, B., Clarke, A. J., & Wood, P. (1975). Tissue concentrations of mercury after chronic dosing of squirrel-monkeys with thiomersal. *Toxicology, 3*(2), 171–176.

Blaylock, R. (2008–2009). Do vaccines work? Retrieved June 10, 2009, from http://poisonevercure.150m.com/vaccines2.htm

Bleuler, E. (1908). Schizoid disorder. In Details recorded by Salman Akhtar in Schizoid Personality Disorder: A Synthesis of Developmental, Dynamic, and Descriptive Features. *American Journal of Psychotherapy, 41,* 499–518.

Block, S. L., Vesikari, T., Goveia, M. G., Rivers, S. B., Adeyi, B. A., Dallas, M. J., Bauder, J., Boslego, J. W., & Heaton, P. M. (2007). Efficacy, immunogenicity, and safety of a pentavalent human-bovine (WC3) reassortant rotavirus vaccine at the end of shelf life. *Pediatrics, 119*(1), 11–18.

Bock, K., & Stauth, C. (2007). *Healing the new childhood epidemics: Autism, ADHD, asthma, and allergies.* New York: Ballantine.

Bodaghi, B., Weber, M. E., Arnoux, Y. V., Jaulerry, S. D., Le Hoang, P., & Colin, J. (2005). Comparison of the efficacy and safety of two formulations of diclofenac sodium 0.1% eyedrops in controlling postoperative inflammation after cataract surgery. *European Journal of Ophthalmology, 15*(6), 702–711.

Boedeker, E. C., & Serna, A. (2008). Pathogenesis and treatment of Shiga toxin-producing *Escherichia coli* infections. *Current Opinion in Gastroenterology, 24*(1), 38–47.

Boisse, L., Gill, M. J., & Power, C. (2008). HIV infection of the central nervous system: Clinical features and neuropathogenesis. *Neurologic Clinics, 2*(3), 799–819.

Borghesi, L., & Milcarek, C. (2006). From B cell to plasma cell: Regulation of V(D)J recombination and antibody secretion. *Immunological Research, 36*(1–3), 27–32.

Bornman, M., Pretorius, E., Marx, J., Smit, E., & van der Merwe, C. (2008). Ultrastructural effects of DDT, DDD, and DDE on neural cells of the chicken embryo model. *Environmental Toxicology, 2*(3), 328–336.

Borsboom, D., Mellenbergh, G. J., & van Heerden, J. (2004). The concept of validity. *Psychological Review, 111,* 1061–1071.

Bothwell, C. M. (2002a, March 17). Docs show Eli Lilly knew mercury in vaccines was known dangerous in 30s. Retrieved June 10, 2009, from http://www.rense.com/general21/vacc.htm

Bothwell, C. M. (2002b, March 17). Press release: Eli Lilly documents reveal dangers of thimerosal. Retrieved June 10, 2009, from http://poisonevercure.150m.com/vaccines/eli_lilly_documents_reveal_dange.htm

Bourke, A., & Rendall, J. (1971, 2009). *A lion called Christian: The true story of the remarkable bond between two friends and a lion.* New York: Broadway Books.

Bourlioux, P., Koletzko, B., Guarner, F., & Braesco, V. (2003, October). The intestine and its microflora are partners for the protection of the host: Report on the Danone Symposium "The Intelligent Intestine," held in Paris, June 14, 2002. *American Journal of Clinical Nutrition, 78*(4), 675–683.

Bower, T. G. R. (1971). The object in the world of the infant. *Scientific American, 225*(4), 30–38.

Bower, T. G. R. (1974). Development of infant behavior. *British Medical Bulletin, 30*(2), 175–178.

Bower, T. G. R. (1982). *Development in infancy.* San Francisco: W. H. Freeman.

Braun, M. M., & Ellenberg, S. S. (1997). Descriptive epidemiology of adverse events after immunization: Reports to the Vaccine Adverse Event Reporting System (VAERS), 1991–1994. *Journal of Pediatrics, 131*(4), 529–535.

Breggin, P. R. (1991). *Toxic psychiatry: Why therapy, empathy and love must replace the drugs, electroshock, and biochemical theories of the "new psychiatry."* New York: St. Martin's Press.

Breggin, P. R. (1998). *Talking back to Ritalin: What doctors aren't telling you about stimulants for children.* Monroe, ME: Common Courage Press.

Brouns, R., Verlinde, P., Lagae, L., De Koster, T., Lemmens, F., & Van de Casseye, W. (2001). Subacute sclerosing panencephalitis in a vaccinated, internationally adopted child. *Acta Neurologica Belgica, 1*(2), 128–130.

Brown, J. (n.d.). Horse therapy—Changing lives: A special report as published in *Your Horse Magazine.* Retrieved June 10, 2009, from http://www.wayofthehorse.org/Articles/horse-therapy.html

Burbacher, T. M., Shen, D. D., Liberato, N., Grant, K. S., Cernichiari, E., & Clarkson, T. W. (2005). Comparison of blood and brain mercury levels in infant monkeys exposed to methylmercury or vaccines containing thimerosal. *Environmental Health Perspectives 113*(8), 1015–1021.

Burton, D. (2002, November 18). Facts and fiction about thimerosal in vaccines. Retrieved June 10, 2009, from http://www.chiropractic.org/index.php?p=news/burton

Bush, G. W. (2002, November 25). Signing of the Homeland Security Act, H. R. 5005. Retrieved July 8, 2008, from http://www.whitehouse.gov/news/releases/2002/11/20021125-6.html

Cabanlit, M., Wills, S., Goines, P., Ashwood, P., & Van de Water, J. V. (2007). Brain-specific in the plasma autoantibodies of subjects with autistic spectrum disorder. In Y. Shoenfeld & M. E. Gershwin (Eds.), *Autoimmunity, Part C—the Mosaic of Autoimmunity*. (Annals of the New York Academy of Sciences, *1107*, 92–103). New York: Wiley-Blackwell.

Cabrera, S., Barden, D., Wolf, M., & Lobner, D. (2007). Effects of growth factors on dental pulp cell sensitivity to amalgam toxicity. *Dental Materials, 23*(10), 1205–1210.

Caby, F., & Katlama, C. (2008). New-generation NNRTIs: Update of clinical trials. *Virologie, 12*, S45–S52.

Campbell, D. B., Sutcliffe, J. S., Ebert, P. J., Militerni, R., Bravaccio, C., Trillo, S. P., et al. (2006). A genetic variant that disrupts MET transcription is associated with autism. *Proceedings of the National Academy of Sciences of the United States of America, 103*(45), 16834–16839.

Campbell, H., Andrews, N., Brown, K. E., & Miller, E. (2007). Review of the effect of measles vaccination on the epidemiology of SSPE. *International Journal of Epidemiology, 3*(6), 1334–1348.

Campbell, S. (2004). Scans uncover secrets of the womb. Video and Audio News (Interview) with the BBC's Vicki Young. Retrieved June 10, 2009, from http://news.bbc.co.uk/2/hi/health/3846525.stm

Cannell, J. J. (2008). Autism and vitamin D. *Medical Hypotheses, 70*(4), 750–759.

Cannino, G., Di Liegro, C. M., & Rinaldi, A. M. (2007). Nuclear-mitochondrial interaction. *Mitochondrion, 7*(6), 359–366.

Carbone, M., & Bedrossian, C. W. M. (2006). The pathogenesis of mesothelioma. *Seminars in Diagnostic Pathology, 23*(1), 56–60.

Carbone, V. (2007). Teaching communication skills to children with autism and other developmental disabilities. Retrieved June 10, 2009, from http://www.autism07.com/index.html

Cardona, F., Ventriglia, F., Cipolla, O., Romano, A., Creti, R., & Orefici, G. (2008). A post-streptococcal pathogenesis in children with tic disorders is suggested by a color Doppler echocardiographic study. *European Journal of Paediatric Neurology, 1*(5), 270–276.

Carlsen, W. (2001). New documents show the monkey virus is present in more recent polio vaccine. *San Francisco Chronicle,* Sunday, July 22, 2001, p. A–6.

Carpi, A. (1999). Atomic structure. Retrieved June 10, 2009, from http://web.jjay.cuny.edu/~acarpi/NSC/3-atoms.htm

Carrico, A., Johnson, M., Moskowitz, J., Neilands, T., Morin, S., Charlebois, E. M., et al. (2008). Affect regulation, stimulant use, and viral load among HIV-positive persons on anti-retroviral therapy. *Psychosomatic Medicine, 6*(8), 785–792.

Carroll, L. (1871). *Through the looking-glass, and what Alice found there*. London: Macmillan.

Carson, M. J. (2002). Microglia as liaisons between the immune and central nervous systems: Functional implications for multiple sclerosis. *Glia, 4*(2), 218–231.

Carson, R. (1962). *Silent spring*. New York: Houghton Mifflin.

Cassel, I. (2008, February). Cluster of "SIDS" deaths in north Idaho prompt parents to blame vaccines; doctors, government deny vaccine link. *Idaho Observer*. Retrieved June 10, 2009, from http://www.proliberty.com/observer/20080214.htm

Cave, S. (2001). *What your doctor may not tell you about children's vaccinations*. New York: Time Warner Books.

CBS News. (2002, December 12). The man behind the vaccine mystery: Dick Armey says he put drug company protection into Homeland Bill. Retrieved June 10, 2009, from http://www.cbsnews.com/stories/2002/12/12/eveningnews/main532886.shtml

Cedrola, S., Guzzi, G., Ferrari, D., Gritti, A., Vescovi, A. L., Pendergrass, J. C., & La Porta, C. A. M. (2003). Inorganic mercury changes the fate of murine CNS stem cells. *FASEB Journal, 17*(3), 869–871.

Celizic, M. (2009, March 18). Christian the lion's owners recall final farewell: Anthony Bourke and John Rendall look back at last goodbye to famous lion. Retrieved June 10, 2009, from http://www.msnbc.msn.com/id/29751849/

Centers for Disease Control and Prevention (CDC). (n.d.). Autism: Learn the signs, act early. Retrieved June 10, 2009, from http://www.cdcfoundation.org/healththreats/autism.aspx

Centers for Disease Control and Prevention (CDC). (1994, February 18). Receipt of well-baby care—Maine, 1988–1992. *Morbidity and Mortality Weekly Report, 43*(6), 105–110. Retrieved June 10, 2009, from http://www.cdc.gov/mmwr/preview/mmwrhtml/00024899.htm

Centers for Disease Control and Prevention (CDC). (1998, November 20). Paralytic poliomyelitis—United States, 1980–1994. *Morbidity and Mortality Weekly Report, 46*(54), 85. Retrieved June 10, 2009, from http://www.cdc.gov/mmwr/preview/mmwrhtml/00045949.htm

Centers for Disease Control and Prevention (CDC). (1999a, April 2). Achievements in public health, 1900–1999: Impact of vaccines universally recommended for children—United States, 1990–1998. *Morbidity and Mortality Weekly Report, 48*(12), 243–248. Retrieved June 10, 2009, from http://www.cdc.gov/mmwr/preview/mmwrhtml/00056803.htm

Centers for Disease Control and Prevention (CDC). (1999b, July 30). Achievements in public health, 1900–1999: Control of infectious diseases. *MMWR, 48*(29), 621–629. Retrieved June 10, 2009, from http://www.cdc.gov/mmwr/preview/mmwrhtml/mm4829a1.htm

Centers for Disease Control and Prevention (CDC). (2000, September). Inter/Intra-Agency Agreement (IAA), Project Title: Vaccine Safety Review Panel, IIA#: 00FED17358.

Centers for Disease Control and Prevention (CDC). (2006, October 23). 50th Anniversary of the Polio Vaccine. Retrieved June 10, 2009, from http://www.cdc.gov/vaccines/events/polio-vacc-50th/default.htm

Centers for Disease Control and Prevention (CDC). (2007a, May 18). Household transmission of vaccinia virus from contact with a military smallpox vaccine—Illinois and Indiana, 2007. *Morbidity and Mortality Weekly Report, 56*(19), 478–481. Retrieved June 10, 2009, from http://www.cdc.gov/mmwr/preview/mmwrhtml/mm5619a4.htm

Centers for Disease Control and Prevention (CDC). (2007b, September 26). Pediarix vaccine: Questions and answers. Retrieved June 10, 2009, from http://www.cdc.gov/vaccines/vpd-vac/combo-vaccines/pediarix/faqs-hcp-pediarix.htm

Centers for Disease Control and Prevention (CDC). (2007c, October 22). Frequently asked questions about cancer, simian virus 40 (SV40), and polio vaccine. Retrieved June 10, 2009, from http://www.cdc.gov/vaccinesafety/concerns/archive/polio_and_cancer.htm

Centers for Disease Control and Prevention (CDC). (2008a). Catch-up immunization schedule: For persons aged 4 months–18 years who start late or who are more than 1 month behind. Retrieved June 10, 2009, from http://www.cdc.gov/vaccines/recs/schedules/downloads/child/2008/08_catch-up_schedule_pr.pdf

Centers for Disease Control and Prevention (CDC). (2008b). Recommended immunization schedule for persons aged 0–6 years. Retrieved June 10, 2009, from http://www.cdc.gov/vaccines/recs/schedules/downloads/child/2008/08_0-6yrs_schedule_pr.pdf (also see the homepage for all the schedules at http://www.cdc.gov/vaccines/recs/schedules/)

Centers for Disease Control and Prevention (CDC). (2008c).Timeline: Thimerosal in vaccines (1999–2008). Retrieved June 10, 2009, from http://www.cdc.gov/vaccinesafety/concerns/thimerosal_timeline.htm

Centers for Disease Control and Prevention (CDC). (2008d, January 30). Prevalence of ASDs. Retrieved June 10, 2009, from http://www.cdc.gov/ncbddd/autism/faq_prevalence.htm

Centers for Disease Control and Prevention (CDC). (2008e, March 27). *Escherichia coli*. Retrieved June 10, 2009, from http://www.cdc.gov/nczved/dfbmd/disease_listing/stec_gi.html#3

Centers for Disease Control and Prevention (CDC). (2008f, October 24). Sudden Infant Death Syndrome (SIDS) and Sudden Unexpected Infant Death (SUID): Home. Retrieved June 10, 2009, from http://www.cdc.gov/sids/

Centers for Disease Control and Prevention (CDC). (2008g, December 23). Measles, Mumps, and Rubella (MMR) vaccine. Retrieved June 10, 2009, from http://www.cdc.gov/vaccinesafety/concerns/mmr_vaccine.htm

Centers for Disease Control and Prevention (CDC). (2009, January 14). Thimerosal in vaccines. Retrieved June 10, 2009, from http://www.fda.gov/cber/vaccine/thimerosal.htm

Centers for Disease Control and Prevention (CDC) Advisory Committee on Immunization Practices. (2006). Thimerosal in vaccines. Retrieved June 10, 2009, from http://www.fda.gov/cber/vaccine/thimerosal.htm#pres

Centers for Disease Control and Prevention (CDC) & Procurements and Grants Office. (2002, September 20). Public Notification of Award of Contract 200-2002-00732, American Association of Health Plans.

Cesaroni, L., & Garber, M. (1991). Exploring the experience of autism through firsthand accounts. *Journal of Autism and Developmental Disorders, 21*(3), 303–313.

Chabon, S. S., Hale, S. T., & Wark, D. J. (2008, February 12). Triangulated ethics: The patient-student-supervisor relationship. *ASHA Leader, 13*(2), 26–27.

Chamberlain, D. (2007). Life before birth. Retrieved June 10, 2009, from http://www.birthpsychology.com/lifebefore/

Chapin, C. V. (1913). Variation in type of infectious disease as shown by the history of smallpox in the United States 1895–1912. *Infectious Disease, 13*, 171–196.

Charman, T., Baron-Cohen, S., Swettenham, J., Baird, G., Cox, A., & Drew, A. (2008). Testing joint attention, imitation, and play as infancy precursors to language and theory of mind. *Cognitive Development, 1*(4), 481–498.

Chen, R. T., Glasser, J. W., Rhodes, P. H., Davis, R. L., Barlow, W. E., Thompson, R. S. C., et al. (1997). Vaccine Safety Datalink project: A new tool for improving vaccine safety monitoring in the United States. *Pediatrics, 99*(6), 765–773.

Chiang, H–M., & Lin, Y–H. (2007). Mathematical ability of students with Asperger syndrome and high-functioning autism—A review of literature. *Autism, 11*(6), 547–556.

Child Health Safety. (2009, February 6). Dr. Andrew Wakefield demolishes ignorant U.S. vaccine lobby. Retrieved June 10, 2009, from http://childhealthsafety.wordpress.com/2009/02/06/andrew-wakefield-demolishes-ignorant-us-vaccine-lobby/

Cho, K., Lee, Y. K., & Greenhalgh, D. G. (2008). Endogenous retroviruses in systemic response to stress signals. *Shock, 3*(2), 105–116.

Chock, K. (2008, February 12). Are vaccines to blame for infant deaths? Retrieved June 10, 2009, from http://www.kxly.com/Global/story.asp?S=7862995

Chomsky, N. A. (1959). A review of B. F. Skinner's *Verbal Behavior. Language, 35*(1), 26–58.

Christian the Lion. (2009, March 18). Final farewell—last journey to Africa. Retrieved June 10, 2009, from http://www.youtube.com/watch?v=zVNTdWbVBgchttp://www.youtube.com/watch?v=qvNlwpK5i44

Churchill, D. W. (1978). Language: The problem beyond conditioning. In M. Rutter & E. Schopler (Eds.), *Autism: A reappraisal of concepts and treatment* (pp. 73–84). New York: Plenum.

Clark, J. F. (2002). *The African stakes in the Congo War.* New York: Palgrave McMillan.

Clarkson, T. W. (2002). The three faces of modern mercury. *Environmental Health Perspectives, 110*(suppls), 11–23.

Clarkson, T. W., & Magos, L. (2006). The toxicology of mercury and its chemical compounds. *Critical Reviews in Toxicology, 36*, 609–662.

Clarkson, T. W., Smith, J. C., & Doherty, R. A. (1973). Methylmercury poisoning in Iraq. *Science, 181*, 230–241.

Clarkson, T. W., & Strain, J. J. (2003, May). Nutritional factors may modify the toxic action of methyl mercury in fish-eating populations. *American Society for Nutritional Sciences Journal of Nutrition, 133*, 1539S–1543S.

Clarkson, T. W., Vyas, J. B., & Ballatorl, N. (2007). Mechanisms of mercury disposition in the body. *American Journal of Industrial Medicine, 50*(10), 757–764.

Clark-Taylor, T., & Clark-Taylor, B. E. (2004). Is autism a disorder of fatty acid metabolism? Possible dysfunction of mitochondrial beta-oxidation by long chain acyl-CoA dehydrogenase. *Medical Hypotheses, 6*(6), 970–975.

Clements, C. J., & McIntyre, P. B. (2006). When science is not enough: A risk/benefit profile of thiomersal-containing vaccines. *Expert Opinion on Drug Safety, 5*(1), 17–29.

CNN. (2008, March 7). Sanjay Gupta interviews Julie Gerberding re Hannah Poling. *House Call with Dr. Sanjay Gupta.* Retrieved September 7, 2008, from http://www.cnn.com/2008/HEALTH/conditions/03/07/autism.vaccines.analysis.ap/#cnnSTCVideo [As of January 31, 2009, the video record of this conversation was no longer available.]

Cogswell, H. D., & Shown, A. (1948). Reaction following the use of tincture of Merthiolate. *Arizona Medicine, 5,* 42–43.

Cohen, J. (1993). HHS: Gallo guilty of misconduct. *Science, 259,* 168–170.

Cohen, S., & Burns, R. C. (2002). *Pathways of the pulp.* 8th ed. St. Louis: Mosby, Inc.

Columbia University Mailman School of Public Health. (2008, September 4). Study shows no connection between MMR vaccine and autism, GI disturbances. Retrieved June 10, 2009, from http://www.pslgroup.com/dg/22ACA6.htm

Comar, M., D'Agaro, P., Luzzati, R., Martini, F., Tognon, M., & Campello, C. (2007). SV40 and HIV sequences in the cerebrospinal fluid of a patient with AIDS dementia complex. *Current HIV Research, 5*(3), 345–347.

Comi, A. M., Zimmerman, A. W., Frye, V. H., Law, P. A., & Peeden, J. N. (1999). Familial clustering of autoimmune disorders and evaluation of medical risk factors in autism. *Journal of Child Neurology, 14,* 388–394.

Congressional Research Service (CRS). (2005, September 23). Homeland Security Act of 2002: Tort liability provisions. Retrieved February 5, 2009, from http://assets.opencrs.com/rpts/RL31649_20050923.pdf

Connor, S. (1993). Gallo guilty of AIDS misconduct. *British Medical Journal, 3*(6871), 161–162.

Cool, H., Ouellette-Kuntz, H., Lloyd, J. E. V., Kasmara, L., Holden, J. J. A., & Lewis, M. E. S. (2007). Trends in autism prevalence: Diagnostic substitution revisited. *Journal of Autism and Developmental Disorders, 38*(6), 1573–3432.

Cooper, L. Z., Larson, H., & Katz, S. L. (2009, February 23). The confidence gap. Retrieved June 10, 2009, from http://www.newsweek.com/id/185986

Cooper, R. P., Abraham, J., Berman, S., & Staska, M. (1997). The development of infants' preference for motherese. *Infant Behavior & Development, 2*(4), 477–488.

Correia, C., Coutinho, A. M., Diogo, L., Grazina, M., Marques, C., Miguel, T. M., et al. (2006). Brief report: High frequency of biochemical markers for mitochondrial dysfunction in autism: No association with the mitochondrial aspartate/glutamate carrier SLC25A12 gene. *Journal of Autism and Developmental Disorders, 36*(8), 1137–1140.

Cosford, R. (2008, October 27). Occult infections, *Streptococcus,* biofilms, PANDAS, MINDDD in autism. Presentation at the Defeat Autism Now! (DAN!) Conference in San Diego, CA.

Costa, A., Branca, V., Pigatto, P. D., & Guzzi, G. (2008). ALS, mercury exposure, and chelation therapy. *Clinical Neurology and Neurosurgery, 1*(3), 319–320.

Cote, P., Baril, J. G., Hebert, M., Klein, M., Lalonde, R., Poliquin, M., et al. (2007). Management and treatment of hepatitis C virus in patients with HIV and hepatitis C virus co infection: A practical guide for health care professionals. *Canadian Journal of Infectious Diseases & Medical Microbiology, 18*(5), 293–303.

Counter v. Lilly. (2002). Legal matters: Eli Lilly and Thimerosal, Case No. 15285. Retrieved January 26, 2009, from http://www.whale.to/v/elililly.html

Counter, S. A., & Buchanan, L. H. (2004). Mercury exposure in children: A review. *Toxicology and Applied Pharmacology, 198*(2), 209–230.

Counter, S. A., Buchanan, L. H., Ortega, F., & Laurell, G. (2002). Elevated blood mercury and neuro-otological observations in children of the Ecuadorian gold mines. *Journal of Toxicology and Environmental Health A, 65,*149–163.

Cox, C., Marsh, D., Myers, G., & Clarkson, T. W. (1995). Analysis of data on delayed development from the 1971–1972 outbreak of methylmercury poisoning in Iraq: Assessment of influential points. *NeuroToxicology, 16*(4), 727–730.

Crespo-Lopez, M. E., de Sa, A. L., Herculano A. M., Burbano, R. R., & do Nascimento, J. L. M. (2007). Methylmercury genotoxicity: A novel effect in human cell lines of the central nervous system. *Environment International, 33*(2), 141–146.

Cutting Edge Information. (n.d.). Retrieved June 10, 2009, from http://www.cuttingedgeinfo.com/

Da Costa, S. L., Malm, O., & Dorea, J. G. (2005). Breast-milk mercury concentrations and amalgam surface in mothers from Brasilia, Brazil. *Biological Trace Element Research, 106*(2), 145–151.

Dahhan, S. S., & Orfaly, H. (1962). Mercury poisoning and electorcardiographic changes. *Journal of the Faculty of Medicine Baghdad, 4*, 104–111.

Dales, L. (2001). [memo]. Retrieved July 1, 2008, from http://www.putchildrenfirst.org/intro.html

Dales, L., Hammer, S. J., & Smith, N. J. (2001). Time trends in autism and in MMR immunization coverage in California. *Journal of the American Medical Association, 285*(9), 1183–1185.

Dally, A. (1997). The rise and fall of pink disease. *Social History of Medicine, 10*(2), 291–304.

Damlugi, S. (1962). Mercurial poisoning with fungicide Granosan M. *Journal of the Faculty of Medicine Baghdad, 4*, 83–103.

Daubert v. Merrell Dow Pharmaceuticals, (92–102), 509 U.S. 579 (1993). Retrieved June 10, 2009, from http://en.wikipedia.org/wiki/Daubert_Standard; also from http://straylight.law.cornell.edu/supct/html/92-102.ZS.html

Davis, T. C., Fredrickson, D. D., Kennen, E. M., Arnold, C., Shoup, E., Sugar, M. A., et al. (2004). Childhood vaccine risk/benefit communication among public health clinics: A time-motion study. *Public Health Nursing, 21*(3), 228–236.

de Cock, K. M. (2001). Book reviews: *The eradication of smallpox: Edward Jenner and the first and only eradication of a human infectious disease. Nature Medicine, 7*, 15–16. Retrieved June 10, 2009, from http://www.nature.com/nm/journal/v7/n1/full/nm0101_15b.html

Deer, B. (n.d.). The MMR–autism crisis: Our story so far. An investigation by Brian Deer. Retrieved June 10, 2009, from http://briandeer.com/mmr/lancet-summary.htm

Defeat Autism Now! (DAN!). (2009). Retrieved June 10, 2009, from http://www.defeatautismnow.com/

DeLong, G. R. (1991). Autism, amnesia, hippocampus, and learning. *Neuroscience and Behavioral Reviews, 16*, 63–70.

DeNoon, D. J. (2005, July 12). New intensity to debate over autism cause: Parents and researchers grapple with claims that autism is linked to thimerosal in vaccines. Retrieved June 10, 2009, from http://www.webmd.com/brain/autism/news/20050712/new-intensity-to-debate-over-autism-cause

DeNoon, D. J. (2006, April 3). Researchers question autism "epidemic" on FoxMD Watch, Monday, April 3, 2006, by Daniel J. DeNoon, WebMD. Retrieved June 2, 2009, from http://www.foxnews.com/story/0,2933,190393,00.html

Deppe, J. (2008, September 2). State of the states in 2008: Successes despite touch economy. *ASHA Leader, 13*(12), 1, 8–9.

Derban, L. K. (1974). Outbreak of food poisoning due to alkyl-mercury fungicide on southern Ghana state farm. *Archives of Environmental Health, 28*, 49–52.

DeRouen, T. A., Martin, M. D., Leroux, B. G., Townes, B. D., Woods, J. S., Leitão, J., et al. (2006). Neurobehavioral effects of dental amalgam in children: A randomized clinical trial. *Journal of the American Medical Association, 295*(15), 1784–1792.

DeStefano, F. (2007). Vaccines and autism: Evidence does not support a causal association. *Clinical Pharmacology & Therapeutics, 82*(6), 756–759.

DeStefano, F., Bhasin, T. K., Thompson, W. W., Yeargin-Allsopp, M., & Boyle, C. (2004). Age at first measles-mumps-rubella vaccination in children with autism and school-matched control subjects: A population-based study in metropolitan Atlanta. *Pediatrics, 1*(2), 259–266.

Deth, R. (2007). Update on methionine synthase, adaptive enzyme functioning, cobalamin, and methylation of phospholipids at the D4 receptor. In Pangborn and Baker (2007), pp. 41–48.

Deth, R., Muratore, C., Benzecry, J., Power-Charnitsky, V. A., & Waly, M. (2008). How environmental and genetic factors combine to cause autism: A redox/methylation hypothesis. *Neurotoxicology, 29*(1), 190–201.

Dietert, R. R., & Dietert, J. M. (2008). Potential for early-life immune insult including developmental immunotoxicity in autism and autism spectrum disorders: Focus on critical windows of immune vulnerability. *Journal of Toxicology and Environmental Health, Part B—Critical Reviews, 1*(8), 660–680.

DiLuzio, W. (2009, April 29). *Escherichia coli* swimming in a microchannel. Retrieved June 10, 2009, from http://www.nsf.gov/news/news_videos.jsp?org=EHR&cntn_id=104283&preview=false&media_id=55634

Domingo, J. L. (2006). Aluminum and other metals in Alzheimer's disease: A review of potential therapy with chelating agents. *Journal of Alzheimer's Disease, 10*(2–3), 331–341.

Dorea, J. G. (2007). Exposure to mercury during the first six months via human milk and vaccines: Modifying risk factors. *American Journal of Perinatology, 24*(7), 387–400.

Dorea, J. G., & Marques, R. C. (2008). Modeling neurodevelopment outcomes and ethylmercury exposure from thimerosal-containing vaccines. *Toxicological Sciences, 103*(2), 414–415.

Douglas, G. (2001, May 2). Strategic planning for the Vaccine Research Center, NIH. Retrieved June 10, 2009, from http://www.nomercury.org/science/documents/Lecture_11_Dr_Douglas__Princeton.PDF

D'Souza, Y., Fombonne, E., & Ward, B. J. (2006). No evidence of persisting measles virus in peripheral blood mononuclear cells from children with autism spectrum disorder. *Pediatrics, 118*(4), 1664–1675.

Duff, P. A., Wong, P., & Early, M. (2000). Learning language for work and life: The linguistic socialization of immigrant Canadians seeking careers in healthcare. *Modern Language Journal, 86*(3), 397–422.

Dunning, J. (2005). *The sign of the book.* New York: Simon and Schuster.

Edelson, S. M., Edelson, M. G., Kerr, D. C. R., & Grandin, T. (1999). Behavioral and physiological effects of deep pressure on children with autism: A pilot study evaluating the efficacy of Grandin's hug machine. *American Journal of Occupational Therapy, 53,* 145–152.

Edlich, R. F., Cochran, A. A., Cross, C. L., Wack, C. A., Long, W. B., & Newkirk, A. T. (2008). Legislation and informed consent brochures for dental patients receiving amalgam restorations. *International Journal of Toxicology, 27*(4), 313–316.

Edlich, R. F., Greene, J. A., Cochran, A. A., Kelley, A. R., Gubler, K. D., Olson, B. M., et al. (2007). Need for informed consent for dentists who use mercury amalgam restorative material as well as technical considerations in removal of dental amalgam restorations. *Journal of Environmental Pathology Toxicology and Oncology, 26*(4), 305–322.

Edlich, R. F., Son, D. M., Olson, B. M., Greene, J. A., Gubler, K. D., Winters, K. L. B., et al. (2007). Update on the national vaccine injury compensation program. *Journal of Emergency Medicine, 33*(2), 199–211.

Edwardes, M., & Baltzan, M. (2001). MMR immunization and autism. *Journal of the American Medical Association, 2*(22), 2852.

Eisele, K., Lang, P. A., Kempe, D. S., Klarl, B. A., Niemoller, O., Wieder, T. F., et al. (2006). Stimulation of erythrocyte phosphatidylserine exposure by mercury ions. *Toxicology and Applied Pharmacology, 210*(1–2), 116–122.

Ejiri, K. (1998). Synchronization between preverbal vocalizations and motor actions in early infancy I: Pre-canonical babbling vocalizations synchronize with rhythmic body movements before the onset of canonical babbling. *Japanese Journal of Psychology, 68,* 433–440.

Eke, D., & Celik, A. (2008). Genotoxicity of thimerosal in cultured human lymphocytes with and without metabolic activation sister chromatid exchange analysis proliferation index and mitotic index. *Toxicology in Vitro, 22*(4), 927–934.

Elbajir, N. (2008, March 6). Broadcast: Lead Story, Series 17, Episode 38. Retrieved June 10, 2009, from http://www.abc.net.au/foreign/content/2008/s2259102.htm

Elliot, K. (2008, June 21). Video clips of two interviews with Ray Moynihan, visiting editor of Feature: Drug marketing: Key opinion leaders: Independent experts or drug representatives in disguise? *British Medical Journal, 336,* 1402–1403. Retrieved June 10, 2009, from http://www.bmj.com/cgi/content/short/336/7658/1402

Ellis, F. A. (1943). Possible danger in use of merthiolate ophthalmic ointment. *Archives of Ophthalmology, 30,* 265–266.

Ellis, F. A. (1947). The sensitizing factor in merthiolate. *Journal of Allergy, 18,* 212–213.

Engler, R. (1985, April 27). Technology out of control. *The Nation, 240,* 488–500.

Engley, F. B. (1950). Evaluation of mercurial compounds as antiseptics. *Annals of the New York Academy of Sciences, 53,* 197–206.

Engley, F. B. (1956). Mercurials as disinfectants: Evaluation of mercurial antimicrobic action and comparative toxicity for skin tissue cells. Chicago: 42nd Mid-Year Meeting of the Chemical Specialties Manufacturer's Association.

Enserink, M. (2002). Biowarfare. Did bioweapons test cause a deadly smallpox outbreak? *Science, 296*(5576), 2116–2117.

Environmental Protection Agency (EPA). (2007, September 21). DDT ban takes effect. Retrieved June 10 2009, from http://www.epa.gov/history/topics/ddt/01.htm

Epstein, R. M., Alper, B. S., & Quill, T. E. (2004). Communicating evidence for participatory decision making *Journal of the American Medical Association, 291*(19), 2359–2366.

Escherichia coli. (2009, February 6). Retrieved June 10, 2009, from http://en.wikipedia.org/wiki Escherichia_coli

Evans, M. (Director), & Pell, A. (Writer). (2006). *Snow Cake* [Motion picture]. United States: Revolution Films. Retrieved June 10, 2009, from http://www.youtube.com/watch?v=aqv5gmsikIQ&feature=related

Evans, T. A., Siedlak, S. L., Lu, L., Fu, X., Wang, Z., McGinnis, W. R., et al. (2008). The autistic phenotype exhibits remarkably localized modification of brain protein by products of free radical-induced lipid oxidation *American Journal of Biotechnology and Biochemistry, 4*(2), 61–72.

Fagan, D. G., Pritchard, J. S., Clarkson, T. W., & Greenwood, M. R. (1977, December). Organ mercury level in infants with omphaloceles treated with organic mercurial antiseptic. *Archives of Disease in Childhood 52*(12), 962–964.

Fanning, L. J., Connor, A. M., & Wu, G. E. (1996). Development of the immunoglobulin repertoire. *Clinical Immunology and Immunopathology, 79*(1), 1–14.

Faria, M. A. (2002). Medical history—Hygiene and sanitation. *Medical Sentinel, 7*(4), 122–123. Retrieved June 10, 2009, from http://www.haciendapub.com/faria5.html

Faria, M. A., Jr. (2007a). Part I: Public health, social science, and the scientific method. *Surgical Neurology 67*(2), 211–214.

Faria, M. A., Jr. (2007b). Part II: Public health, social science, and the scientific method. *Surgical Neurology 67*(3), 318–322.

Federal Autism Insurance Reform Bill. (n.d.). Autism treatment acceleration act of 2008. Retrieved June 10 2009, from http://www.autismvotes.org/atf/cf/%7B2A179B73-96E2-44C3-8816-1B1C0BE5334B%7D Obama%20federal%20autism%20reform.pdf

Feinberg, D. (2007). Foreword. In J. McCarthy, *Louder than words: A mother's journey in healing autism* (pp ix–xiii). New York: Dutton.

Field, T. (1995). Massage therapy for infants and children. *Journal of Developmental and Behavioral Pediatrics 1*(2), 105–111.

Field, T., & Diego, M. (2008). Vagal activity, early growth and emotional development. *Infant Behavior & Development, 3*(3), 361–373.

Ferreira, S. T., Vieira, M. N. N., & De Felice, F. G. (2007). Soluble protein oligomers as emerging toxins in Alzheimer's' and other amyloid diseases. *IUBMB LIFE, 59*(4–5), 332–345.

Fiers, W., Contreras, R., Haegeman, G., Rogiers, R., Vandevoorde, A., Vanheuverswyn, H., Vanherreweghe, J. Volckaert, G., & Ysebaert, M. (1978). Complete nucleotide-sequence of SV40 DNA, *Nature, 273* 113–120.

Fighting Autism. (2009). Retrieved June 10, 2009, from http://www.fightingautism.org/idea/autism.php?

Filipek, P. A., Juranek, J., Smith, M., Mays, L. Z., Ramos, E. R., Bocian, M., et al. (2003). Mitochondrial dysfunction in autistic patients with 15q inverted duplication. *Annals of Neurology, 53*(6), 801–804.

Film Scouts. (1994–2008). Producer: Jonathan Shestack. Retrieved June 10, 2009, from http://www.filmscouts. com/scripts/matinee.cfm?Film=air-for&File=filmmkrs

Fischer, C., Fredriksson, A., & Eriksson, P. (2008). Neonatal co-exposure to low doses of an ortho-PCB (PCB 153) and methyl mercury exacerbate defective developmental neurobehavior in mice. *Toxicology, 2*(2–3), 157–165.

Fisher, B. L. (2001, January 11). Agenda. Retrieved June 10, 2009, from http://www.blogger.com/profile/ 02404025666100094471

Fisher, B. L. (2002, November). Power grab by federal government sets stage for forced vaccination in America: Drug companies get liability protection in Homeland Security Bill. Retrieved June 10, 2009, from http:// www.nvic.org/Issues/homeland%20security.htm

Fisher, B. L. (2009). Barbara Loe Fisher is co-founder and president of the National Vaccine Information Center (NVIC). Retrieved June 10, 2009, from http://www.nvic.org/about/barbaraloefisher.aspx

Fisher, E. S. (2008). Learning to deliver better health care. *Issues in Science and Technology, 24*(3), 58–62.

Fogel, A., & Hannan, T. E. (1985). Manual actions of nine-to-fifteen-week-old human infants during face-to-face interaction with their mothers. *Child Development, 56,* 1271–1279.

Foley, S. (n.d.). Mercury poisoning in Iraq—1971. Retrieved June 10, 2009, from http://toxipedia.org/display/toxipedia/Mercury+Poisoning+in+Iraq+-+1971)

Fombonne, E. (1996). Is the prevalence of autism increasing? *Journal of Autism and Developmental Disorders, 26*(6), 673–676.

Fombonne, E. (1999). The epidemiology of autism: A review. *Psychological Medicine, 29,* 769–786.

Fombonne, E. (2001). Is there an epidemic of autism? *Pediatrics, 107,* 411–413.

Fombonne, E. (2003a). Epidemiological surveys of autism and other pervasive developmental disorders: An update. *Journal of Autism and Developmental Disorders, 33*(4), 365–382.

Fombonne, E. (2003b). The prevalence of autism. *Journal of the American Medical Association, 289*(1), 88–89.

Fombonne, E. (2008). Thimerosal disappears but autism remains. *Archives of General Psychiatry, 65,* 15–16.

Fombonne, E., Zakarian, R., Bennett, A., Meng, L. Y., & McLean-Heywood, D. (2006). Pervasive developmental disorders in Montreal, Quebec, Canada: Prevalence and links with immunizations. *Pediatrics, 118*(1), E139–E150.

Food and Drug Administration (FDA)/Center for Biologics Evaluation and Research (CBER). (2008, July 22). Center for Biologics Evaluation and Research: Frequently asked questions. Retrieved February 3, 2009, from at http://www.fda.gov/cber/faq.htm#6

Food and Drug Administration (FDA)/Center for Biologics Evaluation and Research (CBER). (2009, January 14). Thimerosal in vaccines. Retrieved February 3, 2009, from http://www.fda.gov/cber/vaccine/thimerosal.htm#pres

Food and Drug Administration (FDA)/Department of Health and Human Services (DHHS). (1998, April 22). Status of certain additional over-the-counter drug category II and III active ingredients. 21 CFR Part 310, [Docket Nos. 75N–183F, 75N–183D, and 80N–0280] RIN 0910–AA01. *Federal Register, 63*(77), 19799–19802. Retrieved June 10, 2009, from http://www.fda.gov/ohrms/dockets/98fr/042298a.pdf

Foundation for Autism Information and Research. (2007a, April 19). David Kirby interviews Katie Wright! Part 1. Retrieved June 10, 2009, from http://www.youtube.com/watch?v=IUNO25l1zFs&feature=related

Foundation for Autism Information and Research. (2007b, April 19). David Kirby interviews Katie Wright! Part 2. Retrieved June 10, 2009, from http://www.youtube.com/watch?v=_dHY5K_MP7w

Fox, M. (2009, February 12). U.S. vaccine court denies family's autism case. Retrieved June 10, 2009, from http://www.reuters.com/article/lifestyleMolt/idUSTRE51B4AN20090212

Franco, J. L., Teixeira, A., Meotti, F. C., Ribas, C. M., Stringari, J., Pomblum, S. C. G. M., et al. (2006). Cerebellar thiol status and motor deficit after lactational exposure to methylmercury. *Environmental Research, 102*(1), 22–28.

Francois, G., Duclos, P., Margolis, H., Lavanchi, D., Siegrist, C. A., Meheus, A., et al. (2005). Vaccine safety controversies and the future of vaccination programs. *Pediatric Infectious Disease Journal, 24*(11), 953–961.

Freedom of Information Act (1966–2007). 5 U.S.C. § 552, as amended by, Public Law No. 104-231, 110 Stat. 3048, and by the Open Government Act of 2007, S. 2488 Public Law 110-81, 121 Stat. 735, enacted September 14, 2007. Retrieved June 10, 2009, from http://www.usdoj.gov/oip/foi-upd.htm

Freud, S. (1924). *A general introduction to psychoanalysis* (J. Riviere, Trans.). New York: Boni and Liveright. (Original work published 1915–1917)

Freud, S. (1975). *The psychopathology of everyday life* (A. Tyson, Trans.). Harmondsworth, England: Penguin. (Original work published 1901)

Frye v. United States 54 App. D. C. 46, 47, 293 F. 1013, 1014 (D.C. Cir. 1923).

Fuentes, A. (2003, November 11). Eli Lilly and thimerosal. Retrieved June 10, 2009, from http://www.inthesetimes.com/article/649/

Fugh–Berman, A., & Ahari, S. (2007). Following the script: How drug reps make friends and influence doctors. *Plos Medicine, 4*(4), e150, 0621–0625.

Gallo, R. C., Salahuddin, S. Z., Popovic, M., Shearer, G. M., Kaplan, M., Haynes, B. F., et al. (1984). Frequent detection and isolation of cytopathic retroviruses (HTLV-III) from patients with AIDS and at risk for AIDS. *Science, 224*, 500–502.

Gagnon, M.–A., & Lexchin, J. (2008). The cost of pushing pills: A new estimate of pharmaceutical promotion expenditures in the United States. *PLoS Med* 5(1): E1. doi:10.1371/journal.pmed.005000. Retrieved June 10, 2009, from http://www.plosmedicine.org/article/info:doi/10.1371/journal.pmed.0050001

Geier, D. A., & Geier, M. R. (2005). A case-control study of serious autoimmune adverse events following hepatitis B immunization. *Autoimmunity, 38*(4), 295–301.

Geier, D. A., & Geier, M. R. (2006a). An assessment of downward trends in neurodevelopmental disorders in the United States following removal of thimerosal from childhood vaccines. *Medical Science Monitor, 12*(6) CR231–CR239.

Geier, D. A., & Geier, M. R. (2006db). A meta-analysis epidemiological assessment of neurodevelopmental disorders following vaccines administered from 1994 through 2000 in the United States. *Neuroendocrinology Letters, 27*(4), 401–413.

Geier, D. A., & Geier, M. R. (2006c). A prospective assessment of porphyrins in autistic disorders: A potential marker for heavy metal exposure. *Neurotoxicity Research, 10*(1), 57–63.

Geier, D. A., & Geier, M. R. (2007). A prospective study of mercury toxicity biomarkers in autistic spectrum disorders. *Journal of Toxicology and Environmental Health: Part A: Current Issues, 70*(20), 1723–1730.

Geier, D. A., Mumper, E., Gladfelter, B., Coleman, L., & Geier, M. R. (2008). Neurodevelopmental disorders, maternal Rh-negativity, and Rho(D) immune globulins: A multi-center assessment. *Neuroendocrinology Letters, 29*(2), 272–280.

Geier, D. A., Sykes, L. K., & Geier, M. R. (2007). A review of thimerosal (merthiolate) and its ethylmercury breakdown product: Specific historical considerations regarding safety and effectiveness. *Journal of Toxicology and Environmental Health: Part B: Critical Reviews, 10*(8), 575–596.

George, G. N., Prince, R. C., Gailer, J., Buttigieg, G. A., Denton, M. B., Harris, H. H., & Pickering I. J. (2004). Mercury binding to the chelation therapy agents DMSA and DMPS and the rational design of custom chelators for mercury. *Chemical Research in Toxicology, 17*(8), 999–1006.

Gerberding, J. (2008, March 7). Vaccine settlement complex, may not be first. Retrieved April 14, 2008, from http://www.cnn.com/2008/HEALTH/conditions/03/07/autism.vaccines.analysis.ap/ [No longer accessible on February 4, 2009. But see Adventures in Autism, 2009.]

Gernsbacher, M. A., Dawson, M., & Goldsmith, H. H. (2005). Three reasons not to believe in an autism epidemic. *Current Directions in Psychological Science, 14*(2), 55–59.

Gershon, M. D. (2000). *The second brain.* New York: Harper.

Ghanizadeh, A. (2008). A preliminary study on screening prevalence of pervasive developmental disorder in schoolchildren in Iran. *Journal of Autism and Developmental Disorders, 38*(4), 759–763.

Ghosh, S. K., Chaudhuri, J., Gachhui, R., Mandal, A., & Ghosh, S. (2007). Effect of mercury and organomercurials on cellular glucose utilization: A study using resting mercury-resistant yeast cells. *Journal of Applied Microbiology, 102*(2), 375–383.

Gillberg, C. (1999). Prevalence of disorders in the autism spectrum. *Infants and Young Children, 12*(2), 64–74.

Gillberg, C., Cederlund, M., Lamberg, K., & Zeijlon, L. (2006). Brief report: The autism epidemic. The registered prevalence of autism in a Swedish urban area. *Journal of Autism and Developmental Disorders, 36*(3), 429–435.

Giordano, G., Afsharinejad, Z., Guizzetti, M., Vitalone, A., Kavanagh, T. J., & Costa, L. G. (2007). Organophosphorus insecticides chlorpyrifos and diazinon and oxidative stress in neuronal cells in a genetic model of glutathione deficiency. *Toxicology and Applied Pharmacology, 219*(2–3), 181–189.

Girard, M. (2007). When evidence-based medicine (EBM) fuels confusion: Multiple sclerosis after hepatitis B vaccine as a case in point. *Medical Veritas, 4*, 1436–1451.

GlaxoSmithKline. (2008, October). Pediarix: Prescribing information. Retrieved June 10, 2009, from http://us.gsk.com/products/assets/us_pediarix.pdf

Glutathione. (2009, February 4). Retrieved June 10, 2009, from http://en.wikipedia.org/wiki/Glutathione

Glutathione peroxidase. (2009, February 4). Retrieved June 10, 2009, from http://en.wikipedia.org/wiki/Glutathione_peroxidase

Goff, S. L., Mazor, K. M., Meterko, V., Dodd, K., & Sabin, J. (2008). Patients' beliefs and preferences regarding doctors' medication recommendations. *Journal of General Internal Medicine, 23*(3), 236–241.

Golan, O., Baron-Cohen, S., & Golan, Y. (2008). The "Reading the mind in films" task [child version]: Complex emotion and mental state recognition in children with and without autism spectrum conditions. *Journal of Autism and Developmental Disorders, 38*(8), 1534–1541.

Golse, B., Debray-Ritzen, P., Durosay, P., Puget, K., & Michelson, A.M. (1978). Alterations in two enzymes: Superoxide dismutase and glutathione peroxidase in developmental infantile psychosis (infantile autism). *Revue Neurologique (Paris), 134,* 699–705.

Goncharuk, G. A. (1971). Experimental investigations of the effect of organomercury pesticides on generative functions and on progeny. *Hygiene and Sanitation, 36,* 40–43.

Gordon, J. N. (2008). Foreword. In J. McCarthy, *Mother warriors* (pp. xiii–xviii). New York: Dutton.

Gould, H. J., & Sutton, B. J. (2008). IgE in allergy and asthma today. *Nature Reviews Immunology, 8*(3), 205–217.

Gould, H. J., Sutton, B. J., Beavil, A. J., Beavil, R. L., McCloskey, N., Coker, H. A., Fear, D., & Smurthwaite, L. (2003). The biology of IgE and the basis of allergic disease. *Annual Review of Immunology, 21,* 579–628.

Government Relations News. (2009). Retrieved June 10, 2009, from http://www.autismspeaks.org/government_affairs/index.php?WT.svl=Text_Links

Grandin, T. (1992). Calming effects of deep touch pressure in patients with autistic disorder, college students, and animals. *Journal of Child and Adolescent Psychopharmacology, 2*(1), 359–374. Retrieved June 10, 2009, from http://www.grandin.com/inc/squeeze.html

Gray, F., Adle-Biassette, H., Chrétien, F., Lorin de la Grandmaison, G., Force, G., & Keohane, C. (2001). Neuropathology and neurodegeneration in human immunodeficiency virus infection. Pathogenesis of HIV-induced lesions of the brain, correlations with HIV-associated disorders and modifications according to treatments. *Clinical Neuropathology, 20*(4), 146–155.

Gupta, S. (2008, April 1). Vaccine-autism test case: Video of Michelle Cedillo. Retrieved June 10, 2009, from http://www.cnn.com/2008/HEALTH/conditions/03/24/autism.vaccines/#cnnSTCVideo

Gupta, S. (2009, February 12). Vaccines didn't cause autism, court rules. Retrieved June 10, 2009, from http://www.cnn.com/2009/HEALTH/02/12/autism.vaccines/index.html#cnnSTCVideo

Guzzi, G., Fogazzi, G. B., Cantù, M., Minoia, C., Ronchi, A., Pigatto, P. D., & Severi, G. (2008). Dental amalgam, mercury toxicity, and renal autoimmunity. *Journal of Environmental Pathololology, Toxicology, and Oncology, 27*(2), 147–155.

Haas, R. H., Parikh, S., Falk, M. J., Saneto, R. P., Wolf, N. I., Darin, N., & Cohen, B. H. (2007). Mitochondrial disease: A practical approach for primary care physicians. *Pediatrics, 120*(6), 1326–1333.

Haddon, M. (2003). *The curious case of the dog in the night-time.* New York: Doubleday.

Hadwen, W. (1896, January 25). The case against vaccination: Verbatim report of an address by Walter Hadwen at Goddard's Assembly Rooms, Gloucester, England. (During the Gloucester Smallpox Epidemic). Retrieved June 10, 2009, from http://www.whale.to/v/hadwen.html

Hagerman, R. J. (2006). Lessons from fragile X regarding neurobiology, autism, and neurodegeneration. *Journal of Developmental and Behavioral Pediatrics, 2*(1), 63–74.

Haley, B. (2006, November 2). Mercury toxicity & autism. Parts 1–4. Retrieved June 10, 2009, from http://www.youtube.com/watch?v=GQYISvsgq6s&feature=related (also available May 19, 2009, at http://www.autismmedia.org/media2.html)

Hall, L., & Case-Smith, J. (2008). The effect of sound-based intervention on children with sensory processing disorders and visual-motor delays. *American Journal of Occupational Therapy, 6*(2), 209–215.

Halvorsen, R. (2007). *The truth about vaccines: How we are used as guinea pigs without knowing it.* London: Gibson Square Books.

Harman, D. (1956). Aging: A theory based on free radical and radiation chemistry. *Journal of Gerontology, 11*(3), 298–300.

Harman, D. (1981, November). The aging process. *Proceedings of the National Academy of Sciences Unite* *States of America, 78*(11), 7124–7128.

Harman, D. (2003). The free radical theory of aging. *Antioxidants & Redox Signaling, 5*(5), 557–561.

Harman, H. H. (1976). *Modern factor analysis.* (3rd ed.). Chicago: University of Chicago Press.

Harris, C. E., Biggs, J. C., Concannon, A. J., & Dodds, A. J. (1990). Peripheral-blood and bone-marrow finding in patients with Acquired-Immune-Deficiency-Syndrome. *Pathology, 2*(4), 206–211.

Hauser, K. F., Hahn, Y. K., Adjan, V. V., Zou, S. P., Buch, S. K., Nath, A., Bruce-Keller, A. J., & Knapp, P. E (2009). HIV-1 Tat and morphine have interactive effects on oligodendrocyte survival and morphology. *Glia* 5(2), 194–206.

Hay, W. H. (1937, December 21). Address of William Howard Hay, M.D., Pocono, PA, on June 25, 1937 before the Medical Freedom Society. Retrieved June 10, 2009, from http://www.whale.to/vaccines/hay.htm

Hayes, W. J., Jr., & Laws, E. R. (Eds.). (1991). *Handbook of pesticide toxicology.* San Diego: Academic Press

Hedges, P. (Director/Writer), & Gardner, P. (Writer). (2007). *Dan in Real Life* [Motion picture]. United States Touchstone Pictures.

Heinonen, O. P., Slone, D., & Shapiro, S. (1977). *Birth defects and drugs in pregnancy.* Littleton, MA: Publish ing Sciences Group.

Helper T-cells. (n.d.). Cardiff University T cell research. Retrieved June 10, 2009, from http://www.tcells.org helpertcells.html

Hepper, P. G. (2007). The effect of maternal consumption of alcohol on the behavior of the human fetus A review. *International Journal on Disability and Human Development, 6*(2), 153–159.

Hepper, P. G., Dornan, J. C., & Little, J. F. (2005). Maternal alcohol consumption during pregnancy may dela the development of spontaneous fetal startle behavior. *Physiology & Behavior, 8*(5), 711–714.

Herbert, M. R., Russo, J. P., Yang, S., Roohi, J., Blaxill, A., Kahler, S. G. E., et al. (2006). Autism and envi ronmental genomics. *Neurotoxicology, 27*(5), 671–684.

Herdman, M. L., Marcelo, A., Huang, Y., Niles, R. M., Dhar, S., & Kiningham, K. K. (2006). Thimerosa induces apoptosis in a neuroblastoma model via the cJun N-terminal kinase pathway. *Toxicological Sciences* 92(1), 246–253.

Herman, L. M., Uyeyama, R. K., & Pack, A. A. (2008). Bottlenose dolphins understand relationships betweer concepts. *Behavioral and Brain Sciences, 3*(2), 139–140.

Hertz-Picciotto, I., Croen, L. A., Hansen, R., Jones, C. R., van de Water, J., & Pessah, I. N. (2006). The CHARGE study: An epidemiologic investigation of genetic and environmental factors contributing to autism. *Environmental Health Perspectives, 114*(7), 1119–1125.

Hess, K. L., Morrier, M. J., Heflin, L. J., & Ivey, M. L. (2008). Autism treatment survey: Services received by children with autism spectrum disorders in public school classrooms. *Journal of Autism and Developmenta Disorders, 3*(5), 961–971.

Higgins, C. M. (1920). *Horrors of vaccination exposed and illustrated. Petition to the President to Abolish Compulsory Vaccination in Army and Navy.* Brooklyn, NY: Chas M. Higgins.

Hill, J. (Director), Adamson, J. (Writer), Cole, L. (Screenplay). (1966). *Born free* [Motion picture]. Kenya: Atlas.

HLA-DR4. (2008, June 29). Retrieved June 10, 2009, from http://en.wikipedia.org/wiki/HLA-DR4

Hoffman, R. (2008). Anaphylactic children: Canaries in the public health mine shaft? Are vaccines responsible for the epidemic of anaphylaxis in young children today? Retrieved June 10, 2009, from http://www.vran. org/vaccines/anaphylaxis/ana-vac.htm

Hogan, B. (2002, January 3). Environment U.S. experts deployed in Uzbekistan to address bioweapons threat. Retrieved June 10, 2009, from http://www.eurasianet.org/departments/environment/articles/eav010302. shtml#

Holland, J. G., & Skinner, B. F. (1961). *The analysis of behavior: A program for self-instruction.* New York: McGraw-Hill. Retrieved June 10, 2009, from http://www.bfskinner.org/educational.html

Holmes, A. S., Blaxill, M. F., & Haley, B. E. (2003). Reduced levels of mercury in first baby haircuts of autistic children. *International Journal of Toxicology, 22*(4), 277–285.

Homer. (ca. 1178 BC). *The Odyssey* (A. Pope, Trans.) Retrieved June 10, 2009, from http://ebooks.adelaide. edu.au/h/homer/h8op/book17.html

Hornig, M., Chian, D., & Lipkin, W. I. (2004). Neurotoxic effects of postnatal thimerosal are mouse strain dependent. *Molecular Psychiatry*, *9*(9), 833–845.

Horvath, K., Papadimitriou, J. C., Rabsztyn, A., Drachenberg, C., & Tildon, J. T. (1999). Gastrointestinal abnormalities in children with autistic disorder. *Journal of Pediatrics*, *1*(5), 559–563.

Horvath, K., & Perman, J. A. (2002). Autistic disorder and gastrointestinal disease. *Current Opinion in Pediatrics*, *14*(5), 583–587.

House Call with Dr. Sanjay Gupta. (2008, March 29). Unraveling the mystery of autism; Talking with the CDC director; Stories of children with autism; Aging with autism. Retrieved June 10, 2009, from http://transcripts.cnn.com/TRANSCRIPTS/0803/29/hcsg.01.html

Howe, S. G. (2009). Samuel Gridley Howe [1801–1876]. Retrieved June 10, 2009, from http://en.wikipedia.org/wiki/Samuel_Gridley_Howe

Hrdlicka, M. (2008). EEG abnormalities, epilepsy and regression in autism: A review. *Neuroendocrinology Letters*, *2*(4), 405–409.

Hughes, J. R. (2008). A review of recent reports on autism: 1000 studies published in 2007. *Epilepsy & Behavior*, *1*(3), 425–437.

Human Genome Project. (2008, October 15). Retrieved February 6, 2009, from http://www.ornl.gov/sci/techresources/Human_Genome/home.shtml; also see http://en.wikipedia.org/wiki/Genome_project

Human leukocyte antigen. (2009, February 6). Retrieved June 10, 2009, from http://en.wikipedia.org/wiki/Human_leukocyte_antigen

Human Microbiome Project. (2008, August 12). Retrieved June 10, 2009, from http://en.wikipedia.org/wiki/Human_microbiome

Humphrey, M. L., Cole, M. P., Pendergrass, J. C., & Kiningham, K. K. (2005). Mitochondrial mediated thimerosal-induced apoptosis in a human neuroblastoma cell line (SK-N-SH). *Neurotoxicology*, *26*(3), 407–416.

Hunt, D. L., & Rai, S. N. (2008). Interlitter response variability in a threshold dose-response model. *Communications in Statistics—Theory and Method*, *3*(1), 2304–2314.

Hyman, M. (2008). Why current thinking about autism is completely wrong. Retrieved June 10, 2009, from http://www.youtube.com/watch?v=vOEXldRNxcA&feature=related; http://www.youtube.com/user/ultrawellness

Hyson, M. T. (n.d.). Dolphins, therapy and autism. Retrieved June 10, 2009, from http://www.planetpuna.com/dolphin-paper-html/dolphin-paper.htm

Ichim, T. E., Solano, F., Glenn, E., Morales, F., Smith, L., Zabrecky, G., & Riordan, N. H. (2007, June 27). Stem cell therapy for autism. *Journal of Translational Medicine*, *5*, 1–9. Article 30.

Illustrated London News. (1853). Smallpox vaccination becomes compulsory in Britain. Retrieved June 10, 2009, from http://www.iln.org.uk/iln_years/year/1853.htm

Institute for Vaccine Safety. (2009, January 7). Thimerosal content in some US licensed vaccines. Retrieved June 10, 2009, from http://www.vaccinesafety.edu/thi-table.htm

Institute of Medicine (IOM). (2005). *Vaccine safety research, data access, and public trust.* Washington, DC: Committee on the Review of the National Immunization Program's Research Procedures and Data Sharing Program. Board on Health Promotion and Disease Prevention; National Academies Press. Retrieved June 10, 2009, from http://books.nap.edu/openbook.php?record_id=11234&page=R1

Institute of Medicine (IOM)—Immunization Safety Review Committee. (2001a, January 12). *Transcript of Closed Meeting: On file in the US District Court of Texas, Eastern District; Case #5:03-CV-141.* Retrieved June 10, 2009, from http://www.nomercury.org/iom.htm

Institute of Medicine (IOM)—Immunization Safety Review Committee. (2001b, July 16). *Thimerosal-containing vaccines and neurodevelopmental outcomes public meeting.* Retrieved June 10, 2009, from http://www.iom.edu/Object.File/Master/8/176/Transcript7-16.pdf#search=%22Rogam%20%26%20thimerosal%22

Institute of Medicine (IOM)—Immunization Safety Review Committee. (2004, February 9). Meeting nine: Vaccines and autism. Retrieved June 10, 2009, from http://www.iom.edu/?id=53422

International Academy of Oral Medicine and Toxicology (IAOMT). (2008). Safe removal of amalgam fillings. Retrieved June 10, 2009, from http://www.iaomt.org/articles/category_view.asp?intReleaseID=288&catid=30; also see Koral (2002, 2007).

Itoi, M., Ishii, Y., & Kaneko, N. (1972). Teratogenicities of antiviral ophthalmics on experimental animals Japanese Journal of Clinical Ophthalmology, 26, 631–640.

Iwaniuk, A. N., Koperski, D. T., Cheng, K. M., Elliott, J. E., Smith, L. K., Wilson, L. K., & Wylie, D. R. W (2008). The effects of environmental exposure to DDT on the brain of a songbird: Changes in structure associated with mating and song. Behavioural Brain Research, 1(1), 1–10.

Jabarra, A. (1999, July 31). Letter from John Jabarra, VP and Vaccines Director for SmithKline Beecham, t Dr. Jeffrey Koplan, Director of CDC. Retrieved June 10, 2009, from http://www.putchildrenfirst.org media/2.4.pdf

Jalili, M. A., & Abbasi, A. H. (1961). Poisoning by ethyl mercury toluene sulphonanilide. British Journal c Internal Medicine, 18, 303–308.

James, S. J., Cutler, P., Melnyk, S., Jernigan, S., Janak, L., Gaylor, D. W., & Neubrander, J. A. (2004). Metaboli biomarkers of increased oxidative stress and impaired methylation capacity in children with autism. America Journal of Clinical Nutrition, 80(6), 1611–1617.

James, S. J., Melnyk, S., Fuchs, G., Reid, T., Jernigan, S., Pavliv, O., et al. (2009). Efficacy of methylcobalami and folinic acid treatment on glutathione redox status in children with autism. American Journal of Clinica Nutrition, 8(1), 425–430.

James, S. J., Melnyk, S., Jernigan, S., Cleves, M. A., Halsted, C. H., & Wong, D. H. W. (2006). Metaboli endophenotype and related genotypes are associated with oxidative stress in children with autism. America Journal of Medical Genetics B, 141, 947–956.

James, S. J., Slikker, W., Melnyk, S., New, E., Pogribna, M., & Jernigan, S. (2005). Thimerosal neurotoxicit is associated with glutathione depletion: Protection with glutathione precursors. Neurotoxicology, 26 1–8.

Jefferson, T., Price, D., Demicheli, V., & Bianco, E. (European Research Program for Improved Vaccines) (2003). Unintended events following immunization with MMR: A systematic review. Vaccine, 2(25–26) 3954–3960.

Jepson, B. (2007a, November 6). An interview with Dr. Brian Jepson about his new book, Changing the cours of autism. Dr. Bryan Jepson. Part 1: Background. Retrieved June 10, 2009, from http://www.youtube.com watch?v=RmnlaFypfv0&feature=related

Jepson, B. (2007b, November 6). An interview with Dr. Brian Jepson about his new book, Changing the cours of autism. Dr. Bryan Jepson. Part 2: Background. Retrieved June 10, 2009, from http://www.youtube.com watch?v=g-2TdyN20Ww&feature=related

Jepson, B., & Johnson, J. (2007). Changing the course of autism: A scientific approach for parents and physi cians. Boulder, CO: Sentient.

Johnson, C. P., & Myers, S. M. (2007). Identification and evaluation of children with autism spectrum disorders Pediatrics, 120(5), 1183–1215.

Jyonouchi, H., Sun, S., & Le, H. (2001). Proinflammatory and regulatory cytokine production associate with innate and adaptive immune responses in children with autism spectrum disorders and developmenta regression. Journal of Neuroimmunology, 120, 170–179.

Kadane, J. B. (2008). Statistics in the law. New York: Oxford University Press.

Kanner, L. (1943). Autistic disturbances of affective contact. Nervous Child, 2, 217–250.

Kanner, L. (1944). Early infantile autism. Journal of Pediatrics, 25, 211–217.

Kanner, L. (1946). Irrelevant and metaphorical language in early infantile autism. American Journal of Psychia try, 103, 242–246.

Kanner, L. (1949). Problems of nosology and psychodynamics of early infantile autism. American Journal c Orthopsychiatry, 19, 416–426.

Kanner, L., & Eisenberg, L. (1956). Early infantile autism 1943–1955. American Journal of Orthopsychiatry 26, 556–66.

Karamouzi, A., Kovachev, D., Karamouzis, I., Antontadou-Hitoglou, M., Tsikoulas, M., & Aggelopoulou Sakadami, N. (2007). Saliva levels of 15-F-2t-isoprostane as biomarker of lipid peroxidation in autisti children. European Journal of Inflammation, 5(3), 141–144.

Kartzinel, J. J. (2007). Introduction. In J. McCarthy, Louder than words: A mother's journey in healing autisn (pp. xv–xvii). New York: Dutton.

Kastrup, O., Wanke, I., & Maschke, M. (2008). Neuroimaging of infections of the central nervous system. *Seminars in Neurology*, 2(4), 511–522.

Kaye, K. L., & Bower, T. G. R. (1994). Learning and intermodal transfer of information in newborns. *Psychological Reports*, 5, 286–288.

Keisler, P. D., Garren, T. P., Rogers, M. W., Matanoski, V. J., Renzi, L. S., & Ricciardella, L. E. (2008). Hannah Poling Case Record in the United States Court of Federal Claims, Office of Special Masters. Reprinted in D. Kirby (2008a). Retrieved June 10, 2009, from http://www.huffingtonpost.com/david-kirby/the-vaccineautism-court-_b_88558.html

Kendrick, D. B. (1989). *Blood program in World War II*. Washington, DC: Office of the Surgeon General, Department of the Army.

Kennedy, D. (2007, January 30). Smoking teeth = poison gas. Retrieved June 10, 2009, from http://www.youtube.com/watch?v=9ylnQ-T7oiA; http://iaomt.org/videos/

Kennedy, D. (2008, July 27). Poison in your dentist's office. Retrieved June 10, 2009, from http://www.youtube.com/watch?v=rxL8ScRvpaQ

Kennedy, R. F., Jr. (2005, June 22). Tobacco science and the thimerosal scandal. Retrieved June 10, 2009, from http://www.robertfkennedyjr.com/docs/ThimerosalScandalFINAL.PDF

Kennedy, R. F., Jr. (2006, March 1). Time for CDC to come clean. Retrieved June 10, 2009, from http://www.huffingtonpost.com/robert-f-kennedy-jr/time-for-cdc-to-come-clea_b_16550.html

Kennedy, R. F., Jr. (2007, June 19). Attack on mothers. Retrieved June 11, 2009, from http://www.huffingtonpost.com/robert-f-kennedy-jr/attack-on-mothers_b_52894.html

Kennedy, R. F., Jr., & Kirby, D. (2009, February 24). Vaccine court: Autism debate continues. Retrieved June 11, 2009, from http://www.huffingtonpost.com/robert-f-kennedy-jr-and-david-kirby/vaccine-court-autism-deba_b_169673.html

Kern, J. K., & Jones, A. M. (2006). Evidence of toxicity, oxidative stress, and neuronal insult in autism. *Journal of Toxicology and Environmental Health, Part B—Critical Reviews*, 9(6), 485–499.

Kharasch, M. S. (1928, June 5). Alkyl mercuric sulphur compound and process of producing it. United Stated Patent No. 1,672,615. Retrieved June 11, 2009, from http://v3.espacenet.com/origdoc?DB=EPODOC&IDX=US1672615&QPN=US1672615

Kharasch, M. S. (1932). Stabilized bactericide and process of stabilizing it. U.S. Patent 1,862,896.

Kharasch, M. S. (1935). Stabilized organo-meruri-sulphur compounds. U.S. Patent 2,012,820.

Kharasch, Morris. (2008, June 25). Retrieved June 10, 2009, from http://en.wikipedia.org/wiki/Morris_S._Kharasch

Kharasch, M. S., & Mayo, F. R. (1933). The peroxide effect in the addition of reagents to unsaturated compounds. I. The addition of hydrogen bromide to alkyl bromide. *Journal of the American Chemical Society*, 55, 2468–2496.

Kharasch, M. S., McBay, H. C., & Urry, W. H. (1945). Reactions of atoms and free radicals. 7. Diacetyl peroxide as an agent for linking alpha-carbon to alpha-carbon atoms in organic esters. *Journal of Organic Chemistry*, 10(5), 394–400.

Kim, H. L., Donnelly, J. H., Tournay, A. E., Book, T. M., & Filipek, P. (2006). Absence of seizures despite high prevalence of epileptiform EEG abnormalities in children with autism monitored in a tertiary care center. *EPILEPSIA*, 47(2), 394–398.

Kimmel, S. R. (2002). Vaccine adverse events: Separating myth from reality. *American Family Physician*, 66(11), 2113–2120.

Kinney, D. K., Munir, K. M., Crowley, D. J., & Miller, A. M. (2008). Prenatal stress and risk for autism. *Neuroscience and Biobehavioral Reviews*, 3(8), 1519–1532.

Kinsella, R. A. (1941). Chemotherapy of bacterial endocarditis. *Annals of Internal Medicine*, 15, 982–986.

Kirby, D. (2005). *Evidence of harm: Mercury in vaccines and the autism epidemic: A medical controversy*. New York: St. Martin's Press.

Kirby, D. A. (2007, April 12). Mercury, vaccines and autism: Is there a link? Keynote lecture presented at the Sertoma International Conference on Autism Spectrum Disorders (Autism07) at the Cajundome Convention Center, Lafayette, LA.

Kirby, D. (2008a, February 26). The vaccine–autism court document every American should read. Retrieved June 10, 2009, from http://www.huffingtonpost.com/david-kirby/the-vaccineautism-court-_b_88558.html

Kirby, D. (2008b, March 20). Give us answers on vaccines. Retrieved June 10, 2009, from http://www.ajc.com/opinion/content/opinion/2008/03/19/autismed_0320.html

Kirby, D. (2008c, April 27). The next vaccine–autism newsmaker: Not isolated, not unusual. Retrieved June 10, 2009, from http://www.huffingtonpost.com/david-kirby/the-next-vaccine-autism-n_b_98807.html

Kline, E. R., Bassit, L., Hernandez-Santiago, B. I., Detorio, M. A., Liang, B., Kleinhenz, D. J., et al. (2009). Long-term exposure to AZT, but not d4T, increases endothelial cell oxidative stress and mitochondrial dysfunction. *Cardiovascular Toxicology*, 9(1), 1–12.

Knox, K. K., & Carrigan, D. R. (1996). Active HHV-6 infection in the lymph nodes of HIV-infected patients: In vitro evidence that HHV-6 can break HIV latency. *Journal of Acquired Immune Deficiency Syndromes and Human Retrovirology*, 1(4), 370–378.

Koch, M., & Trapp, R. (2006). Ethyl mercury poisoning during a protein A immunoadsorption treatment. *American Journal of Kidney Disease*, 47(2), e31–e34.

Koch, R. (1905). The Nobel Prize in Physiology or Medicine 1905. Retrieved June 10, 2009, from http://nobelprize.org/nobel_prizes/medicine/laureates/1905/koch-bio.html

Koch, W. F. (1961). *The survival factor in neoplastic and viral diseases*. Detroit, MI: Author. Retrieved June 10, 2009, from http://www.rexresearch.com/koch/survival/survcont.htm

Kokayi, K., Altman, C. H., Callely, R. W., & Harrison, A. (2006). Findings of and treatment for high levels of mercury and lead toxicity in Ground Zero rescue and recovery workers and Lower Manhattan residents. *Explore*, 2(5), 400–407.

Koplan, J. (1999, November 26). Letter from CDC director to Merck and SmithKline Beecham rejecting offer of immediate thimerosal removal from vaccines. Retrieved June 10, 2009, from http://www.putchildrenfirst.org/media/2.17.pdf

Kopnisky, K. L., Bao, J., & Lin, Y. W. (2008). Neurobiology of HIV, psychiatric and substance abuse comorbidity research: Workshop report. *Brain Behavior and Immunity*, 2(4), 428–441.

Koral, S. M. (2002, 2007). Safe removal of amalgam fillings. Retrieved June 10, 2009, from http://www.iaomt.org/articles/files/files288/Safe%20Removal%20of%20Amalgam%20Fillings.pdf

Kuhn, T. S. (1962). *The structure of scientific revolutions*. Chicago: University of Chicago Press.

Kumar, R. A., & Christian, S. L. (2008). Genetics of autism spectrum disorders. *Current Neurology and Neuroscience Reports*, 9(3), 188–197.

Kurlan, R., Johnson, D., & Kaplan, E. L. (2008). Streptococcal infection and exacerbations of childhood tics and obsessive–compulsive symptoms: A prospective blinded cohort study. *Pediatrics*, 1(6), 1188–1197.

Kurtz, S. (n.d.) Ethan now. [Video]. Retrieved June 10, 2009, from http://www.childrenscornerschool.com/recoveries_new.html

Kurtz, S. (2005–2008a). Methylcobalamin recovery (vitamin MB12). Retrieved June 10, 2009, from http://www.autismrecoveryvideos.org/autism/methylcobalamin-vitamin-b12.html

Kurtz, S. (2005–2008b). Stan's son Ethan and his recovery from autism: Ethan's recovery. Retrieved June 10, 2009, from http://www.autismrecoveryvideos.org/autism/ethans-autism-recovery.html

Kurtz, S. (2007). A comprehensive antiviral approach. [Draft document: written July 3, 2007; updated August 27, 2007.] Retrieved June 10, 2009, from http://www.stankurtz.org/biomedical/comprehensive-antiviral-approach.html

Kurtz, S. (2008). Dental fillings/mercury amalgams. Retrieved June 10, 2009, from http://www.youtube.com/watch?v=730QNlAmLnM

Kvito, E. (2001, November 13). Smallpox: As bad a weapon: An interview with General Pyotr Burgasov (in Russian), *Moskovskie Novosti* [Moscow News], November 13, 2001. As reported by Tucker & Zilinskas (2002, p. 21).

Laidler, J. R. (2004, September 15). The "refrigerator mother" hypothesis of autism. Retrieved June 10, 2009, from http://www.autism-watch.org/causes/rm.shtml

Landers, S. J. (2008, February 4). Vaccines get a boost: Global market increases profitability of making vaccine Retrieved June 10, 2009, from http://www.ama-assn.org/amednews/2008/02/04/hlsa0204.htm

Lane, H. L. (1976). *The wild boy of Aveyron*. Cambridge, MA: Harvard University Press.

Lapointe, L., & Katz, R. C. (2002). Neurogenic disorders of speech in adults. In *Human communication disorders: An introduction* (pp. 472–509). Boston: Allyn and Bacon.

Larry King Live. (2007, September 25). Autism. Retrieved June 10, 2009, from http://www.cnn.com/video/#/video/bestoftv/2007/09/27/lkl.autism.treatments.cnn?iref=videosearch

Larry King Live. (2008a, March 7). The autism vaccine debate. Retrieved March 8, 2008, from http://www.cnn.com/video/#/video/bestoftv/2008/03/07/lkl.autism.vaccine.long.cnn?iref=videosearch [No longer accessible on February 4, 2009.]

Larry King Live. (2008b, April 2). Jenny McCarthy on *Larry King Live*: Parts 1–5. Retrieved June 10, 2009, from http://www.youtube.com/watch?v=vPDDzwhu–s&feature=related

Larry King Live. (2009, April 3). Jim Carrey and Jenny McCarthy on autism controversy: Parts 1–5. Retrieved June 10, 2009, from http://www.nowpublic.com/health/jenny-mccarthy-tries-save-children-autism

Lash, J. P. (1980). *Helen and Teacher: The story of Helen Keller and Anne Sullivan Macy*. New York: Delacorte Press.

Latour, B., & Levine, A. (1993). Translation into English of Pasteur (1864). Retrieved June 10, 2009, from http://shell.cas.usf.edu/~alevine/pasteur.pdf

Lawrence, M. (Director/Writer). (2002). *Two weeks notice* [Motion picture]. Castle Rock Entertainment. Cited clip retrieved June 10, 2009, from http://www.imdb.com/video/screenplay/vi1742733593/

Lawton, G. (2005). The autism myth. *New Scientist, 187*(2512), 36–40.

Le Couteur, A., Haden, G., Hammal, D., & McConachie, H. (2006). Diagnosing autism spectrum disorders in pre-school children using two standardized assessment instruments: The ADI-R and the ADOS. *Journal of Autism and Developmental Disorders, 3*(2), 362–372.

Leary, M. A., & Hill, D. (1996). Moving on: Autism and movement disturbance. *Mental Retardation, 34*, 39–53.

Lee, L. C., Zachary, A. A., Leffell, M. S., Newschaffer, C. J., Matteson, K. J., Tyler, J. D., & Zimmerman, A. W. (2006). HLA-DR4 in families with autism. *Pediatric Neurology, 35*(5), 303–307.

Lee, S., Mian, M. F., Lee, H. J., Kang, C. B., Kim, J. S., Ryu, S. H., et al. (2006). Thimerosal induces oxidative stress in HeLaS epithelial cells. *Environmental Toxicology and Pharmacology, 22*(2), 194–199.

Leimbach, M. (2006). *Daniel isn't talking*. New York: Anchor Books.

Leong, C. C. W., Syed, N. I., & Lorscheider, F. L. (2001). Retrograde degeneration of neurite membrane structural integrity of nerve growth cones following in vitro exposure to mercury. *Neuroreport, 12*(4), 733–737.

Leslie, D. L., Kozma, L., Martin, A., Landeros, A., Katsovich, L., King, R. A., & Leckman, J. F. (2008). Neuropsychiatric disorders associated with streptococcal infection: A case-control study among privately insured children. *Journal of the American Academy of Child and Adolescent Psychiatry, 4*(10), 1166–1172.

Lessac, M. (Director/Writer), & Litz, R. J. (Story). (1993). *House of Cards* [Motion picture]. United States: A&M Films.

Leung, R. (2004, September 29). When Jerry met Mary. Retrieved June 10, 2009, from http://www.cbsnews.com/stories/2004/09/29/60II/main646311.shtml

Levine, R. S. (2008, September 3). Study firmly shows no connection between measles, mumps, rubella (MMR) vaccine and autism. Retrieved June 10, 2009, from http://www.mailmanschool.org/news/display.asp?id=666

Levy, S. E., Souders, M. C., Ittenbach, R. F., Giarelli, E., Mulberg, A. E., & Pinto-Martin, J. A. (2007). Relationship of dietary intake to gastrointestinal symptoms in children with autistic spectrum disorders. *Biological Psychiatry, 61*, 492–497.

Liang, H., Wang, X., Chen, H., Song, L., Ye, L., Wang, S. H., Wang, Y. J., Zhou, L., & Ho, W. Z. (2008). Methamphetamine enhances HIV infection of macrophages. *American Journal of Pathology, 1*(6), 1617–1624.

Lieberman, S. (2003, February 6). Homeland security vs. vaccine immunity. Retrieved June 10, 2009, from http://realtytimes.com/rtpages/20030206_homeland.htm

Lienhard, J. H. (1988–1997). Engines of ingenuity, No. 622: Ignaz Philipp Semmelweis. Retrieved June 10, 2009, from http://www.uh.edu/engines/epi622.htm

Lima, P. D. L., Leite, D. S., Vasconcellos, M. C., Cavalcanti, B. C., Santos, R. A., Costa-Lotufo, L. V., et al. (2007). Genotoxic effects of aluminum chloride in cultured human lymphocytes treated in different phases of cell cycle. *Food and Chemical Toxicology, 45*(7), 1154–1159.

Lincoln, A. (1861). Annual Message to Congress. Retrieved June 10, 2009, from http://www.infoplease.com/t hist/state-of-the-union/73.html

Lonsdale, D. (2001). Sudden infant death syndrome requires genetic predisposition, some form of stress and marginal malnutrition. *Medical Hypotheses, 57*(3), 382–386.

Loren, K., & D. B. Harris (1998, January). Interview with Denham Harman. Retrieved June 10, 2009, from http://www.karlloren.com/biopsy/p61.htm

Lovely, T. J., Levin, D. E., & Klekowski, E. (1982). Light-induced genetic toxicity of thimerosal and benzalko nium chloride in commercial contact-lens solutions. *Mutation Research, 101*(1), 11–18.

Lowe, T. L., Cohen, D. J., Miller, S., & Young, J. G. (1981). Folic-acid and B-12 in autism and neuropsychiatric disturbances of childhood. *Journal of the American Academy of Child and Adolescent Psychiatry, 20*(1), 104–111.

Lower, R., Lower, J., & Kurth, R. (1996). The viruses in all of us: Characteristics and biological significance of human endogenous retrovirus sequences. *Proceedings of the National Academy of Sciences of the United States of America, 9*(11), 5177–5184.

Mahmoud, A. A. F. (1999, July 7). Letter from Merck's president to CDC director to Dr. Jeffrey P. Koplan. Retrieved June 10, 2009, from http://www.putchildrenfirst.org/media/2.3.pdf

Makani, S., Gollapudi, S., Yel, L., Chiplunkar, S., & Gupta, S. (2002). Biochemical and molecular basis of thimerosal-induced apoptosis in T cells: AA major role of mitochondrial pathway. *Genes and Immunity, 3*(5), 270–278.

Mal'tsev, P. V. (1972). Granosan poisoning in children. *Feldsher Akush, 37*, 14–16.

Mamishi, S., Shahmahmoudi, S., Tabatabaie, H., Teimourian, S., Pourakbari, B., Gheisari, Y., et al. (2008). Novel BTK mutation presenting with vaccine-associated paralytic poliomyelitis. *European Journal of Pediatrics, 1*(11), 1335–1338.

Manzi, B., Loizzo, A. L., Giana, G., & Curatolo, P. (2008). Autism and metabolic diseases. *Journal of Child Neurology, 2*(3), 307–314.

Marks, H. H., Powell, H. M., & Jamieson, W. A. (1932). Merthiolate as a skin disinfecting agent. *Journal of Laboratory and Clinical Medicine, 18*, 443–449.

Marn-Pernat, A., Buturovic-Ponikvar, J., Logar, M., Horvat, M., & Ponikvar, R. (2005). Increased ethyl mercury load in protein A immuno adsorption. *Therapeutic Apheresis and Dialysis, 9*(3), 254–257.

Marques, R. C., Dorea, J. G., Fonseca, M. F., Bastos, W. R., & Malm, O. (2007). Hair mercury in breast-fed infants exposed to thimerosal-preserved vaccines. *European Journal of Pediatrics, 166*(9), 935–941.

Marr, J. S. (2005). Book review, *War epidemics: An historical geography of infectious diseases in military conflict and civil strife, 1850–2000.* Retrieved June 10, 2009, from http://www.medscape.com/viewarticle/ 500064

Marsh, D. O., Clarkson, T. W., Cox, C., Myers, G. J., Aminzaki, L., & Altikriti, S. (1987). Fetal methylmercury poisoning: Relationship between concentration in single strands of maternal hair and child effects. *Archives of Neurology, 44*(10), 1017–1022.

Masataka, N. (1995). The relation between index-finger extension and the acoustic quality of cooing in 3-month old infants. *Journal of Child Language, 22*, 247–257.

Matheson, D. S., Clarkson, T. W., & Gelfand, E. W. (1980). Mercury toxicity (acrodynia) induced by long term injection of gammaglobulin. *Journal of Pediatrics, 97*, 153–155.

Matsumoto, H., & Takeuchi, T. (1965). Fetal Minamata disease.: A neurological study of two cases of intrau terine intoxication by a methyl mercury compound. *Journal of Neuropathology & Experimental Neurology 24*, 563–574.

McCarthy, J. (2007a, September 18). Jenny McCarthy talks to Oprah about autism and her book *Louder than words: A mother's journey in healing autism.* New York: Dutton.

McCarthy, J. (2007b). Retrieved June 10, 2009, from http://www.livevideo.com/video/IndependentFreePress/ 8722430613AA40E2BDCAE75A699302D6/jenny-mccarthy-and-holly-peete.aspx; still pictures retrieved June 10, 2009, from http://www.oprah.com/dated/oprahshow/oprahshow_20070918

McCarthy, J. (2007c, September 26). Talk About Curing Autism (TACA): An introduction for new parents. Retrieved June 10, 2009, from http://www.youtube.com/watch?v=zVZDPrgwZ78&NR=1

McCarthy, J. (2007d, November 10). Take the Crap Out of Vaccines. Retrieved June 10, 2009, from http://www.youtube.com/watch?v=Tah7PLj8sAk&feature=user

McCarthy, J. (2008). *Mother warriors: A nation of parents healing autism against all odds*. New York: Dutton.

McCarthy, J., & Kartzinel, J. (2009). *Healing and preventing autism*. New York: Penguin Group.

McComsey, G. A., Libutti, D. E., O'Riordan, M., Shelton, J. M., Storer, N., Ganz, J., et al. (2008). Mitochondrial RNA and DNA alterations in HIV lipoatrophy are linked to antiretroviral therapy and not to HIV infection. *Antiviral Therapy, 1*(5), 715–722.

McDonald, K. L., Huq, S. I., Lix, L. M., Becker, A. B., & Kozyrskyj, A. L. (2008). Delay in diphtheria, pertussis, tetanus vaccination is associated with a reduced risk of childhood asthma. *Journal of Allergy and Clinical Immunology, 1*(3), 626–631.

McElwain, J. (2006, February 27). Jason McElwain autistic basketball player. Retrieved June 10, 2009, from http://www.youtube.com/watch?v=1fw1CcxCUgg

McGovern, C. (2006). *Eye contact*. New York: Penguin.

McHugh, L., Barnes-Holmes, Y., & Barnes-Holmes, D. (2004). Perspective-taking as relational responding: A developmental profile. *Psychological Record, 5*(1), 115–144.

McMahon, A. W., Iskander, J. K., Haber, P., Braun, M. M., & Ball, R. (2008). Inactivated influenza vaccine (IIV) in children <2 years of age: Examination of selected adverse events reported to the Vaccine Adverse Event Reporting System (VAERS) after thimerosal-free or thimerosal-containing vaccine. *Vaccine, 26*(3), 427–429.

Medical Hypotheses. (2009). Science Direct Web site. Retrieved June 10, 2009, from http://www.sciencedirect.com/science/journal/03069877

Melchart, D., Vogt, S., Kohler, W., Streng, A., Weidenhammer, W., Kremers, L., et al. (2008). Treatment of health complaints attributed to amalgam. *Journal of Dental Research, 8*(4), 349–353.

Mercola, J. (2009, April 23). Drug company had hit list for doctors who criticized them. Retrieved June 10, 2009, from http://articles.mercola.com/sites/articles/archive/2009/04/23/Drug-Company-Had-Hit-List-for-Doctors-Who-Criticized-Them.aspx

Mercury element. (2009). Retrieved June 10, 2009, from http://en.wikipedia.org/wiki/Mercury_(element)

Micali, N., Chakrabarti, S., & Fombonne, E. (2004). The broad autism phenotype: Findings from an epidemiological survey. *Autism, 8*(1), 21–37.

Miller, G. A. (1956). The magical number 7, plus or minus 2: Some limits on our capacity for processing information. *Psychological Review, 63*, 81–97. Retrieved June 10, 2009, from http://www.musanim.com/miller1956/

Miller, G. M. (Director/Writer), & Enright, N. (Writer). (1992). *Lorenzo's oil* [Motion picture]. Universal Pictures.

Miller, H., Zhang, J., KuoLee, R., Patel, G. B., & Chen, W. (2007, March 14). Intestinal M cells: The fallible sentinels? *World Journal of Gastroenterology, 13*(10), 1477–1486.

Minamata disease. (2009). Retrieved June 10, 2009, from http://en.wikipedia.org/wiki/Minamata_disease

Minami, T., Oda, K., Gima, N., & Yamazaki, H. (2007). Effects of lipopolysaccharide and chelator on mercury content in the cerebrum of thimerosal-administered mice. *Environmental Toxicology and Pharmacology, 24*(3), 316–320.

Ming, X., Stein, T. P., Brimacombe, M., Johnson, W. G., Lambert, G. H., & Wagner, G. C. (2005). Increased excretion of a lipid peroxidation biomarker in autism. *Prostaglandins Leukotrienes and Essential Fatty Acids, 73*(5), 379–384.

Mintz, M. (1994). Clinical comparison of adult and pediatric neuroAIDS. *Advances in Neuroimmunology, 4*(3), 207–221.

Mitchell, J. (2008, November 22). Insurance coverage: Salvation or harm for autistics? Retrieved May 26, 2009, from http://autismgadfly.blogspot.com/2008/11/insurance-coverage-salvation-or-harm.html

Mitchell, S. (2007, February 8). Global vaccine market to top 23 billion dollars. Terra Daily: News about Planet Earth. United Press International. Retrieved June 11, 2009, from http://www.terradaily.com/reports/Global_Vaccine_Market_To_Top_23_Billion_Dollars_999.html

Money, J., Bobrow, N. A., & Clarke, C. F. (1971). Autism and autoimmune disease: A family study. *Journal o Autism and Childhood Schizophrenia, 1,* 146–160.

Moore, V. (2007, May 4). Christian, the lion who lived in my London living room. Retrieved June 10, 2009 from http://www.dailymail.co.uk/femail/article-452820/Christian-lion-lived-London-living-room.html

Morris, C. W. (1958). Words without meaning: A review of B. F. Skinner's *Verbal behavior. Contemporar Psychology, 3,* 212–214.

Morton, D. (2008). Deafness and autism. *Odyssey: New Directions in Deaf Education, 9*(1), 4–5.

Morton, H. E., North, L. L., & Engley, F. B. (1948). The bacteriostatic and bactericidal actions of some mercu rial compounds on hemolytic streptococci: In vivo and in vitro studies. *Journal of the American Medica Association, 136,* 37–41.

Mosmann, T. R., Cherwinski, H., Bond, M. W., Giedlin, M. A., & Coffman, R. L. (1986, April 1). Two type of murine helper T cell clone. I. Definition according to profiles of lymphokine activities and secreted proteins *Journal of Immunology, 136*(7), 2348–2357.

Mostaghimi, A., Levison, J. H., Leffert, R., Ham, W., Nathoo, A., Halamka, J., et al. (2006). The doctor's new black bag: Instructional technology and the tools of the 21st century physician. *Medical Education Onlin [serial online], 11.* Retrieved June 10, 2009, from http://www.med-ed-online.org

Moumen, R., Nouvelot, A., Duval, D., Lechevalier, B., & Viader, F. (1997). Plasma superoxide dismutase and glutathione peroxidase activity in sporadic amyotrophic lateral sclerosis. *Journal of the Neurological Sciences 151*(1), 35–39.

Mouridsen, S. E., Hansen, H. B., Rich, B., & Isager, T. (2008). Mortality and causes of death in autism spectrum disorders: An update. *Autism, 1*(4), 403–414.

Mouridsen, S. E., Rich, B., Isager, T., & Nedergaard, N. J. (2008). Psychiatric disorders in the parents o individuals with infantile autism: A case-control study. *Psychopathology, 4*(3), 166–171.

Moy, S. S., & Nadler, J. J. (2008). Advances in behavioral genetics: Mouse models of autism. *Molecula Psychiatry, 13*(1), 4–26.

Moynihan, R. (2008, June 21). Drug marketing: Key opinion leaders: Independent experts or drug representa tives in disguise? *British Medical Journal, 336,* 1402–1403. Retrieved June 10, 2009, from http://www.bmj com/cgi/content/short/336/7658/1402

MSNBC *Nightly News.* (2008). Autism: The hidden epidemic. Search for a cure (featuring Jonathan Shestacl and Dov). Retrieved June 10, 2009, from http://www.msnbc.msn.com/id/21134540/vp/7013684#7013684

MSNBC.com News Services. (2007, May 18). Destruction of smallpox virus delayed again: U.N. won't decide on fate of remaining stockpiles for at least four years. Retrieved June 10, 2009, from http://www.msnbc.msn com/id/18737208/

Muhle, R., Trentacoste, S. V., & Rapin, I. (2004). The genetics of autism. *Pediatrics, 113*(5), E472-E486.

Mukai, N. (1972). An experimental study of alkylmercurial encephalopathy. *Acta Neuropathologica, 72* 102–109.

Mukhtarova, N.D. (1977). Late sequelae of nervous system pathology caused by the action of low concentra tions of ethyl mercury chloride. *Gigiena Truda I Professionalnye Zabolevaniia, 3,* 4–7.

Müller, P. H. (1948). Nobel Prize in Physiology or Medicine 1948: For his discovery of the high efficiency o DDT as a contact poison against several arthropods. Retrieved June 10, 2009, from http://nobelprize.org nobel_prizes/medicine/laureates/1948/

Munoz, A., Abarca, K., Jimenez, J., Luchsinger, V., O'Ryan, M., Ripoll, E. R., et al. (2007). Safety of thimerosa containing vaccines. Statement of the Consultive Committee of Immunizations on behalf of the Chilear Infectious Diseases Society. *Revista Chilena de Infectologia, 24*(5), 372–376.

Mutter, J., Naumann, J., & Guethlin, C. (2007). Comments on the article "The toxicology of mercury and its chemical compounds" by Clarkson and Magos (2006). *Critical Reviews in Toxicology, 37*(6), 537–549.

Mutter, J., Naumann, J., Sadaghiani, C., Walach, H., & Drasch, G. (2004). Amalgam studies: Disregarding basic principles of mercury toxicity. *International Journal of Hygiene and Environmental Health, 207*(4) 391–397.

Mutter, J., Naumann, J., Schneider, R., Walach, H., & Haley, B. (2005). Mercury and autism: Accelerating evidence? *Neuroendocrinology Letters, 26*(5), 439–446.

Mutter, J., Naumann, J., Walach, H., & Daschner, F. (2005). Amalgam risk assessment with coverage of references up to 2005. *Gesundheitswesen, 67*(3), 204–216.

The Myelin Project. (2009). Retrieved June 10, 2009, from http://www.myelin.org/en/cms/?14

Nash, A. G. (1973). Diathermy burn hazard. *British Medical Journal, 4*(5895), 783.

Nash, J. F. (2002). Interview with John Nash: Misconceptions about mental illness. Retrieved June 10, 2009, from http://www.pbs.org/wgbh/amex/nash/sfeature/sf_nash_07.html

Nash, J. F. (2009). Portrayal in *A Beautiful Mind* (film). Retrieved June 10, 2009, from http://en.wikipedia.org/wiki/A_Beautiful_Mind_(film)

Nataf, R., Skorupka, C., Amet, L., Lam, A., Springbett, A., & Lathe, R. (2006). Porphyrinuria in childhood autistic disorder: Implications for environmental toxicity. *Toxicology and Applied Pharmacology, 214,* 99–108.

National Institute of Allergy and Infectious Diseases (NIAID). (2008, March). Research on thimerosal. Retrieved June 10, 2009, from http://www.niaid.nih.gov/factsheets/thimerosal.htm

National Institute of Mental Health (NIMH). (2008, April 3). Autism spectrum disorders (pervasive developmental disorders). Retrieved June 10, 2009, from http://www.nimh.nih.gov/health/publications/autism/complete-index.shtml

National Public Radio (NPR). (2007, August 16). Parents fight for autism insurance coverage. Retrieved June 10, 2009, from http://www.npr.org/templates/story/story.php?storyId=12829221

National Vaccine Injury Compensation Program. (n.d.). Retrieved June 10, 2009, from http://www.hrsa.gov/vaccinecompensation/persons_eligible.htm

NBC6.net. (2008, March 31). Children with autism swim with dolphins. Retrieved February 6, 2009, from http://www.nbc6.net/autism/15734230/detail.html

Needleman, H. L. (2006). Mercury in dental amalgam—A neurotoxic risk? *Journal of the American Medical Association, 2*(15), 1835–1836.

Nelson, E. A., & Gottshall, R. Y. (1967). Enhanced toxicity for mice of pertussis vaccines when preserved with Merthiolate. *Applied Microbiology, 15,* 590–593.

Ness, P. (Director), & Bass, R. (Writer). (2005). *Mozart and the Whale* [Motion Picture]. United States: Big City Pictures.

Newschaffer, C. J. (2006). Diagnostic substitution and autism prevalence trends. *Pediatrics, 117*(4), 1436–1437.

Newschaffer, C. J., Falb, M. D., & Gurney, J. G. (2005). National autism prevalence trends from United States special education data. *Pediatrics, 115*(3), e277–e282.

Nielsen, J. B., & Andersen, O. (1995). A comparison of the lactational and transplacental deposition of mercury in offspring from methylmercury-exposed mice: Effect of seleno-l-methionine. *Toxicology Letters, 76*(2), 165–171.

Nierenberg, D. W., Nordgren, R. E., Cang, M. B., Siegler, R. W., Blayney, M. G., Hochberg, F. W., et al. (1998). Delayed cerebellar disease and death after accidental exposure to dimethylmercury. *New England Journal of Medicine, 338,* 1672–1675.

Nishida, H., Kushida, M., Nakajima, Y., Ogawa, Y., Tatewaki, N., Sato, S., & Konishi, T. (2007). Amyloid-beta-induced cytotoxicity of PC-12 cell was attenuated by Shengmai-san through redox regulation and outgrowth induction. *Journal of Pharmacological Sciences, 104*(1), 73–81.

Nizov, A. A., & Shestakov, H. M. (1971). Contribution to the clinical aspects of Granosan poisoning. *Soviet Medicine, 11,* 150–152.

Novella, S. (2008, February 29). Has the government conceded vaccines cause autism? Published by Steven Novella under Neuroscience, Science and Medicine. Retrieved June 10, 2009, from http://www.theness.com/neurologicablog/index.php?p=203

Nuland, S. B. (2003). *The doctors' plague: Germs, childbed fever and the strange story of Ignac Semmelweis.* New York: W. W. Norton.

Nunnally, J. C. (1967). *Psychometric theory.* New York: McGraw-Hill.

O'Connor, A. M., Wennberg, J. E., Legare, F., Llewellyn-Thomas, H. A., Moulton, B. W., Sepucha, K. R. S., et al. (2007). Toward the "tipping point": Decision aids and informed patient choice. *Health Affairs, 26*(3), 716–725.

Odone, A. (2007–2009). The myelin project. Retrieved June 10, 2009, from http://www.myelin.org/

O'Garra, A., Stockinger, B., & Veldhoen, M. (2008, June). Differentiation of human T-H-17 cells does require TGF-beta! *Nature Immunology*, 9(6), 588–590.

Office of Environmental Management/Risk Assessment Information System. (2005, March 17). Toxicity summary for mercury. Retrieved June 10, 2009, from http://rais.ornl.gov/tox/profiles/mercury_f_V1.shtml

Office of Special Masters. (OSM). (2002, July 3). Autism General Order # 1. Retrieved June 10, 2009, from http://www.uscfc.uscourts.gov/sites/default/files/autism/Autism+General+Order1.pdf

Office of Special Masters (OSM). (2007, July 20). Bailey Banks, by his father, Kenneth Banks v. Secretary of Health and Human Services (02-0738V). Retrieved June 10, 2009, from http://www.uscfc.uscourts.gov/docket-omnibus-autism-proceeding

Office of Special Masters (OSM). (2008a, April 10). Hannah Poling, a minor, by her parents and natural guardians, Terry Poling v. Secretary of Health and Human Services (02-146V). Retrieved June 10, 2009, from http://www.uscfc.uscourts.gov/sites/default/files/CAMPBELL-SMITH.POLING041008.pdf

Office of Special Masters (OSM). (2008b, August 29). Docket of Omnibus Autism Proceeding. Retrieved June 10, 2009, from http://www.uscfc.uscourts.gov/docket-omnibus-autism-proceeding

Office of Special Masters (OSM). (2009, April 23). Docket of Omnibus Autism Proceeding. Retrieved June 10, 2009, from http://www.uscfc.uscourts.gov/sites/default/files/autism/master_autism_4_23_09.pdf

Offit, P. A. (2007). Thimerosal and vaccines: A cautionary tale. *New England Journal of Medicine*, 357(13) 1278–1279.

Offit, P. A. (2008). *Autism's false prophets: Bad science, risky medicine, and the search for a cure*. New York Columbia University Press. Review by himself, retrieved August 3, 2009, from http://www.youtube.com/watch?v=MTr-HLz7dPc

Offit, P. A. & Jew, R. K. (2003). Addressing parents' concerns: Do vaccines contain harmful preservatives, adjuvants, additives, or residuals? *Pediatrics*, 112(6), 1394–1397.

Offit, P. A., Quarles, J., Gerber, M. A., Hackett, C. J., Marcuse, E. K., Kollman, T. R. S., et al. (2002). Addressing parents' concerns: Do multiple vaccines overwhelm or weaken the infant's immune system? *Pediatrics* 109(1), 124–129.

Oharazawa, H. (1968). Effect of ethylmercuric phosphate in the pregnant mouse on chromosome abnormalities and fetal malformation. *Journal of the Japanese Obstetrics & Gynecological Society*, 20 1479–1487.

Oliveira, G., Ataide, A., Marques, C., Miguel, T. S., Coutinho, A. M., Mota-Vieira, L. M., et al. (2007) Epidemiology of autism spectrum disorder in Portugal: Prevalence, clinical characterization, and medical conditions. *Developmental Medicine and Child Neurology*, 49(10), 726–733.

Oliveira, G., Diogo, L., Grazina, M., Garcia, P., Ataide, A., Marques, C. R., et al. (2005). Mitochondrial dysfunction in autism spectrum disorders: A population-based study. *Developmental Medicine and Child Neurology*, 47(3), 185–189.

Olivieri, G., Novakovic, M., Savaskan, E., Meier, F., Baysang, G., Brockhaus, M., & Muller-Spahn, F. (2002). The effects of beta-estradiol on SHSY5Y neuroblastoma cells during heavy metal induced oxidative stress, neurotoxicity and beta-amyloid secretion. *Neuroscience*, 113(4), 849–855.

Oller, D. K., Eilers, R. E., & Basinger, D. (2001). Intuitive identification of infant vocal sounds by parents. *Developmental Science*, 4(1), 49–60.

Oller, D. K., & Lynch, M. P. (1992). Infant vocalizations and innovations in infraphonology: Toward a broader theory of development and disorders. In C. F. Ferguson, L. Menn, & C. S. Gammon (Eds.), *Phonological development: Models, research, implications* (pp. 509–536). Timonium, MD: York.

Oller, J. W., Jr. (1993). Reasons why some methods work. In J. W. Oller, Jr. (Ed.), *Methods that work: Ideas for literacy and language teachers* (pp. 374–385). Boston, MA: Heinle and Heinle.

Oller, J. W., Jr. (1996a). How grammatical relations are determined. In B. Hoffer (Ed.), *The 22nd Linguistic Association of Canada and the United States (LACUS) forum, 1995* (pp. 37–88). Chapel Hill, NC: Linguistic Association of Canada and the United States.

Oller, J. W., Jr. (1996b). Semiotic theory applied to free will, relativity, and determinacy: Or why the unified field theory sought by Einstein could not be found. *Semiotica*, 108(3/4), 199–244.

Oller, J. W., Jr., & Chen, L. (2007). Episodic organization in discourse and valid measurement in the sciences. *Journal of Quantitative Linguistics*, 14(2&3), 127–144.

Oller, J. W., Jr., Chen, L., Oller, S. D., & Pan, N. (2005). Empirical predictions from a general theory of signs. *Discourse Processes, 40*(2), 115–144.

Oller, J. W., Jr., & Giardetti, J. R. (1999). *Images that work: Creating successful messages in marketing and high stakes.* Westport, CT: Quorum Books.

Oller, J. W., Jr., Oller, S. D., & Badon, L. C. (2010). *Cases: Introducing communication disorders across the life span.* San Diego: Plural.

Oller, J. W., Jr., Oller, S. D., & Badon, L. C. (2006). *Milestones: Normal speech and language development across the life span.* San Diego: Plural.

Oller, J. W., Jr., & Rascón, D. (1999). Applying sign theory to autism. *Clinical Linguistics and Phonetics, 13*(2), 77–112.

Oller, S. D. (2005). Meaning matters: An application of a general theory of signs to language intervention. *Journal of Communication Disorders, 38*(5), 359–373.

Oller, S. D., & Oller, S. A. (2008a, November). Assessing ASDs using the individual's representational capacity: Reliability based on student and SLP ratings. Short course presented at the American Speech-Language and Hearing Association Annual Meeting in Chicago.

Oller, S. D., & Oller, S. A. (2008b, November). Intervention for ASDs using an individual's representational capacity: Working within the zone of proximal development. Short course presented at the American Speech-Language and Hearing Association Annual Meeting in Chicago.

Olsen, G. L. (2005). *Confessions of an Rx drug pusher: God's call to loving arms.* Lincoln, NE: Universe Books.

Olsen, G. L. (2007). Ex drug rep manipulating doctors. Retrieved June 10, 2009, from http://www.youtube.com/watch?v=kOW8LNU2hFE

Onal, A. E., Gurses, C., Direskeneli, G. S., Yilmaz, G., Demirbilek, V., Yentur, S. P., et al. (2006). Subacute sclerosing panencephalitis surveillance study in Istanbul. *Brain & Development, 2*(3), 183–189.

Orenstein, W. A. (2001). Immunization Safety Review Committee Institute of Medicine: Charge to the committee. Retrieved June 10, 2009, from http://www.iom.edu/Object.File/Master/7/743/Orenstein%20IOMSafetyReviewCharge.pdf

Oshinsky, D. M. (2005). *Polio: An American story.* New York: Oxford University Press.

Oshinsky, D. M., & Dentzer, S. (2005, April 12). *PBS Online NewsHour*: The battle against polio. Retrieved June 10, 2009, from http://www.pbs.org/newshour/bb/health/jan-june06/polio_4-24.html

Oskarsson, A., Schutz, A., Skerfving, S., Hallen, I. P., & Lagerkvist, B. J. (1996). Total and inorganic mercury in breast milk and blood in relation to fish consumption and amalgam fillings in lactating women. *Archives of Environmental Health, 51*(3), 234–241.

Oslejskova, H., Dusek, L., Makovska, Z., Dujickova, E., Autrata, R., & Slapak, I. (2008a). Complicated relationship between autism with regression and epilepsy. *Neuroendocrinology Letters, 2*(4), 558–570.

Oslejskova, H., Dusek, L., Makovska, Z., Dujickova, E., Autrata, R., & Slapak, I. (2008b). The incidence of epileptic seizures and/or epileptiform EEG abnormalities in children with childhood and atypical autism. *Ceska a Slovenska Neurologie a Neurochirurgie, 7*(4), 435–444.

Owhadi, H., & Boulos, A. (2008). Bistable equilibrium points of mercury body burden. *Journal of Biological Systems, 16*(1), 139–150.

Oxford University Press. (2006, April 20). Oshinsky wins the Pulitzer Prize for History. Retrieved June 10, 2009, from http://www.oup.co.uk/news/archive/oshinsky

Pabello, N. G., & Lawrence D. A. (2006). Neuroimmunotoxicology: Modulation of neuroimmune networks by toxicants. *Clinical Neuroscience Research, 6*(1–2), 69–85.

Palkovicova, L., Ursinyova, M., Masanova, V., Yu, Z. W., & Hertz-Picciotto, I. (2008). Maternal amalgam dental fillings as the source of mercury exposure in developing fetus and newborn. *Journal of Exposure Science and Environmental Epidemiology, 18*(3), 326–331.

Palomo, T., Archer, T., Beninger, R. J., & Kostrzewa, R. M. (2004). Gene–environment interplay in neurogenesis and neurodegeneration. *Neurotoxicity Research, 6*(6), 415–434.

Palomo, T., Beninger, R. J., Kostrzewa, R. M., & Archer, T. (2003). Brain sites of movement disorder: Genetic and environmental agents in neurodevelopmental perturbations. *Neurotoxicity Research, 5*(1–2), 1–26.

Palop, J. J., Chin, J., & Mucke, L. (2006). A network dysfunction perspective on neurodegenerative disease. *Nature, 4*(7113), 768–773.

Pan, N., & Chen, L. (2005). Phonological/phonemic awareness and reading: A crosslinguistic perspective. *Journal of Multilingual Communication Disorders, 3*(2), 145–152.

Pangborn, J. (2005). Molecular aspects of autism. In J. Pangborn & S. M. Baker, *Autism: Effective biomedical treatments—Have we done everything we can for this child? Individuality in an epidemic* (pp. 149–188). San Diego, CA: Autism Research Institute.

Pangborn, J. (2007). Autism in perspective. In J. Pangborn & S. M. Baker, 2007 Supplement to 2005 Edition of *Autism: Effective biomedical treatments—Have we done everything we can for this child? Individuality in an epidemic* (pp. 35–37). San Diego, CA: Autism Research Institute.

Pangborn, J., & Baker, S. M. (2005). *Autism: Effective biomedical treatments—Have we done everything we can for this child? Individuality in an epidemic.* San Diego, CA: Autism Research Institute.

Pangborn, J., & Baker, S. M. (2007). Supplement to *Autism: Effective biomedical treatments—Have we done everything we can for this child? Individuality in an epidemic.* San Diego, CA: Autism Research Institute.

Papadopulos-Eleopulos, E., Turner, V. F., & Papadimitriou, J. M. (1993). Has Gallo proven the role of HIV in AIDS? *Emergency Medicine, 5*(2), 113–123.

Pardo, C. A., & Eberhart, C. G. (2007). The neurobiology of autism. *Brain Pathology, 17*(4), 434–447.

Parker, S. K., Schwartz, B., Todd, J., & Pickering, L. K. (2004). Thimerosal-containing vaccines and autistic spectrum disorder: A critical review of published original data. *Pediatrics, 114*(3), 793–804.

Parran, D. K., Barker, A., & Ehrich, M. (2005). Effects of thimerosal on NGF signal transduction and cell death in neuroblastoma cells. *Toxicological Science, 1*, 132–140.

Parry, L. A. (1928, January 21). Fatality rates of small-pox in the vaccinated and unvaccinated. *British Medical Journal, 1*, 116. Retrieved June 10, 2009, from http://www.bmj.com/cgi/reprint/1/3498/116

Pasca, S. P., Nemes, B., Vlase, L., Gagyi, C. E., Dronca, E., Miu, A. C., & Dronca, M. (2006). High levels of homocysteine and low serum paraoxonase 1 arylesterase activity in children with autism. *Life Sciences 78*(19), 2244–2248.

Pasteur, L. (n.d.). Reflections on my life. Retrieved June 10, 2009, from http://www.woodrow.org/teachers/ci/1992/Pasteur.html

Pasteur, L. (1864, April 23). On spontaneous generation: An address delivered by Louis Pasteur at the "Sorbonne Scientific Soirée" of April 7, 1864. *Revue des cours scientifics, I* (1863–1864,) 257–264. English translation incorporating Pasteur's handwritten corrections commissioned 1993 by Bruno Latour and copyrighted 1993 by Alex Levine. Retrieved June 10, 2009, from http://shell.cas.usf.edu/~alevine/pasteur.pdf

Patel, R. J., Patel, G. C., Patel, M. M., & Patel, N. J. (2007). HIV infection and tuberculosis. *Indian Journal of Pharmaceutical Education and Research, 4*(2), 95–101.

Pausch, R. (2007, September 18). The "last lecture." Retrieved June 10, 2009, from http://download.srv.cs.cmu.edu/~pausch/

PBS. (1995). Plague war interview: Dr. Kantjan Alibekov. Retrieved June 10, 2009, from http://www.pbs.org/wgbh/pages/frontline/shows/plague/interviews/alibekov.html

Pearce, R. K. B., Owen, A., Daniel, S., Jenner, P., & Marsden, C. D. Alterations in the distribution of glutathione in the substantia nigra in Parkinson's disease. *Journal of Neural Transmission, 104*(6–7), 661–677.

Peirce, C. S. (1897). The logic of relatives. *The Monist, 7*, 161–217. Also in C. Hartshorne & P. Weiss (Eds.) (1932), *Collected Papers of C. S. Peirce* (Vol. 2, pp. 288–345). Cambridge, MA: Harvard University Press.

Pereira, C. F., & Oliveira, C. R. (2000). Oxidative glutamate toxicity involves mitochondrial dysfunction and perturbation of intracellular Ca2+ homeostasis. *Neuroscience Research, 37*(3), 227–236.

Pertussis. (2009, February 3). Retrieved June 10, 2009, from http://en.wikipedia.org/wiki/Pertussis

Pesticide Action Network of North America. (2006). PAN pesticides database—California pesticide use. Retrieved June 10, 2009, from http://www.pesticideinfo.org/Search_Use.jsp

Phillips, M. (2009, February 27). Another ruling in the US vaccine court. Retrieved June 10, 2009, from http://www.spectator.co.uk/melaniephillips/3395891/another-ruling-in-the-us-vaccine-court.thtml

Pier, G. B., Lyczak, J. B., & Wetzler, L. M. (2004). *Immunology, infection, and immunity.* Washington, DC: ASM Press.

Platt, J. R. (1964). Strong inference. *Science, 146*(3642), 348–353. Retrieved June 10, 2009, from http://256.com/gray/docs/strong_inference.html

Pliny the Younger. (AD 62?–ca. AD 113). To Caninus. In *Letters: The Harvard Classics* (1909–1914), CVII. Retrieved June 10, 2009, from http://www.bartleby.com/9/4/1107.html

Pomeroy, J. C., Friedman, C., & Stephens, L. (1991). Autism and Asperger's: Same or different? *Journal of the Academy of Child and Adolescent Psychiatry, 29,* 152.

Popovic, M., Sarngadharan, M. G., Read, E., & Gallo, R. C. (1984). Detection, isolation, and continuous production of cytopathic retroviruses (HTLV-III) from patients with AIDS and pre-AIDS. *Science, 224,* 497–500.

Popper, K. (1959). *The logic of scientific discovery.* New York: Harper.

Posserud, M. B., Lundervold, A. J., & Gillberg, C. (2006). Autistic features in a total population of 7–9-year-old children assessed by the ASSQ (Autism Spectrum Screening Questionnaire). *Journal of Child Psychology and Psychiatry, 47*(2), 167–175.

Pouchet, F., & Houzeau, M. (1858). Expériences sur les générations spontanées: Deuxième partie: Développement de certains proto-organismes dans l'air artificiel. [Experiments on spontaneous generation: Part 2: Development of certain proto-organisms in artificial air.] *Comptes Rendus de l'Académie des Sciences, 47,* 982–984.

Powell, H. M., & Jamieson, W. A. (1931). Merthiolate as a germicide. *American Journal of Hygiene, 13,* 296–310.

Premack, D. G., & Woodruff, G. (1978). Does the chimpanzee have a theory of mind? *Behavioral and Brain Sciences, 1,* 515–526.

Public Law 94–142 (S. 6). (1975, November 29). Education for All Handicapped Children. Retrieved June 10, 2009, from http://users.rcn.com/peregrin.enteract/add/94-142.txt; also see http://www.ed.gov/policy/speced/leg/idea/history.html

Putchildrenfirst.org. (2009). Introduction [and linked documents]. Retrieved June 10, 2009, from http://www.putchildrenfirst.org/intro.html

Rampersad, G. C., Suck, G., Sakac, D., Fahim, S., Foo, A., Denomme, G. A., et al. (2005). Chemical compounds that target thiol-disulfide groups on mononuclear phagocytes inhibit immune mediated phagocytosis of red blood cells. *Transfusion, 45*(3), 384–393.

Rapin, I., & Tuchman, R. F. (2008). Autism: Definition, neurobiology, screening, diagnosis. *Pediatric Clinics of North America, 5*(5), 1129–1146.

Razagui, I. B. A., & Haswell, S. J. (2001). Mercury and selenium concentrations in maternal and neonatal scalp hair: Relationship to amalgam-based dental treatment received during pregnancy. *Biological Trace Element Research, 81*(1), 1–19.

Redhead, K., Sesardic, D., Yost, S. E., Attwell, A. M., Watkins, J., Hoy, C. S. J., et al. (1994). Combination of DTP and *Haemophilus influenzae* type B conjugate vaccines can affect laboratory evaluation of potency and immunogenicity. *Biologicals, 22*(4), 339–345.

Reuters. (2008, 23 April). Acambis PLC—ACAM2000 U.S. Government Contract. RNS Number 90205. Retrieved June 10, 2009, from http://www.reuters.com/article/pressRelease/idUS62089+23-Apr-2008+RNS20080423

Richardson, M., Elliman, D., Maguire, H., Simpson, J., & Nicoll, A. (2001). Evidence base of incubation periods, periods of infectiousness and exclusion policies for the control of communicable diseases in schools and preschools. *Pediatric Infectious Disease Journal, 2*(4), 380–391.

Richet, C. (1913). Charles Richet: The Nobel Prize in Physiology or Medicine 1913: Nobel Lecture, December 11, 1913. Retrieved June 10, 2009, from http://nobelprize.org/nobel_prizes/medicine/laureates/1913/richet-lecture.html

Richler, J., Luyster, R., Risi, S., Hsu, W. L., Dawson, G., Bernier, R., et al. (2006). Is there a "regressive 'phenotype'" of autism spectrum disorder associated with the measles–mumps–rubella vaccine? A CPEA study. *Journal of Autism and Developmental Disorders, 3*(3), 299–316.

Rimland, B. (1964). *Infantile autism: The syndrome and its implications for a neural theory of behavior.* New York: Appleton-Century-Crofts.

Rimland, B. (1978). Inside the mind of the autistic savant. *Psychology Today, 12*(3), 69–90.

Rimland, B. (2000). The autism increase: Research needed on the vaccine connection. *Autism Research Review International, 14*(1), 3–6.

Rimland, B. (2005). The history of the Defeat Autism Now! (DAN!) project: How it got started, and why i got started. In J. Pangborn & S. M. Baker, *Autism: Effective biomedical treatments—Have we done everything we can for this child? Individuality in an epidemic* (pp. 6–10). San Diego, CA: Autism Research Institute.

Risk, W. S., & Haddad, F. S. (1979). The variable natural history of subacute sclerosing panencephalitis *Archives of Neurology, 36*, 610–614.

Ritvo, R. A., Ritvo, E. R., Guthrie, D., & Ritvo, M. J. (2008). Clinical evidence that Asperger's disorder is a mild form of autism. *Comprehensive Psychiatry, 49*(1), 1–5.

Ritvo, R. A., Ritvo, E. R., Guthrie, D., Yuwiler, A., Ritvo, M. J., & Weisbender, L. (2008). A scale to assist the diagnosis of autism and Asperger's disorder in adults (RAADS): A pilot study. *Journal of Autism and Developmental Disorders, 38*(2), 213–223.

Roberts, E. M., English, P. B., Grether, J. K., Windharn, G. C., Somberg, L., & Wolff, C. (2008). Maternal residence near agricultural pesticide applications and autism spectrum disorders among children in the California Central Valley. *Environmental Health Perspectives, 1*(10), 1482–1489.

Rock, A. (2004, March/April). Toxic tipping point: Are the CDC, the FDA, and other health agencies covering up evidence that a mercury preservative in childrens' vaccines caused a rise in autism? *Mother Jones* Retrieved June 10, 2009, from http://www.motherjones.com/news/feature/2004/03/02_354.html

Rohyans, J., Walson, P. D., Wood G. A., & Macdonald, W. A. (1984). Mercury toxicity following merthiolate ear irrigations. *Journal of Pediatrics, 104*(2), 311–313.

Rones, N. (2008a, May). What autism does to a mother. *Redbook Magazine*, 172–176.

Rones, N. (2008b, July). We need to pull Ryan into this world. *Redbook Magazine*, 158–162, 166–167.

Rosas, L. G., & Eskenazi, B. (2008). Pesticides and child neurodevelopment. *Current Opinion in Pediatrics 2*(2), 191–197.

Rosenblum, W. I., Nishimura, H., Ellis, E. F., & Nelson, G. H. (1992). The endothelium-dependent effects o thimerosal on mouse pial arterioles invivo: Evidence for control of microvascular events by EDRF as well as prostaglandins. *Journal of Cerebral Blood Flow and Metabolism, 12*(4), 703–706.

Rossignol, D. A. (2007). Hyperbaric oxygen therapy might improve certain pathophysiological findings in autism. *Medical Hypotheses, 68*(6), 1208–1227.

Rotig, A., & Munnich, A. (2003). Genetic features of mitochondrial respiratory chain disorders. *Journal of the American Society of Nephrology, 14*, 2995–3007.

Rout, M. (2009, April 1). Vioxx maker Merck and Company drew up doctor hit list. *The Australian*. Retrieved June 10, 2009, from http://www.infowars.com/merck-drew-up-hit-list-of-doctors-to-be-neutralized/

Ruata, C. (1898, November). Vaccination in Italy [a public lecture at the University of Perugia, Italy]. Retrieved June 10, 2009, from http://www.whale.to/vaccines/ruata_h.html

Ruata, C. (1899, May 10). [Letter written on this date.] Retrieved June 11, 2009, from http://www.whale.to/vaccines/ruata_h.html

Rusiecki, J. A., Baccarelli, A., Bollati, V. Tarantini, L., Moore, L. E., & Bonefeld-Jorgensen, E. C. (2008). Global DNA hypomethylation is associated with high serum-persistent organic pollutants in Greenlandic Inuit *Environmental Health Perspectives, 1*(11), 1547–1552.

Russell, C. A. (2004). Advances in organic chemistry over the last 100 years. *Annual Reports on the Progress of Chemistry Section B (Organic Chemistry), 100*, 3–31.

Rutter, M. (1978). Diagnosis and definition of childhood autism. *Journal of Autism and Developmental Disorders, 8*, 139–161.

RxList. (2009). DTP drug description. Retrieved June 10, 2009, from http://www.rxlist.com/cgi/generic/dtp.htm

Ryan, K. J., & Ray, C. G. (Eds.). (2004). Enteroviruses. *Sherris Medical Microbiology* (4th ed., pp. 535–537). New York: McGraw-Hill.

Sacks, O. W. (1990). *The man who mistook his wife for a hat and other clinical tales*. New York: Harper Perennial Library.

Sacks, O. W. (1993, December 27–1994, January 3). A neurologist's notebook: An anthropologist on Mars. *The New Yorker*, 107–125.

Safeminds.org. (2009). Simpsonwood conference transcript. Retrieved June 10, 2009, from http://www.safeminds.org/legislation/foia/Simpsonwood_Transcript.pdf

Saley, P. L. (1970). Evaluation of slaughter products from Granosan-poisoned animals. *Veterinariya, 46,* 102–103.

Salle, A. J., & Lazarus, A. S. (1935). A comparison of the resistance of bacteria and embryonic tissue to germicidal substances. *Proceedings of the Society for Experimental Biology and Medicine, 32,* 665–667.

Sanford, J. (2005). *Genetic entropy and the mystery of the genome.* San Diego, CA: Ivan.

Sapir, E. (1921). *Language: An introduction to the study of speech.* New York: Harcourt, Brace.

Sarngadharan, M. G., Popovic, M., Bruch, L., Schupbach, J., & Gallo, R. C. (1984). Antibodies reactive to human T-Lymphotrophic retroviruses (HTLV-III) in the serum of patients with AIDS. *Science, 224,* 506–508.

Sass, J. E. (1937). Histological and cytological studies of ethyl mercury phosphate poisoning in corn seedlings. *Phytopathologia, 27,* 95–99.

Schanen, N. C. (2006). Epigenetics of autism spectrum disorders. *Human Molecular Genetics, 15*(2), R138–R150.

Schellenberg, G. D., Dawson, G., Sung, Y. J., Estes, A., Munson, J., Rosenthal, E., et al. (2006). Evidence for multiple loci from a genome scan of autism kindreds. *Molecular Psychiatry, 11*(11), 1049–1060.

Schopenhauer, A. (ca. 1860). Arthur Schopenhauer [1788–1860]. Retrieved June 10, 2009, from http://www. encyclopedia.com/doc/1B1-377961.html

Schupbach, J., Popovic, M., Gilden, R. V., Gonda, M. A., Sarngadharan, M. G., & Gallo, R. C. (1984). Serological analysis of a subgroup of human T-lymphotrophic retroviruses (HTLV-III) associated with AIDS. *Science, 224,* 503–505.

Sears, B. (2009, May 15). Return of separate measles, mumps, rubella vaccines planned for 2011. Retrieved June 10, 2009, from http://www.askdrsears.com/thevaccinebook/

Segarra, A. R., & Murphy, T. K. (2008). Cardiac involvement in children with PANDAS. *Journal of the American Academy of Child and Adolescent Psychiatry, 4*(5), 603–604.

Segura-Aguilar, J., & Kostrzewa, R. M. (2006). Neurotoxins and neurotoxicity mechanisms: An overview. *Neurotoxicity Research, 10*(3–4), 263–287.

Sell, J. Z. (2006). Vaccine litigation update: Althen & beyond. Retrieved June 10, 2009, from http://www. autismone.org/download2006.cfm

Semmelweis, Ignaz. (2009, February 5). Retrieved June 10, 2009, from http://en.wikipedia.org/wiki/ Ignaz_Semmelweis.

Semmelweis, I. P. (1861). *Etiology, concept and prophylaxis of childbed fever [Die Ätiologie, der Begriff und die Prophylaxis des Kindbettfiebers].* (Trans. K. C. Carter). Madison, WI: University of Wisconsin Press.

Semmelweis, I. P. (1862). *Open letter to all professors of obstetrics [Offener Brief an sämtliche Professoren der Geburtshilfe].* Retrieved July 22, 2009, from http://en.wikipedia.org/wiki/File:Ignaz_Semmelweis_1862_ Open_letter.jpg (Originally published in Ofen [Budapest], Hungary: Royal Hungarian University of Buchdruckerei).

Semmelweis Society International. (2009). Retrieved July 22, 2009, from http://www.semmelweis.org/about/ dr-semmelweis-biography/

Servais, V. (2008). Some comments on context embodiment in zootherapy: The case of the Autidolfijn project. *Anthrozoos, 1*(1), 5–15.

Setz, J. M., van der Linde, A. A. A., Gerrits, G. P. J. M., & Meulstee, J. (2008). EEG findings in an eleven-year-old girl with mercury intoxication. *Clinical EEG and Neuroscience, 39*(4), 210–213.

Shanahan, L. (2005–2008). About Stan Kurtz. Retrieved June 10, 2009, from http://www.stankurtz.org/about/ about-stan-kurtz.html

Sharma, S. K., Goloubinoff, P., & Christen, P. (2008). Heavy metal ions are potent inhibitors of protein folding. *Biochemical and Biophysical Research Communications, 372*(1), 341–345.

Shattuck, P. T. (2006). The contribution of diagnostic substitution to the growing administrative prevalence of autism in US special education. *Pediatrics, 117*(4), 1028–1037.

Shaw, G. M., Harper, M. E., Hahn, B. H., Epstein, L. G., Gajdusek, D. C., Price, R. W., et al. (1985). HTLV-III infection in brains of children and adults with AIDS encephalopathy. *Science, 227,* 177–182.

Shestack, J. (2003). The face of autism. Presentation at the Autism Summit Conference in Washington, DC. Retrieved June 10, 2009, from http://www.tvworldwide.com/events/nimh/031119/agenda.cfm

Shevell, M., & Fombonne, E. (2006). Autism and MMR vaccination or thimerosal exposure: An urban legend? *Canadian Journal of Neurological Sciences*, *33*(4), 339–340.

Shi, X. B., Xue, L. R., Tepper, C. G., Gandour-Edwards, R., Ghosh, P., Kung, H. J., & White, R. W. D. (2007). The oncogenic potential of a prostate cancer–derived androgen receptor mutant. *Prostate*, *67*(6), 591–602.

Shustov, V. I. A., & Syganova, S. I. (1970). Clinical aspects of subacute intoxication with *Granosan. Kazanskii Meditsinskii Zhurnal*, *2*, 78–79.

Siegel, M., Fuerst, H. T., & Guinee, V. F. (1971). Rubella epidemicity and embryopathy. Results of a long-term prospective study. *American Journal of Diseases in Children*, *121*(6), 469–473.

Sierles, F. S., Brodkey, A. C., Cleary, L. M., McCurdy, F. A., Mintz, M., Frank, J., Lynn, J., Chao, J., Morgenstern, B. Z., Shore, W., & Woodard, J. L. (2005). Medical students' exposure to and attitudes about drug company interactions: A national survey. *JAMA*, *294*, 1034–1042. Retrieved June 10, 2009, from http://jama.ama-assn.org/cgi/content/short/294/9/1034

Silva, L. M. T., Ayres, R., & Schalock, M. (2008). Outcomes of a pilot training program in a qigong massage intervention for young children with autism. *American Journal of Occupational Therapy*, *6*(5), 538–546.

Silverman, C., & Brosco, J. P. (2008). Understanding autism—Parents and pediatricians in historical perspective. *Archives of Pediatrics & Adolescent Medicine*, *1*(4), 392–398.

Silvers, L. E., Ellenberg, S. S., Wise, R. P., Varricchio, F. E., Mootrey, G. T., & Salive, M. E. (2001). The epidemiology of fatalities reported to the Vaccine Adverse Event Reporting System 1990–1997. *Pharmacoepidemiology and Drug Safety*, *1*(4), 279–285.

Silvers, L. E., Varricchio, F. E., Ellenberg, S. S., Krueger, C. L., Wise, R. P., & Salive, M. E. (2002). Pediatric deaths reported after vaccination: The utility of information obtained from parents. *American Journal of Preventive Medicine*, *22*(3), 170–176.

Simon, M. A. (2008). Polyomaviruses of nonhuman primates: Implications for research. *Comparative Medicine*, *5*(1), 51–56.

Simpson, D. (2001, June 11). Email to Larry Pickering about DTP Coverage and autism caseload on California—Time trend data. Retrieved June 10, 2009, from http://www.putchildrenfirst.org/media/4.6.pdf

Simpsonwood Conference. (2000). Transcript of the scientific review of Vaccine Safety Datalink Information, June 7–8, 2000, Simpsonwood Retreat Center, Norcross, Georgia. Retrieved June 10, 2009, from http://www.putchildrenfirst.org/media/2.9.pdf

Sinclair, I. (1992–1993). Smallpox. In *Vaccination: The hidden facts*. Ryde, NSW, Australia: Author. Retrieved June 10, 2009, from http://www.whale.to/vaccines/sinclair.html

Singer, H. S., Gause, C., Morris, C., & Lopez, P. (2008). Serial immune markers do not correlate with clinical exacerbations in pediatric autoimmune neuropsychiatric disorders associated with streptococcal infections. *Pediatrics*, *1*(6), 1198–1205.

Skinner, B. F. (1957). *Verbal behavior*. New York: Appleton-Century-Crofts.

Skladal, D., Halliday, J., & Thorburn, D. R. (2003). Minimum birth prevalence of mitochondrial respiratory chain disorders in children. *Brain*, *126*, 1905–1912.

Slavin, B. (2004, September 9). Powell accuses Sudan of genocide. *USA Today*. Retrieved June 10, 2009, from http://www.usatoday.com/news/washington/2004-09-09-sudan-powell_x.htm

Slotkin, T. A., Oliver, C. A., & Seidler, F. J. (2005). Critical periods for the role of oxidative stress in the developmental neurotoxicity of chlorpyrifos and terbutaline, alone or in combination. *Developmental Brain Research*, *157*(2), 172–180.

Smallman-Raynor, M. R., & Cliff, A. D. (2004). *War epidemics: An historical geography of infectious diseases in military conflict and civil strife, 1850–2000*. New York: Oxford University Press.

Smallshop Africa News. (2009, April 16). Chad refugee camps foster Dharfur rebels. Retrieved June 10, 2009, from http://africa.smallshop.com/2009/04/chad-refugee-camps-foster-darfur-rebels.html

Smith, A. M. (2001, July 1). The photograph "Tomoko and Mother in the Bath." Retrieved June 10, 2009, from http://aileenarchive.or.jp/aileenarchive_en/aboutus/aboutphoto.html

Smith, A. M. (2004). Minamata: Ailene archive. Retrieved June 10, 2009, from http://aileenarchive.or.jp/minamata_en/slides/swf.html; also see http://www.aileenarchive.or.jp/aileenarchive_en/index.html

Smith, E. W., & Smith, A. M. (1975). *Minamata: Words and photos*. New York: Holt, Rinehart, and Winston.

Smith, L., & Smith, H. (2001–2010). Death from Ritalin: The truth behind ADHD. Retrieved June 10, 2009, from http://www.ritalindeath.com/

Smithburn, K. C., Kempf, G. F., Zerfas, L. G., & Gilman, L. H. (1930). Meningococcic meningitis: A clinical study of one-hundred and forty-four epidemic cases. *Journal of the American Medical Association, 95,* 776–780.

Snopes.com. (2008, July 7). Lion hug. Retrieved February 6, 2009, from http://www.snopes.com/photos/animals/christian.asp

Sodium chloride. (2009, February 3). Retrieved June 10, 2009, from http://www.britannica.com/EBchecked/topic/519712/salt; also see http://en.wikipedia.org/wiki/Sodium_chloride

Soontornniyomkij, V., & Wiley, C. A. (1998). HIV quantification in the central nervous system. *NeuroAIDS, 1*(1). Retrieved June 10, 2009, from http://aidscience.org/neuroaids/articles/Neuro1(1).asp

Spitzer, R. L. (1980). Introduction. In the American Psychiatric Association, 1980, *Diagnostic and Statistical Manual of Mental Disorders (3rd edition)* (pp. 1–12). Washington, DC: APA.

Spitzer, R. L., & Williams, J. B. W. (1987). Introduction. In American Psychiatric Association, *Diagnostic and Statistical Manual of Mental Disorders, third edition revised (DSM-III-R).* Washington, DC: Author.

Springer. (2009). *Journal of Autism and Developmental Disorders*: Description. Retrieved June 10, 2009, from http://www.springer.com/psychology/child+%26+school+psychology/journal/10803

Stapleton, A., & Brodsky, L. (2008). Extra-esophageal acid reflux induced adenotonsillar hyperplasia: Case report and literature review. *International Journal of Pediatric Otorhinolaryngology, 72*(3), 409–413.

Stevens-Johnson Syndrome Foundation. (2001). The official site. Retrieved June 10, 2009, from http://www.sjsupport.org/

Steyaert, J. G., & De la Marche, W. (2008). What's new in autism? *European Journal of Pediatrics, 1*(10), 1091–1101.

Stott, C., Blaxill, M., & Wakefield, A. J. (2004). MMR and autism in perspective: The Denmark story. *Journal of American Physicians and Surgeons, 3,* 70–75.

Subcommittee on Human Rights and Wellness, Government Reform Committee. (2003, May 21). *Mercury in medicine report.* Washington, DC: Congressional Record: E1011–E1030.

Sullivan, A. (ca. 1925). Anne Sullivan explains how Helen [Keller] learned to speak. Retrieved June 10, 2009, from http://www.afb.org/braillebug/hkgallery.asp?tpid=3

Sullivan, M. W., & Lewis, M. (2003). Emotional expressions of young infants and children: A practitioner's primer. *Infants and Young Children, 16*(2), 120–142.

Sundberg, J., Jonsson, S., Karlsson, M. O., & Oskarsson, A. (1999). Lactational exposure and neonatal kinetics of methylmercury and inorganic mercury in mice. *Toxicology and Applied Pharmacology, 154*(2), 160–169.

Suzuki, T., Takemoto, T. L., Kashiwazaki, H., & Miyama, T. (1973). Metabolic fate of ethylmercury salts in man and animals. In M. W. Miller & T. W. Clarkson (Eds.), *Mercury, mercurials, mercaptans* (pp. 209–240). Springfield, IL: Charles C. Thomas.

Swain, A. R., Dutton, S. P., & Truswell, A. S. (1985). Salicylates in foods. *Journal of the American Diet Association, 85*(8), 950–960. Listed and tabled and retrieved June 10, 2009, from http://www.plantpoisonsandrottenstuff.info/content/elimination-diet/salicylates.aspx

Swedo, S. E., Leonard, H. L., Mittleman, B. B., Allen, A. J., Rapoport, J. L., Dow, S. P., et al. (1997). Identification of children with pediatric autoimmune neuropsychiatric disorders associated with streptococcal infections by a marker associated with rheumatic fever. *American Journal of Psychiatry, 154*(1), 110–112.

Sweet, B. H., & Hilleman, M. R. (1960, November). The vacuolating virus, SV40. *Proceedings of the Society of Experimental Biological Medicine, 105,* 420–427.

Sweeten, T. L., Bowyer, S. L., Posey, D. J., Halberstadt, G. M., & McDougle, C. J. (2003). Increased prevalence of familial autoimmunity in probands with pervasive developmental disorders. *Pediatrics, 112,* e420.

T helper cell. (2009, February 3). Retrieved June 10, 2009, from http://en.wikipedia.org/wiki/T_helper_cell

TACA. (2008). Jenny McCarthy and *Louder than words: A mother's journey in healing autism.* Retrieved June 10, 2009, from http://www.talkaboutcuringautism.org/jenny/jenny-mccarthy-autism.htm

TACA. (2009). Autism: Hope after diagnosis. Retrieved June 10, 2009, from http://www.talkaboutcuringautism.org/video/hope-video.htm

Tantam, D. (1988). Annotation: Asperger's syndrome. *Journal of Child Psychology and Psychiatry, 29,* 245–255.

Tarski, A. (1949/1944). The semantic conception of truth. In H. Feigl & W. Sellars (Eds. & Trans.), *Readings in philosophical analysis* (pp. 341–374). New York: Appleton.

Tarski, A. (1956/1936). The concept of truth in formalized languages. In J. J. Woodger (Ed. & Trans.), *Logic semantics, and metamathematics* (pp. 152–278). Oxford, UK: Oxford University Press.

Temin, H. M. (1975). The Nobel Prize in Physiology or Medicine 1975. Retrieved June 10, 2009, from http://nobelprize.org/nobel_prizes/medicine/laureates/1975/temin-autobio.html

Temin, H. M., & Mizutani, S. (1970). RNA-dependent DNA polymerase in virions of Rous sarcoma virus *Nature, 226,* 1211–1213.

Theoharides, T. C. (1990). Mast cells: The immune gate to the brain. *Life Sciences, 46,* 607–617.

Theoharides, T. C., & Doyle, R. (2008). Autism, gut–blood–brain barrier, and mast cells. *Journal of Clinica Psychopharmacology, 2*(5), 479–483.

Theoharides, T. C., Doyle, R., Francis, K., Conti, P., & Kalogeromitros, D. (2008). Novel therapeutic target for autism. *Trends in Pharmacological Sciences, 29*(8), 375–430.

Thiomersal. (2009). Retrieved June 10, 2009, from http://en.wikipedia.org/wiki/Thiomersal

Thoughtful House. (2009). Past publications specific to childhood developmental disorders. Retrieved February 4, 2009, from http://www.thoughtfulhouse.org/publications.htm

Tillberg, A., Marell, L., Berglund, A., & Eriksson, N. (2008). Replacement of restorations in subjects with symptoms associated with dental restorations; a follow-up study. *European Journal of Oral Sciences, 1*(4) 362–368.

Titzer, R. C. (2009). Your baby can read. Retrieved June 10, 2009, from http://www.yourbabycanread.com/ce-y-about.aspx

Tobacco mosaic virus. (2006–2008). Retrieved June 10, 2009, from http://www.biotecnika.org/microbiology/virus/plant-virus/tobacco-mosaic-virus/

Tocopherol. (2009, February 6). Retrieved June 10, 2009, from http://en.wikipedia.org/wiki/Tocopherol

Today in History. (1971, April 6). U.S. enters World War I. Retrieved June 10, 2009, from http://lcweb2.loc gov/ammem/today/apr06.html

Tokuomi, H., Okajima, T., et al. (1962). Neuroepidemiology of Minamata disease [article in Japanese]. *Advances in Neurological Science, 7,* 276–289.

Ton, C., Lin, Y. X., & Willett, C. (2008). Zebrafish as a model for developmental neurotoxicity testing. *Birth Defects Research Part A—Clinical and Molecular Teratology, 7*(7), 553–567.

Tosteson, D. C., Adelstein, S. J., & Carver, S. T. (1994). *New pathways to medical education.* Cambridge, MA Harvard University Press.

Trakhtenberg, I. M. (1950). The toxicity of vapors of organic mercury compounds (ethylmercuric phosphate and ethylmercuric chloride) in acute and chronic intoxication (experimental data). *Gigiena I Sanitariia, 6,* 13–17.

Treffert, D. A., & Wallace, G. L. (2002). Islands of genius. *Scientific American, 286*(6), 76–85.

Trevelyan, B., Smallman-Raynor, M., & Cliff, A. D. (2005, June). The spatial dynamics of poliomyelitis in the United States: From epidemic emergence to vaccine-induced retreat, 1910–1971. *Annual Association of American Geography, 95*(2), 269–293. Retrieved June 10, 2009, from http://www.pubmedcentral.nih.gov/articlerender.fcgi?tool=pubmed&pubmedid=16741562

Troese, M., Fukumizu, M., Sallinen, B. J., Gilles, A. A., Wellman, J. D., Paul, J. A., et al. (2008). Sleep fragmentation and evidence for sleep debt in alcohol-exposed infants. *Early Human Development, 8*(9), 577–585.

Truffaut, F. (Director/Screenplay), & Itard, J. (Novel). (1969). *L'enfant sauvage* [Motion picture]. France: Les Films du Carrosse.

Tryphona, L., & Nielsen, N. O. (1973). Pathology of chronic alkylmercurial poisoning in swine. *American Journal of Veterinary Research, 34*(3), 379–392.

Tsai, L. Y. (1999). Psychopharmacology in autism. *Psychosomatic Medicine, 61*(5), 651–665.

Tsao, C. Y., & Mendell, J. R. (2007). Autistic disorder in 2 children with mitochondrial disorders. *Journal of Child Neurology, 22*(9), 1121–1123.

Tucker, J. B., & Zilinskas, R. A. (Eds.). (2002, July). *The 1971 smallpox epidemic in Aralsk, Kazakhstan, and the Soviet Biological Warfare Program. Occasional Paper No. 9.* Monterey, CA: Monterey Institute of International Studies, Center for Nonproliferation Studies. Retrieved June 10, 2009, from http://cns.miis.edu/pubs/opapers/op9/op9.pdf

Uebersax, J. S. (1988). Validity inferences form interobserver agreement. *Psychological Bulletin, 104,* 405–416.

Uebersax, J. S. (1992). A review of modeling approaches for the analysis of observer agreement. *Investigative Radiology, 27,* 738–743.

Underdown, B., & Schiff, J. (1986). Immunoglobulin A: Strategic defense initiative at the mucosal surface. *Annual Review of Immunology, 4,* 389–417.

University of Maryland Medical Center. (2008). Beta carotene. Retrieved June 10, 2009, from http://www.umm.edu/altmed/ConsSupplements/BetaCarotenecs.html#Dietary

U.N. Wire. (2002, November 6). United States says four countries hold covert stockpiles. Retrieved June 10, 2009, from http://www.unwire.org/unwire/20021106/30138_story.asp

U.S. Census Bureau. (2000, June 28). Historical national population estimates 1900–1999. Retrieved June 10, 2009, from http://www.census.gov/popest/archives/1990s/popclockest.txt

U.S. Congress Consolidated Appropriations Resolution. (2003). P. L. 108-7. Retrieved June 11, 2009, from http://frwebgate.access.gpo.gov/cgi-bin/getdoc.cgi?dbname=108_cong_bills&docid=f:hj2enr.txt.pdf

U.S. Court of Federal Claims. (2007, June 11). Transcript of day 1 in the *Omnibus Autism Proceeding.* Retrieved June 10, 2009, from ftp://autism.uscfc.uscourts.gov/autism/transcripts/day01.pdf

U.S. Government Printing Office. (2006, December 1). *The federal rules of evidence.* Retrieved June 10, 2009, from http://www.uscourts.gov/rules/Evidence_Rules_2007.pdf

U.S. Office of Special Education Programs. (ca. 2000). History: Twenty-five years of progress in educating children with disabilities through IDEA. Retrieved June 10, 2009, from http://www.ed.gov/policy/speced/leg/idea/history.pdf

Valicenti-McDermott, M. D., McVicar, K., Cohen, H. J., Wershil, B. K., & Shinnar, S. (2008). Gastrointestinal symptoms in children with an autism spectrum disorder and language regression. *Pediatric Neurology, 3*(6), 392–398.

Valicenti-McDermott, M., McVicar, K., Rapin, I., Wershil, B. K., Cohen, H., & Shinnar, S. (2006). Frequency of gastrointestinal symptoms in children with autistic spectrum disorders and association with family history of autoimmune disease. *Journal of Developmental and Behavioral Pediatrics, 27*(2 suppl), S128–S136.

Van de Water, J. V. (2008, October). *Immunologic abnormalities in ASD.* Paper presented at Defeat Autism Now!, San Diego, CA.

Van Der Linde, A. A. A., Pillen, S., Gerrits, G. P. M., & Bavinck, J. N. B. (2008). Stevens-Johnson syndrome in a child with chronic mercury exposure and 2,3-dimercaptopropane-1-sulfonate (DMPS) therapy. *Clinical Toxicology, 4*(5), 479–481.

Van Horn, D. L., Edlehauser, H. F., Prodanovich, G., Eiferman, R., & Pederson, H. J. (1977). Effect of ophthalmic preservative thimerosal on rabbit and human corneal endothelium. *Investigative Ophthalmology and Visual Science, 16,* 273–280.

Van Krevelen, D. A. (1971). Early infantile autism and autistic psychopathy. *Journal of Autism and Childhood Schizophrenia, 1,* 82–86.

Vargas, D. L., Nascimbene, C., Krishnan, C., Zimmerman, A. W., & Pardo, C. A. (2005). Neuroglial activation and neuroinflammation in the brain of patients with autism. *Annals of Neurology, 57*(2), 304.

Veldhoen, M., Hirota, K., Westendorf, A. M., Buer, J., Dumoutier, L., Renauld, J. C., & Stockinger, B. (2008, May 1). The aryl hydrocarbon receptor links T(H)17-cell-mediated autoimmunity to environmental toxins. *Nature, 453*(7191), 106–109.

Vennemann, M. M. T., Hoffgen, M., Bajanowski, T., Hense, H. W., & Mitchell, E. A. (2007). Do immunisations reduce the risk for SIDS? A meta-analysis. *Vaccine, 25*(26), 4875–4879.

Verstraeten, T. (1999, December 17). Email to Robert Davies and Frank DeStefano: It won't go away. Retrieved June 10, 2009, from http://www.putchildrenfirst.org/media/2.7.pdf

Verstraeten, T., Davis, R. L., DeStefano, F., Lieu, T. A., Rhodes, P. H., Black, S. B., et al. (2003). Safety of thimerosal-containing vaccines: A two-phased study of computerized health maintenance organization databases. *Pediatrics, 112*(5), 1039–1048.

Viel, A., Lue, R. A., & Liebler, J. (2007). Inner life of the cell animation. [Conception and scientific content by Alain Viel and Robert A. Lue: Animation by John Liebler/XVIVO.] Retrieved June 10, 2009, from http://multimedia.mcb.harvard.edu/anim_innerlife.html

Vighi, G., Marcucci, F., Sensi, L., Di Cara, G., & Frati, F. (2008). Allergy and the gastrointestinal system. *Clinical and Experimental Immunology, 153*(suppl 1), 3–6.

Vitamin C. (2009, February 5). Retrieved June 10, 2009, from http://en.wikipedia.org/wiki/Vitamin_C

Vojdani, A., Campbell, A. W., Anyanwu, E., Kashanian, A., Bock, K., & Vojdani, E. (2002). Antibodies to neuron-specific antigens in children with autism: Possible cross-reaction with encephalitogenic proteins from milk, *Chlamydia pneumoniae* and *Streptococcus* group A. *Journal of Neuroimmunology, 129,* 168–177.

Vojdani, A., Pangborn, J. B., Vojdani, E., & Cooper, E. L. (2003). Infections, toxic chemicals and dietary peptides binding to lymphocyte receptors and tissue enzymes are major instigators of autoimmunity in autism. *International Journal of Immunopathology and Pharmacology, 16*(3), 189–199.

Von Burg, R. (1995). Toxicology update: Inorganic mercury. *Journal of Applied Toxicology, 15,* 483–493.

Vygotsky, L. S. (1962). *Thought and language* (E. Hanfmann & G. Vakar, Ed. and Trans.). Cambridge, MA: Harvard University Press.

Vygotsky, L. S. (1978/ca. 1934). *Mind in society: The development of higher psychological processes* (Michael Cole, Vera John-Steiner, Sylvia Scribner, & Ellen Souberman, Eds.). Cambridge, MA: Harvard University Press.

Wagner, J. (1996). Foreign language acquisition through interaction: A critical review of research on conversational adjustments. *Journal of Pragmatics, 2*(2), 215–235.

Wainwright, M., & Swan, H. T. (1986). C. G. Paine and the earliest surviving clinical records of penicillin therapy. *Medical History, 30,* 42–56.

Wakefield, A. J. (2000). Enterocolitis in children with developmental disorders. *American Journal of Gastroenterology, 95,* 2285.

Wakefield, A. J. (2005, November 17). The seat of the soul: The origins of the autism epidemic. Presentation by Andrew Wakefield at the Carnegie Mellon Institute together with Vicky Debold, Edward Yazbak, Debbie Darnley-Fisch, & Arthur Krigsman. Retrieved June 10, 2009, from http://www.chem.cmu.edu/wakefield/

Wakefield, A. J. (2006). The significance of ileocolonic lymphoid nodular hyperplasia in children with autistic spectrum disorder—Reply. *European Journal of Gastroenterology & Hepatology, 18,* 571.

Wakefield, A. J. (2007). Autistic enterocolitis: Is it a histopathological entity? Reply. *Histopathology, 50*(3), 380–384.

Wakefield, A. J. (2008, July). *Thoughtful House Newsletter.* Retrieved June 10, 2009, from http://thoughtfulhouse.org/newsletters/2008-07.pdf

Wakefield, A. J., Anthony, A., Murch, S. H., Thomson, M., Montgomery, S. M., Davies, S., et al. (2000). Enterocolitis in children with developmental disorder. *American Journal of Gastroenterology, 95*(9), 2285–2295.

Wakefield, A. J., Ashwood, P., Limb, K., & Anthony, A. (2005). The significance of ileo-colonic lymphoid nodular hyperplasia in children with autistic spectrum disorder. *European Journal of Gastroenterology & Hepatology, 17*(8), 827–836.

Wakefield, A. J., Blaxill, M., Haley, B., Ryland, A., Hollenbeck, B. S., Johnson, C. et al. (2009). Response to Dr. Ari Brown and the Immunization Action Coalition. *Medical Veritas, 6,* 1907–1924.

Wakefield, A. J., Murch, S. H., Anthony, A., Linnell, J., Casson, D. M., Malik, M., et al. (1997). Ileal lymphoid nodular hyperplasia (LNH), non-specific colitis and regressive behavioural disorder in children. *Gut, 41,* (Suppl. 3), A119.

Wakefield, A. J., Murch, S. H., Anthony, A., Linnell, J., Casson, D. M., Malik, M., et al. (1998). Ileal-lymphoid-nodular hyperplasia, non-specific colitis, and pervasive developmental disorder in children. *Lancet, 351*(9103), 637–641 [Retracted 2004, *Lancet, 353,* 750.].

Wakefield, A. J., Stott, C., & Krigsman, A. (2008). Getting it wrong. *Archives of Disease in Childhood, 93*(10), 905–906.

Wakefield, A. J., Stott, C., & Limb, K. (2006). Gastrointestinal comorbidity, autistic regression and measles-containing vaccines: Positive re-challenge and biological gradient. *Medical Veritas, 3,* 796–802.

Walton, G. E., & Bower, T. G. R. (1993). Newborns form prototypes in less than 1 minute. *Psychological Science, 4*(3), 203–205.

Ward, J. P. T., Clarke, R., Clarke, R. W., & Linden, R. W. A. (2005). *Physiology at a glance.* Boston: Blackwell.

Waters, M. (Director), Lucas, J. (Writer), & Moore, S. (Writer). (2009). *Ghosts of girlfriends past* [Motion picture]. Boston: New Line Cinema.

Weiss, B., Clarkson, T. W., & Simon, W. (2002, October). Silent latency periods in methylmercury poisoning and in neurodegenerative disease. *Environmental Health Perspectives, 110*(suppl 5), 851–854.

Welch, H. (1939). Mechanism of the toxic action of germicides on whole blood measured by the loss of phago-cytic activity of leucocytes. *Journal of Immunology, 37,* 525–533.

Welch, H., & Hunter, A. C. (1940). Method for determining the effect of chemical antisepsis on phagocytosis. *American Journal of Public Health, 30,* 129–137.

Werker, J. F., & Tees, R. C. (1999) Influences on infant speech processing: Toward a new synthesis. *Annual Review of Psychology, 50,* 509–535.

West, J. (1999). A critique of scientific literature: Pesticides and polio. Retrieved June 10, 2009, from http://www.wellwithin1.com/overview.htm

West, J. (2003, February 8). Pesticides and polio: A critique of the scientific literature. Retrieved June 10, 2009, from http://www.westonaprice.org/envtoxins/pesticides_polio.html

Westheimer, F. H. (1960). *Morris Selig Kharasch 1895–1957: A biographical memoir.* Washington, DC: National Academy of Sciences. Retrieved June 10, 2009, from http://books.nap.edu/html/biomems/mkharasch.pdf

Westphal, G. A., Asgari, S., Schutz, T. G., Bunger, J., Muller, M., & Hallier, E. (2003). Thimerosal induces micronuclei in the cytochalasin B block micronucleus test with human lymphocytes. *Archives of Toxicology, 77*(1), 50–55.

White, M. K., Gordon, J., Reiss, K., Del Valle, L., Croul, S., Giordano, A. K., et al. (2005). Human polyoma-viruses and brain tumors. *Brain Research Reviews, 50*(1), 69–85.

Whitman, W. B., Coleman, D. C., & Wiebe, W. J. (1998). Prokaryotes: The unseen majority. *Proceedings of the National Academy of Sciences USA, 95,* 6578–6583.

Willman, D. (2008a, June 28). U.S. settles with anthrax mailings subject Steven Hatfill for $5.82 million. Retrieved June 10, 2009, from http://articles.latimes.com/2008/jun/28/nation/na-anthrax28

Willman, D. (2008b, August 1). Apparent suicide in anthrax case. *Los Angeles Times.* Retrieved August 7, 2008, from http://www.latimes.com/news/printedition/front/la-na-anthrax1-2008aug01,0,3772533.story?page=2 [No longer available there.]. Retrieved, however, on June 10, 2009, from http://www.ph.ucla.edu/epi/bioter/suicideanthraxcase.html

Wills, S., Cabanlit, M., Bennett, J., Ashwood, P., Amaral, D., & Van de Water, J. V. (2007). Autoantibodies in autism spectrum disorders (ASD). In Y. Shoenfeld & M. E. Gershwin (Eds.), *Autoimmunity, Part C— the Mosaic of Autoimmunity.* (Annals of the New York Academy of Science). (pp. 79–91). New York: Wiley-Blackwell.

Wing, L. (1981a). Asperger's syndrome: A clinical account. *Psychological Medicine, 11,* 115–129.

Wing, L. (1981b). Language, social, and cognitive impairments in autism and severe mental retardation. *Journal of Autism and Developmental Disorders, 11,* 31–44.

Wise, R. P., Iskander, J., Pratt, R. D., Campbell, S., Ball, R., Pless, R. P., & Braun, M. M. (2004). Postlicensure safety surveillance for 7-valent pneumococcal conjugate vaccine. *JAMA—Journal of the American Medical Association, 292*(14), 1702–1710.

Wojcik, D. P., Godfrey, M. E., Christie, D., & Haley, B. E. (2006). Mercury toxicity presenting as chronic fatigue, memory impairment and depression: Diagnosis, treatment, susceptibility, and outcomes in a New Zealand general practice setting (1994–2006). *Neuroendocrinology Letters, 27*(4), 415–423.

Wolff, S., & Barlow, A. (1979). Schizoid personality in childhood: A comparative study of schizoid, autistic and normal children. *Journal of Child Psychology and Psychiatry, 20,* 29–46.

Woods, J. S., Martin, M. D., Leroux, B. G., DeRouen, T. A., Bernardo, M. F., Luis, H. S. M., et al. (2008). Biomarkers of kidney integrity in children and adolescents with dental amalgam mercury exposure: Findings from the Casa Pia children's amalgam trial. *Environmental Research, 1*(3), 393–399.

Woods, J. S., Martin, M. D., Leroux, B. G., DeRouen, T. A., Leitão, J. G., Bernardo, M. F. Y., et al. (2007). The contribution of dental amalgam to urinary mercury excretion in children. *Environmental Health Perspectives, 1*(10), 1527–1531.

World Federation of Occupational Therapists. (2004). Retrieved June 10, 2009, from http://www.wfot.org/information.asp

World Health Organization (WHO). (1957). *International statistical classification of diseases, injuries, and causes of death,* 7th Revision. Geneva: Author.

World Health Organization (WHO). (1996–2009). *International statistical classification of diseases and related health problems*, 10th Revision. Geneva: Author.

World Health Organization (WHO). (2003). Concise international chemical assessment document 50. Retrieved June 10, 2009, from http://www.who.int/ipcs/publications/cicad/en/cicad50.pdf

World Health Organization (WHO). (2005, August). Mercury in health care: Policy paper. Retrieved June 10, 2009, from http://www.who.int/water_sanitation_health/medicalwaste/mercurypolpaper.pdf

World Health Organization (WHO). (2008a). History of vaccines. Retrieved April 10, 2008, from www.who.int/gpv-dvacc/history/history.htm

World Health Organization (WHO). (2008b). Smallpox. Retrieved June 10, 2009, from http://www.who.int/mediacentre/factsheets/smallpox/en/

World Now & KLXY. (2009). Are vaccines to blame for infant deaths? Retrieved June 10, 2009, from http://www.kxly.com/Global/story.asp?S=7862995

Wrangham, T. (n.d.). Revelations in vaccine safety. Retrieved May 22, 2009, from http://www.safeminds.org/legislation/Govt%20Affairs%20Activity/RevelationsinVaccineSafety.html

Wright, K. (2007). Foreword. In B. Jepson & J. Johnson (Eds.), *Changing the course of autism* (pp. xiii–xx). Boulder, CO: Sentient Publications.

Wright, P. W. D., Wright, P. D., & Heath, S. W. (2008). No Child Left Behind—Wrightslaw. Retrieved June 10, 2009, from http://www.wrightslaw.com/nclb/

Wu, X., Liang, H., O'Hara, K. A., Yalowich, J. C., & Hasinoff, B. B. (2008). Thiol-modulated mechanisms of the cytotoxicity of thimerosal and inhibition of DNA topoisomerase II alpha. *Chemical Research in Toxicology*, 21(2), 483–493.

Xiong, Y., Lee, C. P., & Peterson, P. L. (2001). Mitochondrial dysfunction following traumatic brain injury. In L. P. Miller, R. L. Hayes, & J. K. Newcomb (Eds.), *Head trauma: Basic, preclinical, and clinical directions* (pp. 257–280). New York: John Wiley and Sons.

Yan, R. (2009). *Assessing English language proficiency in international aviation: Issues of reliability, validity, and aviation safety*. Saarbrücken, Germany: VDM Verlag.

Yole, M., Wickstrom, M., & Blakley, B. (2007). Cell death and cytologic effects in YAC-1 lymphoma cells following exposure to various forms of mercury. *Toxicology*, 231(1), 40–57.

Yorbik, O., Sayal, A., Akay, C., Akbiyik, D. I., & Sohmen, T. (2002). Investigation of antioxidant enzymes in children with autistic disorder. *Prostaglandins, Leukotrienes and Essential Fatty Acids*, 67, 341–343.

Yoshida, K. A., Fennell, C. T., Swingley, D., & Werker, J. F. (2009). Fourteen-month-old infants learn similar-sounding words. *Developmental Science*, 12(3), 412–418.

Young, H. A., Geier, D. A., & Geier, M. R. (2008). Thimerosal exposure in infants and neurodevelopmental disorders: An assessment of computerized medical records in the Vaccine Safety Datalink. *Journal of the Neurological Sciences*, 271(1–2), 110–118.

Yrigollen, C. M., Han, S. S., Kochetkova, A., Babitz, T., Chang, J. T., Volkmar, F. R., et al. (2008). Genes controlling affiliative behavior as candidate genes for autism. *Biological Psychiatry*, 6(10), 911–916.

Zahir, F., Rizwi, S. J., Haq, S. K., & Khan, R. H. (2005). Low dose mercury toxicity and human health. *Environmental Toxicology and Pharmacology*, 20(2), 351–360.

Zamula, E. (1991, June). A new challenge for former polio patients. *FDA Consumer*, 25, 21–25.

Zecavati, N., & Spence, S. J. (2009). Neurometabolic disorders and dysfunction in autism spectrum disorders. *Current Neurology and Neuroscience Reports*, 9(2), 129–136.

Zentz, D. R. (2006, September 6). Comments of Dr. Ronald R. Zentz, RPh, DDS, to Joint Meeting of the Dental Products Panel of the Medical Devices Advisory Committee of the Center for Devices and Radiological Health and the Peripheral and Central Nervous System Drugs Advisory Committee of the Center for Drug Evaluation and Research. Chicago, IL: American Dental Association. Retrieved June 10, 2009, from http://www.ada.org/public/media/presskits/fillings/testimony_zentz.pdf

Zhang, J. (1984). Clinical observations in ethyl mercury chloride poisoning. *American Journal Indian Medicine*, 5, 251–258.

Zimmerman, O. T., & Lavine, I. (1946). *DDT, killer of killers*. Dover, NH: Industrial Research Service.

Index